IMMUNO BIOLOGY

THE IMMUNE SYSTEM IN HEALTH AND DISEASE

SECOND EDITION

IMMUNO BIOLOGY

THE IMMUNE SYSTEM IN HEALTH AND DISEASE

SECOND EDITION

Charles A. Janeway, Jr.
Yale University Medical School

Paul Travers
Birkbeck College, London University

CURRENT
BIOLOGY
LIMITED ■

Current Biology Ltd
London, San Francisco and Philadelphia

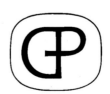

Garland Publishing Inc
New York and London

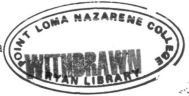

Text editors: Miranda Robertson, Eleanor Lawrence
Project editors: Emma Hunt, Emma Dorey
Illustrator: Matthew McClements
Layout: Huw Woodman
Production: Kate Oldfield
Software support: Gary Brown
Proofreader: Melanie Paton
Indexer: Maija Hinkle

Distributors
Inside North America: Garland Publishing Inc., 717 Fifth
Avenue, New York, NY 10022, USA.
Inside Japan: Nankodo Co. Ltd., 42-6, Hongo 3-Chome,
Bunkyo-ku, Tokyo 113, Japan.
Outside North America and Japan: Churchill Livingstone,
Robert Stevenson House, 1-3 Baxter's Place, Leith Walk,
Edinburgh, EH1 3AF.

ISBN 0-8153-2044-2 (paperback) Garland
ISBN 0-443-05658-7 (paperback) Churchill Livingstone
ISBN 0-443-05659-5 (paperback) International Student Edition

A catalog record for this book is available from the British
Library.

Library of Congress Cataloging-in-Publication Data
Janeway, Charles.
   Immunobiology: the immune system in health and disease/
   Charles A. Janeway, Jr., Paul Travers.—Second ed.
      p. cm.
   Includes bibliographical references and index.
   ISBN 0-8153-2044-2 (pbk.).
   1. Immunity. 2. Immune System. I. Travers, Paul, 1956- .
II. Title
QR181.J37 1996
616. 07'9—dc20
                                        95-49564
                                          CIP

This book was produced using Corel Ventura Publisher 5.0
and CorelDRAW 5.0.

Printed in Singapore by Stamford Press.

Published by Current Biology Ltd., Middlesex House, 34-42
Cleveland Street, London W1P 5FB, UK and Garland
Publishing Inc., 717 Fifth Avenue, New York, NY 10022, USA.

Preface for the first edition

This book is intended as an introductory text for use in immunology courses for medical students, advanced undergraduate biology students, and graduate students. It attempts to present the field of immunology from a consistent viewpoint, that of the host's interaction with an environment containing myriad species of potentially harmful microbes. The justification for this particular approach is that the absence of components of the immune system is virtually always made clinically manifest by an increased susceptibility to infection. Thus, first and foremost, the immune system exists to protect the host from infection, and its evolutionary history must have been shaped largely by this challenge. Other aspects of immunology, such as allergy, autoimmunity, graft rejection, and immunity to tumors are treated as variations on this basic protective function in which the nature of the antigen is the major variable.

We have attempted to structure the book logically, focusing mainly on the adaptive immune response mediated by antigen-specific lymphocytes operating by clonal selection. The first part of the book summarizes our understanding of immunology in conceptual terms and introduces the main players — the cells, tissues, and molecules of the immune system. It also contains a 'toolbox' of experiments and techniques that form the experimental basis of immunology. The middle three parts of the book deal with three main aspects of adaptive immunity: how the immune system recognizes and discriminates among different molecules; how individual cells develop so that each bears a unique receptor directed at foreign, and not at self, molecules; and how these cells are activated when they encounter microbes whose molecular components bind their receptors, and the effector mechanisms that are used to eliminate these microbes from the body.

Having described the major features of lymphocytes and of adaptive immune responses, the last part of the book integrates this material at the level of the intact organism, examining when, how, and where immune responses occur, and how they fail in some instances. In this part of the book we also consider those aspects of host defense that do not involve clonal selection of lymphocytes, known as innate immunity or natural resistance. We then look at the role of the immune system in causing rather than preventing disease, focusing on allergy, autoimmunity, and graft rejection as examples. Finally, we consider how the immune system can be manipulated to the benefit of the host, emphasizing endogenous regulatory mechanisms and the possibility of vaccinating not only against infection, but also against cancer and immunological diseases. The book also contains a glossary of key terms, biographical notes on some immunologists, and summary tables of key molecules.

In preparing this textbook, we have striven for a coherent overall presentation of concepts supported by experiment and observation. We have had the chapters read by experts (see page ix) who have helped us to eliminate errors of fact and conclusion, to improve presentation, and to achieve better balance; we are sincerely grateful to them for their hours of hard work. Any shortcomings of the book are not their fault, but ours. We plan to keep this material current by revising the book each year, again relying on a panel of experts for each chapter. But the greatest help in improving the value of the book will come from its readers; we welcome your comments and criticisms, and we will work to incorporate your ideas into each new update. Thus, we plan to make this the first current textbook: we are attempting to do this because we believe that the field of immunology is advancing so rapidly at present that annual updating is essential.

There is no doubt that we have both omitted and included too much; the field of immunology covers such a broad area of interest that one of the most daunting challenges in writing this book has been in deciding what has to be discussed and what can be ignored. The judgements we have made are personal and so will not be shared exactly by anyone else. Again, we welcome your input and suggestions about places where this judgement is in clear error.

Finally, we want to thank the many people who have worked so hard to make this book possible. Our illustrator, Celia Welcomme, has brought her extraordinary talents to bear on the figures, while the book itself was edited by three highly skilled and knowledgeable individuals, Miranda Robertson, Rebecca Ward, and Eleanor Lawrence; led by Miranda, they questioned every word, sentence, comma and figure in the book, and made us tear our hair out in trying to be clear and accurate at the same time. If we have failed, it is not their fault. Peter Newmark and Vitek Tracz have provided intelligent and even inspirational guidance, motivated in no small part by the memory of our original publisher, the remarkable Gavin Borden, who sadly died young and never saw this book, into which he put so much, in print. Nothing would have been achieved without the diligence of Becky Palmer, who kept all of us organized over a long period, with the help of Emma Dorey, Sylvia Purnell, Gary Brown, and many other people at Current Biology Ltd. Charlie Janeway wants to thank several patient secretaries, especially Liza Cluggish, Anne Brancheau, Susan Morin, and Kara McCarthy for all their help. Finally, our families have suffered more than we have, from neglect, absence and fits of ill temper. Thus, we thank Kim Bottomly, Katie, Hannah and Megan Janeway, and Rose Zamoyska for their forbearance and support.

Charles A. Janeway Jr.
Yale University School of Medicine
Howard Hughes Medical Institute

Paul Travers
Birkbeck College
University of London

April 1994

Preface for the second edition

The field of immunobiology is moving at an astonishing rate, and it is difficult to conceive of, let alone assimilate, the amount of material that needs to be mastered to comprehend the progress that has taken place in the year and a half since publication of the first edition of this book. We have made extensive revisions in this second edition, and we hope we have included the most important advances. The basic structure of the book remains the same, but we have completely rewritten certain parts, modified others, and scrapped or changed many figures where new information has compelled us to do so. Our aim in working on this revision has been to improve the book as well as to update it. We ask each reader to contact us about any errors of commission or omission that you may (and surely will) find here.

We have been helped greatly in preparing this edition by a team of experts who read the chapters of the first edition, critiqued them, and sent us many valuable suggestions for changes. One of our advisors even drafted a revised version of one section. Their names can be found on page ix.

Again, as for the first edition, we have a team of talented and patient people to thank. Good books often owe much to their editors, and Miranda Robertson has again distinguished herself in this area, where she has served not only as a gadfly but also as a friend, writer and editor. Eleanor Lawrence has again kept us on the editorial straight and narrow in text, figures, and glossary. We were much helped by the work of Matthew McClements, who took over from Celia Wellcome as lead illustrator of the text for this edition. Emma Hunt has worked diligently on the accurate reproduction of often illegible scratches in the margins of page proofs, and was ably assisted in the earlier phases of this edition by Emma Dorey. Finally, we would like to thank our publishers for putting up with us: Libby Borden of Garland Publishing has been very supportive of this effort, filling her late husband Gavin's shoes admirably, while Vitek Tracz and Peter Newmark, of Current Biology Ltd, have provided encouragement, logistical support, and sage advice.

Charlie Janeway would particularly like to take this opportunity to thank his family for all their support in the past year, and also to thank all those who communicated their wishes for his speedy recovery from a very scary episode, whether they wrote, phoned, or just thought of him. He would also like to thank Kara McCarthy for her constant efforts of the past year, especially those that coincided with her own family illness and attendant difficulties. Paul Travers wants to thank Rose Zamoyska for her continuing encouragement and support.

It is also appropriate this year that we should mark the bicentenary of Edward Jenner's first use of cowpox (vaccinia) to induce immunity to smallpox, and the origin of the term vaccination. This experiment is generally accepted as the birth of the discipline of immunology. Vaccination has completely eliminated the disease of smallpox but, as yet, it is the only disease to have been so eliminated. Jenner's vaccine, the vaccinia virus itself, through modern techniques of genetic engineering is today being developed to induce immunity to other widespread diseases such as malaria and hepatitis. His bold experiment continues to bear fruit. At the time of Jenner's experiment, an alternative protective treatment of inoculating smallpox itself (variolation) was already in use, but with the risk of leading to full-blown smallpox. The contemporary dispute between the proponents of vaccination and variolation has resonances today, where the efficacy of mass vaccination has reduced the incidence of many diseases, especially in the developed countries, to the level where the risks of vaccine-related pathology appear to many to outweigh the risks of the diseases themselves. One need only look at the continuing toll of disease in countries lacking vaccination programs to realize that this is not so.

We hope that you enjoy reading this book, and that the effort of trying to stay up-to-date in this area will have proved worthwhile.

Charles A. Janeway Jr.   Paul Travers
Yale University School of Medicine   Birkbeck College
Howard Hughes Medical Institute   University of London

November 1995

Acknowledgements

Text

We would like to thank the following experts who read parts or the whole of the chapters indicated and provided us with invaluable advice.

Chapter 1: J.J. Cohen, University of Colorado; K. Grimnes, Alma College, Alma. E. Rothenberg, California Institute of Technology.

Chapter 2: H. Acha-Orbea, Ludwig Institute for Cancer Research; J. Gooding, Emory University of Medicine, Atlanta; R. Hardy, Institute of Cancer Research, Philadelphia; J. Ledbetter, Bristol Myers Squibb Pharmaceutical Research Institute; D.B. Murphy, New York State Department of Health.

Chapter 3: F. Alt, Howard Hughes Medical Institute, Columbia University College of Physicians and Surgeons; D. Fearon, University of Cambridge; A. de Franco, University of California, San Francisco; H. Gould, Randall Institute, University of London; M. Neuberger, MRC Center, Cambridge; R. Poljak, Institute Pasteur, Paris; I. Tomlinson, MRC Center, Cambridge; I. Wilson, Scripps Research Institute.

Chapter 4: P. Cresswell, Howard Hughes Medical Institute, Yale University School of Medicine; M. Davis, Howard Hughes Medical Institute, Stanford University; R.N. Germain, National Institute of Allergy and Infectious Diseases; B. Malissen, INSERM-CNRS de Marseille-Luminy; A. Weiss, Howard Hughes Medical Institute, SanFrancisco; I. Wilson, Scripps Research Institute.

Chapter 5: F. Alt, Howard Hughes Medical Institute, Columbia University College of Physicians and Surgeons; C. Goodnow, Howard Hughes Medical Institute, Stanford University; P. Kincade, Oklahoma Medical Research Council; K. Rajewsky, University of Cologne; D. Schatz, Howard Hughes Medical Institute, Yale University School of Medicine; A. Strasser, Walter and Eliza Hall Institute, Melbourne.

Chapter 6: M.J. Bevan, Howard Hughes Medical Institute, University of Washington; E.J. Jenkinson, University of Birmingham, U.K.; D.H. Raulet, University of California, Berkeley.

Chapter 7: J.P. Allison, University of California, Berkeley; M. Davis, Howard Hughes Medical Institute, Stanford University; S. Gillis, Immunex Research and Development Corporation; P. Golstein, INSERM-CNRS de Marseille-Luminy; S. Gordon, University of Oxford; W.E. Paul, National Institute of Allergy and Infectious Diseases, Bethesda;

D. Paulnock, University of Wisconsin Medical School; A. Sher, National Institute of Allergy and Infectious Diseases, Bethesda; T. Springer, Harvard University Medical School.

Chapter 8: D.T. Fearon, University of Cambridge; H. Gould, Randall Institute, University of London; J-P. Kinet, National Institute of Allergy and Infectious Diseases, Bethesda; I.C.M. MacLennan, University of Birmingham, U.K.; I. Mellman, Yale University School of Medicine; R.J. Noelle, Dartmouth Medical School; K. Rajewsky, University of Cologne; K.B.M. Reid, University of Oxford.

Chapter 9: P. Beverley, Ludwig Institute for Cancer Research; L. Gooding, Emory University School of Medicine, Atlanta; K. Karre, Karolinska Institute, Stockholm; L. Picker, University of Texas Southwestern Medical Centre; S. Shaw, National Cancer Institute, Bethesda; J. Sprent, Scripps Research Institute, California; T. Springer, Harvard Medical School; S. Wright, Rockefeller University.

Chapter 10: T. Fauci, National Institute of Allergy and Infectious Diseases, Bethesda; M. Feinberg, Office of AIDS Research, Bethesda; K. Joiner, Yale University School of Medicine; C. Kinnon, Institute of Child Health, London; T.B. Nutman, National Institute of Allergy and Infectious Diseases, Bethesda; D. Richman, University of California, San Diego; F. R. Rosen, Harvard Medical School; S. Wain Hobson, Unite de Retrovirologie Moleculaire; M. Walport, Royal Postgraduate Medical School, University of London.

Chapter 11: R. Geha, Boston Children's Hospital; P. Holt, West Australian Research Institute for Child Health; N.R. Rose, John Hopkins University School of Hygiene and Public Health, Baltimore; D.H. Sachs, Massachussetts General Hospital; D. Wraith, University of Bristol.

Chapter 12: B.R. Bloom, Howard Hughes Medical Institute, Albert Einstein College of Medicine, New York; T. Boon, Ludwig Institute for Cancer Research; R. Corley, Duke University Medical Center, Durham, N.C.; G. Crabtree, Howard Hughes Medical Institute, Stanford University; D. Pardoll, John Hopkins University School of Medicine; E. Sercarz, University of California, Los Angeles; H. Waldmann, University of Oxford.

Appendix: N. Barclay, MRC Center, Univeristy of Oxford; S. Gillis, Immunex Research and Development Corporation.

First edition A.K. Abbas, Harvard Medical School; K. Arai, University of Tokyo; F.M. Brodsky, University of California, San Francisco; M.P. Cancro, University of Pennsylvania School of Medicine; S. Corey, Walter and Eliza Hall Institute, Melbourne; A. Coutinho, Institute Pasteur, Paris; S.C. Crebe, The American University, Washington, D.C.; W. Dunnick, University of Michigan; A. Gann, Ludwig Institute for Cancer Research, London; D. Gray, Royal Postgraduate Medical School, London; J. Groopman, New England Deaconess Hospital, Boston; R. Handschumacher, Yale University of Medicine; E.R. Heise, Bowman Gray School of Medicine, Winston-Salem; J. Howard, Babraham Institute, Cambridge, U.K.; G. Kelsoe, University of Maryland; B. Moss, National Institute of Allergy and Infectious Diseases, Bethesda; P. Parham, Stanford University Medical Center; B. M. Peterlin, Howard Hughes Medical Institute, University of California, San Francisco; G.A. Petsko, Brandeis University; S.K. Pierce, Northwestern University; M. Ptashne, Harvard University; J.J. van Rood, University Hospital, Leiden; R. Steinman, Rockefeller University; J. W. Streilein, University of Miami School of Medicine; J. Tooze, Imperial Cancer Research Fund, London; J. Uhr, University of Texas Southwestern Medical School; H. Weiner, Harvard Medical School.

Photographs

The following photographs have been reproduced with the kind permission of the journal in which they were originally published.

Chapter 1.

Fig. 1.18 middle panels from *Proc Natl Acad Sci USA* 1988, **85**:5210–5214. Bottom left panel from *J Exp Med* 1972, **135**:200–219. By copyright permission of the Rockefeller University Press.
Fig. 1.23 from *J Exp Med* 1989, **169**:893–907. By copyright permission of the Rockefeller University Press.

Chapter 3.

Fig. 3.5 from *Adv Immunol* 1969, **11**:1–30.
Fig. 3.9 panel a from *Science* 1990, **248**:712–719. © 1990 by the AAAS. Panel b from *Structure* 1993, **1**:83–93.
Fig. 3.10 from *Science* 1985, **229**:1358–1365. © 1985 by the AAAS.
Fig. 3.13 from *Science* 1986, **233**:747–753. © 1986 by the AAAS.
Fig. 3.31 top panel from *Eur J Immunol* 1988, **18**:1001–1008.

Chapter 4.

Fig. 4.5 panel a from *J Biochem* 1988, **263**:10541–10544.
Fig. 4.6 panel a from *Nature* 1987, **329**:506–512. Panel b from *Nature* 1991, **353**:321–325. Both © 1987 by Macmillan Magazines Ltd.
Fig. 4.15 from *Science* 1994, **266**:1566–1569. © 1994 by the AAAS.

Chapter 6.

Fig. 6.5 from *Nature* 1994, **372**:100–103. © 1994 by Macmillan Magazines Ltd.
Fig. 6.20 from *Science* 1990, **250**:1720–1723. © 1990 by the AAAS.

Chapter 7.

Fig. 7.29 panel c from *Second International Workshop on Cell Mediated Cytotoxicity*. Eds. P.A. Henkart and E. Martz. New York: Plenum Press 1985, 99–119.

Fig. 7.36 from *Eur J Immunol* 1989, **19**:1253–1259.
Fig. 7.37 panels a and b from *Second International Workshop on Cell Mediated Cytotoxicity*. Eds. P.A. Henkart and E. Martz. New York: Plenum Press 1985, 99–119. Panel c from *Immunol Today* 1985, **6**:21–27.

Chapter 8.

Fig. 8.18 from *Nature* 1994, **372**:336-383. © 1994 by Macmillan Magazines Ltd.
Fig. 8.35 from *Essays in Biochem* 1986, **22**:27–68.
Fig. 8.36 (planar conformation) from *Eur J Immunol* 1988, **18**:1001–1003.
Fig. 8.50 from *Blut* 1990, **60**:309–318.

Chapter 9.

Fig. 9.15 top panel from *Nature* 1994, **367**:338–345. © 1994 by Macmillan Magazines Ltd. Bottom panel from *J Immunol* 1990, *144*:2287–2294. © 1990, The Journal of Immunology.
Fig. 9.33 panel a from *J Immunol* 1985, **134**:1349–1359. © 1985, The Journal of Immunology.
Fig. 9.33 panels a, b, and c from *Annu Rev Immunol* 1989, **7**:91–109. © 1989 by Annual Reviews Inc.

Chapter 10.

Fig. 10.5 top left panel from *Int Rev Exp Pathology* 1986, **28**:45–78. © courtesy of Academic Press.

Chapter 11.

Fig. 11.26 left panel from *Cell* 1989, **59**:247. © by Cell Press.
Fig. 11.37 from *J Exp Med* 1992, **176**:1355–1364. By copyright permission of the Rockefeller University Press.

Chapter 12.

Fig. 12.22 from *Mechanisms of Cytotoxicity by Natural Killer Cells*. R.B. Herberman (Ed.) Academic Press, New York. 1985, pp 195. © courtesy of Academic Press.

CONTENTS

List of Headings

Part II	THE RECOGNITION OF ANTIGEN

Chapter 3:   Structure of the Antibody Molecule and Immunoglobulin Genes

Part IV   THE ADAPTIVE IMMUNE RESPONSE

Chapter 7:   T-cell Mediated Immunity

Part IV   THE ADAPTIVE IMMUNE RESPONSE

Chapter 12: Control and Manipulation of the Immune Response

PART I

AN INTRODUCTION TO IMMUNOBIOLOGY

Basic Concepts in Immunology

1

Immunology is a relatively new science. Its origin is usually attributed to Edward Jenner (Fig. 1.1) who discovered 200 years ago, in 1796, that cowpox or vaccinia induced protection against human smallpox, an often fatal disease. Jenner called his procedure **vaccination**, and this term is still used to describe the inoculation of healthy individuals with weakened or attenuated strains of disease-causing agents to provide protection from disease. Although Jenner's bold experiment was successful, it took two centuries for smallpox vaccination to become

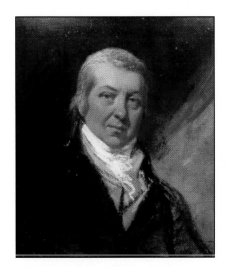

Fig. 1.1 Edward Jenner. Portrait by John Raphael Smith. Reproduced courtesy of Yale Historical Medical Library.

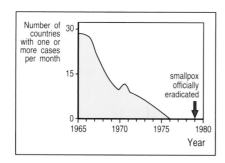

Fig. 1.2 The eradication of smallpox by vaccination. After a period of three years in which no cases of smallpox were recorded, The World Health Organization was able to announce in 1979 that smallpox had been eradicated.

universal, an advance that enabled the World Health Organization to announce in 1979 that smallpox had been eradicated (Fig. 1.2), arguably the greatest triumph of modern medicine.

When Jenner introduced vaccination he knew nothing of the infectious agents that cause disease: it was not until late in the 19th century that Robert Koch proved that infectious diseases were caused by **microorganisms**, each one responsible for a particular disease, or **pathology**. We now recognize four broad categories of disease-causing microorganisms, or **pathogens**: these are **viruses**, **bacteria**, pathogenic **fungi**, and other relatively large and complex eukaryotic organisms collectively termed **parasites**.

The discoveries of Koch and other great 19th century microbiologists made the development of immunology possible, and extended the example of Jenner's vaccination to other diseases. In the 1880s, Louis Pasteur devised a vaccine against cholera in chickens, and developed a rabies vaccine that proved a spectacular success upon its first trial use in a boy bitten by a rabid dog. These practical triumphs led to a search for the mechanism of protection. In 1890, Emil von Behring and Shibasaburo Kitasato discovered that the serum of vaccinated individuals contained substances — which they called **antibodies** — that specifically bound to the relevant pathogen.

A specific **immune response**, such as the production of antibodies to a particular pathogen, is known as an **adaptive immune response**, because it occurs during the lifetime of an individual as an adaptive response to infection with that pathogen. In many cases, an adaptive immune response confers lifelong protective **immunity** to re-infection with the same pathogen. This distinguishes such responses from **innate immunity**, which, at the time von Behring and Kitasato discovered antibodies, was known chiefly through the work of the great Russian immunologist Elie Metchnikoff. Metchnikoff discovered that many microorganisms could be engulfed and digested by **phagocytic cells**, which he called **macrophages**. These cells are immediately available to combat a wide range of bacteria without requiring prior exposure, and act in the same way in all normal individuals. Antibodies, by contrast, are produced only in response to specific infections, and the antibodies present in a given individual directly reflect the infections to which he or she has been exposed.

Indeed, it quickly became clear that specific antibodies can be induced against a vast range of substances, known as **antigens** because they can *gen*erate *anti*bodies, although we shall see that not all adaptive immune responses entail the production of antibodies, and the term antigen is now used in a rather broader sense, to describe any substance capable of being recognized by the adaptive immune system.

Both innate immunity and adaptive immune responses depend upon the activities of white blood cells, or **leukocytes**. Innate immunity is mediated largely by **granulocytes**, so called because they contain prominent cytoplasmic granules. They are a diverse collection of cells, many of which are phagocytic and are thus able to engulf and destroy microorganisms. Adaptive immune responses are mediated by **lymphocytes**, which provide the lifelong immunity that can follow exposure to disease or vaccination. The innate and adaptive immune systems together provide a remarkably effective defense system that ensures that although we spend our lives surrounded by potentially pathogenic microorganisms we become ill only relatively rarely, and when infection does occur it is usually successfully met and is followed by lasting immunity.

The main focus of this book will be on the diverse mechanisms of adaptive immunity, whereby specialized classes of lymphocytes recognize and target pathogenic microorganisms or cells infected with them. We shall see, however, that all the cells that mediate innate immune responses also participate in adaptive immune responses, and indeed most of the actions of the adaptive immune system depend upon them.

In this chapter, we first introduce the cells of the immune system, and the tissues in which they develop and through which they circulate or migrate. In later sections, we outline the specialized functions of the different types of cells and the mechanisms whereby they eliminate infection.

The components of the immune system.

The cells of the immune system originate in the **bone marrow**, where many of them also mature. They then migrate to patrol the tissues, circulating in the blood and in a specialized system of vessels called the **lymphatic system**.

1-1	**The white blood cells of the immune system derive from precursors in the bone marrow.**

All the cellular elements of blood, including the red blood cells that transport oxygen, the platelets that trigger blood clotting in damaged tissues, and the white blood cells of the immune system, derive ultimately from the same **progenitor** or precursor cells, the **hematopoietic stem cells** in the bone marrow. Because these stem cells can give rise to all of the different types of blood cells, they are often known as pluripotent hematopoietic stem cells. They give rise in turn to stem cells of more limited potential, which are the immediate progenitors of red blood cells, platelets, and the two main categories of white blood cells. The different types of blood cells and their lineage relationships are summarized in Fig. 1.3. We shall be concerned here only with the cells derived from the **myeloid progenitor** and the **common lymphoid progenitor**.

The myeloid progenitor is the precursor of the granulocytes and **macrophages** of the immune system. Macrophages are one of the two types of phagocytes of the immune system and are widely distributed in the body tissues where they play a critical part in innate immunity. They are the mature form of **monocytes**, which circulate in the blood and differentiate continuously into macrophages upon migration into the tissues.

The granulocytes are so called because they have densely staining granules in their cytoplasm; they are also sometimes called **polymorphonuclear leukocytes** because of their oddly shaped nuclei. There are three types of granulocytes. **Neutrophils**, which comprise the other phagocytic cell of the immune system, are the most numerous and are the most important cellular component of the innate immune response: hereditary deficiencies in neutrophil function lead to overwhelming bacterial infection which is fatal if untreated. **Eosinophils** are thought to be important chiefly in defense against parasitic infections; they are activated by the lymphocytes of the adaptive immune

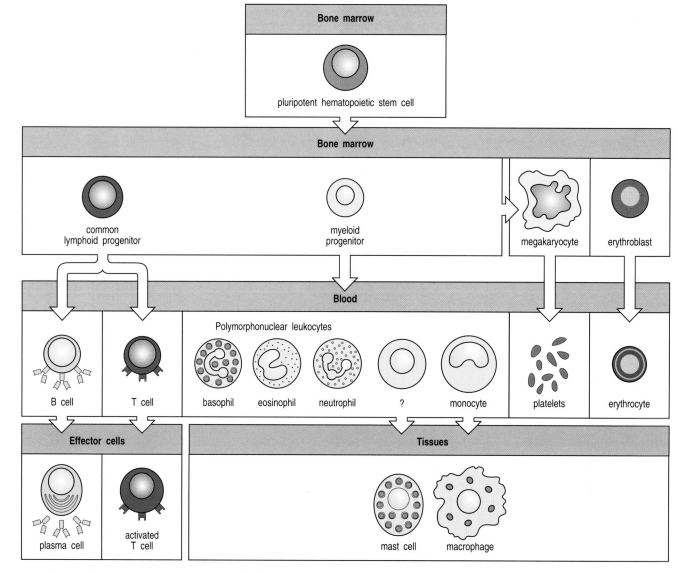

Fig. 1.3   All the cellular elements of blood, including the lymphocytes of the adaptive immune system, arise from hematopoietic stem cells in the bone marrow. These pluripotent cells divide to produce two more specialized types of stem cells, a lymphoid stem cell (or progenitor), which gives rise to T and B lymphocytes, and a myeloid stem cell (or progenitor), which gives rise to leukocytes, erythrocytes (red blood cells that carry oxygen) and the megakaryocytes that produce platelets, which are important in blood clotting. We have illustrated only one progenitor cell for both T and B lymphocytes, but an alternative that has not been ruled out is that both T and B cell lineages arise directly from the pluripotent stem cell. The T and B lymphocytes are distinguished by their site of differentiation, T cells in the thymus and B cells in the bone marrow, and by their antigen receptors. B lymphocytes differentiate on activation into antibody-secreting plasma cells, and T lymphocytes

differentiate into cells that can kill infected cells or activate other cells of the immune system. The leukocytes that derive from the myeloid stem cell are the monocytes, and the basophils, eosinophils, and neutrophils, which are collectively termed either poly-morphonuclear leukocytes, because of their irregularly shaped nuclei, or granulocytes, because of the cytoplasmic granules whose characteristic staining gives them a distinctive appearance in blood smears. Monocytes differentiate into macrophages in the tissues where they are the main phagocytic cells of the immune system. Neutrophils and eosinophils are also phagocytic cells with functions similar to those of macrophages; basophils are found in blood and are similar in some ways to mast cells but arise from a separate lineage. Mast cells also arise from precursors in bone marrow but complete their maturation in tissues, although it is not known how they migrate there; they are important in allergic responses.

response and we shall discuss their functions in Chapter 8. The function of **basophils** is probably similar to that of **mast cells**, which are believed to play a part in protecting the mucosal surfaces of the body and are the cells that release histamine in allergic responses. The cells of the myeloid lineage are shown in Fig. 1.4.

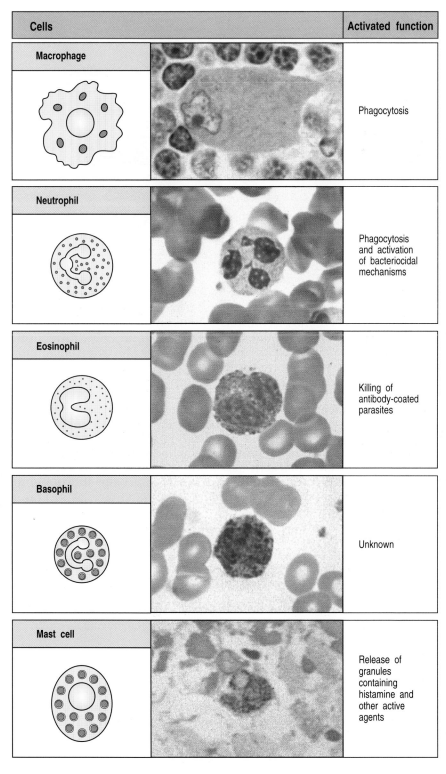

Cells		Activated function
Macrophage		Phagocytosis
Neutrophil		Phagocytosis and activation of bacteriocidal mechanisms
Eosinophil		Killing of antibody-coated parasites
Basophil		Unknown
Mast cell		Release of granules containing histamine and other active agents

Fig. 1.4 Myeloid cells in innate and adaptive immunity. Several different cell types of the myeloid lineage perform important functions in the immune response; these cells are shown schematically in the left column in the form in which they will be represented throughout the rest of the book. A photomicrograph of each cell type is shown in the center column. Macrophages and neutrophils, or polymorpho-nuclear neutrophilic leukocytes, are primarily phagocytic cells that engulf antibody-coated pathogens, which they destroy in intracellular vesicles after pathogen uptake. The other myeloid accessory effector cells are primarily secretory cells that release the contents of their prominent granules upon binding to antibody-coated particles. Eosinophils are thought to be involved in attacking large parasites such as worms, while the function of basophils is unclear. Mast cells are tissue cells that trigger a local inflammatory response by releasing vasoactive substances when they are activated by antigen binding to IgE. Photographs courtesy of N Rooney.

The common lymphoid progenitor gives rise to the lymphocytes, with which most of this book will be concerned. There are two major types of lymphocytes: **B lymphocytes** or **B cells**, which when activated differentiate into **plasma cells** which secrete antibodies; and **T lymphocytes** or **T cells**, of which there are two main classes: one includes the cytotoxic T cells, which kill cells infected with viruses, and the second includes both helper and inflammatory T cells, which activate other cells such as B cells and macrophages.

Fig. 1.5 Small lymphocytes are cells whose main feature is inactivity. The left panel shows a light micrograph of a small lymphocyte. Note the condensed chromatin of the nucleus, indicating little transcriptional activity, the relative absence of cytoplasm, and the small size. The right panel shows a transmission electron micrograph of a small lymphocyte. Note the condensed chromatin, the scanty cytoplasm and the absence of rough endoplasmic reticulum and other evidence of functional inactivity. Photographs courtesy of N Rooney.

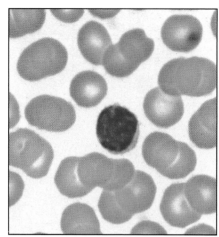
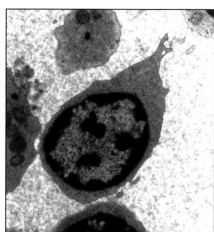

Most lymphocytes are small, featureless cells with much of the chromatin in the nucleus in the condensed state and few cytoplasmic organelles (Fig. 1.5). This appearance is typical of inactive cells and it is not surprising that textbooks as recently as the early 1960s could describe these cells, now the central focus of immunology, as having no known function. Indeed, lymphocytes have no functional activity until they encounter antigen, which is necessary to trigger their proliferation and specialized actions.

Both T and B lymphocytes bear on their surface highly diverse **receptors**, each of which is specific for a particular antigen, and which together are capable of recognizing a wide diversity of antigens. The **antigen receptor** of B lymphocytes is a membrane-bound form of the antibody that they will secrete when activated. Antibody molecules as a class are now generally known as **immunoglobulins**, usually shortened to **Ig**, and the antigen receptor of B lymphocytes is known as **surface immunoglobulin**. Immunoglobulin molecules, how they function and how they are generated, are the subject of Chapter 3. The antigen receptor of T lymphocytes is related to immunoglobulin but quite distinct from it, and we shall describe the T-cell receptor for antigen in detail in Chapter 4.

1-2 Lymphocytes mature in the bone marrow or the thymus.

The **lymphoid organs** are organized tissues where lymphocytes interact with non-lymphoid cells that are important either to their maturation or to the initiation of adaptive immune responses. They can be broadly divided into primary or **central lymphoid organs**, where lymphocytes are generated, and secondary or **peripheral lymphoid organs**, where adaptive immune responses are initiated. The central lymphoid organs are the bone marrow and the **thymus**, a large organ in the upper chest: the location of the thymus, with the other lymphoid organs, is shown schematically in Fig. 1.6.

Both B and T lymphocytes originate in the bone marrow, but only B lymphocytes mature there: T lymphocytes migrate to the thymus to undergo maturation. Thus B lymphocytes are so called because they are bone-marrow derived, and T lymphocytes because they are thymus-derived. Once they have completed their maturation, both types of lymphocytes enter the bloodstream, from which they migrate to the peripheral lymphoid organs.

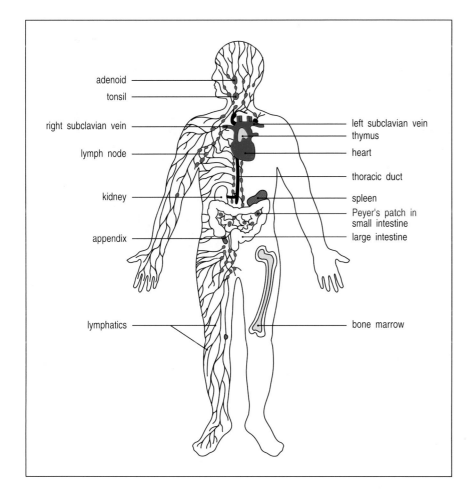

Fig. 1.6 The distribution of lymphoid tissues in the body. Lymphocytes arise from stem cells in bone marrow, and differentiate in the central lymphoid organs (yellow): B cells in bone marrow and T cells in the thymus. They migrate from these tissues through the bloodstream to the peripheral lymphoid tissues (blue), the lymph nodes, spleen, and lymphoid tissues associated with mucosa, like the gut-associated lymphoid tissues such as tonsils, Peyer's patches, and appendix. These are the sites of lymphocyte activation by antigen. Lymphatics drain extracellular fluid as lymph through the lymph nodes and into the thoracic duct, which returns the lymph to the bloodstream by emptying into the left subclavian vein. Lymphocytes that circulate in the bloodstream enter the peripheral lymphoid organs, and are eventually carried by lymph to the thoracic duct where they re-enter the bloodstream. Lymphoid tissue is also associated with other mucosa such as the bronchial linings (not shown).

1-3 | **The peripheral lymphoid organs are specialized to trap antigen and allow the initiation of adaptive immune responses.**

Once lymphocytes are mature, they leave the central lymphoid organs and are now capable of responding to antigen. But before they can respond to an antigen they must first find it. As the total number of small lymphocytes in an individual is very large, a lymphocyte able to recognize a particular antigen will be rare in the pool of naive lymphocytes. Pathogens can enter the body by many routes and set up infections anywhere, but antigen and lymphocytes will eventually encounter each other in the peripheral lymphoid organs — the lymph nodes, the spleen, and various lymphoid tissues associated with mucosal surfaces (see Fig. 1.6). Naive lymphocytes are continually recirculating through these tissues, to which antigen is also carried from all sites of infection and where it is trapped by specialized cells.

The **lymph nodes** are highly organized lymphoid structures that are the sites of convergence of an extensive system of vessels that collect the extracellular fluid from tissues and return it to the blood. The fluid is called **lymph**, and the vessels that carry it **lymphatic vessels**, or sometimes just **lymphatics** (see Fig. 1.6). The **afferent lymphatic vessels** which drain fluid from the tissues also carry antigens from sites of infection in most parts of the body to the lymph nodes, where they are trapped. In the lymph nodes, B lymphocytes are localized in **follicles**, with T cells more diffusely distributed in

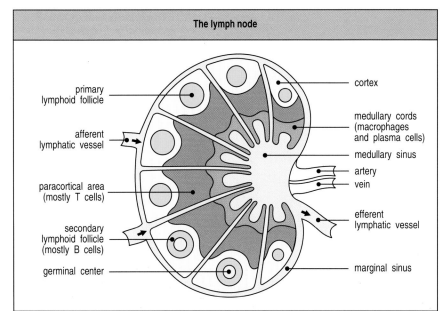

The lymph node

primary lymphoid follicle

afferent lymphatic vessel

paracortical area (mostly T cells)

secondary lymphoid follicle (mostly B cells)

germinal center

cortex

medullary cords (macrophages and plasma cells)

medullary sinus

artery

vein

efferent lymphatic vessel

marginal sinus

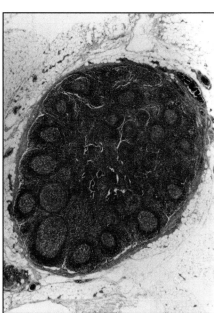

Fig. 1.7   A schematic view and a light micrograph of a lymph node. A lymph node consists of an outermost cortex and an inner medulla. The cortex is composed of an outer cortex of B lymphocytes organized into lymphoid follicles, and deep or paracortical areas made up mainly of T lymphocytes. Some of the B-cell follicles contain central areas of intense B-cell proliferation called germinal centers. These follicles are known as secondary lymphoid follicles. Lymph draining the extracellular spaces of the body carries antigens from the tissues to the lymph node via the afferent lymphatics. Lymph leaves by the efferent lymphatic in the medulla. The medulla consists of strings of macrophages and antibody-secreting plasma cells known as the medullary cords. Naive lymphocytes enter the node from the bloodstream through specialized post-capillary venules (not shown) and leave with the lymph through the efferent lymphatic. The photograph shows a section through a lymph node, with prominent follicles containing germinal centers. Photograph (x 7) courtesy of N Rooney.

surrounding **paracortical areas**. Some of the B-cell follicles contain central areas called **germinal centers**, where B cells are undergoing intense proliferation after encountering antigen (Fig. 1.7). B and T lymphocytes are segregated in a similar fashion in the other peripheral lymphoid tissues, and we shall see when we come to discuss the adaptive immune response that this organization promotes the crucial interactions that occur between B and T cells on encounter with antigen.

The **spleen** is a fist-sized organ just behind the stomach (see Fig. 1.6) that collects antigen from the blood. It also collects and disposes of senescent red blood cells. Its organization is shown schematically in Fig. 1.8. The bulk of the spleen is composed of **red pulp**, which is the site of red blood cell disposal. The lymphocytes surround the arterioles entering the organ, forming areas of **white pulp**, the inner region of which is divided into a **periarteriolar lymphoid sheath (PALS)** containing mainly T cells, and a flanking **B-cell corona**.

The **gut-associated lymphoid tissues (GALT)**, which include the **tonsils**, **adenoids**, and **appendix**, and specialized structures called **Peyer's patches** in the small intestine, collect antigen from the epithelial surfaces of the gastrointestinal tract. In Peyer's patches, which are the most important and highly organized of these tissues, the antigen is collected by specialized epithelial cells called M cells. The lymphocytes form a follicle consisting of a large central dome of B lymphocytes surrounded by smaller numbers of T lymphocytes

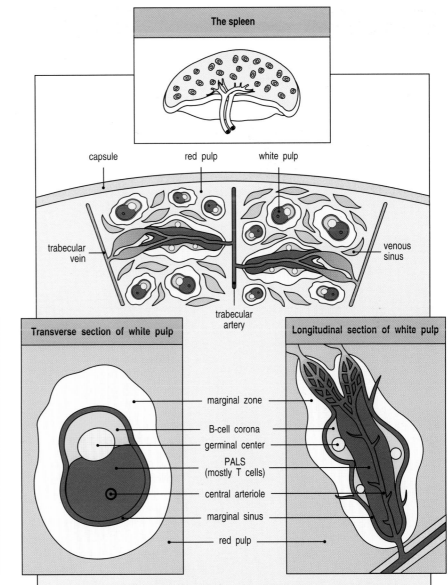

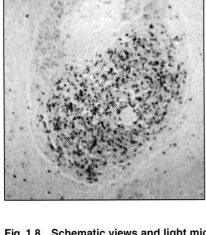

Fig. 1.8 Schematic views and light micrograph of a section of spleen. The spleen consists of red pulp (pink areas), which is a site of red blood cell destruction, interspersed with lymphoid white pulp (yellow and blue areas in the lower panels). The center panel shows an enlargement of a small section of the spleen showing the arrangement of discrete areas of white pulp around central arterioles. Most of the white pulp is shown in transverse section, with one portion shown in longitudinal section. The bottom two diagrams show enlargements of a transverse section (lower left) and longitudinal section (lower right) of white pulp. In each area of white pulp, blood carrying lymphocytes and antigen flows from a trabecular artery into a central arteriole and a marginal sinus and drains into a trabecular vein. The marginal sinus is surrounded by a marginal zone of lymphocytes. Within the marginal sinus and surrounding the central arteriole is the periarteriolar lymphoid sheath (PALS), made up of T cells (stained darkly in the micrograph, which shows a transverse section of white pulp). The lymphoid follicles consist mainly of B cells (lightly stained), including germinal centers (the unstained cells lying between the B- and T-cell areas in the micrograph). While the organization of the spleen is similar to that of a lymph node, antigen enters the spleen from the blood rather than from the lymph. Photograph courtesy of J Howard.

(Fig. 1.9). Similar but more diffusely organized aggregates of lymphocytes protect the respiratory epithelium, where they are known as **bronchial-associated lymphoid tissue** (**BALT**) and other mucosa, where they are simply known as **mucosal-associated lymphoid tissue** (**MALT**).

Fig. 1.9 Typical gut-associated lymphoid tissue in schematic and light microscopic views. The antigen enters across a specialized epithelium made up of so-called M cells. The bulk of the lymphoid tissue is B cells, organized in a large and highly active domed follicle. T cells occupy the areas between follicles. Although this tissue looks very different from other lymphoid organs, the basic divisions are maintained. The photograph shows a section of the gut wall. The dome of gut-associated lymphoid tissue can be seen lying beneath the epithelial tissues. Photograph (x 16) courtesy of N Rooney.

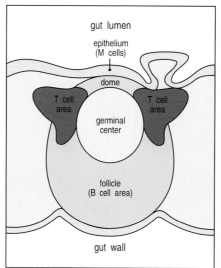
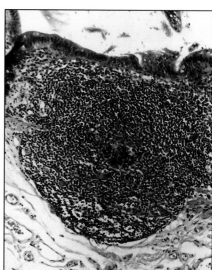

Although remarkably different in appearance, the lymph nodes, spleen, and gut-associated lymphoid tissues all share the same basic architecture. Each of these tissues operates on the same principle, trapping antigen from sites of infection and presenting it to migratory small lymphocytes, thus inducing adaptive immune responses.

| 1-4 | Lymphocytes circulate between blood and lymph. |

Small T and B lymphocytes that have matured in the bone marrow and thymus but have not yet encountered antigen are referred to as **naive lymphocytes**. These cells circulate continually from the blood into the peripheral lymphoid tissues, which they enter by means of specialized adhesive interactions with the capillaries supplying these tissues that allow them to squeeze between the endothelial cells. They are then returned to the blood via the lymphatic vessels (Fig. 1.10). In the presence of an infection, lymphocytes that recognize the infectious agent are arrested in the lymphoid tissue where they proliferate and differentiate into **effector cells** capable of combating the infection.

If an infection occurs in the periphery, for example, antigens drain from the site of infection through the afferent lymphatic vessels into the lymph nodes (Fig. 1.10). In the lymph nodes the antigen is trapped by specialized cells that display them to recirculating lymphocytes which they also help to activate. Once the lymphocytes have undergone a period of proliferation and differentiation, they leave the lymph nodes as effector cells through the **efferent lymphatic vessel** (see Fig. 1.7).

All the lymphoid tissues operate on the same principle, trapping antigen from sites of infection and presenting it to migratory small lymphocytes to stimulate adaptive immune responses. The lymphoid tissues are thus not static structures, but vary quite dramatically depending upon whether infection is present. The diffuse mucosal lymphoid tissues may appear and disappear in response to infection, while the architecture of the more organized tissues changes in a defined way during an infection. For example, the B-cell follicles of the lymph nodes expand as B lymphocytes proliferate to form germinal centers (see Fig. 1.7), and the entire lymph node enlarges, a phenomenon familiarly known as 'swollen glands'.

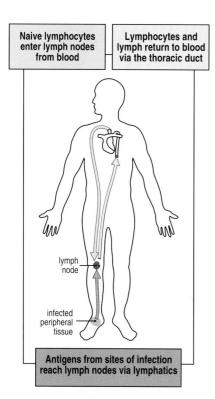

Fig. 1.10 Circulating lymphocytes encounter antigen in peripheral lymphoid tissues.

Summary.

Immune responses are mediated by leukocytes which derive from precursors in the bone marrow. These give rise to the polymorpho-nuclear leukocytes and the macrophages of the innate immune system, and the lymphocytes of the adaptive immune system. There are two major types of lymphocytes: B lymphocytes, which mature in the bone marrow, and T lymphocytes, which mature in the thymus. The bone marrow and thymus are thus known as the central lymphoid organs. Once they have matured, macrophages and mast cells migrate to the body tissues, but all the other cells of the immune system circulate in the blood. Lymphocytes continually recirculate from the bloodstream through the peripheral lymphoid organs, where antigen is trapped, returning to the bloodstream through the lymphatic vessels. The three major types of peripheral lymphoid tissue are the spleen, which collects antigens from the blood, the lymph nodes, which collect antigen from sites of infection in the tissues, and the gut-associated lymphoid tissue, which collects antigens from the gut. Other epithelia also have diffuse lymphoid tissue associated with them: these are known as bronchial-associated lymphoid tissue and mucosal-associated lymphoid tissue. Adaptive immune responses are initiated in the peripheral lymphoid tissues.

Principles of innate and adaptive immunity.

The phagocytes of the innate immune system provide a first line of defense against many common microorganisms and are essential to the control of common bacterial infections. However, they cannot always eliminate infectious organisms, and there are many pathogens that they cannot recognize. The lymphocytes of the adaptive immune system have evolved to provide a more versatile means of defense that, in addition, provides an increased level of protection to a subsequent re-infection with the same pathogen. The cells of the innate immune system play a crucial part in the initiation and subsequent direction of adaptive immune responses. Moreover, since there is a delay of four to five days before the initial adaptive immune response takes effect, the innate immune response has a critical role in controling infections during this period.

1-5 Many bacteria activate phagocytes and trigger inflammatory responses.

Macrophages and neutrophils have surface receptors that have evolved to recognize and bind common constituents of many bacterial surfaces. Bacterial molecules binding to these receptors trigger the cells to engulf the bacterium and also induce the secretion of **cytokines** and other chemical mediators by macrophages. Cytokines are chemical mediators released by cells that affect the behavior of other cells. The cytokines released by macrophages in response to bacterial constituents have a range of effects that are collectively known as **inflammation**. Inflammation is traditionally defined by the four Latin words *dolor, rubor, calor,* and *tumor,* meaning pain, redness, heat, and swelling, all of which reflect the effects of cytokines on the local blood vessels

Fig. 1.11 Bacterial infection triggers an inflammatory response. Macrophages encountering bacteria in the tissues are increase the permeability of blood vessels, allowing fluid and proteins to pass into the tissues. The stickiness of the endothelial cells of the blood vessels is also changed, so that cells adhere to the blood vessel wall and are able to crawl through it: macrophages and neutrophils are shown here entering the infected tissue from a blood vessel. The accumulation of fluid and cells at the site of infection causes the swelling, heat, and pain that are collectively known as inflammation. Macrophages and neutrophils are the principal inflammatory cells. Later in an immune response, activated lymphocytes may also contribute to inflammation.

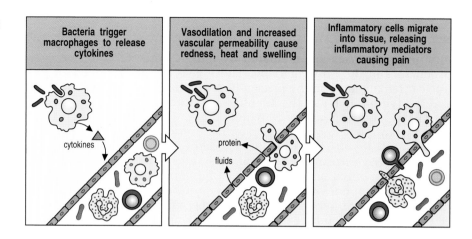

(Fig. 1.11). Dilation and increased permeability of the blood vessels lead to increased local blood flow and the leakage of fluid, and account for the heat, redness and swelling. Cytokines also have important effects on the adhesive properties of the endothelium, causing circulating leukocytes to stick to the endothelial cells of the blood vessel wall and migrate through them to the site of infection, to which they are attracted by yet other cytokines. The migration of cells into the tissue and their local actions account for the pain. The main cell types seen in an inflammatory response in its initial phases are neutrophils, followed by macrophages, which mature from their precursor monocytes; these are therefore known as **inflammatory cells**.

Inflammatory responses later in an infection involve the lymphocytes making an adaptive immune response, which meanwhile is being activated by antigen draining from the site of infection via the lymphatics to the local lymph node. Bacterial constituents induce changes in the surface molecules expressed by macrophages that are critical to the central part played by these cells in the induction of adaptive immune responses; we shall discuss them in detail in Chapter 9.

1-6 Lymphocytes are activated by antigen to give rise to clones of antigen-specific cells that mediate adaptive immunity.

The defense systems of innate immunity are effective in combating many bacterial pathogens, but they are limited to those bacteria bearing surface molecules that are common to many bacteria and that have remained unchanged in the course of evolution so that they can be recognized by neutrophils and macrophages. Not surprisingly, many bacteria have evolved capsules that enable them to conceal these molecules and thereby avoid provoking phagocytic cells. Viruses carry no such unvarying molecules and are never recognized by phagocytic cells. Moreover, the surface molecules of pathogens evolve much faster than could any ordinary vertebrate recognition system. The recognition mechanism used by the lymphocytes of the adaptive immune response has evolved to overcome these problems.

Instead of bearing several receptors each specifically recognizing a conserved surface molecule of a pathogen, each naive lymphocyte entering the bloodstream bears receptors of only a single specificity. However, the specificity of these receptors is determined by a unique genetic mechanism that operates during the development of lymphocytes in the bone marrow and thymus to generate hundreds of different variants of the genes encoding the receptor molecules. Thus, although the individual

Fig. 1.12 The clonal selection hypothesis. During its normal course of development, each lymphocyte progenitor is able to give rise to a number of lymphocytes, each bearing a distinct antigen receptor. Lymphocytes with receptors that bind self antigens are eliminated early in development before they become able to respond, assuring tolerance of self. When antigen interacts with the receptor on a mature lymphocyte, that cell is activated to become a blast cell (lymphoblast) and then starts to divide. It gives rise to a clone of identical progeny, all of whose receptors bind the same antigen. Antigen specificity is thus maintained as the progeny proliferate and differentiate into effector cells. Once antigen is eliminated by these effector cells, the immune response ceases.

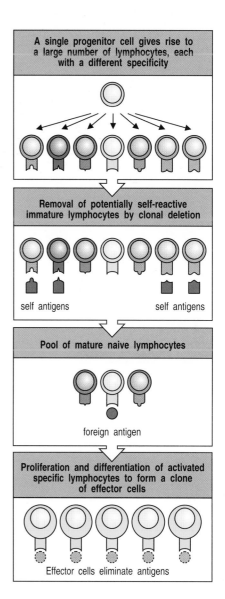

A single progenitor cell gives rise to a large number of lymphocytes, each with a different specificity

Removal of potentially self-reactive immature lymphocytes by clonal deletion

self antigens   self antigens

Pool of mature naive lymphocytes

foreign antigen

Proliferation and differentiation of activated specific lymphocytes to form a clone of effector cells

Effector cells eliminate antigens

lymphocyte carries receptors of only one specificity, the specificity of each lymphocyte is different, and thus the millions of lymphocytes in the body give rise to millions of different specificities (Fig. 1.12). These lymphocytes then undergo a process akin to natural selection during the lifetime of an individual: only those lymphocytes that encounter an antigen to which their receptor binds will be activated to proliferate and differentiate into effector cells.

This selective mechanism was first proposed in the 1950s by F. McFarlane Burnet to explain why antibodies, which can be induced in response to virtually any antigen, are produced in each individual only to those antigens to which he or she is exposed. He postulated the pre-existence in the body of many different potential antibody-producing cells, each having the ability to make antibody of a different specificity and displaying on its surface a membrane-bound version of the antibody serving as a receptor for antigen. On binding antigen, the cell is activated to proliferate and produce many identical progeny, known as a **clone**, which now secrete antibodies with a specificity identical to that of the surface receptor. McFarlane Burnet called this the **clonal selection theory**.

| 1-7 | **Clonal selection of lymphocytes is the central principle of adaptive immunity.** |

Remarkably, at the time that McFarlane Burnet formulated his theory, nothing was known of the antigen receptors of lymphocytes and indeed the function of lymphocytes themselves was still obscure. Lymphocytes did not take center stage until the early 1960s, when James Gowans discovered that removal of the small lymphocytes from rats resulted in the loss of all known immune responses. The immune responses were restored when the lymphocytes were replaced. This led to the realization that lymphocytes must be the units of clonal selection and their biology became the focus of the new field of **cellular immunology**.

Clonal selection of lymphocytes with diverse receptors elegantly explained adaptive immunity, but it raised one significant intellectual problem. If the antigen receptors of lymphocytes are randomly generated during the lifetime of an individual, how are lymphocytes prevented from recognizing antigens on the tissues of the body and attacking them? Peter Medawar had shown in 1953 that if exposed to foreign tissues during embryonic development, animals will become immunologically tolerant to these tissues and will not subsequently make immune responses to them. Burnet proposed that developing lymphocytes that are potentially self-reactive are removed before they can mature. He has since been proved right in this too, although the

Fig. 1.13 The four basic principles of the clonal selection theory.

Postulates of the clonal selection hypothesis
Each lymphocyte bears a single type of receptor of a unique specificity
Interaction between a foreign molecule and a lymphocyte receptor capable of binding that molecule with high affinity leads to lymphocyte activation
The differentiated effector cells derived from an activated lymphocyte will bear receptors of identical specificity to those of the parental cell from which that lymphocyte was derived
Lymphocytes bearing receptors specific for self molecules are deleted at an early stage in lymphoid cell development and are therefore absent from the repertoire of mature lymphocytes

mechanisms of **tolerance** are still being worked out, as we shall see when we discuss the development of lymphocytes in Chapters 5 and 6.

Clonal selection of lymphocytes is the single most important principle in adaptive immunity. It is shown schematically in Fig. 1.12, and its four basic postulates are listed in Fig. 1.13. The last of the problems posed by the clonal selection theory — that of how the diversity of lymphocyte antigen receptors is generated — was solved in the 1970s when advances in molecular biology made it possible to clone the genes encoding antibody molecules.

variable regions (antigen-binding sites)

constant region (effector function)

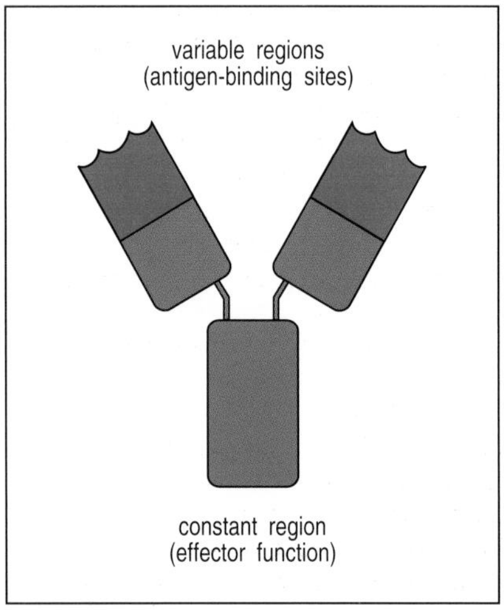

Fig. 1.14 Structure of the antibody molecule. The two arms of the Y-shaped antibody molecule contain the variable regions that form the two identical antigen-binding sites. The stem can take one of only a limited number of forms and is known as the constant region. It is the region that engages the effector mechanisms that antibodies activate to eliminate pathogens.

1-8   The structure of antibody molecules illustrates the problem of lymphocyte antigen receptor diversity.

Antibodies, as discussed above, are the secreted form of the B-cell receptor for antigen. Because they are produced in very large quantities in response to antigen, they can be studied by traditional biochemical techniques and their structure was understood long before recombinant DNA technology made it possible to study the membrane-bound antigen receptors of lymphocytes. The startling feature that emerged from the biochemical studies was that antibody molecules as a class are composed of two distinct regions: a **constant region**, that can take one of only four or five biochemically distinguishable forms; and a **variable region** that can take an apparently infinite variety of subtly different forms that allow it to bind specifically to an equally vast variety of different antigens.

This division is illustrated in the simple schematic diagram in Fig. 1.14, where the antibody is depicted as a Y-shaped molecule with the constant region shown in blue and the variable region in red. The variable region determines the antigen-binding specificity of the antibody, and the constant region determines how the antibody disposes of the antigen once it is bound.

Each of the two antigen-binding regions of the antibody molecule is in fact composed of two chains, each having both a constant and a variable region; the variable regions combine to form the antigen-binding site and both chains contribute to the antigen-binding specificity of the antibody molecule. The antibody molecule itself, therefore, is composed of four chains. The structure of antibody molecules will be described in detail in Chapter 3, where we shall also discuss the structural and genetic basis for the different functional properties of antibodies conferred by their constant regions. For the time being we are concerned only with the properties of immunoglobulin molecules as antigen receptors. The antigen receptors of T cells, which we discuss in detail in Chapter 4, show many similarities to the B-cell antigen receptor and have both a variable, antigen-binding part, and a constant part.

This organization of the antigen receptors, however, highlighted an important problem in immunology; namely, how was the diversity in the receptors generated? The receptors of each lymphocyte are different, and there are many millions of lymphocytes in the body. The great question then was whether this implied that there must be millions of genes each encoding the same constant region, and a slightly different variable region, or whether there was some special mechanism that allowed diversity to be created with a very much smaller number of genes.

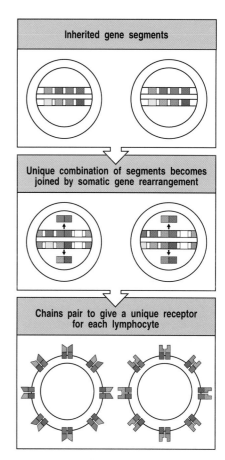

| 1-9 | **Each developing lymphocyte generates a unique receptor by rearranging its receptor genes.** |

The question of how antigen receptors with an almost infinite range of specificities could be encoded by a finite number of genes was answered in 1976, when Susumu Tonegawa discovered that the genes for immunoglobulin variable regions are inherited as sets of **gene segments**, each of which encodes a part of the variable region of one of the polypeptide chains that makes up an immunoglobulin molecule (Fig. 1.15). As B lymphocytes differentiate in the bone marrow, these gene segments are joined to form a stretch of DNA that codes for an entire variable region. Because different gene segments are joined in different cells, each cell generates a unique gene for the variable region of each chain of the antibody molecule.

This mechanism has three important consequences. First, it enables a limited number of gene segments to generate a very diverse set of proteins. Second, as each cell assembles a different set of gene segments to encode its antigen receptor, each cell expresses a unique receptor specificity. Third, as gene rearrangement involves an irreversible change in a cell's DNA, all the progeny of that cell will inherit genes encoding the same receptor specificity.This general scheme was later confirmed for the genes encoding the antigen receptor on T lymphocytes. The main distinctions between B and T lymphocyte receptors are that the cell-surface immunoglobulin molecule that serves as the B-cell receptor has two identical antigen recognition sites and can be secreted, while the **T-cell receptor** has a single antigen recognition site, and is always a cell-surface molecule. We shall see later that these receptors also recognize antigen in very different ways.

The potential diversity of lymphocyte receptors generated in this way is enormous. Just a few hundred different gene segments can combine in different ways to generate thousands of different receptor chains. The diversity of lymphocyte receptors is further amplified by the fact that each receptor is made by pairing two different variable chains, each encoded in distinct sets of gene segments. A thousand different chains of each type could generate 10^6 distinct antigen receptors through this **combinatorial diversity**. Thus a small amount of genetic material can encode a truly staggering diversity of receptors; there are at least 10^8 different lymphocytes in an individual. Once gene rearrangement is complete, the antigen receptor is expressed on the surface of the developing lymphocyte, which is now ready to interact with antigen.

Fig. 1.15 The diversity of lymphocyte antigen receptors is generated by somatic gene rearrangements. Different parts of the variable region of antigen receptors are encoded by sets of gene segments. During a lymphocyte's development, one member of each set of gene segments is randomly joined together by an irreversible process of DNA recombination. The juxtaposed gene segments make up a complete gene encoding the variable part of one chain of the receptor, which is unique to that cell. This random process is repeated for the other set of gene segments, giving rise to the other chain. The expressed rearranged genes produce the two types of polypeptide chains that come together to form the unique antigen receptor on the lymphocyte surface. Once the two required recombination events have occurred, further gene rearrangement is prohibited. Thus, the receptor specificity of a lymphocyte cannot change once it has been determined, and the lymphocyte can only express one receptor specificity. Each lymphocyte bears many copies of its unique receptor.

Lymphocytes proliferate in response to antigen in peripheral lymphoid tissue.

Because each lymphocyte has a different antigen-binding specificity, the number of lymphocytes that can bind and respond to any given antigen is very small. To generate sufficient specific effector lymphocytes to fight an infection, an activated lymphocyte must proliferate before its progeny finally differentiate into effector cells. This **clonal expansion** is a feature of all adaptive immune responses.

Lymphocyte activation and proliferation is initiated in the lymphoid tissues where antigen is trapped by specialized cells. These display the antigen to the naive recirculating lymphocytes as they migrate through

Fig. 1.16 Transmission electron micrographs of lymphocytes at various stages of activation to effector function. Small resting lymphocytes (upper panel) have not yet encountered antigen. Note the small amount of cytoplasm, with no rough endoplasmic reticulum, indicating an inactive cell. This cell could be either a T cell or a B cell. Small circulating lymphocytes are trapped in lymph nodes when their receptors encounter antigen displayed on the surface of specialised cells known as antigen-presenting cells. Stimulation by antigen induces the lymphocyte to become an active lymphoblast. This cell undergoes clonal expansion by repeated division, which is followed by differentiation to effector function. The central micrograph shows an activated lymphoblast responding to antigen. Note the large size, the nucleoli, the enlarged nucleus with diffuse chromatin, and the active cytoplasm; again, T and B lymphoblasts are similar in appearance. The lower panels show effector T and B lymphoblasts. Note the large amount of cytoplasm, the nucleus with prominent nucleoli, abundant mitochondria and the presence of rough endoplasmic reticulum, all hallmarks of active cells. The rough endoplasmic reticulum is especially prominent in antibody-secreting B cells, usually called plasma cells, which synthesize and secrete very large amounts of antibody protein. Photographs courtesy of N Rooney.

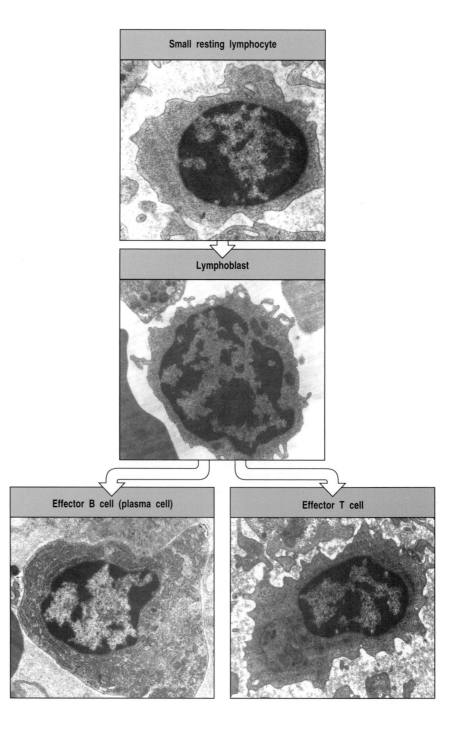

the lymphoid tissue before returning to the bloodstream via the lymph. On recognizing its specific antigen, the small lymphocyte stops migrating and enlarges. The chromatin in its nucleus becomes less dense, nucleoli appear, the volume of cytoplasm increases, and new RNA and protein synthesis are induced. Within a few hours, the cell looks completely different, and activated cells at this stage are called **lymphoblasts** (Fig. 1.16).

The cell now begins to divide, normally duplicating two to four times every 24 hours for three to five days, so that the original lymphocyte gives rise to a clone of around 1 000 daughter cells of identical specificity. These then differentiate into effector cells able to secrete antibody, in the case of B cells, or in the case of T cells, to destroy infected cells or activate other cells of the immune system. These changes also affect the recirculation of lymphocytes: because of changes in the expression of specialized adhesion molecules on their surface, they cease circulating through the blood and lymph and instead migrate through the endothelial cells at sites of infection, signaled by the cytokines released by inflammatory cells at these sites.

After a lymphocyte has been activated, it takes four to five days before clonal expansion is complete and the lymphocytes have differentiated into effector cells. That is why adaptive immune responses occur only after a delay. Some of the antigen-specific cells generated by the clonal expansion of small lymphocytes persist after the antigen has been eliminated. These are the basis of **immunological memory**, which ensures a more rapid and effective response on a second encounter with a pathogen and thereby provides lasting immunity.

The characteristics of immunological memory are readily observed by comparing the antibody response of an individual to a first or **primary immunization** with the response elicited in the same individual by a **secondary** or **booster immunization** with the same antigen. As detailed in Fig. 1.17, the **secondary antibody response** occurs after a shorter lag phase, achieves a markedly higher plateau level, and produces antibodies of higher affinity. We shall describe the mechanisms of these remarkable changes in Chapters 8 and 9. The cellular basis of immunological memory is the clonal expansion and clonal differentiation of cells specific for the eliciting antigen, and it is therefore entirely antigen specific.

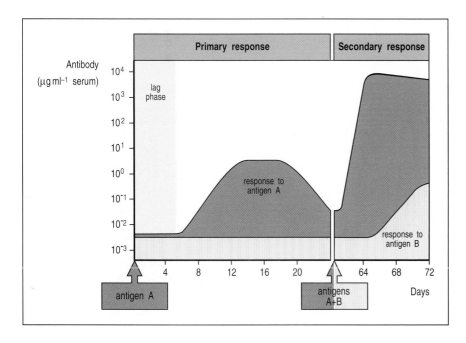

Fig. 1.17 The course of a typical antibody response. Antigen A introduced at time zero encounters little specific antibody in the serum. After a lag phase, antibody to antigen A (blue) appears and its concentration rises to a plateau, and then declines. When the serum is tested for antibody against another antigen, B (yellow), there is none present, demonstrating the specificity of the antibody response. When the animal is later challenged with a mixture of antigens A and B, a very rapid and intense response to A occurs. This illustrates immunological memory, the ability of the immune system to make a second response to the same antigen more efficiently and effectively, providing the host with specific defense against infection. Note that the response to B resembles the initial or primary response to A, as this is the first encounter of the host with antigen B.

It is immunological memory that allows successful vaccination and prevents re-infection with pathogens that have been successfully repelled by an adaptive immune response. Immunological memory is perhaps the most important biological consequence of the development of adaptive immunity based on clonal selection, although its cellular and molecular basis is still not fully understood, as we shall see in Chapter 9.

1-11	**Interactions with other cells as well as with antigen are necessary for lymphocyte activation.**

Secondary lymphoid tissues are specialized not only to trap antigen but also to promote the interactions between cells that are necessary for the initiation of adaptive immune responses. The spleen and lymph nodes in particular are highly organized for the latter function.

We have already mentioned that one of the functions of T cells is to stimulate the production of antibody by B cells. In fact all lymphocyte responses to antigen require a second signal from another cell. For most B-cell responses the signal comes from a T cell (Fig. 1.18, left panel); for T cells (Fig. 1.18, right panel), the second signal may be delivered by any of three cell types: **dendritic cells**, macrophages and B cells. Dendritic cells are cells with a distinctive branched morphology found exclusively in the T-cell areas of lymphoid tissue. These cells trap and present antigens to T cells, and because of this and their ability to deliver activating signals, they are known as **professional antigen-presenting cells**, or often just **antigen-presenting cells**. The three cell types that present antigen to T cells are illustrated in Fig. 1.19. Dendritic cells are probably the most important antigen-presenting cell of the three. They therefore play a central part in the initiation of adaptive immune responses while macrophages directly mediate innate immune responses and make a crucial contribution to the effector phase of the adaptive immune response.

Antigen may be swept into the spleen by the blood or into the lymph nodes by the lymph, or be taken up by the M cells of the gut-associated lymphoid tissue and trapped by antigen-presenting cells already present in these tissues. Antigen may also be imported into lymphoid tissues by dendritic cells, which migrate there after trapping antigen in the periphery. It is thought that some or all dendritic cells originate as migratory cells that trap antigen in the periphery before settling in the lymphoid tissues where they interact with T cells.

Fig. 1.18 Two signals are required for lymphocyte activation. As well as receiving a signal through their antigen receptor, mature lymphocytes must also receive a second signal in order to become activated. For B cells (left panel), the second signal is usually delivered by a T cell. For T cells (right panel) it is delivered by a professional antigen-presenting cell, shown here as a dendritic cell.

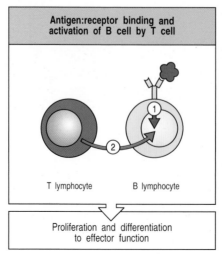

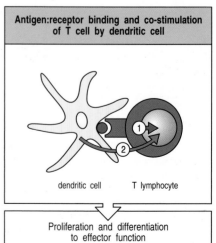

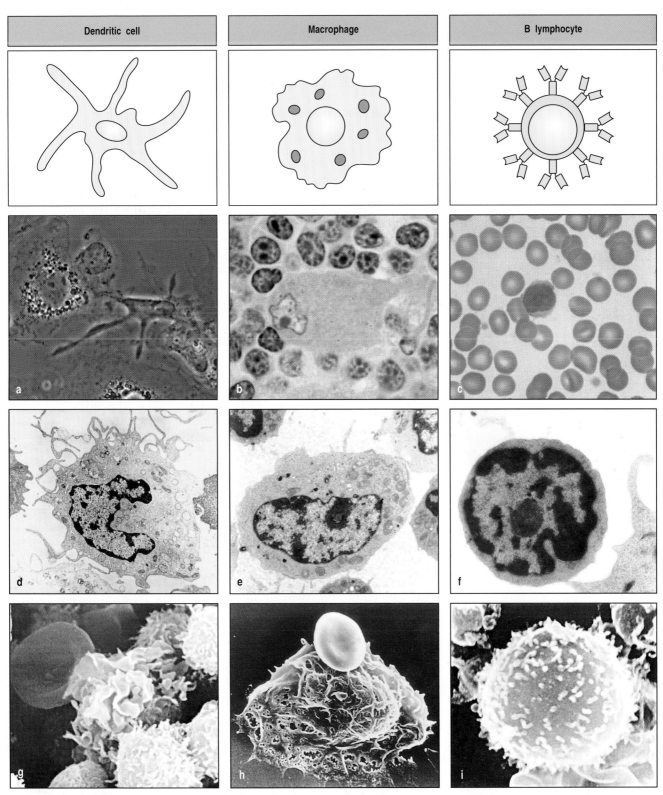

| Dendritic cell | Macrophage | B lymphocyte |

Fig. 1.19 The professional antigen-presenting cells. The three types of professional antigen-presenting cells are shown in the form in which they will be depicted throughout this book (top row), as they appear in the light microscope (second row), and as they appear by transmission electron microscopy (third row) and scanning electron microscopy (bottom row). Dendritic cells are found in lymphoid and other tissues where they constitutively express co-stimulatory activity; they are thought to have a critical role in immunity to viruses. Macrophages are specialized to internalize and present particulate antigens and they can also be induced to express co-stimulatory activity. B cells have antigen-specific receptors that allow them to internalize large amounts of specific antigen and they can be induced to express co-stimulatory activity. Photographs courtesy of R Steinman (a); N Rooney (b, c, e, f); S Knight (d, g); P Heap (h, i).

Summary.

The early innate systems of defense, which depend on invariant responses to common features of pathogens, are important but they cannot confer protection from novel types of pathogens and do not lead to immunological memory. These are the unique features of adaptive immunity based on clonal selection of lymphocytes bearing specific receptors.

The clonal selection of lymphocytes provides a theoretical framework for understanding all the key features of adaptive immunity. Each lymphocyte carries cell-surface receptors of a single specificity, generated by random recombination of variable receptor gene segments and the pairing of different variable chains. This produces lymphocytes each bearing a distinct receptor, so that the total **repertoire** of receptors can recognize virtually any antigen. If the receptor on a lymphocyte is specific for a ubiquitous self antigen, the cell is eliminated by encountering the antigen early in development. When a recirculating lymphocyte encounters foreign antigen in lymphoid tissues, it is induced to proliferate and its progeny to differentiate into effector cells that can eliminate a specific infectious agent. A subset of these proliferating lymphocytes differentiates into memory cells, ready to respond rapidly to the same pathogen if encountered again. The details of these processes of recognition, development, and differentiation form the main material of the middle three parts of this book.

Recognition and effector mechanisms of adaptive immunity.

Clonal selection describes the basic operating principle of the adaptive immune response, but not its mechanisms. In the last section of this chapter, we outline the mechanisms by which pathogens are detected by lymphocytes and eventually destroyed in a successful adaptive immune response. Different pathogens have distinct lifestyles that require different mechanisms not only to ensure their destruction but also for their detection and recognition (Fig. 1.20). We have already seen that

Fig. 1.20 The major pathogen types confronting the immune system and some of the diseases they cause.

The immune system protects against four classes of pathogens		
Type of pathogen	Examples	Diseases
Extracellular bacteria, parasites, fungi	*Streptococcus pneumoniae* *Clostridium tetani* *Trypanosoma brucei*	Pneumonia Tetanus Sleeping sickness
Intracellular bacteria, parasites	*Mycobacterium leprae* *Listeria monocytogenes* *Leishmania donovani*	Leprosy Listeriosis Leishmaniasis
Viruses (intracellular)	Variola Influenza Varicella	Smallpox Flu Chickenpox
Parasitic worms (extracellular)	*Ascaris* *Schistosoma*	Ascariasis Schistosomiasis

there are two different kinds of antigen receptors: the surface immuno-globulin of B cells, and the smaller antigen receptor of T cells. These surface receptors are adapted to recognize antigen in two different ways: B cells recognize antigen outside cells, where for example most bacteria are found; T cells by contrast can detect antigens generated inside cells, for example by viruses.

The **effector mechanisms** that operate to eliminate pathogens in an adaptive immune response are essentially identical to those of innate immunity. Indeed it seems likely that specific recognition by clonally distributed receptors evolved as a late addition to existing innate effector mechanisms to produce the present-day adaptive immune response. We begin by outlining the effector actions of antibodies, which depend almost entirely on recruiting cells and molecules of the innate immune system.

1-12   Extracellular pathogens and their toxins are eliminated by antibodies.

Antibodies, which were the first specific product of the immune response to be identified, are found in the fluid component of blood, or **plasma**, and in extracellular fluids. Because body fluids were once known as humors, immunity mediated by antibody is known as **humoral immunity**.

As we have seen in Fig. 1.14, antibodies are Y-shaped molecules whose arms form two identical antigen-binding sites that are highly variable from one molecule to another, providing the diversity required for specific antigen recognition. The stem of the Y, which defines the **class** of the antibody and determines its functional properties, takes one of only five major forms, or **isotypes**. Each of the five antibody classes engages a distinct set of effector mechanisms for disposing of antigen once it is recognized. We shall describe the isotypes and their actions in detail in Chapters 3 and 8.

The simplest way in which antibodies can protect from pathogens or their toxic products is by binding to them and thereby blocking their access to cells they may infect or destroy (Fig. 1.21, left panels). This is known as **neutralization** and is important for protection against bacterial toxins and against pathogens such as viruses, which can thus be prevented from entering cells and replicating.

Binding by antibodies, however, is not sufficient on its own to arrest the replication of bacteria that multiply outside cells. In this case, one role of antibody is to enable a phagocytic cell to ingest and destroy the bacterium. This is important for the many bacteria that are resistant to direct recognition by phagocytes: instead, the phagocytes recognize the constant region of the antibodies coating the bacterium (Fig. 1.21, middle panels). The coating of pathogens and foreign particles in this way is known as **opsonization**.

The third function of antibodies is to activate a system of plasma proteins known as **complement**. The complement system, which we shall discuss in detail in Chapter 8, can directly destroy bacteria, and this is important in a few bacterial infections (Fig. 1.21, right panels). Its main function, however, like that of antibodies themselves, is to enable phagocytes to engulf and destroy bacteria they would otherwise not recognize. Complement also enhances the bacteriocidal actions of phagocytes; indeed it is so called because it complements the activities of antibodies.

Fig. 1.21 Antibodies can participate in host defense in three main ways.
The left-hand column shows antibodies binding to and neutralizing a bacterial toxin, preventing it from interacting with host cells and causing pathology. Unbound toxin can react with receptors on the host cell, whereas the toxin: antibody complex cannot. Antibodies also neutralize complete virus particles and bacterial cells by binding to them and inactivating them. The antigen: antibody complex is eventually scavenged and degraded by macrophages. Antibodies coating an antigen render it recognizable as foreign by phagocytes (macrophages and polymorphonuclear leukocytes), which then ingest and destroy it; this is called opsonization. The central column shows opsonization and phagocytosis of a bacterial cell. The right-hand column shows activation of the complement system by antibodies coating a bacterial cell. Bound antibodies form a receptor for the first protein of the complement system, which eventually forms a protein complex on the surface of the bacterium that in some cases, can kill the bacterium directly, but more generally favors the uptake and destruction of the bacterium by phagocytes. Thus, antibodies target pathogens and their products for disposal by phagocytes.

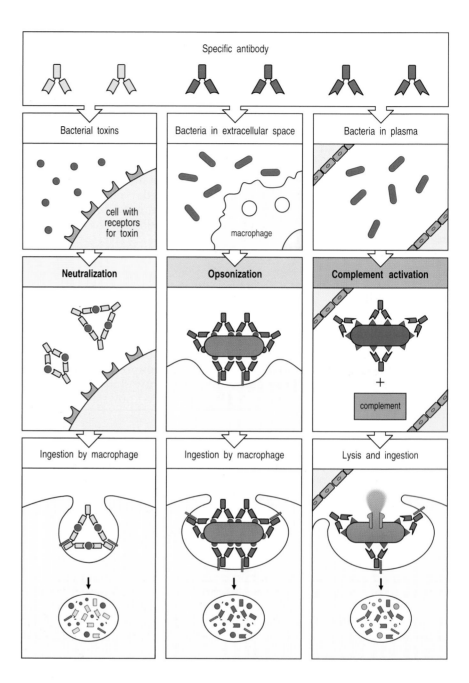

Antibodies of different isotypes are found in different compartments of the body and differ in the effector mechanisms they recruit, but all pathogens and particles bound by antibody are eventually delivered to phagocytes for ingestion, degradation and removal from the body (Fig. 1.21, bottom panels).

The complement system and the phagocytes that antibodies recruit are not themselves antigen specific; they depend upon antibody molecules to mark the particles as foreign. Antibodies are the sole contribution of B cells to the adaptive immune response. T cells by contrast have a variety of effector actions.

1-13 **T cells are needed to control intracellular pathogens and to activate B-cell responses to most antigens.**

Pathogens are accessible to antibodies only in the blood and the extracellular spaces. However, some bacterial pathogens and parasites, and all viruses, replicate inside cells where they cannot be detected by antibodies. The destruction of these invaders is the function of the T lymphocytes, or T cells, which are responsible for the **cell-mediated immune responses** of adaptive immunity.

Cell-mediated reactions depend on direct interactions between T lymphocytes and cells bearing the antigen the T cells recognize. The actions of **cytotoxic T cells** are the most direct. These cells recognize body cells infected with viruses, which replicate inside cells using the synthetic machinery of the cell itself, and eventually kill the cell, releasing the new virus particles. Antigens derived from the replicating virus are meanwhile displayed on the surface of infected cells. Here they are recognized by cytotoxic T cells, which control the infection by killing the cell before viral replication is complete (Fig. 1.22).

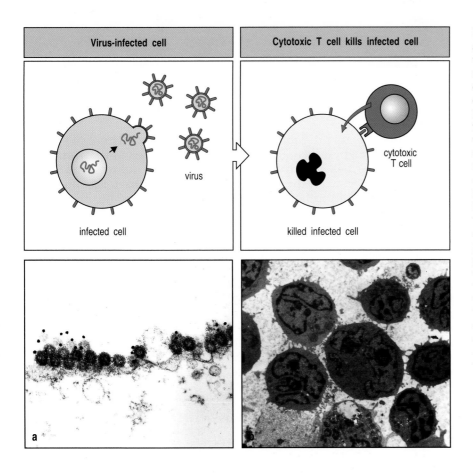

| Virus-infected cell | Cytotoxic T cell kills infected cell |

virus

infected cell

cytotoxic T cell

killed infected cell

a

Fig. 1.22 Mechanism of host defense against intracellular infection by viruses. Cells infected by viruses are recognized by specialized T cells called cytotoxic T cells, which kill the infected cells directly. The killing mechanism involves the activation of nucleases in the infected cell, which cleave host and viral DNA. Panel a is a transmission electron micrograph showing the plasma membrane of a Chinese hamster ovary (CHO) cell infected with influenza virus. Many virus particles can be seen budding from the cell surface. Some of these have been labeled by a monoclonal antibody that is specific for a viral protein and that is coupled to gold particles, which appear as the solid black dots in the micrograph. Panel b is a transmission electron micrograph of a virus-infected cell surrounded by reactive T lymphocytes. Note the close apposition of the membranes of the virus-infected cell and the T cell in the upper left corner of the micrograph, and the clustering of the cytoplasmic organelles between the nucleus and the point of contact with the infected cell. Panel a courtesy of M Bui and A Helenius. Panel b courtesy of N Rooney.

T lymphocytes are also important in the control of intracellular bacterial infections. Some bacteria grow only in the vesicles of macrophages: an important example is *Mycobacterium tuberculosis*, the pathogen that causes tuberculosis (Fig. 1.23). Bacteria entering macrophages are usually destroyed in the lysosomes, which contain a variety of enzymes and bacteriocidal substances. Intracellular bacteria survive because the

Fig. 1.23 Mechanism of host defense against intracellular infection by mycobacteria. Mycobacteria infect macrophages and live in cytoplasmic vesicles that resist fusion with lysosomes and consequent destruction of the bacteria by macrophage bacteriocidal activity. However, when the appropriate T cell, an inflammatory T cell (T$_H$1), recognizes an infected macrophage it releases macrophage-activating molecules or cytokines that induce lysosomal fusion and the activation of macrophage bacteriocidal activities. The elimination of mycobacteria from the vesicles of activated macrophages can be seen in the light micrographs (bottom row) of resting (left) and activated (right) macrophages infected with *M. tuberculosis*. The cells have been stained with an acid-fast red dye to reveal the presence of the mycobacteria, which are prominent in the resting macrophages but have been eliminated from the activated macrophages. Photographs courtesy of G Kaplan.

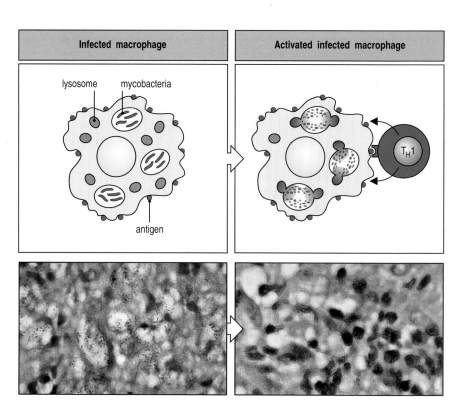

vesicles they occupy do not fuse with the lysosomes. These infections can be controlled by a second type of T cell, known as an **inflammatory T cell**, or a **T$_H$1** cell, which activates macrophages, inducing the fusion of their lysosomes with the vesicles containing the bacteria and at the same time stimulating other antibacterial mechanisms of the phagocyte.

T cells destroy intracellular pathogens by killing infected cells and by activating macrophages, but they also play a central part in the destruction of extracellular pathogens by activating B cells. This is the specialized role of a third subset of T cells, called **helper T cells** or **T$_H$2 cells**. We shall see in Chapter 8 when we discuss the humoral immune response in detail that only a few antigens, which have special properties, are capable of activating naive B lymphocytes on their own. Most require a signal from T$_H$2 cells before they will proliferate and differentiate into cells capable of secreting antibody (see Fig. 1.18 top panel). Before it was recognized that the T cells that activate macrophages (the T$_H$1 cells) are distinct from those that help activate B cells (the T$_H$2 cells), both these types of T cell were called helper T cells. To avoid confusion, we will, in the remainder of this book, reserve the term helper T cells for T$_H$2 cells, and call T$_H$1 cells inflammatory T cells.

1-14 | **T cells are specialized to recognize foreign antigens as peptides bound to proteins of the major histocompatibility complex.**

All the effects of T lymphocytes depend upon interactions with cells containing foreign proteins. In the case of cytotoxic T cells and inflammatory T cells, the proteins are those produced by pathogens infecting the target cell. Helper T cells, on the other hand, recognize and interact with B cells that have bound and internalized foreign antigen via their surface immunoglobulin. In all cases, T cells recognize their targets by detecting peptide fragments derived from these foreign proteins and bound to specialized cell-surface molecules on the infected host cells or B cells. The molecules that display peptide antigen to T cells are membrane glycoproteins encoded in a cluster of genes bearing the cumbersome name **major histocompatibility complex**, abbreviated **MHC**.

The human **MHC molecules** were first discovered as the result of attempts to use skin grafts from donors to repair badly burned pilots and bomb victims during World War II. The patients rejected the grafts, and eventually genetic experiments on inbred mice led to the identification of a complex of genes that would cause the rejection of skin grafts between mice that differed only at these genetic loci and at no other. Because they control the compatibility of tissue grafts, these genes, of which there is an analogous set in humans, became known as the histocompatibility complex of genes. It is called the major histocompatibility complex because proteins encoded by other genes can have minor effects on tissue compatibility, for reasons we shall discuss when we deal with antigen recognition by T cells in Chapter 4. The physiological function of the proteins encoded by the MHC did not emerge until many years after their discovery.

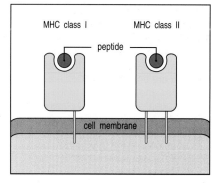

Fig. 1.24 MHC molecules display peptide fragments of antigens on the surface of cells. MHC molecules are membrane proteins whose outer extracellular domains form a cleft in which a peptide fragment can bind. These fragments, which are derived from proteins degraded inside the cell, including foreign protein antigens, are bound by the newly synthesized MHC molecule before it reaches the surface. There are two kinds of MHC molecules, MHC class I molecules and MHC class II molecules, which differ in structure and function.

1-15	**Two major types of T cells recognize peptides bound by two different classes of MHC molecule.**

It is now known that there are two types of MHC molecules, called class I and class II, which differ in subtle ways but share most of their major structural features. The most important of these structural features is an outer extracellular domain that forms a long cleft in which peptide fragments are trapped during the synthesis of the MHC molecule inside the cell. The MHC molecule bearing its cargo of peptide is then transported to the cell surface where it displays the bound peptide to T cells (Fig. 1.24). The antigen receptors of T lymphocytes are specialized to recognize antigenic peptide fragments bound to an MHC molecule.

The most important differences between the two classes of MHC molecules lie not in their structure but in the source of the peptides they trap and carry to the cell surface. **MHC class I molecules** collect peptides derived from proteins synthesized in the cytosol, and thus display fragments of viral proteins on the cell surface (Fig. 1.25).

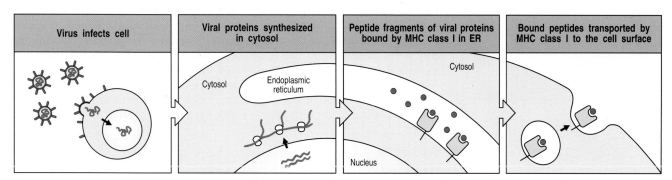

Fig. 1.25 MHC class I molecules present antigen derived from proteins in the cytosol. In cells infected with viruses, viral proteins are synthesized in the cytosol. Peptide fragments of viral proteins are transported into the endoplasmic reticulum where they are bound by MHC class I molecules, which then deliver the peptides to the cell surface.

Fig. 1.26   MHC class II molecules present antigen originating in intracellular vesicles. Some bacteria infect cells and grow in intracellular vesicles. Peptides derived from such bacteria are bound by MHC class II molecules and transported to the cell surface (top row). MHC class II molecules also bind and transport peptides derived from antigen that has been bound and internalized by endocytosis into intracellular vesicles (bottom row).

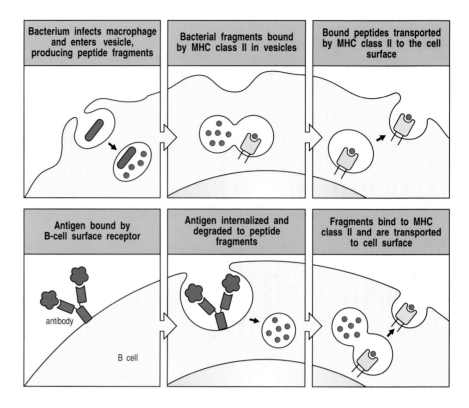

Bacterium infects macrophage and enters vesicle, producing peptide fragments	Bacterial fragments bound by MHC class II in vesicles	Bound peptides transported by MHC class II to the cell surface

Antigen bound by B-cell surface receptor	Antigen internalized and degraded to peptide fragments	Fragments bind to MHC class II and are transported to cell surface

antibody

B cell

MHC class II molecules bind peptides derived from proteins in intracellular membrane-bound vesicles, and thus display peptides derived from antigens engulfed by macrophages or internalized by B cells (Fig. 1.26). We shall see in Chapter 4 exactly how peptides from these different origins are made differentially accessible to the two types of MHC molecules.

Once they reach the cell surface with their cargo of antigenic peptides, the two classes of MHC molecules are recognized by different functional classes of T cells. MHC class I molecules bearing viral peptides are recognized by cytotoxic T cells which kill the infected cell (Fig. 1.27); MHC class II molecules bearing peptides derived from antigens in the vesicles of macrophages or B cells are recognized by inflammatory and helper T cells, respectively (Fig. 1.28). How the differential recognition of the two types of MHC molecules becomes coupled to the distinct functions of the different classes of T cells during their development is a central problem in immunology and will be a major topic of Chapter 6.

On recognizing their targets, the three types of T cells are stimulated to release different sets of effector molecules that directly affect their target cells in ways we shall discuss in Chapter 7, and help to recruit other effector cells, as we shall see in Chapter 9 where we discuss the integration of the response to infection. We shall see that many **cytokines** are included in these effector molecules; they play a crucial part in clonal expansion of lymphocytes as well as in innate immune responses and in the effector actions of most immune cells, and are thus central to the understanding of the immune system.

Cytotoxic T cell recognizes complex of viral fragment with MHC class I and kills infected cell

kills

Tc

MHC class I

Fig. 1.27   Cytotoxic T cells recognize antigen presented by MHC class I molecules and kill the cell. The peptide:MHC class I complex on virus-infected cells is detected by antigen-specific cytotoxic T cells. Cytotoxic T cells kill other cells by releasing molecules that penetrate infected cells and activate the process of programmed cell death or apoptosis in those cells. The T cell itself is unaffected and can move on to kill many more infected cells.

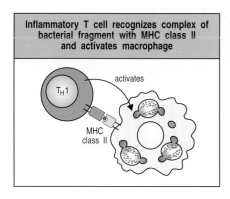

Inflammatory T cell recognizes complex of bacterial fragment with MHC class II and activates macrophage

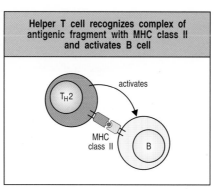

Helper T cell recognizes complex of antigenic fragment with MHC class II and activates B cell

Fig. 1.28 Inflammatory and helper T cells recognize antigen presented by MHC class II molecules. Inflammatory and helper T cells (T_H1 and T_H2) both recognize peptides bound to MHC class II molecules. On recognition of their specific antigen on infected macrophages, inflammatory T cells activate the macrophage, leading to the destruction of the intracellular bacteria (left panel). When they recognize antigen on B cells, helper T cells activate these cells to proliferate and differentiate into antibody-producing plasma cells (right panel).

1-16   **Specific infectious diseases result from immune deficiencies or specialized strategies of pathogens.**

We tend to take for granted the ability of our immune systems to free our bodies of infection and prevent its recurrence. In some people, however, parts of the immune system fail. In the most severe of these **immunodeficiency diseases**, adaptive immunity is completely eliminated, and death occurs in infancy from overwhelming infection unless heroic measures are taken. Other less catastrophic failures lead to specific recurrent infections, and much has been learned about the functions of the different components of the immune system through the study of these diseases.

Recently, a devastating form of immunodeficiency has appeared, the **acquired immune deficiency syndrome**, or **AIDS**, which is itself caused by an infectious agent. This disease destroys the helper and inflammatory T cells that play a central part in most immune responses, leading to infections caused by intracellular bacteria and other pathogens normally controlled by macrophages activated by these T cells. Such infections are the major cause of death from this increasingly prevalent immunodeficiency disease.

AIDS is caused by a virus, the **human immunodeficiency virus**, or **HIV**, that has evolved a number of strategies whereby it not only evades but also subverts the protective mechanisms of the adaptive immune response. We discuss in Chapter 10 the devices that have evolved to allow many bacteria and parasites, as well as viruses, to avoid destruction by the immune system. The conquest of many of the world's leading causes of disease, including malaria and the various diarrheal diseases (the leading killers of children), as well as of the more recent threat from AIDS, may depend upon a better understanding of the interactions of these pathogens with the cells of the immune system.

1-17   **Understanding adaptive immune responses is important for the control of allergies, autoimmune disease, and organ graft rejection.**

Many medically important diseases are associated with immune responses directed against inappropriate antigens, in the absence of infectious disease. Normal immune responses in the absence of infection occur in **allergy**, where the antigen is an innocuous foreign substance, in **autoimmune disease**, where the response is to a self antigen, and in **graft rejection**, where the antigen is borne by a foreign cell. What

Fig. 1.29 Immune responses can be beneficial or harmful depending on the nature of the antigen. Beneficial responses are shown in white, harmful responses in shaded boxes. Where the response is beneficial, its absence is harmful.

Antigen	Effect of response to antigen	
	Normal response	Deficient response
Infectious agent	Protective immunity	Recurrent infection
Innocuous substance	Allergy	No response
Grafted organ	Rejection	Acceptance
Self organ	Autoimmunity	Self tolerance
Tumor	Tumor immunity	Cancer

we call an immune response or its failure, and whether the response is considered harmful or beneficial to the host, depends not on the response itself but on the nature of the antigen (Fig. 1.29).

Allergies, which include asthma, are an increasingly common cause of disability in the developed world, and many important diseases are now recognized as autoimmune. An autoimmune response directed against pancreatic β cells is the leading cause of diabetes in the young. In allergies and autoimmune diseases, the powerful protective mechanisms of the adaptive immune response are the cause of serious damage to the host.

Immune responses to harmless antigens, to body tissues, or to organ grafts, like all other immune responses, are highly specific. At present, the usual way to treat these responses is with **immunosuppressive drugs**, which inhibit all immune responses, desirable or undesirable. If, instead, it were possible to suppress only those lymphocyte clones responsible for the unwanted response, the disease could be cured (or the grafted organ protected) without impeding protective immune responses. Antigen-specific suppression of immune responses can be induced experimentally, but the molecular basis of suppression is not known. If one could achieve control of the immunoregulatory apparatus, then the dream of antigen-specific **immunoregulation** to control unwanted immune responses could become a reality. We shall see in Chapter 7 and Chapter 9 how the mechanisms of immune regulation are beginning to emerge from a better understanding of the functional subsets of lymphocytes and the cytokines that control them, and we shall discuss the present state of understanding of allergies and autoimmune disease and of immunosuppressive drugs in Chapters 11 and 12.

1-18   Specific stimulation of adaptive immune responses is the most effective way to prevent infectious disease and may be effective in cancer therapy.

While the specific suppression of immune responses must await advances in basic research on immune regulation and its application, immunology has in the two centuries since Jenner's pioneering experiment achieved its greatest practical successes in the results of vaccination. Mass immunization programs have led to the virtual eradication of several diseases that used to be associated with significant mortality and morbidity (Fig. 1.30). Immunization is considered so safe and so important that most states in the USA require children to be immunized against several different diseases (Fig. 1.31). Impressive as these accomplishments

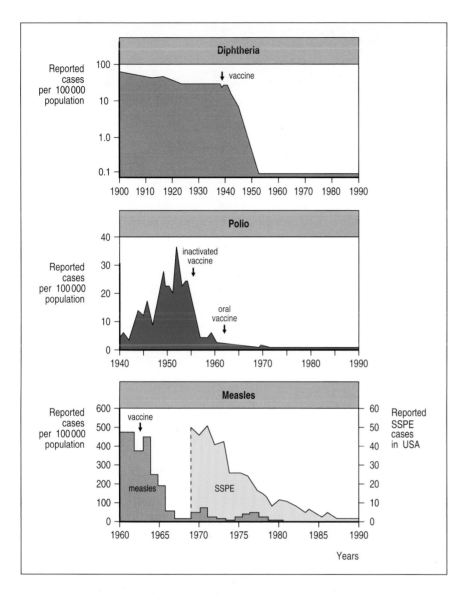

Fig. 1.30 Successful vaccination campaigns. Diphtheria, polio, and measles and its consequences have been virtually eliminated in the USA as shown in these three graphs. SSPE stands for subacute sclerosing panencephalitis, a brain disease that is a late consequence of measles infection in a few patients. When measles was prevented, SSPE disappeared 10–15 years later. However, as these diseases have not been eradicated worldwide, immunization must be maintained in a very high percentage of the population to prevent their reappearance.

Fig. 1.31 Childhood vaccination schedules (in red) in the USA.

Current immunization schedule for children (USA)								
Vaccine given	2 months	4 months	6 months	15 months	18 months	24 months	4–6 years	14–15 years
Diphtheria-pertussis-tetanus (DPT)	■	■	■		■		■	
Trivalent oral polio (TVOP)	■	■			■		■	
Measles				■				
Rubella				■				
Mumps				■				
Haemophilus B polysaccharide						■		
Diphtheria-tetanus toxoids								■

Fig. 1.32 Diseases for which
effective vaccines are still needed.
*Current measles vaccines are effective
but heat sensitive, which makes their use
difficult in tropical countries.

Some diseases for which effective vaccines are not yet available		
Disease	Annual mortality	Annual incidence
Malaria	1 500 000	150 000 000
Schistosomiasis	330 000	10 000 000
Worm infestation	50 000	4 900 000 000
Tuberculosis	3 000 000	10 000 000
Diarrhea	4 300 000	28 000 000
Respiratory disease	10 000 000	15 000 000
AIDS	100 000	750 000
Measles*	2 000 000	67 000 000

Fig. 1.32 Diseases for which effective vaccines are still needed. *Current measles vaccines are effective but heat sensitive, which makes their use difficult in tropical countries.

are, there are still many diseases for which we lack effective vaccines, as shown in Fig. 1.32. Even where a vaccine against diseases such as measles or polio can be used effectively in developed countries, technical and economic problems may prevent its widespread use in developing countries, where mortality from these diseases is still high. The tools of modern immunology and molecular biology are being applied to develop new vaccines and improve old ones, and we shall discuss these advances in Chapter 12. The prospect of controlling these important diseases is tremendously exciting. The guarantee of good health is a critical step towards population control and economic development. At a cost of pennies per person, great hardship and suffering can be alleviated.

In the case of cancer, many scientists believe that tumor cells express antigens recognizable by the immune system, and that disease results because the immune response to these antigens does not occur or is not successful in eliminating the tumor. The goal of research in **tumor immunology** is to identify and induce such responses in order to cure cancer. To date, a few successes and many failures have been recorded. A general method for inducing immunity to specific cancers would have the most profound impact on therapy in this disease, since it would be physiological and presumably non-toxic to the host, while virtually all current cancer therapy is highly toxic.

Summary.

Lymphocytes have two distinct recognition systems specialized for detection of extracellular and intracellular pathogens. B cells have cell-surface immunuglobulin molecules as receptors for antigen and, upon activation, secrete the immunoglobulin as soluble antibody that provides defense against pathogens in the extracellular spaces of the body. T cells have receptors that recognize peptide fragments of intracellular pathogens transported to the cell surface by the glycoproteins of the major histocompatibility complex (MHC). Two classes of MHC molecules transport peptides from different intracellular compartments to present them to distinct types of effector T cells: cytotoxic T cells that kill infected target cells, and inflammatory and helper T cells that activate macrophages and B cells, respectively. Thus, T cells are crucially important for both the humoral and cell-mediated responses of adaptive immunity. The adaptive immune response appears to have engrafted specific antigen recognition by highly diversified receptors onto innate defense systems that play a central part in the effector actions of both B and T lymphocytes. The antigen-specific suppression of adaptive immune responses is the goal of treatment for important diseases caused by allergic or autoimmune responses. The specific stimulation of adaptive immune responses is the basis of successful vaccination campaigns.

Summary to Chapter 1.

The immune system defends the host against infection. Innate immunity serves as a first line of defense, but lacks the ability to recognize certain pathogens and to provide specific protective immunity that prevents re-infection. Adaptive immunity is based on the clonal selection of lymphocytes bearing highly diverse antigen-specific receptors that allow the immune system to recognize any foreign antigen. In the adaptive immune response, antigen-specific lymphocytes proliferate and differentiate into effector cells that eliminate pathogens. Host defense requires different recognition systems and a wide variety of effector mechanisms to seek out and destroy the wide variety of pathogens in their various habitats within the body and at its surfaces. Not only can the adaptive immune response eliminate a pathogen, but in the process it also generates increased numbers of differentiated memory lymphocytes through clonal section, and this allows a more rapid and effective response upon re-infection. The regulation of immune responses, whether to suppress them when unwanted or to stimulate them in the prevention of infectious disease, is the major medical goal of research in immunology.

General References.

Historical background

Silverstein, A.M.: *History of Immunology*, 1st edn. London, Academic Press, 1989.

Landsteiner, K.: *The Specificity of Serological Reactions*, 3rd edn. Boston, Harvard University Press, 1964.

Burnet, F.M.: *The Clonal Selection Theory of Acquired Immunity*. London, Cambridge University Press, 1959.

Metchnikoff, E.: *Immunity in the Infectious Diseases*, 1st edn. New York, Macmillan Press, 1905.

Biological background

Alberts, B., Bray, D., Lewis, J., Raff, M., Roberts, K., and Watson, J.D.: *Molecular Biology of the Cell*, 3rd edn. New York, Garland Publishing, 1994.

Davis, B.D., Dulbecco, R., Eisen, H.N., and Ginsberg, H.S.: *Microbiology*, 4th edn. Philadelphia, J.B. Lippincott, 1990.

Stryer, L.: *Biochemistry*, 3rd edn. New York, Freeman, 1994.

Watson, J.D., Hopkins, N.H., Roberts, J.W., Steitz, J.A., and Weiner, A.M.: *Molecular Biology of the Gene*, 4th edn. Menlo Park, CA., W.A. Benjamin, Cummings Publishing, 1987.

Primary journals devoted solely or primarily to immunology

Immunity
Journal of Immunology
European Journal of Immunology
International Immunology
Journal of Experimental Medicine
Immunology
Thymus
Clinical and Experimental Immunology
Regional Immunology
Comparative and Developmental Immunology
Infection and Immunity
Immunogenetics
Autoimmunity

Primary journals with frequent papers in immunology

Nature
Science
Proceedings of the National Academy of Sciences, USA
Cell
EMBO Journal
Journal of Clinical Investigation
Journal of Cell Biology
Journal of Biological Chemistry
Molecular Cell Biology

Review journals in immunology

Current Opinion in Immunology
Immunological Reviews
Annual Reviews in Immunology

The Immunologist
Immunology Today
Seminars in Immunology
International Reviews in Immunology
Contemporary Topics in Microbiology and Immunology
Research in Immunology
Proceedings of the International Congress of Immunology. Progress in Immunology, Vol 1–8, 1971–1992, issued every three years.

Advanced textbooks in immunology, compendia, etc.

Paul, W.E., (ed): *Fundamental Immunology*, 3rd edn, New York, Raven Press, 1993.

Roitt, I.M., and Delves, P.J. (eds): Encyclopedia of Immunology, 3rd edn. London/San Diego, Academic Press, 1992.

Sampter, M. (ed.): *Immunological Diseases*, 4th edn. Boston, Little, Brown, 1988.

Stiehm, E.R. (ed.): *Immunologic Disorders in Infants and Children*, 3rd edn. Philadelphia, W.B. Saunders, 1989.

The Induction, Measurement, and Manipulation of the Immune Response

2

 Before you read further, a word from the authors about this chapter. We have written it to be read when it is needed to understand a particular method; later chapters reference Chapter 2 as appropriate. Although it is also written so that it can be read from start to finish, most students will want to dip into this toolbox of methods when they encounter a reference to it in later chapters, rather than tackling it now. To make the sections relevant to later chapters easy to identify, the edges of the paper in this chapter are colored, and the most useful methods for any part of the book are color coded to the part in which it is needed. However, we recommend that you read the first six sections of Chapter 2 before continuing with the rest of the book.

The description of the immune system outlined in Chapter 1 is drawn from the results of many different kinds of experiment and from the study of human disease. Immunologists have devised a wide variety of techniques for inducing, measuring, and characterizing immune responses, and for altering the immune system through cellular, molecular, and genetic manipulation. Before we examine the cellular and molecular basis of host defense that occupies the rest of this book, we shall look at how the immune system is studied and introduce the specialized language of immunology. In this chapter we also describe many basic immunological phenomena that experimental immunologists seek to explain in terms of the cellular and molecular features of the immune system. Because genetics plays an important role in the analysis of the immune system and of human disease, the genetic analysis of the immune system is discussed here, including recently developed techniques for genetic manipulation that have had a tremendous impact on all areas of biology. We also describe clinical tests used to assess immune function in patients with immunological disorders.

Immunological techniques are also widely applied in many other areas of biology and medicine. The use of antibodies to detect specific molecules in complex mixtures and in tissues is of particular importance. We therefore devote an entire section of this chapter to the antibody-based methods used by immunologists, by basic scientists in many other biological disciplines, and by clinicians. These methods illustrate the specificity and utility of antibodies, whose structure and generation form an important theme in subsequent parts of this book.

Related
to Part I

The induction and detection of immune responses.

Most of the material in this book focuses on **adaptive immunity**, that is, on immune responses of lymphocytes to foreign materials, most importantly the antigens borne by various pathogenic microorganisms. However, experimental immunologists have mainly examined responses induced by simple non-living antigens in developing our understanding of the immune response. Thus, we shall begin our consideration of how the immune system is studied by discussing how such adaptive immune responses are induced and detected. The deliberate induction of an immune response is known as **immunization**. Experimental immunizations are carried out routinely by injecting the test antigen into the animal or human subject, and we shall see that the route, dose, and form in which antigen is administered can profoundly affect whether a response occurs and the type of response that is produced. To determine whether an immune response has occurred and to follow its course, the immunized individual is monitored for the appearance of one of many different immune reactions directed at the specific antigen. Monitoring often involves analysis of relatively crude preparations of **antiserum** (plural: **antisera**). This is the fluid phase of clotted blood (the **serum**), which in an immunized individual, contains the specific antibodies as well as other soluble serum proteins. Immune responses to most antigens elicit the production of both specific antibodies and specific effector T cells. To study immune responses mediated by T cells, blood lymphocytes or cells from lymphoid organs are tested; T-cell responses are more commonly studied in experimental animals than in humans.

Any substance that can elicit an immune response is said to be **immunogenic** and is called an **immunogen**. There is a clear operational distinction between an immunogen and an antigen. An **antigen** is defined as any substance that can bind to a specific antibody. All antigens therefore have the potential to elicit specific antibodies but some need to be attached to an immunogen in order to do so. This means that although all immunogens are antigens, not all antigens are immunogenic.

The following sections describe some of the most commonly used techniques for inducing, detecting, and measuring adaptive immune responses. These techniques are used to address many questions in immunology. What determines whether a particular substance will be immunogenic or not? How does one raise antibodies against substances that are not by themselves immunogenic? And what determines which type of response will be provoked by a particular immunization? We shall first examine the nature of antigens and the features that make a substance immunogenic, before turning to a general consideration of how the response is detected.

2-1   Antibodies can be produced against almost any substance.

When antibodies were first discovered as the agents of resistance to infection, it was thought likely that their ability to bind pathogens had been selected over evolutionary time because of their importance to survival. However, Karl Landsteiner soon showed that antibodies could be elicited against a virtually limitless range of molecules, including synthetic chemicals never found in the natural environment. This demonstrated unequivocally that the repertoire of possible antibodies in any individual is essentially unlimited and that the genes encoding

Fig. 2.1 Antibodies can be elicited by small chemical groups called haptens only when the hapten is linked to a protein carrier. Three types of antibodies are produced. One set (blue) binds the carrier protein alone and is called carrier-specific. One set (red) binds to the hapten on any carrier or free in solution and is called hapten-specific. One set (purple) only binds the specific conjugate of hapten and carrier used for immunization, apparently binding to sites at which the hapten joins the carrier, and is called conjugate-specific. The amount of antibody of each type in this serum is shown schematically in the graphs at the bottom; note that the original antigen binds more antibody than the sum of anti-hapten and anti-carrier owing to the additional binding of conjugate-specific antibody.

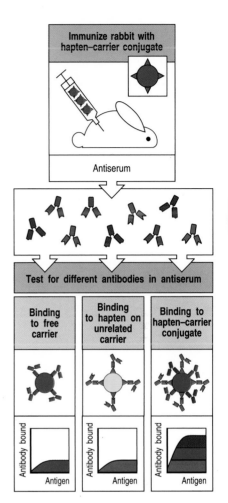

Related to Part I

individual antibodies could not have been selected for their action against pathogens. This radically changed the way that immunologists thought about the antibody response, forcing them to the conclusion that evolution must have selected not for specific antibody structures but rather for the ability to generate an open repertoire of antibodies of diverse structure, a subject we shall focus on in Chapter 3. It also alerted immunologists to the potential utility of antibodies for detecting and measuring almost any substance in a complex mixture of molecules.

In order to determine the range of antibodies that could be produced, Landsteiner studied the immune response to small organic molecules such as arsonates and nitrophenyls. These simple structures do not provoke antibodies when injected by themselves, but Landsteiner found that antibodies could be raised against them if the molecule was covalently attached to a protein carrier. He therefore termed them **haptens** (from the Greek *haptein*, to fasten). Animals immunized with a hapten–carrier conjugate produced three distinct sets of antibodies (Fig. 2.1). One set comprised hapten-specific antibodies that reacted with the hapten on any carrier as well as with free hapten. The second set of antibodies reacted with the unmodified carrier protein. Finally, some antibodies reacted only with the specific conjugate of hapten and carrier used for immunization. Landsteiner studied mainly the antibody response to the hapten, as these small molecules could be synthesized in a great variety of closely related forms. As can be seen in Fig. 2.2, antibodies raised against a particular hapten bind that hapten but in general fail to bind even very closely related chemical structures. The binding of haptens by anti-hapten antibodies has played an important part in defining the precision of antigen binding by antibody molecules. Anti-hapten antibodies are also important medically as they mediate allergic reactions to penicillin and other compounds that elicit antibody responses when they attach to self proteins (see Section 11-5).

Antisera contain many different antibody molecules that bind to the immunogen in slightly different ways (see Fig. 2.1 and Fig. 2.2). Some of these antibodies also cross-react with related antigens (see Fig. 2.2), and even in some cases with antigens having no clear relationship to the

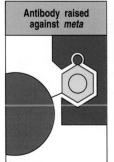

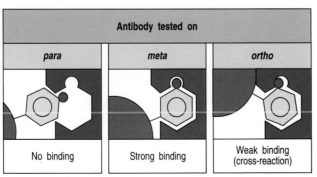

Fig. 2.2 Anti-hapten antibodies can distinguish small changes in hapten structure. Antibodies raised to the *meta* substituted azobenzenearsonate ring react predominantly with the *meta* form, and have limited cross-reactivity with the *para* and *ortho* forms. The particular antibody shown here fits the *meta* form perfectly, weakly binds to the *ortho* form, and does not bind the *para* form.

Related to Part I

immunogen. These cross-reacting antibodies can create problems when the antiserum is used for detection of specific antigen using the techniques outlined in the next part of this chapter. They can be removed from an antiserum by **absorption** with the cross-reactive antigen, leaving behind the antibodies that bind only to the immunogen. The problems resulting from the heterogeneity of the antibodies present in an antiserum can be avoided by making monoclonal antibodies, which are homogeneous antibodies derived from a single antibody-producing cell (see Section 2-11).

The antigens used most frequently in experimental immunology are proteins, and antibodies to proteins are of enormous utility in experimental biology and medicine. Therefore, we will focus in this chapter on the production and use of anti-protein antibodies. While antibodies can also be made to haptens, to carbohydrates, to nucleic acids, and to other structural classes of antigen (see Chapter 8), their induction generally requires the attachment of the antigen to a protein carrier. Thus, the immunogenicity of protein antigens determines the outcome of virtually every immune response.

2-2 The immunogenicity of a protein reflects both its intrinsic properties and host factors.

Although any structure can be recognized as an antigen, only proteins elicit fully developed adaptive immune responses because only proteins can engage the T lymphocytes required for immunological memory. This occurs because T cells recognize antigens only as peptide fragments of proteins bound to self MHC molecules (see Section 1-14). An adaptive immune response that includes immunological memory can only be induced by other classes of antigen when they are attached to a protein carrier that can engage the necessary T cells. Thus, immunogenicity must be defined in respect of the response to protein antigens. When proteins or hapten–protein conjugates are used for immunization, immunological memory is produced as a result of the initial or **primary immunization**. This is also known as **priming**, as the animal or person is now primed to mount a more potent response to subsequent challenges with the same antigen. The response to each challenge is increasingly intense, so that **secondary**, **tertiary**, and subsequent responses are of increasing magnitude. Repetitive injection of antigen to achieve a heightened state of immunity is known as **hyperimmunization**.

Certain properties of a protein that favor an adaptive immune response have been defined by studying antibody responses to simple natural proteins like hen egg-white lysozyme and, more importantly, to synthetic polypeptide antigens (Fig. 2.3). Antibody responses to most protein

Fig. 2.3 Intrinsic properties of proteins that affect immunogenicity.

Intrinsic properties of protein antigens that influence immunogenicity		
Parameter	**Increased immunogenicity**	**Decreased immunogenicity**
Size	Large	Small (MW<2500)
Composition	Complex	Simple
Similarity to self protein	Multiple differences	Few differences
Interaction with host MHC	Effective	Ineffective

Related
to Part I

antigens require activation of T cells, which require the antigen to be presented to them by specialized antigen-presenting cells (see Section 1-11) so a full understanding of immunogenicity will become evident only when the priming of T cells is described in Chapter 7. Briefly, the antigen-presenting cell degrades the protein antigen into peptides that bind to specialized cell-surface molecules called MHC class II molecules for presentation to the T cell. Antigen-presenting cells preferentially take up aggregated or particulate antigens, and the larger and more complex a protein, and the more distant its relationship to self proteins, the more likely it is to contain peptides that will bind to MHC molecules and be distinguishable from self peptides. In addition, as we shall see in Sections 2-3 and 2-4, the immunogenicity of proteins can be enhanced greatly by the way in which they are administered.

2-3 Immunogenicity can be enhanced by administration of proteins in adjuvants.

Most proteins are poorly immunogenic or non-immunogenic when administered by themselves. Strong adaptive immune responses to protein antigens almost always require that the antigen be injected in a mixture known as an adjuvant. An **adjuvant** is any substance that enhances the immunogenicity of substances mixed with it. Adjuvants differ from protein carriers in that they do not form stable linkages with the immunogen. Furthermore, adjuvants are needed primarily in initial immunizations, whereas carriers are required to elicit not only primary but also subsequent responses to haptens. Commonly used adjuvants are listed in Fig. 2.4.

Adjuvants can enhance immunogenicity in two different ways. First, adjuvants convert soluble protein antigens into particulate material, which is more readily ingested by antigen-presenting cells such as

Adjuvants that enhance immune responses		
Adjuvant name	Composition	Mechanism of action
Incomplete Freund's adjuvant	Oil-in-water emulsion	Delayed release of antigen; enhanced uptake by macrophages
Complete Freund's adjuvant	Oil-in-water emulsion with dead mycobacteria	Delayed release of antigen; enhanced uptake by macrophages; induction of co-stimulators in macrophages
Freund's adjuvant with MDP	Oil-in-water emulsion with muramyldipeptide (MDP), a constituent of mycobacteria	Similar to complete Freund's adjuvant
Alum (aluminum hydroxide)	Aluminum hydroxide gel	Delayed release of antigen; enhanced macrophage uptake
Alum plus *Bordetella pertussis*	Aluminum hydroxide gel with killed *B. pertussis*	Delayed release of antigen; enhanced uptake by antigen-presenting cell; induction of co-stimulators
Immune stimulatory complexes (ISCOMs)	Matrix of Quil A containing viral proteins	Delivers antigen to cytosol; allows induction of cytotoxic T cells

Fig. 2.4 Common adjuvants and their use. Adjuvants are mixed with the antigen and usually render it particulate, which helps to retain the antigen in the body and promotes macrophage uptake. Most adjuvants include bacteria or bacterial components that stimulate macrophages, aiding in the induction of the immune response. ISCOMs (immune stimulatory complexes) are small micelles of the detergent Quil A; when viral proteins are placed in these micelles, they apparently fuse with the antigen-presenting cell, allowing the antigen to enter the cytosol and stimulate a response to the protein, much as a virus infecting these cells would stimulate an anti-viral response.

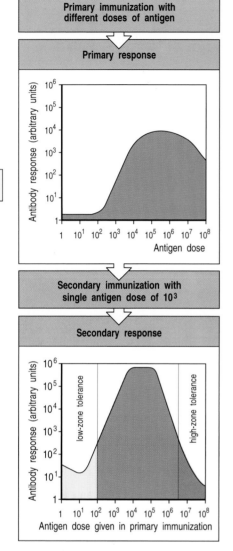

Fig. 2.5   The dose of antigen used in an initial immunization affects the primary and secondary antibody response. The typical antigen dose–response curve shown here illustrates the influence of dose on both a primary antibody response (amounts of antibody produced expressed in arbitrary units) and the effect of the dose used for priming on a secondary antibody response elicited by a dose of antigen of 10^3 arbitrary mass units. Very low doses of antigen do not cause an immune response at all. Slightly higher doses appear to inhibit specific antibody production, an effect known as low-zone tolerance. Above these doses there is a steady increase in the response with antigen dose to reach a broad optimum. Very high doses of antigen also inhibit immune responsiveness to a subsequent challenge, a phenomenon known as high-zone tolerance.

macrophages. The antigen can be adsorbed on particles of the adjuvant (such as alum) or made particulate by emulsification in mineral oils. This enhances immunogenicity somewhat, but such adjuvants are relatively weak unless they also contain bacteria or bacterial products. Although the exact contribution of the microbial constituents to enhancing immunogenicity is not known, they are clearly the more important component of an adjuvant. Microbial products may signal the macrophage to become a more effective antigen-presenting cell, and their role is considered in more detail in Chapter 7. The bacterial constituents in most adjuvants induce potent local inflammatory responses, however, which preclude their use in humans. However, killed cells of the bacterium *Bordetella pertussis*, which is the causal agent of whooping cough, are used as both antigen and adjuvant in the triplex DPT (diphtheria, pertussis, tetanus) vaccine against these diseases.

2-4   The response to a protein antigen is influenced by dose, form, and route of administration.

The magnitude of the immune response depends on the dose of immunogen administered. Below a certain threshold dose, most proteins do not elicit an immune response. Above the threshold dose, there is a gradual increase in the response with increasing dose to a broad plateau level, followed by a decline at very high antigen doses (Fig. 2.5). As most infectious agents enter the body in small numbers, immune responses are generally elicited only by pathogens that multiply to a level sufficient to exceed the antigen dose threshold. The broad response optimum allows the system to respond to infectious agents across a wide range of doses. At very high antigen doses the immune response is inhibited, which may be important in maintaining tolerance to abundant self proteins such as plasma proteins. In general, secondary and subsequent immune responses occur at lower antigen doses and achieve higher plateau values, a sign of immunological memory. However, under some conditions, very low or very high doses of antigen may induce specific unresponsive states, known respectively as acquired **low-zone** or **high-zone tolerance**.

The route by which antigen is administered also affects both the magnitude and the type of response obtained (Fig. 2.6). Antigens injected subcutaneously generally elicit the strongest responses, while antigens injected or transfused directly into the bloodstream, especially those freed of aggregates that are readily taken up by antigen-presenting cells, tend to induce unresponsiveness or tolerance. Antigens administered solely to the gastrointestinal tract have distinctive effects, frequently eliciting a local antibody response in the intestinal lamina propria, while at the same time producing a state of systemic tolerance that manifests as a diminished response to the same antigen if it is administered in immunogenic form elsewhere in the body. This 'split tolerance' may be important in avoiding allergy to antigens in food, as the local response prevents food antigens from entering the body, while the inhibition of systemic immunity helps to prevent formation of IgE antibodies, which are the cause of such allergies (see Chapter 11). By contrast, protein antigens that enter the body through the respiratory epithelium tend to elicit allergic responses, for reasons that are not clear.

The precise means by which the route of antigen administration controls the nature and intensity of the response are not known. Antigens entering the body by different routes encounter distinct types of antigen-presenting cells and enter different lymphoid tissues, and the special characteristics of regional immune systems such as the gut-associated

Factors that influence the response to antigen		
Parameter	**Increased immunogenicity**	**Decreased immunogenicity**
Dose	Intermediate	High or low
Route	Subcutaneous > intraperitoneal > intravenous or intragastric	
Form	Particulate	Soluble
	Denatured	Native
Adjuvants	Slow release	Rapid release
	Bacteria	No bacteria

Fig. 2.6 Factors that influence the adaptive immune response to an antigen. How an antigen is administered has a marked influence on the response obtained. Dose, route, and form of administration are all important, as is the adjuvant used.

Related to Part I

lymphoid tissues (GALT), bronchial-associated lymphoid tissues (BALT), and other mucosal-associated lymphoid tissues (MALT) (see Fig. 1.9), are not yet fully defined. Understanding the differences between these local environments will one day explain the effect of the route of antigen administration on the immune response. In practice, feeding an antigen is a good way to prevent a systemic immune response to it, while subcutaneous injection of an optimal dose of antigen in a suitable adjuvant is the best way to elicit such a response.

2-5   B-cell responses are detected by antibody production.

The response of B cells to an injected immunogen is usually measured by analyzing the specific antibody produced in a **humoral immune response**. This is most conveniently achieved by assaying the antibody that accumulates in the fluid phase of the blood or plasma; such antibodies are known as circulating antibodies. Circulating antibody is usually measured by collecting blood, allowing it to clot, and isolating the serum from the clotted blood. The amount and characteristics of the antibody in the immune serum are then determined using the assays we shall describe in the next part of this chapter.

The most important characteristics of an antibody response are the specificity, amount, isotype (class), and affinity of the antibodies produced. The specificity determines the ability of the antibody to distinguish the immunogen from self and from other non-self antigens. The amount of antibody can be determined in many different ways and is a measure of the number of responding B cells, their rate of antibody synthesis, and the persistence of the antibody after production. Persistence of an antibody in the plasma and extracellular fluid bathing the tissues is determined by the isotypes produced (see Section 3-19); each isotype has a different half-life *in vivo*. The isotypic composition of an antibody response also determines the biological functions these antibodies can perform and the sites in which antibody will be found. For instance, an antibody response dominated by IgE antibodies will lead to an allergic reaction when the antigen is reintroduced. Techniques for identifying isotypes are discussed in Section 2-9. Finally, the strength of binding of the antibody to its antigen is termed its affinity. Binding strength is important, since the higher the affinity of the antibody for its antigen, the less antibody is required to eliminate the antigen, as antibodies

Related to Part I

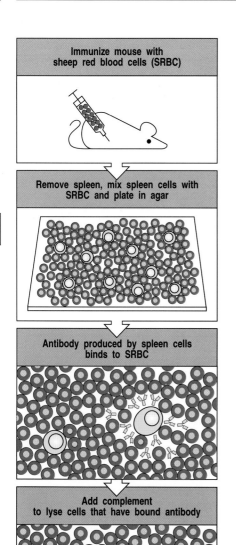

Immunize mouse with sheep red blood cells (SRBC)

Remove spleen, mix spleen cells with SRBC and plate in agar

Antibody produced by spleen cells binds to SRBC

Add complement to lyse cells that have bound antibody

Fig. 2.7 Antibody secretion by single activated B cells can be detected using the Jerne hemolytic plaque assay. Spleen cells making antibody against red blood cells are mixed with red blood cells and placed in a thin agar layer. The antibody secreted by immune B cells binds to red blood cells immediately surrounding the antibody-forming cell. Complement is added, which binds to the antibody coating the red blood cells and causes lysis of the red blood cells, generating a visible hemolytic 'plaque' in the layer of red blood cells. In the center of each plaque is a single antibody-producing cell. The number of antibody-secreting cells can be determined by the number of plaques formed.

with higher affinity will bind at lower antigen concentrations (see Section 2-12). All these parameters of the humoral immune response help to determine the capacity of that response to protect the host from infection.

B-cell responses can be measured by determining directly the number of B cells producing antibody to a given antigen. This can be accomplished by trapping the antibody produced by a single B cell on a sensitive indicator, such as a sheep red blood cell. When complement is added, the red blood cells that have bound antibody are destroyed, creating a clear hemolytic plaque surrounding each antibody-forming cell (Fig. 2.7). By attaching different antigens to the indicator red blood cells, this **hemolytic plaque assay** can be adapted to measure B-cell responses to any antigen.

2-6   T-cell responses are detected by their effects on other cells.

The measurement of antibody responses in humoral immunity is fairly simple; immunity mediated by T cells (**cell-mediated immunity**), by contrast, is technically far more difficult to measure. For example, T cells do not make a secreted antigen-binding product, so there is no simple binding assay for such responses. T-cell activity can be divided into an induction phase, in which T cells are activated, and an effector phase, in which this activation is expressed and detected. Moreover, all T-cell responses require an interaction between two cells, a target cell displaying specific antigen in the form of peptide:MHC complexes and an armed effector T cell that recognizes the antigen on the target cell surface. Most commonly, the presence of T cells that have responded to a specific antigen is detected by their subsequent *in vitro* proliferation when re-exposed to the same antigen. However, T-cell proliferation only indicates that cells able to recognize that antigen have been activated previously; it does not reveal what effector function they mediate. The effector function of a T cell is assayed by its effect on an appropriate target cell. As we learned in Chapter 1, several basic effector functions have been defined for T cells. Cytotoxic CD8 T cells can kill infected target cells, thus preventing further replication of obligate intracellular pathogens, while CD4 T cells have several roles that are determined largely by the cytokines they produce (see Section 7-17).

The different T-cell effector responses that can be elicited by immunization determine the functional outcome of an immune response. To achieve high levels of antibody, for example, it is important to immunize in such a way that helper CD4 T cells are activated. This is especially important in designing vaccines that seek to augment particular kinds of immunity while preventing or diminishing others. However, no general principles have emerged that allow one to predict the type of immune response produced by a particular immunization regimen. Empirical observations on the types of responses elicited by particular antigens or

Influences on the priming of different T-cell subsets in mice		
T-cell subset primed	**Antigen**	**Effect of adjuvant**
Helper CD4 T cells ($T_H2 > T_H1$)	Low antigen dose; extracellular antigen	Marked enhancement of priming; Freund's adjuvant favors IgG2a (T_H1) in mice; alum and *B. pertussis* favors IgG1, IgE (T_H2)
Inflammatory CD4 T cells ($T_H1 \gg T_H2$)	High antigen dose; intracellular antigen in vesicle	Marked enhancement of priming by complete Freund's adjuvant; inhibition by incomplete Freund's adjuvant
Cytotoxic CD8 T cells	Live virus infection; antigen in cytosol	Priming not enhanced by conventional adjuvants; may be enhanced by ISCOMs

Fig. 2.8 Factors that influence priming of different T-cell subsets. The general trends are shown here, but it is difficult to predict how immunization will affect the two CD4 T-cell subsets (T_H1 and T_H2) that activate macrophages and B cells respectively.

Related to Part I

immunization schedules offer some clues but there are no definitive answers. Experimentation remains the best way to determine the optimal immunization procedure for obtaining the required response to a given antigen (Fig. 2.8). The ability to control the type of immune response produced remains a central goal of immunology as we shall see in Chapter 12.

Summary.

Adaptive immunity is studied by eliciting a response through deliberate infection or, more commonly, by injection of antigens in an immunogenic form, and by measuring the outcome in terms of humoral and cell-mediated immunity. Intrinsic properties of the antigen determine its immunogenicity. Furthermore, the elicitation of an immune response is heavily influenced by the dose and route of antigen administration and by the adjuvants used to administer it. The main parameters of the antibody response are the amount, affinity, isotype, and specificity of the antibody produced, the isotype determining the functional capabilities of the humoral immune response to a given antigen. The main parameters of the cell-mediated immune response are the intensity of the response and the functions of the T cells elicited. These fall into three main groups: the ability to activate macrophages and other aspects of inflammation; the ability to kill infected target cells; and the ability to induce antibody production by B cells, also known as T-cell help.

The measurement and use of antibodies.

Antibody molecules are highly specific for their corresponding antigen, being able to detect one molecule of a protein antigen out of more than 10^8 similar molecules. This makes antibodies both easy to isolate and study, and invaluable as probes of biological processes. While standard chemistry would have great difficulty in distinguishing two such closely related proteins as human and pig insulin, antibodies can be made that discriminate between these two structures absolutely. The utility of antibodies as molecular probes has stimulated the development of many sensitive and highly specific techniques to measure their presence, to determine their specificity and affinity for a range of antigens, and to ascertain their functional capabilities. Many standard techniques used throughout biology exploit the specificity and stability of antigen binding by antibodies. Comprehensive guides to the conduct of these antibody assays are available in many books on immunological methodology; we shall illustrate here only the most important techniques, especially those used in studying the immune response itself. These examples also illustrate the unique properties of antibody molecules that are explained by their structure and genetic origin, as we shall see in Chapter 3.

2-7 | **The amount and specificity of an antibody can be measured by direct binding to antigen.**

The presence of specific antibody can be detected using many different assays. Some measure the direct binding of the antibody to its antigen and such assays are based on **primary interactions**; we shall describe several of these assays in this section. Others determine the amount of antibody present by the changes it induces in the physical state of the antigen, such as the precipitation of soluble antigen or the clumping of antigenic particles called **secondary interactions**, and these will be described in the next section. Both types of assay can be used to measure the amount and specificity of the antibodies produced after immunization, and both can be applied to a wide range of other biological problems. Here, we shall describe several of these assays that are commonly used in immunology, biology, and medicine. As such assays were originally conducted using sera from immune individuals, or antisera, they are commonly referred to as **serological assays**, and the use of antibodies is often called **serology**.

Two commonly used direct binding assays are **radioimmunoassay** (**RIA**) and **enzyme-linked immunosorbent assay** (**ELISA**). For these one needs a pure preparation of a known antigen or antibody, or both. In a radioimmunoassay, a pure component (antigen or antibody) is radioactively labeled, usually with ^{125}I. For the ELISA, an enzyme is chemically linked to the antibody or antigen. The unlabeled component (again either antigen or antibody) is attached to a solid support, such as the wells of a plastic multiwell plate, which will adsorb a certain amount of any protein. Most commonly, the antigen is attached to the solid support and the binding of labeled antibody is assayed. The labeled antibody is allowed to bind to the unlabeled antigen, under conditions where non-specific adsorption is blocked, and any unbound material is washed away. Antibody binding is measured directly in terms of the amount of radioactivity retained by the coated wells in radioimmunoassay, while in ELISA, binding is detected by a reaction that converts a colorless substrate into a colored reaction product (Fig. 2.9). The color change can be read directly in the reaction tray, making data collection very easy, and ELISA also avoids the hazards of radioactivity. This makes ELISA the preferred method for most direct-binding assays.

These assays illustrate two crucial aspects of all serological assays. First, at least one of the reagents must be available in a pure, detectable form in order to obtain quantitative information. Second, there must be a means of separating the bound fraction of the labeled reagent from the unbound, free fraction so that specific binding can be determined. Normally, this separation is achieved by having the unlabeled partner trapped on a solid support, allowing unbound material to be washed away before measuring the fraction of the labeled reagent bound to it. In Fig. 2.9, the unlabeled antigen is attached to the well and the labeled antibody is trapped by binding to it. This separation of bound from free is an essential step in every assay that uses antibodies.

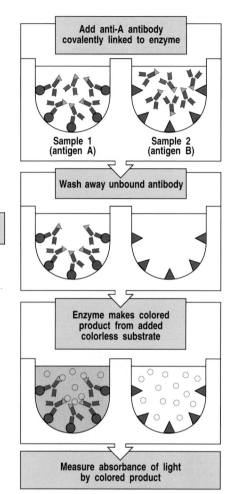

Fig. 2.9   The principle of the enzyme-linked immunosorbent assay (ELISA). To detect antigen A, purified antibody specific for antigen A is linked chemically to an enzyme. The samples to be tested are coated onto the surface of plastic wells to which they bind non-specifically; residual sticky sites on the plastic are blocked by adding irrelevant proteins (not shown). The labeled antibody is then added to the wells under conditions where non-specific binding is prevented, so that only binding to antigen A causes the labeled antibody to be retained on the surface. Unbound labeled antibody is removed from all wells by washing, and bound antibody is detected by an enzyme-dependent color change reaction. This assay allows arrays of wells known as microtiter plates to be read in fiberoptic multichannel spectrometers, greatly speeding the assay. Modifications of this basic assay allow antibody or antigen in unknown samples to be measured as shown in Figs. 2.10 and 2.37 (see also Section 2-9).

Within the figure:
Add anti-A antibody covalently linked to enzyme
Sample 1 (antigen A)   Sample 2 (antigen B)
Wash away unbound antibody
Enzyme makes colored product from added colorless substrate
Measure absorbance of light by colored product

Related to Part II

These assays do not allow one to measure directly the amount of antigen or antibody in a sample of unknown composition, as both depend on binding of a pure labeled antigen or antibody. There are various ways around this problem, one of which is to use a **competitive binding assay**, as shown in Fig. 2.10. In this type of assay the presence and amount of a particular antigen in an unknown sample is determined by its ability to compete with a labeled reference antigen for binding to an antibody attached to a plastic well. By adding varying amounts of a known, unlabeled standard preparation, a standard curve is constructed, and the assay can then measure the amount of antigen in unknown samples by comparison to the standard. Because only identical or closely related molecules will bind to the antibody, this technique allows molecules of antigen present at low concentrations to be detected, such as the hormone insulin in a complex mixture of proteins like serum. Some proteins that are closely related to the reference antigen may cross-react with the antibody; because these generally bind less well, their inhibition curve is flatter, indicating that competitive binding is due to cross-reacting rather than identical antigens. The competitive binding assay can also be used for measuring antibody in a sample of unknown composition by attaching the appropriate antigen to the plate and measuring the ability of the test sample to inhibit the binding of a labeled specific antibody.

An alternative approach to measuring antibody content in an unknown sample is to detect its binding to antigen-coated plastic wells by means

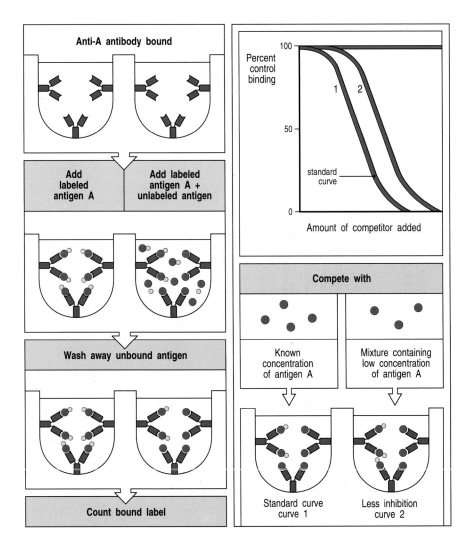

Fig. 2.10 Competitive inhibition immunoassay for antigen in unknown samples. A fixed amount of unlabeled antibody is attached to a set of wells, and a standard reference preparation of a labeled antigen is bound to it. Unlabeled standard or test samples are then added in varying amounts and the displacement of labeled antigen is measured, generating characteristic inhibition curves. A standard curve is obtained using known amounts of unlabeled antigen identical to that used as the labeled species, and comparison with this curve allows the amount of antigen in unknown samples to be calculated. The green line on the graph represents a sample lacking any substance cross-reactive with anti-A antibodies.

Antigen A bound to insoluble beads

Add mixture of antibodies raised in mouse immunized against antigen A

Wash away unbound antibodies

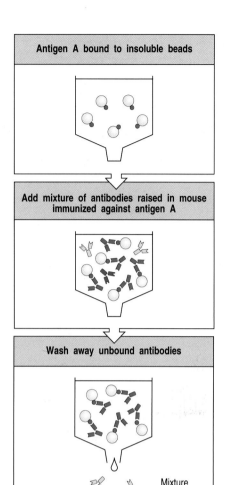

Mixture depleted of anti-A antibodies

Elute bound antibodies

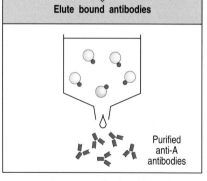

Purified anti-A antibodies

Fig. 2.11 Affinity chromatography uses antigen:antibody binding to purify antibodies or antigens. To purify a specific antibody from serum, antigen is attached to an insoluble matrix, such as chromatography beads, and the serum is passed over the matrix. The specific antibody binds, while other antibodies and proteins are washed away. Specific antibody is then eluted by altering pH or ionic strength, which can frequently disrupt antigen:antibody bonds. In this way, antibodies can be purified from highly complex mixtures of proteins. Antigens can be purified in the same way on beads coupled to antibody (not shown).

of labeled anti-immunoglobulin antibodies specific for constant features on immunoglobulin molecules. The use of anti-immunoglobulin antibodies is described in detail in Section 2-9. An ELISA based on this technique is used to screen human sera for antibodies to human immunodeficiency virus (HIV), a sign that the donor is infected.

All the assays described so far rely on pure preparations of an antibody. However, antibody to any one antigen makes up a very small percentage of the total protein in an antiserum, even after repeated immunizations. Therefore, antibody must be purified before it can be labeled. Specific antibody can be isolated from serum by **affinity chromatography**, in which the specific binding of antibody to antigen held on a solid matrix is exploited (Fig. 2.11). Antigen is covalently bound to small, chemically reactive beads, which are loaded into a long column, and the antiserum is allowed to pass over the beads. The specific antibodies bind, while all the other proteins in the serum, including antibodies to other substances, can be washed away. Typical elution conditions consist of lowering the pH to 2.5 or raising it to greater than 11. This demonstrates that antibodies bind stably under physiological conditions of salt concentration, temperature, and pH, but that the bonds are non-covalent since the binding is reversible. Affinity chromatography can also be used to purify antigens from complex mixtures by coating the beads with specific antibody. The technique is known as affinity chromatography because it separates molecules on the basis of their affinity for one another.

The techniques described in this section involve the primary interaction of antibody with antigen and are in wide use in immunology, clinical medicine, and cell biology. They rely on the specific antigen-binding properties of antibody molecules to directly detect and measure either antigens or antibodies. They also illustrate the specificity and nature of antigen:antibody interactions that result from the unique features of the antibody molecule, as we shall learn in Chapter 3.

2-8 **Antibody binding can be detected by changes in the physical state of the antigen.**

The direct measurement of antibody binding to antigen is used in most quantitative serological assays. However, some important assays are based on the ability of antibody binding to alter the physical state of the antigen it binds to. These secondary interactions can be detected in a variety of ways. For instance, when the antigen is displayed on the surface of a large particle like a bacterium, antibodies can cause the bacteria to clump or **agglutinate**. The same principle applies to the reactions used in blood typing, only here the target antigens are on the surface of red blood cells and the clumping reaction caused by antibodies against them is called **hemagglutination** (from the Greek, *haima*, blood).

This procedure is used to determine the ABO blood group of blood donors and transfusion recipients (Fig. 2.12). The hemagglutination reaction, like the hemolytic plaque assay described in Section 2-5, can be extended to detect antibody to any antigen by attaching it to the red blood cell surface, an assay known as passive hemagglutination. In the case of the ABO blood group antigens, the agglutinating antibodies (agglutinins) anti-A or anti-B bind to the A or B blood group substances, which are arrayed in many copies on the surface of the red blood cell, causing the cells to agglutinate. Since agglutination involves the simultaneous binding of antibody molecules to two identical particles, crosslinking them together, it demonstrates that each antibody molecule has at least two identical antigen-binding sites.

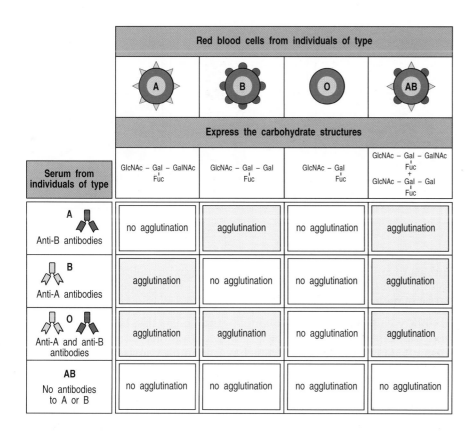

	Red blood cells from individuals of type			
	A	B	O	AB
Serum from individuals of type	Express the carbohydrate structures			
	GlcNAc – Gal – GalNAc Fuc	GlcNAc – Gal – Gal Fuc	GlcNAc – Gal Fuc	GlcNAc – Gal – GalNAc Fuc + GlcNAc – Gal – Gal Fuc
A Anti-B antibodies	no agglutination	agglutination	no agglutination	agglutination
B Anti-A antibodies	agglutination	no agglutination	no agglutination	agglutination
O Anti-A and anti-B antibodies	agglutination	agglutination	no agglutination	agglutination
AB No antibodies to A or B	no agglutination	no agglutination	no agglutination	no agglutination

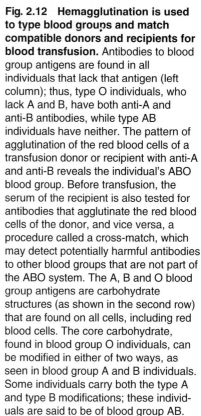

Fig. 2.12 Hemagglutination is used to type blood groups and match compatible donors and recipients for blood transfusion. Antibodies to blood group antigens are found in all individuals that lack that antigen (left column); thus, type O individuals, who lack A and B, have both anti-A and anti-B antibodies, while type AB individuals have neither. The pattern of agglutination of the red blood cells of a transfusion donor or recipient with anti-A and anti-B reveals the individual's ABO blood group. Before transfusion, the serum of the recipient is also tested for antibodies that agglutinate the red blood cells of the donor, and vice versa, a procedure called a cross-match, which may detect potentially harmful antibodies to other blood groups that are not part of the ABO system. The A, B and O blood group antigens are carbohydrate structures (as shown in the second row) that are found on all cells, including red blood cells. The core carbohydrate, found in blood group O individuals, can be modified in either of two ways, as seen in blood group A and B individuals. Some individuals carry both the type A and type B modifications; these individuals are said to be of blood group AB.

When sufficient quantities of antibody are mixed with soluble macromolecular antigens, a visible precipitate consisting of large aggregates of antigen crosslinked by antibody molecules can form. The amount of precipitate depends on the amounts of antigen and antibody, and on the ratio between them (Fig. 2.13). This **precipitin reaction** provided the first quantitative assay for antibody but is now seldom used in immunology. However, it is important to understand the interaction of antigen with antibody that leads to this reaction, as the production of antigen:antibody complexes (**immune complexes**) *in vivo* occurs in almost all immune responses, often causing significant pathology (see Chapter 11).

In the precipitin reaction, varying amounts of soluble antigen are added to a fixed amount of serum containing antibody. As the amount of antigen added increases, the amount of precipitate generated also increases up to a maximum and then declines (see Fig. 2.13). When small amounts of antigen are added, antigen:antibody complexes are formed under conditions of antibody excess so that each molecule of antigen is extensively bound by antibody and crosslinked to other molecules of antigen. When large amounts of antigen are added, only small antigen:antibody complexes can form and these are often soluble in this zone of antigen excess. Between these two zones, all of the antigen and antibody is found in the precipitate, generating a zone of equivalence. At equivalence, very large

Fig. 2.13 Antibody can precipitate soluble antigen to generate a precipitin curve. Different amounts of antigen are added to a fixed amount of antibody, and precipitates form by antibody crosslinking of antigen molecules. The precipitate is recovered and the amount of precipitated antibody measured, while the supernatant is tested for residual antigen or antibody.

This defines zones of antibody excess, equivalence, and antigen excess. At equivalence, the largest antigen:antibody complexes form. In the zone of antigen excess, some of the immune complexes are too small to precipitate. These soluble immune complexes can cause pathological damage to small blood vessels when they form *in vivo* (see Chapter 11).

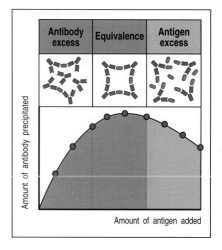

Fig. 2.14 Different antibodies bind to distinct epitopes on an antigen molecule. The surface of an antigen possesses many potential antigenic determinants or epitopes, distinct sites to which an antibody can bind. The number of antibody molecules that can bind to a molecule of antigen at one time defines the antigen's valence. Steric considerations can limit the number of different antibodies that bind to the surface of an antigen at any one time (right panel) so that the number of epitopes on an antigen is always greater than or equal to its valence.

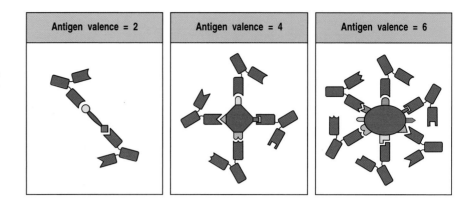

lattices of antigen and antibody are formed by crosslinking. The small, soluble immune complexes formed in the zone of antigen excess are the cause of pathology *in vivo*.

Antibody can only precipitate antigen molecules that have several antibody-binding sites, so that large antigen:antibody complexes can be formed. Macromolecular antigens have a complex surface to which antibodies of many different specificities can bind. The site to which each distinct antibody molecule binds is called an **antigenic determinant** or an **epitope**. Because of the complexity of macromolecular surfaces, a single molecule of antigen has many different epitopes. However, steric considerations limit the number of antibody molecules that can bind to a molecule of antigen at any one time, as antibody molecules binding to epitopes that partially overlap will compete for binding. For this reason, the **valence** of an antigen, which is the number of antibody molecules that can bind to a molecule of the antigen at saturation, is almost always less than the number of epitopes on the antigen (Fig. 2.14, right panel).

The precipitation of antigen by antibody can be exploited to characterize the antigen:antibody mixtures by carrying out the reaction in a clear gel. When antigen is placed in one well cut in the gel and the antibody is placed in an adjacent well, they diffuse into the gel and form a line of visible precipitate where they meet at equivalence (Fig. 2.15). The same principle is used in other assays that we shall learn about in subsequent sections.

Fig. 2.15 Ouchterlony gel-diffusion assay for antigen:antibody binding. Antigen and antibody are placed in different wells of an agar gel. They diffuse toward each other and precipitate where they meet at equivalence, forming a visible band. When samples in two wells are tested against the same well of antigen the relatedness of the samples can be determined by the shape of the precipitin line formed (not shown).

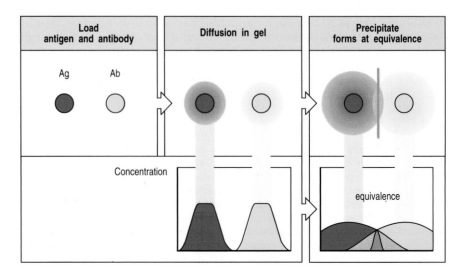

The measurement and use of antibodies.

2-9   Anti-immunoglobulin antibodies are a useful tool for detecting bound antibody molecules.

As we learned in Section 2-7, antibody can be detected by the direct binding of labeled antibody to antigen coated on plastic surfaces. A more general approach that avoids the need to label each antibody molecule is to detect bound, unlabeled antibody with a labeled antibody specific for all immunoglobulins. Immunoglobulins, like all other proteins, are immunogenic when used to immunize individuals of another species. The **anti-immunoglobulin antibodies** raised in this way recognize conserved features of antibodies known as constant domains because they are shared by all immunoglobulin molecules. These anti-immunoglobulin antibodies can be purified by affinity chromatography, labeled, and used as a general probe for bound antibody.

Anti-immunoglobulin antibodies were first developed by Robin Coombs to study **hemolytic disease of the newborn**, or **erythroblastosis fetalis**, and the test for this disease is still called the Coombs test. Hemolytic disease of the newborn occurs when a mother makes IgG antibodies specific for the **Rhesus** or **Rh blood group antigen** expressed on the red blood cells of her fetus. Rh-negative mothers make these antibodies when they are exposed to Rh-positive fetal red blood cells bearing the paternally inherited Rh antigen. Maternal IgG antibodies cross the placenta to the fetus where they normally provide the newborn infant with maternal antibodies that can fight infection. However, IgG anti-Rh antibodies attack the fetal red blood cells instead, causing a hemolytic anemia in the fetus and newborn infant.

For reasons that are not fully understood, antibodies to Rh blood group antigens do not agglutinate red blood cells as do antibodies to the ABO blood group antigens, making their detection difficult. However, maternal IgG antibodies bound to the fetal red blood cells can be detected by washing the cells to remove unbound immunoglobulin in the serum that interferes with detection of bound antibody, and then adding anti-human immunoglobulin antibodies, which agglutinate the antibody-coated red blood cells. This is the **direct Coombs test** (Fig. 2.16), called direct because it detects directly antibody bound to the surface of the patient's red blood cells. An **indirect Coombs test** is used to detect non-agglutinating anti-Rh antibody in serum; the serum is first incubated with Rh-positive red blood cells, which bind the anti-Rh antibody, after which the antibody-coated cells are washed to remove unbound immunoglobulin and are then agglutinated with anti-immunoglobulin antibody (see Fig. 2.16). The indirect Coombs test allows Rh incompatibilities that might lead to hemolytic disease of the newborn to be detected and this knowledge allows the disease to be prevented, as we shall see in Chapter 12.

Related to Part II

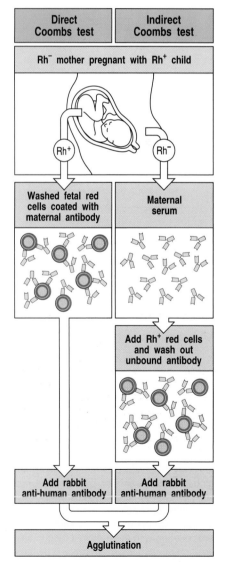

Fig. 2.16 The Coombs direct and indirect anti-globulin tests for antibody to red blood cell antigens. An Rh⁻ mother of an Rh⁺ fetus can become immunized to fetal red blood cells that enter the maternal circulation at the time of delivery. In a subsequent pregnancy with an Rh⁺ fetus, IgG anti-Rh antibodies can cross the placenta and damage the fetal red blood cells. In contrast to anti-Rh antibodies, anti-ABO antibodies are of the IgM isotype and cannot cross the placenta, and so do not cause harm. Anti-Rh antibodies do not agglutinate red blood cells but their presence can be shown by washing the fetal red blood cells and then adding antibody to human immunoglobulin, which agglutinates the antibody-coated cells. The washing removes unrelated immunoglobulins that would otherwise react with the anti-human immuno-globulin antibody. Anti-Rh antibodies can be detected in the mother's serum in an indirect Coombs test; the serum is incubated with Rh⁺ red blood cells, and once the antibody binds, the red cells are treated as in the direct Coombs test.

Anti-immunoglobulin antisera have found many uses in clinical medicine and biological research since their introduction. Labeled anti-immuno-globulin antibodies can be used in radioimmunoassay or ELISA to detect binding of unlabeled antibody to antigen-coated plates. The ability of anti-immunoglobulins to react with antibodies of all specificities demonstrates that antibody molecules have constant features recognizable by the anti-immunoglobulin, in addition to the variability required for antibodies to discriminate between a myriad of antigens. The presence of both constant and variable features in one protein posed a genetic puzzle for immunologists, the solution to which is described in Chapter 3.

Not all anti-immunoglobulin antibodies react with all immunoglobulin molecules. Some react only with immunoglobulins of a single isotype, and it was this property of anti-immunoglobulin antibodies that led to the discovery that several distinct sets of antibodies, the immuno-globulin isotypes, are present in human serum. Human serum proteins can be identified individually by combining electrophoresis, to separate the proteins by charge, with immunodiffusion to detect individual proteins as precipitin arcs. This is done by placing an antiserum against whole human serum in a trough cut parallel to the direction of electro-phoresis, so that each antibody forms an arc of precipitation with a particular serum protein. This technique is called **immunoelectrophoresis** (Fig. 2.17). In the serum from some individuals, who demonstrate increased susceptibility to infections, no precipitin lines appear in the region where immunoglobulins are normally detected.

As proteins migrating in this region of a serum protein electrophoresis were originally called **gamma globulins**, the failure to make immuno-globulins, which is due to a single-gene defect on the X chromosome and

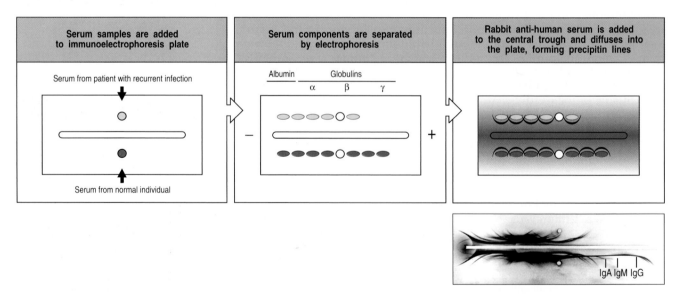

Fig. 2.17 Immunoelectrophoresis reveals the presence of several distinct immunoglobulin isotypes in normal human serum. Serum samples from a normal control and from a patient with recurrent bacterial infection due to an absence of antibody production, as reflected in an absence of gamma globulins, are separated by electrophoresis on an agar-coated slide. Antiserum raised against whole normal human serum and containing antibodies to many of its different proteins is put in a trough down the middle, and each antibody forms an arc of precipitation with the protein it recognizes, as in Fig. 2.15. The position of each arc is determined by the electrophoretic mobility of the serum protein; immunoglobulins migrate to the gamma globulin region of the gel. The absence of immunoglobulins of several different isotypes in a patient who has X-linked agammaglobulinemia, a form of immune deficiency in which no antibodies of any isotype are formed, is shown in the photograph at the bottom, where several arcs are missing from the patient's serum (upper set). These are IgM, IgA, and several subclasses of IgG, each recognized in normal serum (lower set) by antibodies in the antiserum against human serum proteins. Photograph from the collection of the late Dr Charles A Janeway Snr.

so occurs mainly in males, is called **X-linked agammaglobulinemia**; its cause has recently been discovered, as we shall see in Chapter 10. This single-gene defect in antibody production causes the absence of the immunoglobulin isotypes now known as IgM, IgA, and several subclasses of IgG.

Anti-immunoglobulins specific for each isotype can be produced by immunizing an animal of a different species with a pure preparation of one isotype and then absorbing out those antibodies that cross-react with immunoglobulins of other isotypes. Anti-isotype antibodies can be used to measure how much antibody of a particular isotype in an antiserum reacts with a given antigen. This reaction is particularly important for detecting IgE antibodies, which are responsible for most allergies. High levels of IgE binding to an antigen correlate with allergic reactions to that antigen.

An alternative approach to detecting bound antibodies exploits bacterial proteins that bind to immunoglobulins with high affinity and specificity. One of these, **Protein A** from the bacterium *Staphylococcus aureus*, has been exploited widely in immunology for the affinity purification of immunoglobulin and for detection of bound antibody.

All these techniques use the specificity of an antibody binding to its antigen to distinguish the antigen from all the other molecules in the mixture, and they all rely on labeled anti-immunoglobulin or Protein A to detect the bound antibody. This allows great savings in reagent labeling costs and also provides a standard detection system so that results in different assays can be compared directly.

Related to Part II

| 2-10 | **Antisera contain heterogeneous populations of antibody molecules.** |

The antibodies generated in a natural immune response or after immunization in the laboratory are a mixture of molecules of different specificities and affinities. Some of this heterogeneity is due to the production of antibodies that bind to different epitopes on the immunizing antigen, but even antibodies directed at a hapten with a single antigenic determinant can be markedly heterogeneous. This heterogeneity is detectable by **isoelectric focusing**. In this technique, proteins are separated on the basis of their isoelectric point, the pH at which their net charge is zero. By electrophoresing proteins in a pH gradient for long enough, each molecule migrates along the pH gradient until it reaches the pH at which it is neutral, and is thus concentrated (focused) at that point. When antiserum containing anti-hapten antibodies is treated in this way and then transferred to a solid support such as nitrocellulose paper, the anti-hapten antibodies can be detected by their ability to bind labeled hapten (Fig. 2.18). The binding of antibodies of varying isoelectric points to the hapten shows that even antibodies that bind the same antigenic determinant are heterogeneous.

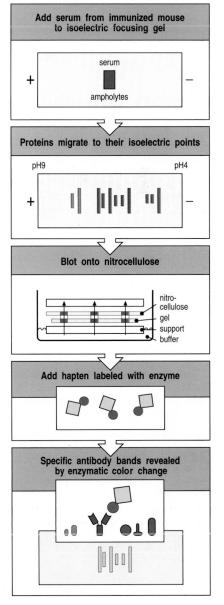

Fig. 2.18 Isoelectric focusing of antiserum reveals the heterogeneity of antibodies specific for a given antigen. The heterogeneity of antibodies specific for a hapten can be shown by gel electrophoresis of antiserum in a pH gradient generated by ampholytes. The serum proteins migrate to a pH equivalent to their isoelectric point, where they become uncharged and cease to migrate. The proteins are transferred to nitrocellulose paper, which is then treated with the enzyme-coupled hapten, which binds the hapten-specific antibodies in the antiserum. These antibodies are then detected by an enzymatic reaction which produces a colored product from a colorless substrate, as in ELISA. Even antibodies to a single hapten can be very heterogeneous, as seen here, because of differences in their amino acid sequence.

Antisera are valuable for many biological purposes but they have certain disadvantages that relate to the heterogeneity of the antibodies they contain. First, each antiserum is different from all other antisera, even if raised in a genetically identical animal using the identical preparation of antigen and the same immunization protocol. Second, antisera can only be produced in limited volumes, and thus it is impossible to use the identical serological reagent in a long or complex series of experiments or clinical tests. Finally, even antibodies purified by affinity chromatography (see Section 2-7) may include minor populations of antibodies that give unexpected cross-reactions, which confound the analysis of experiments. For this reason, an unlimited supply of antibody molecules of homogeneous structure and known specificity would be very desirable. This has been achieved through the production of monoclonal antibodies from hybrid antibody-forming cells or, more recently, by genetic engineering, as we shall see in the next section.

2-11 Monoclonal antibodies have a homogeneous structure and can be produced by cell fusion or by genetic engineering.

Even antibodies specific for the same small defined antigenic determinant are heterogeneous in structure, as shown by their differing isoelectric points, making detailed chemical analysis of such antibodies impossible. In order to examine a homogeneous preparation of antibody, biochemists first analyzed proteins produced by patients with multiple myeloma, a common tumor of plasma cells. It was known that antibodies are normally produced by plasma cells, and, as this disease is associated with the presence of large amounts of a homogeneous gamma globulin called a myeloma protein in the patient's serum, it seemed likely that myeloma proteins would serve as models for normal antibody molecules. Thus, much of the early knowledge of antibody structure came from studies on myeloma proteins. However, these proteins had one major limitation for such studies; the antigen specificity of most myeloma proteins was not known.

This problem was solved by Georges Köhler and César Milstein, who devised a technique for producing a homogeneous population of antibodies of known antigen specificity. They did this by fusing spleen cells from an immunized mouse to cells of a mouse myeloma to produce hybrid cells that both proliferated indefinitely and secreted antibody specific for the antigen

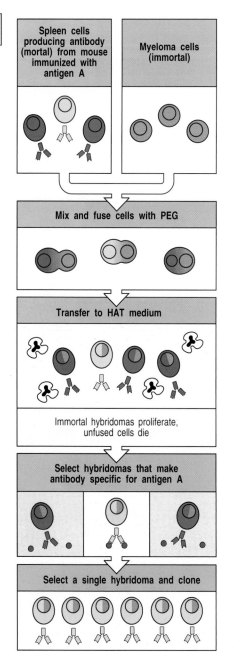

Spleen cells producing antibody (mortal) from mouse immunized with antigen A

Myeloma cells (immortal)

Mix and fuse cells with PEG

Transfer to HAT medium

Immortal hybridomas proliferate, unfused cells die

Select hybridomas that make antibody specific for antigen A

Select a single hybridoma and clone

Fig. 2.19 The production of monoclonal antibodies. Mice are immunized with antigen A and given an intravenous booster immunization three days before they are killed in order to produce a large population of spleen cells secreting specific antibody. Spleen cells die after a few days in culture. In order to produce a continuous source of antibody they are fused with immortal myeloma cells using polyethylene glycol (PEG) to produce a hybrid cell line called a hybridoma. The myeloma cells are selected beforehand to ensure that they are not secreting antibody themselves and that they are sensitive to the hypoxanthine-aminopterin-thymidine (HAT) medium that is used to select hybrid cells because they lack the enzyme hypoxanthine:guanosine phosphoribosyl transferase (HGPRT).

The HGPRT gene contributed by the spleen cell allows hybrid cells to survive in the HAT medium, and only hybrid cells can grow continuously in culture because of the malignant potential contributed by the myeloma cells. Therefore, unfused myeloma cells and unfused spleen cells die in the HAT medium, as shown here by cells with dark, irregular nuclei. Individual hybridomas are then screened for antibody production, and cells that make antibody of the desired specificity are cloned by growing them up from a single antibody-producing cell. The cloned hybridoma cells are grown in bulk culture to produce large amounts of antibody. As each hybridoma is descended from a single cell, all the cells of a hybridoma cell line make the same antibody molecule, which is called a monoclonal antibody.

used to immunize the spleen cell donor. The spleen cell provides the ability to make specific antibody, while the myeloma cell provides the ability to grow indefinitely in culture and secrete immunoglobulin continuously. By using a myeloma cell partner that produces no antibody proteins itself, the antibody produced by the hybrid cells comes only from the immune spleen cell partner. After fusion, the hybrid cells are selected using drugs that kill the myeloma parental cell, while the unfused parental spleen cells have a limited lifespan and soon die, so that only hybrid myeloma cell lines or **hybridomas** survive. Those hybridomas producing antibody of the desired specificity are then identified and cloned by regrowing the cultures from single cells. Since each hybridoma is a **clone** derived from a single B cell, all the antibody molecules it produces are identical in structure, including their antigen-binding site and isotype. Such antibodies are therefore called **monoclonal antibodies** (Fig. 2.19). This technology has revolutionized the use of antibodies by providing a limitless supply of antibody of a single and known specificity and a homogeneous structure. Monoclonal antibodies are now used in most serological assays, as diagnostic probes, and as therapeutic agents.

Recently, a novel technique for producing antibody-like molecules has been introduced. Gene segments encoding the antigen-binding variable or V domains of antibodies are fused to genes encoding the coat protein of a bacteriophage. Bacteriophage containing such gene fusions are used to infect bacteria, and the resulting phage particles have coats that express the antibody-like fusion protein, with the antigen-binding domain displayed on the outside of the bacteriophage. A collection of recombinant phage, each displaying a different antigen-binding domain on its surface, is known as a **phage display library**. In much the same way that antibodies specific for a particular antigen can be isolated from a complex mixture by affinity chromatography (see Section 2-7), phage expressing antigen-binding domains specific for a particular antigen can be isolated by selecting the phage in the library for binding to that antigen. The phage particles that bind are recovered and used to infect fresh bacteria. Each phage isolated in this way will produce a monoclonal antigen-binding particle analogous to a monoclonal antibody (Fig. 2.20). The

Related to Part II

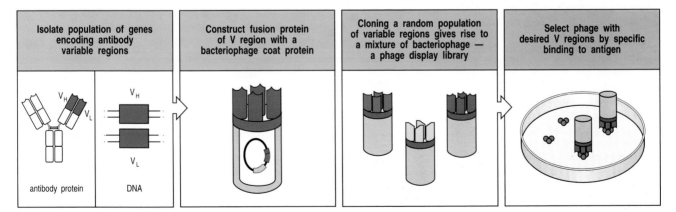

| Isolate population of genes encoding antibody variable regions | Construct fusion protein of V region with a bacteriophage coat protein | Cloning a random population of variable regions gives rise to a mixture of bacteriophage — a phage display library | Select phage with desired V regions by specific binding to antigen |

Fig. 2.20 The production of antibodies by genetic engineering. Short primers to consensus sequences in heavy- and light-chain variable or V regions of immunoglobulin genes are used to generate a library of heavy- and light-chain V-region cDNAs by the polymerase chain reaction (see Fig. 2.48) using spleen mRNA as the starting material. These heavy- and light-chain V-region genes are cloned randomly into a filamentous phage such that each phage expresses one heavy- and one light-chain V region as a surface fusion protein with antibody-like properties. The resulting phage display library is expanded in bacteria, and the phage are then bound to a surface coated with antigen. The unbound phage are washed away, while the bound phage are recovered and again bound to antigen. After a few cycles, only specific, high-affinity antigen-binding phage are left. These can be used like antibody molecules, or their V genes can be recovered and engineered into antibody genes to produce genetically engineered antibody molecules (not shown). This technology may replace the hybridoma technology for producing monoclonal antibodies and has the advantage that any species can be used as the source of the initial mRNA.

genes encoding the antigen-binding site, which are unique to each phage, can then be recovered from the phage DNA and used to construct genes for a complete antibody molecule by joining them to gene segments that encode the invariant parts of an antibody. When these reconstructed antibody genes are introduced into a suitable host cell line, such as the non-antibody producing myeloma cells used for hybridomas, the transfected cells secrete antibodies with all the desirable characteristics of monoclonal antibodies produced from hybridomas. This tecnique may ultimately replace the traditional route of cell fusion for production of monoclonal antibodies.

| 2-12 | **The affinity of an antibody can be determined directly by binding to small ligands.** |

The **affinity** of an antibody is the strength of binding of a monovalent ligand to a single antigen-binding site. The affinity of an antibody that binds small antigens such as haptens that can diffuse freely across a dialysis membrane can be determined directly by the technique of

Fig. 2.21 The affinity and valence of an antibody can be determined by equilibrium dialysis. A known amount of antibody is placed in a dialysis bag and exposed to different amounts of a diffusible monovalent antigen, such as a hapten. At each concentration of antigen added, the fraction of the antigen bound is determined from the difference in concentration of total ligand inside and outside the bag (upper panels). This information can be transformed into a Scatchard plot as shown here. In Scatchard analysis, the ratio of r/c, where r = moles of antigen bound per mole of antibody and c = molar concentration of free antigen, is plotted against r. The number of binding sites per antibody molecule can be determined from the value of r at infinite free antigen concentration, where r/free = 0, in other words at the x-axis intercept. The analysis of an IgG antibody molecule in which there are two identical antigen-binding sites per molecule is shown in the left lower panel. The slope of the line is determined by the affinity of the antibody molecule for its antigen; if all the antibody molecules in a preparation are identical, as for a monoclonal antibody, then a straight line is obtained whose slope is equal to $-K_a$, where K_a is the association (or affinity) constant and the dissociation constant $K_d = 1/K_a$. However, antisera raised even against a simple antigenic determinant like a hapten contain heterogeneous populations of antibody molecules (see Section 2-10). Each antibody molecule would, if isolated, make up part of the total and give a straight line whose x-axis intercept is less than 2, as it contains only a fraction of the total binding sites in the population (right lower panel). As a mixture, they give curved lines with x-axis intercepts of 2 from which an average affinity ($\overline{K}_a$) can be determined from the slope of this line at a concentration of antigen where 50% of the sites are bound, or at x = 1 (central lower panel). The association constant determines the equilibrium state of the reaction Ag + Ab = Ag:Ab, where antigen = Ag and antibody = Ab, and $K_a = $[Ag:Ab]/[Ag][Ab]. This constant reflects the on and off rates for antigen binding to the antibody; with small antigens like haptens, binding is usually as rapid as diffusion allows, while differences in off rates determine the affinity constant. However, with larger antigens the on rate may also vary as the interaction becomes more complex.

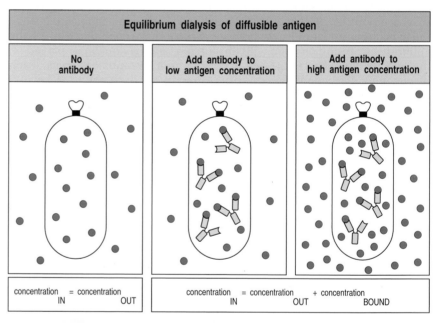

Equilibrium dialysis of diffusible antigen

| No antibody | Add antibody to low antigen concentration | Add antibody to high antigen concentration |

concentration = concentration
    IN   OUT

concentration = concentration + concentration
    IN   OUT   BOUND

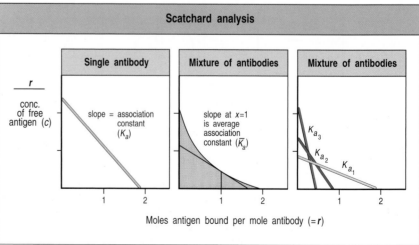

Scatchard analysis

| Single antibody | Mixture of antibodies | Mixture of antibodies |

$\dfrac{r}{\text{conc. of free antigen } (c)}$

slope = association constant (K_a)

slope at x=1 is average association constant ($\overline{K}_a$)

K_{a_3} K_{a_2} K_{a_1}

Moles antigen bound per mole antibody (= r)

equilibrium dialysis. A known amount of antibody, whose molecules are too large to cross a dialysis membrane, is placed in a dialysis bag and offered varying amounts of antigen. Molecules of antigen that bind to the antibody are no longer free to diffuse across the dialysis membrane, so only the unbound molecules of antigen equilibrate across it (Fig. 2.21). By measuring the concentration of antigen inside the bag and in the surrounding fluid, one can determine the amount of the antigen that is bound as well as the amount that is free when equilibrium has been achieved. Given that the amount of antibody present is known, the affinity of the antibody and the number of specific binding sites for the antigen per molecule of antibody can be determined from this information. The data is usually analyzed using **Scatchard analysis** (Fig. 2.21); this type of analysis was used to demonstrate that a molecule of IgG has two identical antigen-binding sites.

While affinity measures the strength of binding of an antigenic determinant to a single antigen-binding site, an antibody reacting with an antigen that has multiple identical epitopes or with the surface of a pathogen will often bind the same molecule or particle with both of its binding sites. This increases the apparent strength of binding, since both binding sites must release at the same time in order for the two molecules to dissociate. This is often referred to as cooperativity in binding, but it should not be confused with the cooperative binding found in a protein such as hemoglobin in which binding of ligand at one site enhances the affinity of a second binding site for its ligand. The overall strength of binding of an antibody molecule to an antigen or particle is called its **avidity** (Fig. 2.22). For IgG antibodies, bivalent binding can significantly increase avidity; in IgM antibodies, which have ten identical antigen-binding sites, the affinity of each site for a monovalent hapten is often quite low, but the avidity of binding of the whole antibody to a surface such as a bacterium that displays multiple identical epitopes can be very high.

Related to Part II

| 2-13 | **Antibodies can be used to identify antigen in cells, tissues, and complex mixtures of substances.** |

Because antibodies bind stably and specifically to antigen, they are invaluable as probes for identifying a particular molecule in cells, tissues, or biological fluids. They are used in this way to study a wide range of biological processes and clinical conditions. In this section, a few techniques that are used to study the immune system, as well as in cell biology generally, will be described; a complete treatment of this subject can be found in one of the excellent methodology books available.

Antibody molecules can be used to locate their target molecules accurately in single cells or in tissue sections by a variety of different labeling techniques. As in all serological tests, the antibody binds stably to its antigen, allowing unbound antibody to be removed by thorough washing. As antibodies to proteins recognize the surface features of the native, folded protein, the native structure of the protein being sought usually needs to be preserved, either by gentle fixation techniques or by using frozen tissue sections that are fixed only after the antibody reaction has been performed. Some antibodies, however, bind proteins even if they are denatured, and such antibodies will bind specifically even to protein in fixed tissue sections.

The bound antibody can be visualized using a variety of sensitive techniques, and the specificity of antibody binding coupled to sensitive detection provides remarkable detail about the structure of cells. One very powerful technique for identifying antibody-bound molecules in cells or tissue sections is **immunofluorescence**, in which a fluorescent

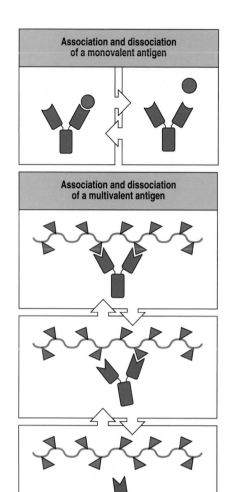

Fig. 2.22 The avidity of an antibody is its strength of binding to intact antigen. When an IgG antibody binds a ligand with multiple identical epitopes, both binding sites can bind the same molecule or particle. The overall strength of binding, called avidity, is greater than the affinity, the strength of binding of a single site, since both binding sites must dissociate at the same time for the antibody to release the antigen. This property is very important in the binding of antibody to bacteria, which usually have multiple identical epitopes on their surfaces.

Related
to Part II

dye is attached directly to the specific antibody. More commonly, bound antibody is detected by fluorescent anti-immunoglobulin, a technique known as **indirect immunofluorescence**. The dyes chosen for immunofluorescence are activated by light of one wavelength, usually ultraviolet, and emit light of a different wavelength in the visible spectrum. By using selective filters, only the light coming from the dye or fluorochrome used is detected in the fluorescent microscope. Albert Coons first devised this technique to identify the plasma cell as the source of antibody, but it can be used to detect the distribution of any protein. By attaching different dyes to different antibodies, the distribution of two or more molecules can be determined in the same cell or tissue section (Fig. 2.23). An alternative method of detecting a protein in tissue sections is to use **immunohistochemistry**, in which the antibody is chemically coupled to an enzyme that converts a colorless substrate into a colored reaction product whose deposition can be directly observed in a light microscope. This technique is analogous to the ELISA assay described in Section 2-7.

The recent development of the confocal fluorescent microscope, which uses computer-aided techniques to produce an ultrathin optical section of a cell or tissue, gives very high resolution immunofluorescence microscopy without the need for elaborate sample preparation. To examine cells at even higher resolution, similar procedures can be applied to ultrathin sections examined in the transmission electron microscope. Antibodies labeled with gold particles of distinct diameter enable two or more proteins to be studied simultaneously. The difficulty with this technique is in staining the ultrathin section, as few molecules of antigen will be present in each section.

In order to raise antibodies against membrane proteins and other cellular structures that are difficult to purify, mice are often immunized with whole cells or crude cell extracts. Antibodies to the individual molecules are then obtained by preparing monoclonal antibodies that bind to the cell used for immunization. To characterize the molecules identified by these antibodies, cells of the same type are labeled with radioisotopes and dissolved in non-ionic detergents that disrupt cell membranes but do not interfere with antigen:antibody interactions so that the labeled protein can be isolated by binding to the antibody. The antibody is usually attached to a solid support such as the beads used in affinity chromatography. Cells can be labeled in two main ways for this **immunoprecipitation analysis**. All of the proteins in a cell can be biosynthetically (metabolically) labeled by growing the cell in radioactive amino acids that are incorporated into cellular protein (Fig. 2.24). Alternatively, one can label only the cell-surface proteins by radioiodination under conditions that prevent iodine from crossing the plasma membrane and labeling proteins inside the cell.

Fig. 2.23 Immunofluorescence microscopy. Antibodies labeled with a fluorescent dye such as fluorescein (green triangle) are used to reveal the presence of their corresponding antigens in cells or tissues. The stained cells are examined in a microscope that exposes them to ultraviolet light to excite the fluorescent dye. This emits light at a characteristic wavelength, which is captured by viewing the sample through a selective filter. This technique is applied widely in biology to determine the location of molecules in cells and tissues. Different antigens can be detected in tissue sections by labeling antibodies with dyes of distinctive color. Here, antibodies to the protein glutamic acid decarboxylase (GAD) coupled to a green dye are shown to stain the β cells of pancreatic islets of Langerhans, while the α cells, labeled with antibodies to the hormone glucagon coupled with an orange fluorescent dye, do not have this enzyme. GAD is an important autoantigen in diabetes, an autoimmune disease in which the insulin-secreting β cells of the islets of Langerhans are destroyed. Photograph courtesy of M Solimena and P De Camilli.

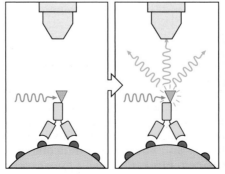
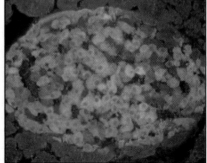

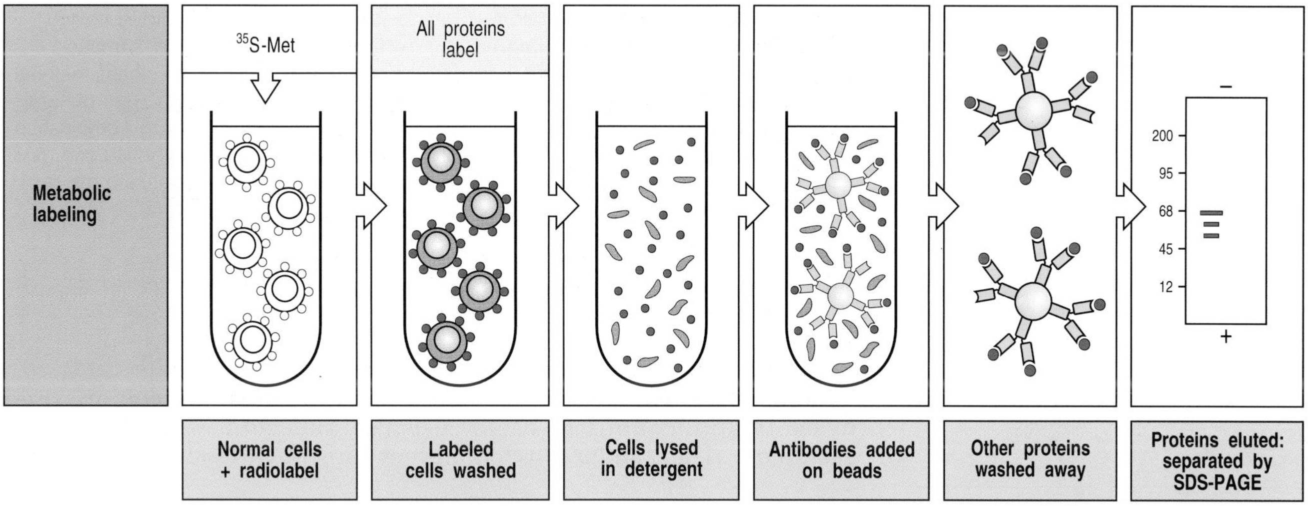

Metabolic labeling

| ³⁵S-Met | All proteins label | | | | |

| Normal cells + radiolabel | Labeled cells washed | Cells lysed in detergent | Antibodies added on beads | Other proteins washed away | Proteins eluted: separated by SDS-PAGE |

200
95
68
45
12

Related to Part II

Fig. 2.24   Cellular proteins reacting with an antibody can be characterized by immunoprecipitation of labeled cell lysates. All actively synthesized cellular proteins can be labeled metabolically by incubating cells with radioactive amino acids (shown here for methionine) or one can label just the cell-surface proteins by using radioactive iodine in a form that cannot cross the cell membrane (not shown). Cells are lysed with detergent and individual labeled cell-associated proteins can be precipitated with a monoclonal antibody attached to beads. After washing away unbound proteins, the bound protein is eluted in the detergent sodium dodecyl sulfate (SDS), which dissociates it from the antibody and also coats the protein with a strong negative charge, allowing it to migrate according to its size in polyacrylamide gel electrophoresis (PAGE). The positions of the radioactively labeled proteins are determined by autoradiography using X-ray film. This technique of SDS-PAGE can be used to determine the molecular weight and subunit composition of a protein. Patterns of protein bands observed using metabolic labeling are usually more complex than those revealed by radioiodination, owing to the presence of precursor forms of the protein (right panel), where the mature, surface form can be identified as being the same size as that detected by surface iodination.

Once the labeled proteins have been isolated by the antibody, they can be characterized in several ways. The most popular is polyacrylamide gel electrophoresis (PAGE) of the proteins once they have been dissociated from antibody in the strong ionic detergent, sodium dodecyl sulfate (SDS), a technique generally abbreviated as **SDS-PAGE**. SDS binds relatively homogeneously to proteins, conferring a charge that allows the electrophoretic field to drive protein migration through the gel. The rate of migration is controlled mainly by protein size (Fig. 2.25). However, this technique does not separate proteins that are of similar size but differ in charge as a result of having different amino acid sequences. Proteins of different charge can be separated by isoelectric focusing (see Section 2-10). MHC proteins from different individuals can vary significantly in amino acid sequence, and hence in their isoelectric point, as can be demonstrated by first running an isoelectric focusing gel in one direction in a narrow tube of polyacrylamide. This first-dimensional isoelectric focusing gel is then placed across the top of an SDS-PAGE slab gel, which is then run vertically to separate the proteins by molecular weight, a procedure known as **two-dimensional gel electrophoresis**. This powerful technique allows many hundreds of proteins in a complex mixture to be distinguished from one another (see Fig. 2.25).

An alternative approach that avoids the problem of radiolabeling cells is to solubilize all cellular proteins by placing unlabeled cells directly in detergent and running the lysate on SDS-PAGE. The proteins are then transferred from the gel to a stable support such as nitrocellulose paper. The proteins are detected by antibodies (mainly those that react with denatured sequences) and the position of the proteins to which the antibodies bind is revealed by anti-immunoglobulin labeled with radioisotopes or an enzyme. This procedure is called **Western blotting** by analogy with the nomenclature for comparable techniques for detecting the other two out of three members in molecular biology, Southern

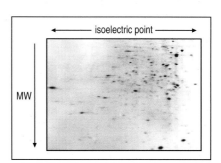

Fig. 2.25   Two-dimensional gel electrophoresis of total cellular proteins. Proteins in spleen cells have been labeled metabolically (see Fig. 2.24), and separated by isoelectric focusing in one direction and SDS-PAGE in a second direction at right angles to the first gel (two-dimensional gel). The separated proteins are detected using autoradiography.

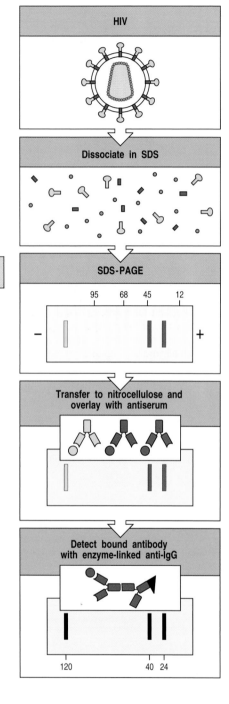

Fig. 2.26 Western blotting is used to identify antibodies to the human immunodeficiency virus (HIV) in serum from infected individuals. The virus is dissociated into its constituent proteins by treatment with the detergent SDS, and its proteins separated by SDS-PAGE. The separated proteins are transferred to a nitrocellulose sheet and reacted with the test serum. Anti-HIV antibodies in the serum bind to the various HIV proteins and are detected using enzyme-linked anti-human immunoglobulin, which deposits colored material from a colorless substrate. This general methodology will detect any combination of antibody and antigen and is used widely, although the denaturing effect of SDS means that the technique works most reliably with antibodies that recognize the antigen when it is denatured.

blotting for DNA and Northern blotting for RNA. Western blots are used in many applications in basic research and clinical diagnosis, for example to detect antibodies to different constituents of HIV (Fig. 2.26).

2-14   Antibodies can be used to isolate protein antigens for further characterization.

Immunoprecipitation and Western blotting are useful for determining the molecular weight and isoelectric point of a protein. These characteristics can then help to distinguish it from other proteins and provide a means of recognizing it on an electrophoretic gel. The protein's abundance, distribution, and whether, for example, it undergoes changes in molecular weight and isoelectric point as a result of processing within the cell can thus be determined. However, these techniques do not provide a definitive characterization of the protein.

To do this, the protein must be isolated and purified. Antibodies specific for the protein can be used to isolate it using affinity chromatography (see Section 2-7), but this does not usually yield sufficient protein for a full characterization. Often, this small amount of purified protein is used to obtain amino acid sequence information from the protein's amino-terminal end or from proteolytic peptide fragments of the protein. These amino acid sequences are used to generate a set of synthetic oligonucleotides of complementary sequence, which are then used as probes to isolate the gene encoding the protein from a complementary DNA (cDNA) or genomic library. The full amino acid sequence of the protein can be deduced from the nucleotide sequence of its cDNA and can sometimes give clues to the type of protein and its biological properties. The nucleotide sequence of the gene and its regulatory regions can be determined from genomic DNA clones. Larger quantities of protein for functional studies can then be produced from genetically engineered cells into which the gene has been introduced by transfection. This approach has been used to identify the genes that encode many immunologically important proteins, such as the MHC glycoproteins.

2-15   Antibodies can be used to identify genes and their products.

An alternative approach uses antibodies directly to identify and isolate a gene encoding a cell-surface protein. A specific antibody is used to detect the expression of the protein on the surface of a cell type that does not normally express it, after the cell has been transfected with the gene in the form of a cDNA. A suitable cDNA library is prepared from total mRNA isolated from a cell type known to express the protein. The cDNA library is then cloned into special vectors, called expression vectors, which are constructed to allow the genes they carry to be expressed upon transfection into cultured mammalian cells. These vectors drive expression of the gene in the transfected cells without integrating into

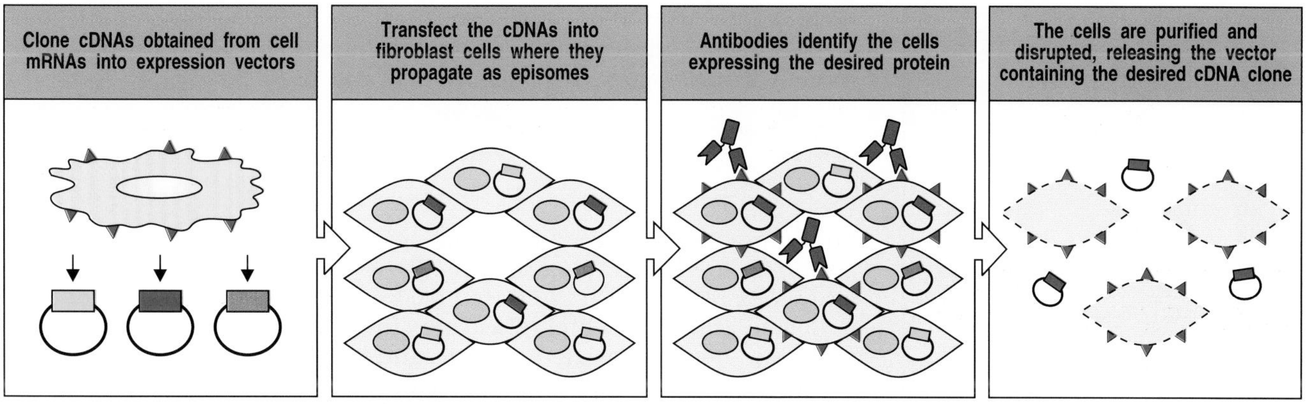

| Clone cDNAs obtained from cell mRNAs into expression vectors | Transfect the cDNAs into fibroblast cells where they propagate as episomes | Antibodies identify the cells expressing the desired protein | The cells are purified and disrupted, releasing the vector containing the desired cDNA clone |

Fig. 2.27   **The gene encoding a cell-surface molecule can be isolated by expressing it in fibroblasts and detecting its protein products with monoclonal antibodies.** Total mRNA from a cell line or tissue expressing the protein is isolated and converted into a cDNA library in a vector that allows direct cDNA expression in fibroblasts. The entire cDNA library is transfected into cultured fibroblasts. Fibroblasts that have taken up cDNA encoding a cell-surface protein express the protein on their surface; they can be isolated by binding a monoclonal antibody against that protein. The vector containing the gene is isolated from these cells and used for more rounds of transfection and re-isolation until uniform positive expression is obtained, ensuring that the correct gene has been isolated. The cDNA insert can then be sequenced to determine the sequence of the protein it encodes and can also be used as the source of material for large-scale expression of the protein for analysis of its structure and function. The method illustrated is limited to cloning genes for single-chain proteins (i.e. those encoded by only one gene) that can be expressed in fibroblasts. It has been used to clone many genes of immunological interest such as that for CD4.

Related to Part II

the host cell DNA. Cells expressing the protein are isolated by binding to antibody (see Section 2-17), and the vector is recovered by lysing the cells (Fig. 2.27).

The vector is then introduced into bacterial cells where it replicates rapidly, and these amplified vectors are used in a second round of transfection in mammalian cells. After several cycles of transfection, isolation, and amplification in bacteria, single colonies of bacteria expressing the vector are picked and used in a final transfection to identify a cloned vector carrying the cDNA of interest, which is then isolated and characterized. This methodology has been used to isolate many genes encoding cell-surface molecules. It cannot, however, be used to isolate genes for proteins that remain within the cell, as these cannot be detected by surface antibody binding, nor can it be used to isolate the genes for proteins that are only expressed on the cell surface as parts of multichain arrays, as these would require the simultaneous expression of several different cDNAs in the same cell to produce a detectable cell-surface molecule.

The converse approach is taken to identify the unknown protein product of a cloned gene. The gene sequence is used to construct synthetic peptides of 10–20 amino acids that are identical to part of the deduced protein sequence, and antibodies are then raised against these peptides by coupling them to carrier proteins; the peptides behave as haptens. These anti-peptide antibodies often bind the native protein and so can be used to identify its distribution in cells and tissues, to isolate it, and to try to ascertain its function (Fig. 2.28). This approach is often called reverse genetics as it works from gene to phenotype rather than from phenotype to gene, which is the classical genetic approach. The great advantage of reverse genetics over the classical approach is that it does not require a phenotypic genetic trait for identifying a gene. The main disadvantage of reverse genetics is that often there is no mutant phenotype of the gene so that its functional importance may be difficult to infer. However, mutant genes can be produced by the technique of *in vitro* mutagenesis and then inserted into cells and animals in order to test for

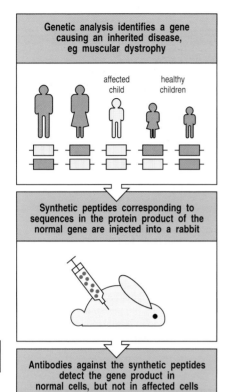

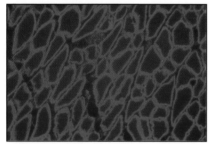

Fig. 2.28   The use of antibodies to detect the unknown protein product of a known gene is called reverse genetics. When the gene responsible for a genetic disorder such as Duchenne muscular dystrophy is isolated, the amino acid sequence of the unknown protein product of the gene can be deduced from the nucleotide sequence of the gene, and synthetic peptides representing parts of this sequence can be made. Antibodies are raised against these peptides and purified from the antiserum by affinity chromatography on a peptide column (see Fig. 2.11). Labeled antibody is used to stain tissue from individuals with the disease and from unaffected individuals to determine differences in the presence, amount, and distribution of the normal gene product. The product of the dystrophin gene is present in normal mouse skeletal muscle cells as shown in the bottom panel (red fluorescence), but is missing in the cells of mice bearing the mutation mdx, the mouse equivalent of Duchenne muscular dystrophy (not shown). Photograph (x 15) courtesy of H Lidov and L Kunkel.

Within the figure:

Genetic analysis identifies a gene causing an inherited disease, eg muscular dystrophy

affected child   healthy children

Synthetic peptides corresponding to sequences in the protein product of the normal gene are injected into a rabbit

Antibodies against the synthetic peptides detect the gene product in normal cells, but not in affected cells

Related to Part III

their effects. In addition, as it is now possible to inactivate genes deliberately in cells and even animals, mutant phenotypes can be generated directly from the gene (see Sections 2-37 and 2-38).

Summary.

The interaction of an antibody molecule with its ligand serves as the paradigm for immunological specificity, an essential concept in immunology. This is best understood by studying the binding of antibodies to antigens, which illustrates their tremendous power to discriminate between related antigens and their high affinity of binding to particular structures. The behavior of antibodies in serological assays shows that antibody molecules are highly diverse, symmetrically bivalent, and have both constant and variable structural features. How the immune system produces the millions of different antibody molecules found in serum while maintaining their overall structural identity that allows anti-immunoglobulin antibodies to detect any antibody molecule, is the main subject of Chapter 3. In Chapter 8 we will learn about the production of antibody by B cells and why the amount, specificity, isotype, and affinity of antibody molecules are important in humoral immunity; here, we have learned how these attributes can be measured in a wide variety of distinct assays, each giving its own type of information about the antibody response. Because antibodies can be raised to any structure, bind it with high affinity and specificity, and be made in unlimited amounts through monoclonal antibody production, they are particularly powerful tools of investigation. Many different techniques using antibodies have been devised and they have played a central role in both clinical medicine and biological research.

The study of lymphocytes.

The analysis of immunological specificity has focused largely on the antibody molecule as the most easily accessible agent of adaptive immunity. However, all adaptive immune responses are mediated by lymphocytes, so an understanding of immunology must be based on an understanding of lymphocyte behavior. To study and assay lymphocyte behavior the cells must be isolated and the distinct functional lymphocyte subpopulations identified and separated. This section emphasizes studies on T lymphocytes, as the only known effector function of B cells is to produce antibodies, the subject of the preceding part of this chapter.

2-16   **Lymphocytes can be isolated from blood, lymphoid organs, epithelia, and sites of inflammation.**

The first step in studying lymphocytes is to isolate them so that their behavior can be analyzed *in vitro*. Human lymphocytes can be isolated most readily from peripheral blood using density centrifugation over a gradient of Ficoll and metrizimide (Hypaque). This yields a population of mononuclear cells at the interface that has been depleted of red blood cells and most polymorphonuclear leukocytes or granulocytes

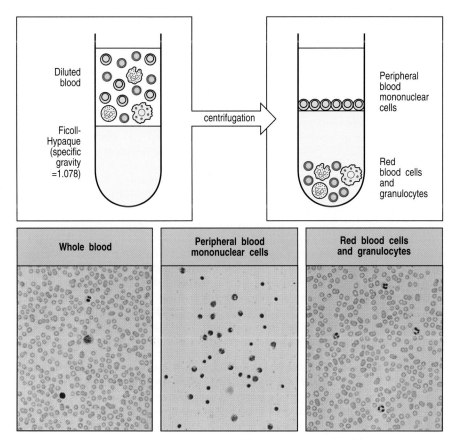

Fig. 2.29 Peripheral blood mononuclear cells can be isolated from whole blood by Ficoll-Hypaque centrifugation. Diluted anti-coagulated blood (bottom left panel) is layered over Ficoll-Hypaque and centrifuged. Red blood cells and polymorphonuclear leukocytes or granulocytes are more dense and centrifuge through the Ficoll-Hypaque, while mononuclear cells consisting of lymphocytes with some monocytes band over it and can be recovered at the interface. Bottom middle and right panels show stained smears of mononuclear cells and the cells from the pellet comprising red blood cells and granulocytes. Photographs courtesy of D Leitenberg and I Visintin.

Related to Part III

(Fig. 2.29). The resulting population, called **peripheral blood mononuclear cells**, consists mainly of lymphocytes and monocytes. Although this population is readily accessible, it is not necessarily representative of the lymphoid system, as only recirculating lymphocytes can be isolated from blood. In experimental animals, and occasionally in humans, lymphocytes can be isolated from lymphoid organs, such as spleen, thymus, lymph nodes, or gut-associated lymphoid tissues, most commonly the palatine tonsils in humans (see Fig. 1.6). A specialized population of lymphocytes resides in surface epithelia; these cells must be isolated by fractionating the epithelial layer after its detachment from the basement membrane. Finally, in situations where local immune responses are prominent, lymphocytes can be isolated from the site of the response itself. For example, in order to study the autoimmune reaction that is thought to be responsible for rheumatoid arthritis, an inflammatory response in joints, lymphocytes are isolated from the fluid aspirated from the inflamed joint space.

2-17 Lymphocyte populations can be purified and characterized by antibodies specific for cell-surface molecules.

Resting lymphocytes present a deceptively uniform appearance to the investigator, all being small round cells with a dense nucleus and little cytoplasm (see Fig. 1.5). However, these cells comprise many functional subpopulations, which are usually identified and distinguished from each other on the basis of their differential expression of cell-surface

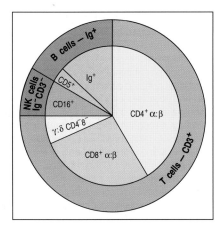

Fig. 2.30 The distribution of lympho-cyte subpopulations in human peripheral blood. As shown on the outside, lymphocytes can be divided into T cells bearing T-cell receptors, detected with anti-CD3 antibodies, B cells bearing immunoglobulin receptors, detected with anti-immunoglobulin, and null cells including natural killer (NK) cells that label with neither. Further divisions of the T-cell and B-cell populations are shown inside. Using anti-CD4 and anti-CD8 antibodies, α:β T cells can be subdivided into two populations, while γ:δ T cells are identified with antibodies against the γ:δ T-cell receptor and mainly lack CD4 and CD8. A minority population of B cells express CD5 on their surface (see Section 5-14).

Related to Part III

proteins, which can be detected using specific antibodies (Fig. 2.30). B and T lymphocytes, for example, are identified unambiguously and separated from each other by antibodies to the constant regions of the B- and T-cell antigen receptors. T cells are further subdivided on the basis of expression of the co-receptor proteins CD4 and CD8.

An immensely powerful tool for defining and enumerating lymphocytes is the **flow cytometer**, which detects and counts individual cells passing in a stream in front of it. A flow cytometer equipped to separate the identified cells is called a **fluorescence-activated cell sorter** (**FACS**). These instruments are used to study the properties of cell subsets identified with monoclonal antibodies to cell-surface proteins. Individual cells within a mixed population are first tagged by treatment with specific monoclonal antibodies labeled with fluorescent dyes. The mixture of labeled cells is then forced with a much larger volume of saline through a nozzle, creating a fine stream of liquid containing cells spaced singly at intervals. As each cell passes in front of a laser beam it scatters the laser light, and any dye molecules bound to the cell will be excited and will fluoresce. Sensitive photomultiplier tubes detect both the scattered light, which gives information on the size and granularity of the cell, and the fluorescence emissions, which give information on the binding of the labeled monoclonal antibodies and hence on the expression of cell-surface proteins by each (Fig. 2.31).

In the cell sorter, the signals passed back to the computer also generate an electric charge, which is passed from the nozzle through the liquid stream to the cell, giving it a charge. Once it has passed a certain point, the stream breaks up into droplets, each containing no more than a single cell; droplets containing a charged cell can then be deflected from the main stream of droplets as it passes between plates of the opposite charge.

When cells are labeled with a single fluorescent antibody, the data from flow cytometry are usually displayed in the form of a histogram of fluorescence intensity versus cell numbers. If two or more antibodies are used, each coupled to different fluorescent dyes, then the data are more usually displayed in the form of a two-dimensional scatter diagram or as a contour diagram, where the fluorescence of one dye-labeled antibody is plotted against that of a second, with the result that a population of cells labeling with one antibody can be further subdivided by its labeling with the second antibody (see Fig. 2.31). By examining large numbers of cells, flow cytometry can give quantitative data on the percentage of cells bearing different molecules, such as surface immunoglobulin, which characterizes B cells, the T-cell receptor-associated molecules known as CD3, and the CD4 and CD8 co-receptor proteins that distinguish the major T-cell subsets. Likewise, FACS analysis has been instrumental in defining stages in the early development of B cells. FACS analysis has been applied to a broad range of problems in immunology; indeed, it played a vital role in the early identification of AIDS as a disease in which T cells bearing CD4 are depleted selectively (see Chapter 10).

Although the FACS is superb for isolating small numbers of cells in pure form, when large numbers of lymphocytes must be prepared quickly, mechanical means of separating cells are preferable. Human T cells were originally separated from other peripheral blood mononuclear cells by their ability to bind selectively to sheep red blood cells, forming **E-rosettes**, so-called to describe the appearance of a lymphocyte surrounded by erythrocytes, which rapidly sediment away from other lymphocytes. A more powerful and accurate way of isolating lymphocyte populations is to expose them to paramagnetic beads coated with monoclonal antibody that recognizes a distinguishing surface molecule. The tube containing the cells is then placed in a strong magnetic field,

Mixture of cells is labeled with fluorescent antibody

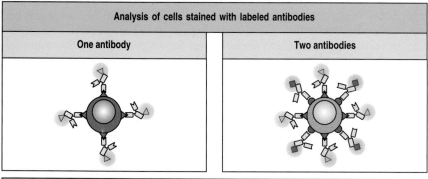

Stream of fluid containing antibody-labeled cells

Green photomultiplier tube (PMT)

Red PMT

Side scatter

Forward scatter

CPU

Laser

Analysis of cells stained with labeled antibodies

One antibody

Two antibodies

One-color histogram displays the amount of fluorescent antibody binding to each cell

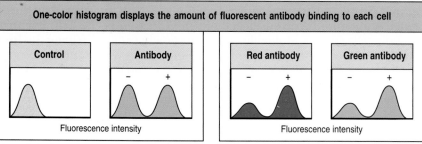

| Control | Antibody | Red antibody | Green antibody |

Fluorescence intensity

Two-color contour diagrams allow multiple populations of cells to be discriminated

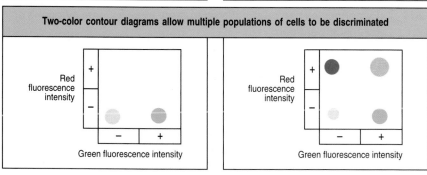

Red fluorescence intensity

Green fluorescence intensity

Fig. 2.31 Flow cytometry allows individual cells to be identified by their cell-surface antigens and to be counted. Cells to be analyzed by flow cytometry are labeled with fluorescent dyes (top panel), usually coupled to antibodies specific for cell-surface antigens. The cells are forced through a nozzle in a single cell stream that passes through a laser beam (second panel). Photomultiplier tubes (PMTs) detect the scattering of light, a sign of cell size and granularity, and emissions from the different fluorescent dyes. This information is analyzed using a computer. By examining many cells in this way, the number of cells with a specific set of characteristics can be counted and levels of expression of various molecules on these cells can be measured. As shown in the bottom left panels, use of a single antibody can indicate the percentage of a cell population bearing the molecule detected by that antibody, and the amount of that molecule expressed by each cell. This information can be presented as a one-color histogram (lower middle panel) or as a two-color contour profile (bottom panel). The latter is used mainly when two or more antibodies are used. The use of two antibodies (bottom right panels) can define four populations of cells: those expressing either molecule alone (red or green), those expressing both (orange), and those expressing neither (gray). The size and intensity of each circle indicates the numbers of cells with these characteristics.

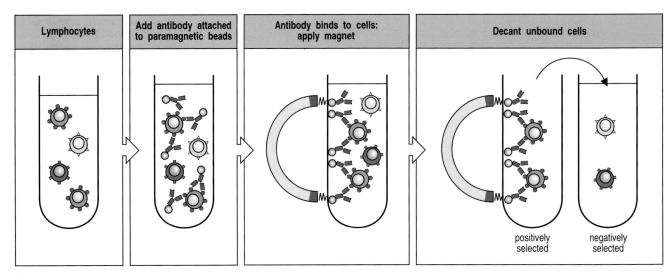

Lymphocytes	Add antibody attached to paramagnetic beads	Antibody binds to cells: apply magnet	Decant unbound cells

positively selected   negatively selected

Fig. 2.32 Lymphocyte subpopulations can be separated physically using antibodies coupled to paramagnetic beads. Lymphocytes bearing a particular cell-surface molecule will bind to paramagnetic beads coupled with a mouse monoclonal antibody. They can be separated from cells that lack the molecule by attraction of the beads to a strong magnet. Unbound cells are decanted to yield a population that is said to be negatively selected for absence of the antigen recognized by the monoclonal antibody. Bound cells are recovered by warming or other treatments that disrupt antigen: antibody binding; they are said to be positively selected for presence of the antigen recognized by the antibody.

Related to Part IV

the cells attached to the beads are retained and cells lacking the surface molecule recognized by the monoclonal antibody can be decanted off, leaving behind only the bound cells that express that protein (Fig. 2.32). The bound cells are positively selected for expression of the determinant, while the unbound cells are negatively selected for its absence. Cells have also been isolated by binding to antibody-coated plastic surfaces, a technique known as panning, or by killing cells bearing a particular molecule with specific antibody and complement (see Fig. 2.42). All these techniques can also be used as a pre-purification step prior to sorting out large numbers of highly purified populations by FACS.

The main conclusion reached from studies on isolated lymphocyte populations is that lymphocytes bearing particular combinations of cell-surface proteins have particular functions, which suggests that these proteins must be involved directly in the function of the cell. For this reason, such surface molecules were originally called **differentiation antigens**. When groups of monoclonal antibodies were found to recognize the same differentiation antigen, they were said to define **clusters of differentiation**, abbreviated to **CD**, followed by an arbitrarily assigned number. This is the origin of the CD nomenclature for lymphocyte cell-surface antigens. The known CD antigens are listed in Appendix I.

2-18 Lymphocytes can be stimulated to grow by polyclonal mitogens or by specific antigen.

To function in adaptive immunity, rare antigen-specific lymphocytes must proliferate extensively before they differentiate into functional effector cells, in order to generate sufficient numbers of effector cells of a particular specificity. Thus, the analysis of induced lymphocyte proliferation is a central issue in their study. However, it is difficult to detect the proliferation of normal lymphocytes in response to specific antigen, because only a minute proportion of cells will be stimulated to divide. Enormous impetus was given to the field of lymphocyte

Mitogen	Abbreviation	Source	Responding cells
Phytohemagglutinin	PHA	*Phaseolus vulgaris* (Red kidney beans)	T cells (human)
Concanavalin A	ConA	*Canavalia ensiformis* (Jack bean)	T cells (mouse)
Pokeweed mitogen	PWM	*Phytolacca americana* (pokeweed)	T and B cells
Lipopolysaccharide	LPS	*Escherichia coli*	B cells (mouse)

Fig. 2.33 Polyclonal mitogens, many of plant origin, stimulate lymphocyte proliferation in tissue culture. Many of these mitogens are used to test the ability of lymphocytes in human peripheral blood to proliferate.

Related to Part IV

culture by the finding that certain substances induce many or all lymphocytes of a given type to proliferate. These substances are referred to collectively as **polyclonal mitogens** because they induce mitosis in lymphocytes of many different specificities or clonal origins (Fig. 2.33). T and B lymphocytes are stimulated by different polyclonal mitogens. Although the polyclonal mitogens probably do not act directly on the antigen-specific receptors of lymphocytes, they seem to trigger essentially the same growth response mechanisms as antigen. Thus, responses to polyclonal mitogens have been very useful in working out the mechanisms of lymphocyte growth in normal cells, and they are still used clinically for assessing the ability of lymphocytes from patients with suspected immunodeficiencies to proliferate in response to a non-specific stimulus.

Lymphocytes normally exist as resting cells in the G_0 phase of the cell cycle. When stimulated with polyclonal mitogens, they rapidly enter the G_1 phase and progress through the cell cycle. This process can be monitored in individual cells using the FACS to analyze their DNA and RNA content as revealed by selective dyes. However, most studies of lymphocyte proliferation simply measure the incorporation of ^{3}H-thymidine into the DNA of cells as a sign of cell growth.

Once lymphocyte culture had been optimized using the proliferative response to polyclonal mitogens as an assay, it became possible to detect antigen-specific T-cell proliferation in culture by measuring ^{3}H-thymidine uptake in response to antigen to which the T cell donor had been previously immunized (Fig. 2.34). This is the assay most commonly used for assessing T-cell responses after immunization but it tells one little about the functional capabilities of the responding T cells. These must be ascertained by functional assays, as described in the next section.

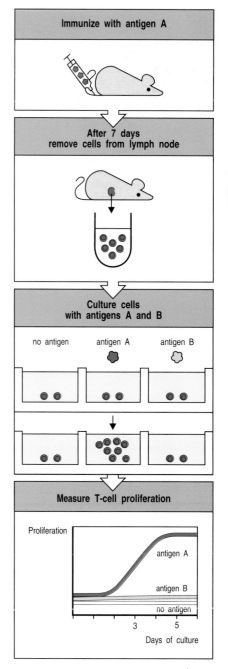

Fig. 2.34 Antigen-specific T-cell proliferation is frequently used as an assay for T-cell responses. T cells from mice or humans that have been immunized with an antigen (A) proliferate when they are exposed to antigen A and antigen-presenting cells but not to unrelated antigens to which they have not been immunized (antigen B). Proliferation can be measured by incorporation of ^{3}H-thymidine into the DNA of actively dividing cells. Antigen-specific proliferation is a hallmark of specific CD4 T-cell immunity.

Related
to Part IV

2-19   T-cell effector functions can be measured in four ways — target-cell killing, macrophage activation, B-cell activation, or lymphokine production.

As we learned in Section 2-6, effector T cells are detected by their effects on target cells displaying antigen. Measuring these effector functions forms the basis for T-cell bioassays used to assess both T-cell specificity for antigen and T-cell effector functions.

CD8 T-cell function is usually determined using the simplest and most rapid T-cell bioassay — the killing of a target cell by a cytotoxic T cell. This is usually detected in a ^{51}Cr-release assay. Live cells will take up, but do not spontaneously release, radioactively labeled sodium chromate, $Na_2^{51}CrO_4$. When these labeled cells are killed, the radioactive chromate is released and its presence in the supernatant of mixtures of target cells and cytotoxic T cells can be measured (Fig. 2.35). In a similar assay, proliferating target cells such as tumor cells can be labeled with ^{3}H-thymidine, which is incorporated into the replicating DNA. On attack by a cytotoxic T cell, the DNA of the target cells is rapidly fragmented and released into the supernatant, and one can measure either the release of these fragments or the retention of ^{3}H-thymidine in chromosomal DNA. These assays provide a rapid, sensitive, and specific measure of the activity of cytotoxic T cells.

Fig. 2.35   Cytotoxic T-cell activity is often assessed by chromium release from labeled target cells. Target cells are labeled with radioactive chromium as $Na_2^{51}CrO_4$ and exposed to cytotoxic T cells. Cell destruction is measured by the release of radioactive chromium into the medium, detectable within four hours of mixing target cells with T cells.

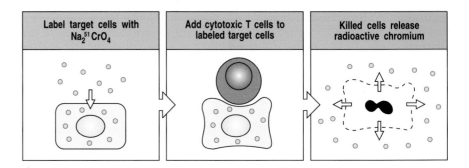

Label target cells with $Na_2^{51}CrO_4$	Add cytotoxic T cells to labeled target cells	Killed cells release radioactive chromium

The fragmentation of the DNA of cells killed by cytotoxic T cells results from the induction of a process of programmed cell death, or apoptosis, within the target cell. The characteristic cleavage of the DNA in cells undergoing programmed cell death has been used as the basis for an assay to identify apoptotic cells *in situ*. Nucleotides can be added to the free 3′ ends of DNA molecules by the enzyme terminal deoxyribonucleotidyl transferase (TdT). If TdT is used to add labeled oligonucleotides, tagged, for example, with biotin, then reporter enzymes coupled to avidin or streptavidin will bind to the tagged nucleotides and can be used to identify apoptotic cells by converting a colorless substrate into a colored insoluble product (Fig. 2.36), in much the same way that such reagents are used in immunohistochemical staining (see Section 2-13). The labeled nucleotide most commonly used in this assay is dUTP, coupled to biotin. Hence the assay is often called the TdT-dependent dUTP–biotin nick end labeling, or **TUNEL assay**.

CD4 T-cell functions involve the activation rather than the killing of cells bearing specific antigen. For example, some CD4 T cells can activate resting macrophages. Normal macrophages will ingest but will not destroy certain bacteria that grow intracellularly, such as *Listeria monocytogenes*. However, macrophages infected with *L. monocytogenes* will kill their intracellular bacteria if exposed to

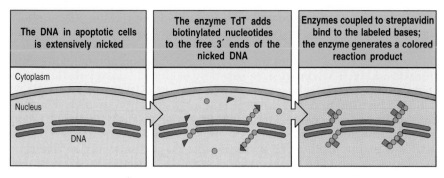

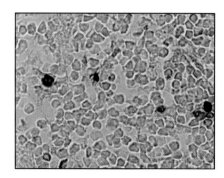

Fig. 2.36 Fragmented DNA can be labeled by terminal deoxynucleotidyl transferase (TdT) to reveal apoptotic cells. When cells undergo programmed cell death, or apoptosis, their DNA becomes fragmented (left panel). The enzyme TdT is able to add nucleotides to the ends of DNA fragments; most commonly in this assay, biotin-labeled nucleotides (usually dUTP) are added (second panel). The biotinylated DNA can be detected using streptavidin, which binds to biotin, coupled to enzymes that convert a colorless substrate into a colored insoluble product (third panel). Cells stained in this way can be detected by light microscopy, as shown in the photograph of apoptotic cells (stained red) in the thymic cortex. Photograph courtesy of R Budd and J Russell.

CD4 T cells from mice immune to *L. monocytogenes* but not if exposed to T cells from uninfected mice. Macrophages can also be activated by T cells that recognize other antigens on the macrophage surface. Activated macrophages can also be detected by their ability to kill certain tumor cells or by the release of toxic chemical mediators such as nitric oxide (NO). Macrophage activation is very important in promoting pathogen destruction, and the loss of this capacity in AIDS patients is probably the reason they die of opportunistic infections. Other CD4 T cells induce B cells to secrete specific antibody, and the production of antibody in the presence of these T cells can serve as an assay for this activity. Such T cells are called helper T cells, and antibody responses to most antigens are absolutely dependent on helper T-cell function (see Fig. 1.28).

T-cell effector functions are mediated in large part by non-specific mediator proteins called cytokines and cytotoxins, which are released by the T cell when it recognizes antigen (see Chapter 7). Thus, T-cell function can also be studied by measuring the type and amount of these released proteins. As different effector T cells release different amounts and types of cytokines or cytotoxins, one can learn about the effector potential of that T cell by measuring the proteins it produces. Cytokines can be detected by their activity in biological assays of cell growth, where they serve either as growth factors or growth inhibitors, or by a modification of ELISA known as a **sandwich ELISA**. In this assay, the cytokine is characterized by its ability to bridge between two monoclonal antibodies reacting with different epitopes on the cytokine molecule (Fig. 2.37). Sandwich ELISA can also be carried out by placing the cells

Related
to Part IV

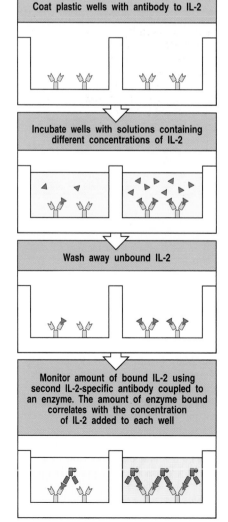

Fig. 2.37 Measurement of interleukin-2 (IL-2) production by sandwich ELISA. When T cells are activated with a mitogen or antigen they usually release the T-cell growth factor IL-2. The IL-2 can be measured by induction of growth of an IL-2 responsive indicator cell (not shown); however, assay for IL-2 by sandwich ELISA is far more accurate and specific. In this assay, one unlabeled anti-IL-2 antibody is attached to the plastic, and then the IL-2-containing fluid is added. After washing, bound IL-2 is detected by binding a second, labeled anti-IL-2 antibody directed at a different epitope. This assay is highly specific because antigens that cross-react with one antibody are very unlikely to cross-react with the other. It can detect and quantify IL-2 with great sensitivity.

themselves on a surface coated with antibody to a cytokine. After a short incubation, the cytokine released by each cell is trapped on the antibody coat and the presence of cytokine-secreting cells can be revealed when the cells are washed off and a labeled second anti-cytokine antibody is added. The cytokine released by each cell makes a distinct spot in this assay, which is therefore known as an **ELISPOT assay**. ELISPOT can also be used to detect specific antibody secretion by B cells, in this case using antigen-coated surfaces to trap specific antibody, and labeled anti-immunoglobulin to detect the bound antibody. Sandwich ELISA avoids a major problem of cytokine bioassays, the ability of different cytokines to stimulate the same response in a bioassay. Bioassays must therefore always be confirmed by inhibition of the response with monoclonal antibodies against the cytokine.

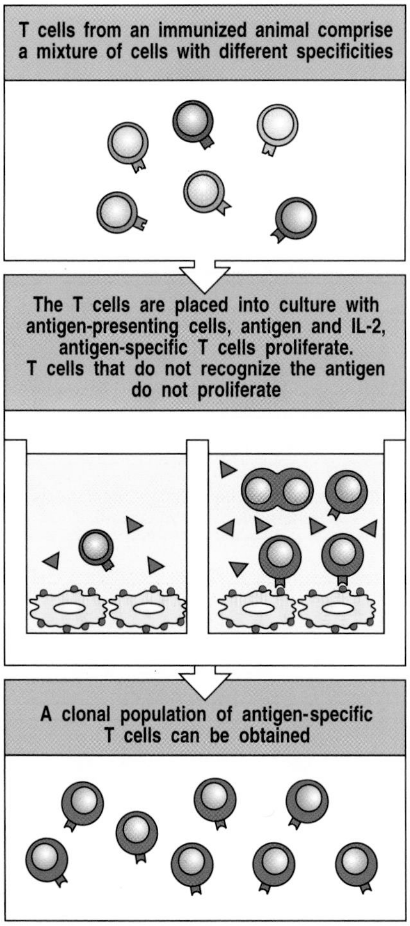

Fig. 2.38   Production of cloned T-cell lines. T cells from an immune donor, comprising a mixture of cells with different specificities, are activated with antigen and antigen-presenting cells. Single responding cells are cultured by limiting dilution (see Fig. 2.40) in the T-cell growth factor interleukin-2 (IL-2). From these single cells, cloned lines specific for antigen are identified and can be propagated by culture with antigen, antigen-presenting cells, and IL-2.

Related to Part IV

2-20   Homogeneous T lymphocytes can be obtained as tumors, T-cell hybrids, or cloned T-cell lines.

Just as the analysis of antibody specificity and structure has been aided greatly by the development of hybridomas making monoclonal antibodies, the analysis of specificity and effector function in T cells has depended heavily on monoclonal populations of T lymphocytes. These can be obtained in three ways. First, as for hybridomas, normal T cells proliferating in response to specific antigen can be fused to malignant T-cell lymphoma lines to generate **T-cell hybrids**. The hybrids express the receptor of the normal T cell, but proliferate indefinitely owing to the cancerous state of the lymphoma parent. T-cell hybrids can be cloned to yield a population of cells all having the same T-cell receptor. These cells can be stimulated by specific antigen to release biologically active mediator molecules such as the T-cell growth factor interleukin-2, and the production of cytokines is used to assess the specificity of the T-cell hybrid.

T-cell hybrids are excellent tools for the analysis of T-cell specificity, as they grow readily in suspension culture. However, they cannot be used to analyze the regulation of specific T-cell proliferation in response to antigen because they are continually dividing. T-cell hybrids cannot be transplanted into an animal to test for function *in vivo* because they would give rise to tumors, and functional analysis of T-cell hybrids is also confounded by the fact that the malignant partner cell affects their behavior in functional assays. Therefore, the regulation of T-cell growth and the effector functions of T cells must be studied using **cloned T-cell lines**, derived from single T cells, whose growth is dependent on periodic restimulation with specific antigen and, frequently, the addition of T-cell growth factors (Fig. 2.38). Such cells are more tedious to grow but, because their growth depends on specific antigen recognition, they maintain antigen specificity, which is often lost in T-cell hybrids. Cloned T-cell lines can be used for studies of effector function both *in vitro* and *in vivo*. In addition, the proliferation of T cells, a critical aspect of clonal selection, can only be characterized in cloned T-cell lines where such growth is dependent on antigen recognition. Thus, both types of monoclonal T-cell line have valuable applications in experimental studies (Fig. 2.39).

In studies of human T cells, T-cell clones have proven of greatest value because a suitable fusion partner for making T-cell hybrids has not been identified. However, a human T-cell lymphoma line, called Jurkat, has been characterized extensively because it secretes interleukin-2 when its antigen receptor is crosslinked with anti-receptor monoclonal

T-cell clone characteristic	Advantages	Disadvantages
Antigen-inducible growth	Selection for growth by antigen; selection for specificity by growth; analysis of growth cycle	Slow growth; need to add feeder cells
Genetic stability	Maintains phenotype	Difficult to select variants
Functional behavior	Maintains function stably	Difficult to select variants; contaminating feeder cells may affect function
T-cell hybrid characteristic	Advantages	Disadvantages
Antigen-independent growth	No feeder cells needed; rapid growth	Frequent loss of specificity; cannot be used to study clonal expansion
Genetic instability	Easy to select variants	Phenotype unstable
Functional behavior	No contaminating cells	Only some functions obtained; function affected by both partners to fusion

Fig. 2.39   The relative merits of cloned T-cell lines and T-cell hybrids in analysis of T-cell specificity and function.

Related to Part IV

antibodies. This simple assay system has yielded much information about signal transduction in T cells. One of the Jurkat cell line's most interesting features, shared with T-cell hybrids, is that it stops growing when its antigen receptor is crosslinked. This has allowed mutants lacking the receptor or having defects in signal transduction pathways to be selected simply by culturing the cells with anti-receptor antibody and selecting those that continue to grow. Thus, T-cell tumors, T-cell hybrids, and cloned T-cell lines all have valuable applications in experimental immunology.

2-21   Limiting dilution measures the frequency of lymphocytes specific for a particular antigen.

The response of a lymphocyte population is a measure of the overall response, but the frequency of specific lymphocytes able to respond to an antigen can only be determined by limiting dilution culture. This assay makes use of the Poisson distribution, a statistical function that describes how objects are distributed at random. For instance, when different numbers of T cells are distributed into a series of culture wells, some wells will receive no specific T cells, some will receive one specific T cell, some two and so on. The T cells are activated with a polyclonal mitogen and growth factors and, after allowing several days for their growth and differentiation, the cells in each well are tested for a response to antigen, such as cytokine release or the ability to kill specific target cells. The proportion of wells in which there is no response is plotted against the number of cells initially added to the well. If cells of one type, typically antigen-specific T cells because of their rarity, are the only limiting factor for obtaining a response, then a straight line is obtained. From the Poisson distribution, it is known that there is on average one antigen-specific cell per well when the proportion of negative wells is 37%. Thus, the frequency of antigen-specific cells in the population equals the reciprocal of the number of cells added to the wells when 37% of the wells are negative. After priming, the frequency of specific cells goes up substantially, reflecting the antigen-driven proliferation of antigen-specific cells. The limiting dilution assay can also be used to measure the frequency of B cells that can make antibody to a given antigen (Fig. 2.40).

Fig. 2.40 The frequency of specific lymphocytes can be determined in limiting dilution assay. Varying numbers of lymphoid cells from normal or immunized mice are added to individual culture wells and stimulated with antigen or polyclonal mitogen. After several days, the wells are tested for a specific response to antigen, such as cytotoxic killing of target cells, or antibody production by purified B cells driven by helper T cells and antigen as shown here. Each well that initially contained a specific B cell will make antibody, and from the Poisson distribution one can determine that when 37% of the cultures are negative, each well contained on average one specific B cell at the beginning of the culture. In the example shown, for the unimmunized mouse 37% of the wells are negative when 12 000 B cells have been added to each well; thus the frequency of antigen-specific B cells is 1 in 12 000. When the mouse is immunized, 37% of the wells are negative when only 2 000 B cells have been added; hence the frequency of specific B cells after immunization is 1 in 2 000.

Related to Part IV

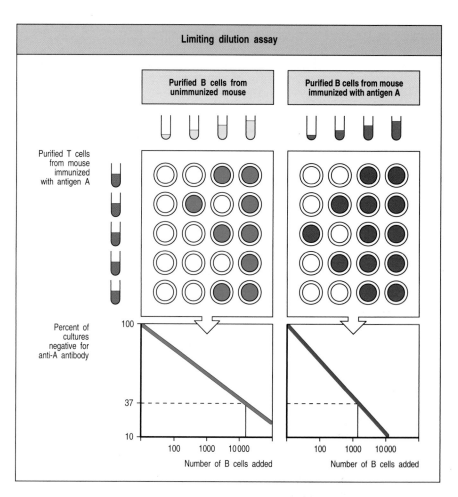

Summary.

The cellular basis of adaptive immunity is the clonal selection of lymphocytes by antigen. Therefore, to study adaptive immune responses, one must isolate lymphocytes and characterize them. Lymphocytes can be divided into subpopulations using antibodies that detect cell-surface molecules expressed selectively on cells of a given type. Subsets defined in this way also differ functionally, suggesting that the cell-surface molecules detected are important for the function of that cell. Antibodies to cell-surface antigens can be used to separate lymphocytes physically, using magnetic beads, or by fluorescence-activated cell sorting, which also allows quantitative analysis of cell distribution. The functional capabilities of these isolated populations can then be tested *in vitro* and *in vivo*. Individual T cells can also be cloned, either as T-cell hybridomas or as continuously growing lines of normal T cells, which are valuable for analyzing the specificity, function, and signaling properties of T cells.

Related to Part II

Immunogenetics: the major histocompatibility complex.

Immunogenetics includes the use of antibodies, and more recently of T cells, to detect genetic differences or polymorphisms within a population. The first polymorphic system to be studied by immunogenetics was the ABO blood group system defined by Karl Landsteiner, and virtually all blood typing is carried out using immunogenetic techniques (see Fig. 2.12). In no area has immunogenetics played such a vital role as in the analysis of the highly polymorphic **major histocompatibility complex (MHC)** of genes (see Chapter 4). As we mentioned in Chapter 1, all T-cell responses involve the recognition of peptide fragments of antigen bound to cell-surface proteins encoded in the MHC (MHC molecules), making the analysis of the MHC a central concern of immunologists. The MHC in humans is the most polymorphic cluster of human genes known, and this polymorphism is of interest to immunologists because it affects antigen recognition by T cells (see Chapter 4). Its role in T-cell development (see Chapter 6), the rejection of tissue grafts (see Chapter 11), and susceptibility to many immunological disorders (see Chapter 11), provides a strong clinical impetus to the analysis of the MHC in humans. The MHC is also of great interest to students of evolution looking at the role of polymorphism in genetic selection. Thus, the analysis of MHC polymorphism is crucial to virtually all aspects of immunological research. Here, we shall look at the techniques used to analyse MHC genetics and function. Analyzing the effects of MHC polymorphism on immune responses requires strains of mice bred to differ only at the MHC. We will start by describing the graft rejection responses that are caused by MHC polymorphism and that first drew the attention of biologists to its existence.

2-22   Tissues grafted between unrelated individuals are rejected.

The existence of a highly polymorphic MHC was first inferred from the rejection of grafted tissues. Blood transfusion had proved very successful once the genetics of the ABO blood group system had been deciphered, and this led to the idea that solid tissues could similarly be replaced by surgical transplantation. The first attempts to do so all failed: graft rejection was rapid and total, most grafts functioning for a brief period before becoming infiltrated with lymphocytes and dying.

Skin was the favored tissue for experimental transplants, as the graft could be examined directly on a regular basis. The genetic basis of graft rejection was first shown by the successful grafting of skin between individuals of an inbred mouse strain. Inbred mice have been specially bred so that they are homozygous at all loci. All members of an inbred strain carry identical alleles at each locus. These mice are equivalent to monozygotic human twins, and tissues can be grafted between monozygotic twins without rejection as well. Skin transplanted to inbred mice from members of other inbred strains or from other species was invariably rejected (Fig. 2.41). It was soon appreciated that the skin graft rejection was caused by an immune response against the grafted tissue. Graft rejection showed specific immunological memory, and immunodeficient mice did not reject grafts. However, the immunological and genetic basis of graft rejection remained to be worked out.

To analyze the genetic basis of this response, two inbred strains that mutually reject skin grafts were bred to each other, so that their F1 hybrid offspring had one set of alleles from each parental strain. When

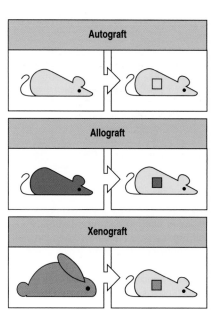

Fig. 2.41 The terminology of transplantation. Grafts from one site to another on the same individual are termed autologous grafts or autografts and are accepted. Grafts between genetically identical individuals, including those between members of the same inbred strain or between identical twins, are called syngeneic grafts and are also accepted. Grafts between genetically non-identical or allogeneic members of the same species are called allografts and are rejected. Grafts between the xenogeneic members of different species are called xenografts and are rejected.

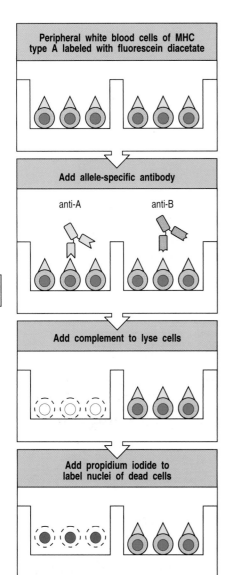

Fig. 2.42 The microcytotoxicity assay is used in histocompatibility testing. Leukocytes labeled with the vital dye fluorescein diacetate, which stains viable cells green, are exposed to antibody specific for allelic variants of MHC proteins and then exposed to complement. If the antibody reacts with the MHC proteins on a cell, this activates the complement so that the cell is killed, as seen by loss of green cells and the appearance of cells labeled by uptake of the dye propidium iodide (red), which only enters dead cells.

grafts were made between the F1 hybrid offspring and the parental strains, the F1 hybrid accepted skin from both parental strains, while the skin of the F1 hybrid was rejected by both parents. This showed that all the antigens involved in transplant rejection are expressed in the F1 hybrid mouse, as both parents reject its skin, and that its immune system is tolerant of all such antigens, as it accepts grafts from both parental strains. What was of particular interest was that half the offspring of F1 mice backcrossed to one parental strain rapidly rejected grafts of the other parental strain, starting about eight days after grafting, indicating that a single genetic locus must control rapid graft rejection. This locus was later found to be composed of a cluster of related genes, and was termed the major histocompatibility complex (MHC) because it is the major determinant of graft survival. The genetic locus determining rapid graft rejection was found to segregate precisely with an antigen detected by an antibody that reacted with mouse blood cells. This antigen was known as antigen-2, and the locus it defined was named histocompatibility-2 or **H-2**, the genetic designation for the mouse MHC. Subsequently, it was discovered that grafts between mice identical at H-2 were also rejected, although rejection generally occurred longer after grafting. These mice were shown to differ at other genetic loci encoding **minor histocompatibility (H) antigens**.

As genetic matching at H-2 led to prolonged survival of tissue grafts, it was believed that identification of a similar genetic complex might allow tissue grafting in humans. The human MHC was studied first using antibody reactions with white blood cells and is now called the human leukocyte antigen, or **HLA**, system (Fig. 2.42). Unfortunately, the remarkable polymorphism of HLA in the outbred human population makes the identification of HLA-identical individuals enormously difficult. Furthermore, the presence of minor H antigens makes the perfect matching available in genetically identical members of an inbred mouse strain possible in humans only when the donor and recipient are monozygotic twins (see Chapter 11).

2-23 | **MHC congenic, mutant, and recombinant inbred mouse strains are essential tools for analyzing MHC function.**

The MHC is a complex of many closely linked genes, and most of the genes that encode MHC molecules that are recognized by T cells are highly polymorphic in both mice and humans. To study the function of the MHC and the effect of MHC polymorphism on immune responses, animals are needed that differ genetically only at the MHC. To produce such animals, George Snell took advantage of the observation that a tumor transplanted from one mouse would grow progressively in another mouse only if the recipient mouse carried the same MHC genes expressed by the tumor. Under these conditions, the recipient is tolerant to the tumor's MHC antigens and fails to reject it, so the tumor grows and kills it. One tumor used by Snell arose in mice of strain A and would therefore grow in and kill any strain A mouse it was injected into, so Snell crossed strain A mice (MHC genotype H-2^a) with mice of a different MHC genotype (such as strain C57BL/6, abbreviated B6, MHC genotype H-2^b) to generate F1 hybrid mice (H-2^{axb}), which were then intercrossed to generate F2 mice. The F2 generation was injected with the tumor, and the one mouse in four that was homozygous (H-2^b) survived because it was intolerant of H-2^a. These mice were then backcrossed to strain A and the progeny again intercrossed and challenged with the tumor. After 10 backcross/intercross generations, Snell obtained a mouse that was genetically 99% strain A but was homozygous for the MHC of the other parent in the initial cross, in this case H-2^b. These mice

Fig. 2.43 The production of MHC congenic mouse strains. Mice of two strains, strain A with MHC genotype a (yellow) and strain B with MHC genotype b (blue) are crossed, and their F1 hybrid offspring, which are heterozygous at all loci including MHC^{axb} (green), are backcrossed to parental strain A. The F1 backcross progeny, which are homozygous A at 50% of their loci (yellow) are selected for expression of the other parental MHC^b and those that are MHC^{axb} are backcrossed again to strain A. This continues for 10 backcross generations, after which the mice are homozygous A at virtually all loci except MHC, where they are a/b (green). These mice are inter-crossed and selected for homozygosity at the MHC for alleles of donor origin (MHC^b) (blue). Virtually all the rest of the genome is derived from strain A to which the MHC genotype MHC^b has been introgressively backcrossed. These mice are strain A co-isogeneic or congenic for MHC^b, and are designated A.B. They can be used to determine if genetic traits that differ between strain A and strain B map to the MHC.

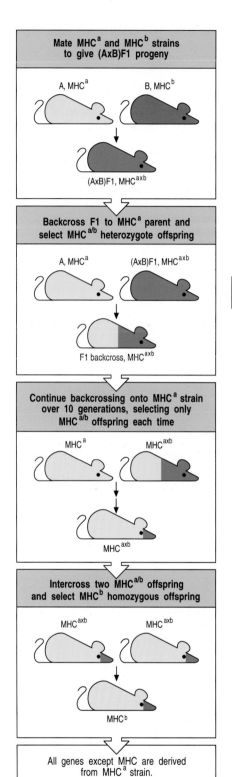

Mate MHC^a and MHC^b strains to give (AxB)F1 progeny

A, MHC^a B, MHC^b

(AxB)F1, MHC^{axb}

Backcross F1 to MHC^a parent and select MHC$^{a/b}$ heterozygote offspring

A, MHC^a (AxB)F1, MHC^{axb}

F1 backcross, MHC^{axb}

Continue backcrossing onto MHC^a strain over 10 generations, selecting only MHC$^{a/b}$ offspring each time

MHC^a MHC^{axb}

MHC^{axb}

Intercross two MHC$^{a/b}$ offspring and select MHC^b homozygous offspring

MHC^{axb} MHC^{axb}

MHC^b

All genes except MHC are derived from MHC^a strain. New strain is termed A.B congenic strain

Related to Part II

are called **congenic resistant** (to the strain A tumor) mice, and are designated A.B, where B denotes the strain designation of the parent donating the MHC genes, in this case B6 (Fig. 2.43). This experiment illustrates not only MHC genetics and function but also that the immune system can combat tumors provided they express recognizable antigens. We shall return to tumor immunity as a potential therapy for naturally occurring cancers in Chapter 12.

Congenic resistant mice have been crucial to our understanding of the role of the MHC in immunobiology. Fortunately there are now easier ways of producing them. For instance, antibodies to allelic variants of MHC proteins can be used to identify offspring that inherit the new MHC genes being bred onto strain A. One can therefore simply select the mice at each backcross generation that carry these genes, speeding the derivation of the new strains by avoiding the intercross generation. During this process, it is also possible to detect mice that have undergone recombination within the MHC, such that only some MHC alleles are inherited from the donor parent. These are called **MHC recombinant strains**. These intra-MHC recombinant mice allow one to map a particular phenotype to a particular region of the MHC, further refining the genetic map. Although the molecular structure of the MHC is now well defined, *in vivo* analysis of MHC function still depends largely on such recombinant and congenic mice. For example, one can map traits to a single locus in the MHC using **congenic** (**co-isogenic**) strains of mice (inbred mice differing only at a single MHC locus), or by using transgenic or gene knock-out mice, as we shall see in Section 2-38.

| 2-24 | **T lymphocytes respond strongly to MHC polymorphisms.** |

Graft rejection is carried out by T cells that recognize foreign MHC molecules and destroy the graft. This process can be studied *in vivo*, but in-depth analysis, especially in humans, required the development of *in vitro* correlates of graft rejection. One such assay is provided by the **mixed lymphocyte reaction** (**MLR**), in which T cells are co-cultured with so-called stimulator cells. These are usually irradiated lymphocytes from an unrelated individual who is therefore likely to be MHC disparate. By studying cultures of lymphocytes obtained from different inbred mouse strains, it was shown that the T cells are stimulated to proliferate and differentiate into effector cells; the irradiation of the stimulator cells prevents them from responding back. The T cells respond because they recognize MHC molecules on the stimulating

Fig. 2.44 The mixed lymphocyte reaction (MLR) can be used for detecting histoincompatibility. Spleens are taken from two mouse strains, and T cells (blue) are isolated from the spleen of one strain and cultured with non-T cells known as stimulator cells from the other strain (yellow). The non-T cells, which will include antigen-presenting cells, are irradiated or treated with the antibiotic mitomycin C before culture to block DNA synthesis and cell division. Three to seven days after mixing the cells, the cultures are assessed for T-cell proliferation by measuring the uptake of ^{3}H-thymidine, and for the generation of cytotoxic T cells by the chromium-release assay on labeled target cells (see Fig. 2.35).

Related to Part II

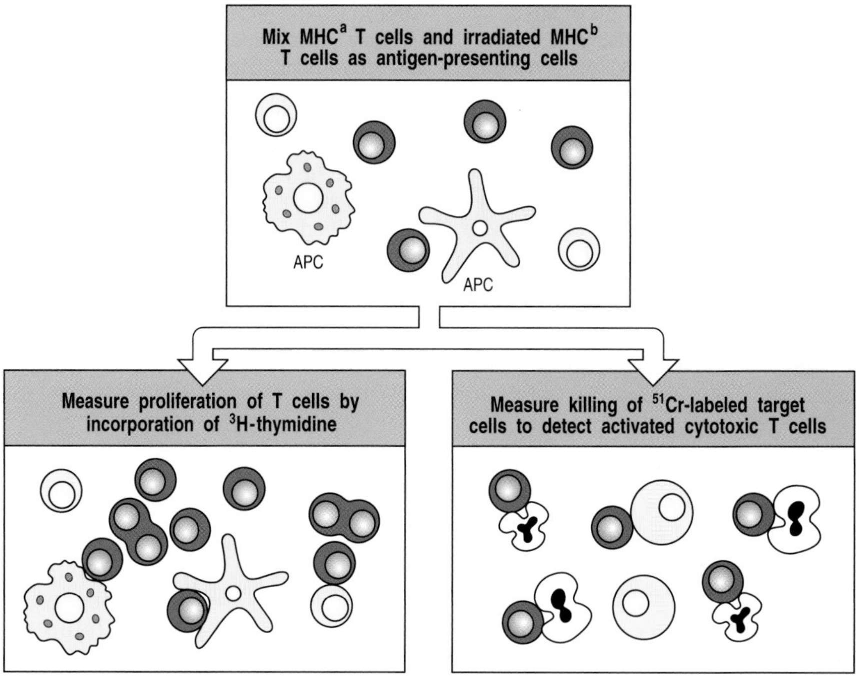

Mix MHC^a T cells and irradiated MHC^b T cells as antigen-presenting cells

Measure proliferation of T cells by incorporation of ^{3}H-thymidine

Measure killing of ^{51}Cr-labeled target cells to detect activated cytotoxic T cells

cells that are different from their own MHC molecules (Fig. 2.44). As we shall see later in the book, MHC gene products can be divided into two types of molecule — MHC class I molecules that are expressed on virtually all cells, and MHC class II molecules that are found only on immune system cells.

The intense proliferative response observed in mixed lymphocyte cultures between cells from unrelated people is largely the result of CD4 T-cell recognition of MHC class II polymorphisms (Fig. 2.45; the HLA-DR antigens of MHC class II molecules), while the cytotoxic T cells that result are predominantly CD8 T cells recognizing MHC class I polymorphisms (the A antigens in Fig. 2.45). This *in vitro* correlate of graft rejection is very useful in screening for histoincompatibility between potential donors and recipients, as it is extremely sensitive and more closely related to the actual graft rejection response than is the microcytotoxicity assay carried out with antibodies (see Fig. 2.42). Unfortunately, it is also more cumbersome and expensive to carry out, and takes several days to produce an answer.

Fig. 2.45 The nature of the MHC disparity between the responding and stimulating cells determines the type of T-cell response obtained in mixed lymphocyte culture. The T-cell response to allogeneic stimulator cells in mixed lymphocyte culture is controlled by the MHC genotype of the two cell types. In a human mixed lymphocyte culture, T-cell proliferation is stimulated largely by differences in MHC class II (HLA-DR) alleles, whereas generation of cytotoxic T cells depends predominantly on differences in MHC class I (HLA-A) alleles. The strongest responses occur when both MHC class I and MHC class II alleles differ between responder and stimulator.

Measure T-cell proliferation and cytotoxicity			
Responding T cell HLA type	Stimulator cell HLA type	Proliferation	Cytotoxicity
A1 DR3	A1 DR3	–	–
A1 DR3	A1 **DR4**	+++	+
A1 DR3	**A2** DR3	+	+++
A1 DR3	**A2 DR4**	++++	++++

Fig. 2.46 Antibody to specific MHC molecules can inhibit the mixed lymphocyte reaction. A CD4 T-cell response to HLA-DR2 is inhibited by anti-HLA-DR2 antibodies, which compete with the T-cell receptor for binding to HLA-DR2. However, anti-HLA-A3 antibodies do not inhibit the response of CD4 T cells to HLA-DR2, even though they bind to the stimulator cell surface. This shows that antibodies inhibit specific recognition events and are not interfering with the response non-specifically.

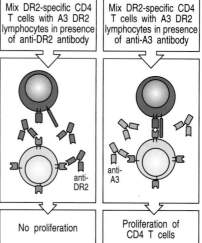

Related to Part II

2-25   **Antibodies to MHC molecules inhibit T-cell responses.**

MHC polymorphism not only accounts for graft rejection but also has profound effects on antigen recognition by T cells, as we shall learn in Chapter 4. As the MHC encodes several different proteins that present antigen to T cells, it is often difficult using genetics alone to determine which MHC molecule a T cell is recognizing.

An alternative approach is to use monoclonal antibodies that bind to a given MHC molecule and prevent its recognition by the T-cell receptor (Fig. 2.46). Thus, proliferative responses of CD4 T cells in mixed lymphocyte reactions are largely inhibited by antibodies to MHC class II molecules, while antibodies to MHC class I molecules block the cytolytic response of CD8 T cells in the same culture. Similarly, antibodies to MHC molecules can be used to define which MHC molecule is presenting peptides to an antigen-specific T cell. Antibodies to other structures crucial for cell interactions likewise inhibit these responses, so the use of monoclonal antibodies to inhibit T-cell responses has played a critical role in our understanding of these processes.

2-26   **Antibodies to MHC molecules can be used to define MHC genotype.**

Although T cells can be used to detect MHC variability, routine genetic typing for MHC uses antibodies that distinguish between the numerous different allelic variants of any MHC molecule. Most of our information about MHC genetics has been and continues to be generated in this way. Antibody typing has defined multiple gene loci within the MHC, each with a large number of alleles in the two species studied most extensively, humans and mice. These loci comprise a tightly linked complex of genes on chromosome 6 in humans and chromosome 17 in mice. As the MHC genes are close together on the chromosome, genetic recombination rarely occurs within the MHC, and most individuals will inherit an intact set of parental alleles from each parent; such a set of linked genes is referred to as a **haplotype**, the MHC genes found in one haploid genome. The tight genetic linkage of MHC genes can be documented readily by genotyping family members (Fig. 2.47).

Even in the case of very closely linked genes, with the passage of millions of years of evolutionary time, one would expect genetic crossover to result in random association of alleles at each locus. However, it is observed that certain MHC alleles are found in particular haplotypes

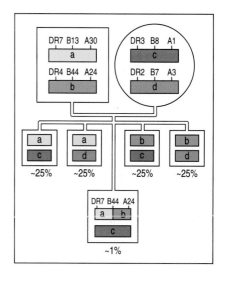

Fig. 2.47 The inheritance of MHC haplotypes in families. Each parent contributes genes from one of their two haplotypes, usually designated as a, b, c, and d. Most offspring inherit a complete MHC haplotype from each parent and can be designated simply a/c, a/d, b/c, or b/d; recombination within MHC haplotypes occurs at a frequency of only 1–2% (bottom panel).

Related
to Part II

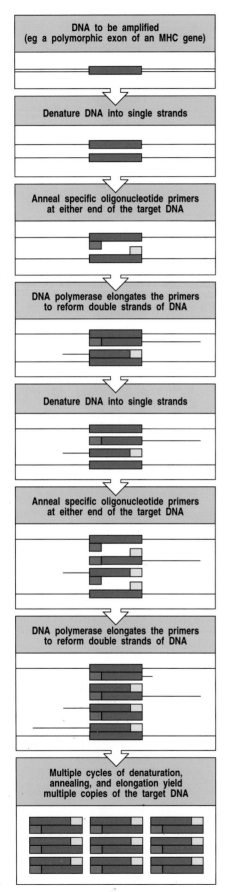

DNA to be amplified
(eg a polymorphic exon of an MHC gene)

Denature DNA into single strands

Anneal specific oligonucleotide primers
at either end of the target DNA

DNA polymerase elongates the primers
to reform double strands of DNA

Denature DNA into single strands

Anneal specific oligonucleotide primers
at either end of the target DNA

DNA polymerase elongates the primers
to reform double strands of DNA

Multiple cycles of denaturation,
annealing, and elongation yield
multiple copies of the target DNA

at frequencies greater or lesser than would be expected if all MHC alleles were at genetic equilibrium. This phenomenon, known as **linkage disequilibrium**, may reflect the recent origin of some alleles, the geographic origins and racial breeding patterns of humans, selection for certain haplotypes over others, or suppression of genetic recombination operating in some haplotypes. Linkage disequilibrium is an important factor in attempting to map susceptibility to diseases (such as autoimmune diseases, see Chapter 11) to a given MHC allele, as alleles of genes in linkage disequilibrium with a susceptibility locus may also appear to be associated with disease susceptibility. As more and more genetic loci are discovered within the MHC, the need grows for correlating disease susceptibility precisely with alleles at a particular locus.

2-27   Accurate MHC genotyping requires direct analysis of DNA sequence.

Although serological analysis is the main method for HLA genotyping humans, the reagents used are not specific enough to determine the precise structural identity of MHC molecules in unrelated individuals, who may have inherited closely related but distinct genes. Thus, while serological typing can accurately genotype family members for shared MHC alleles, the identity of MHC alleles in unrelated individuals can be established only by direct structural analysis of their genes. This is now most conveniently done by the **polymerase chain reaction (PCR)**, a rapid method of selectively replicating a particular stretch of genomic DNA *in vitro* (Fig. 2.48). Once enough DNA is produced from the gene being amplified, it can be sequenced. Sequence analysis has shown that serologically identical alleles actually comprise several closely related alleles. There are now many known sequence variants of most serologically defined MHC alleles, which are quite similar to each other but differ by one or a few amino acids, whereas the proteins of different serologically determined alleles differ from one another by many amino acids.

Once the DNA sequence of a given allele has been determined, oligonucleotide probes can be constructed from the regions where differences from other alleles occur, and these differences can be detected by direct hybridization of the probe to genomic DNA. This provides a rapid, cheap, and sensitive means of defining MHC gene structure. The application of this technique to MHC genetics has allowed the accurate determination of the role of MHC genes in several immunological diseases, and should help ultimately in determining the mechanism by which certain MHC alleles confer genetic susceptibility to particular diseases.

Fig. 2.48 The polymerase chain reaction. To amplify a specific region of genomic DNA, such as a polymorphic exon of an MHC gene, synthetic oligonucleotide primers complementary to the DNA sequence flanking that region are made. The genomic DNA is denatured in the presence of an excess of these two oligonucleotide primers so that after reannealing, the primers have bound their complementary sequence in genomic DNA. The DNA polymerase Taq from the bacterium *Thermus aquaticus*, which is stable at the high temperature used to denature DNA between replication cycles, elongates the primer using the genomic DNA between the two primers as a template. The replicated DNA is separated into single strands by heating and then the mixture is cooled so that a new cycle of primer annealing and replication can commence. The first extension products are random in length but as the reaction continues, products delimited by the primers and hence of the same length, accumulate.

Summary.

The cell-surface glycoproteins encoded by the MHC play a central role in immunology. As we learned in Chapter 1, their main function is to deliver peptide fragments of antigen to the cell surface where the peptide:MHC complex can be recognized by T cells. The MHC was, however, originally discovered as the major genetic barrier to transplantation, because the strong response of T cells to foreign MHC molecules causes graft rejection. T-cell recognition of peptide antigens is also influenced profoundly by MHC polymorphism. Thus, the analysis of this polymorphism is essential in immunology. It is also important in clinical medicine, not only as a way to match graft donors with recipients but also for studying the role of MHC genotype in determining susceptibility to many human allergic and autoimmune diseases. Such studies require reliable genotyping of the MHC in humans, which is carried out by serological analysis, mixed lymphocyte culture, and, most accurately, by DNA analysis. Experimental studies of MHC polymorphism are greatly facilitated by specialized congenic, recombinant, mutant, and recombinant inbred strains of mice. These clinical and experimental tools are essential for examining the impact of MHC polymorphism on immunity and immunological diseases.

Analyzing immune responses in intact organisms.

The ultimate goal of immunology is to understand the immune response *in vivo* and to control it. To do so, techniques to study immunity in live animals and in human patients are essential. The following sections describe how immunity is measured and characterized in the intact organism, be it a mouse or a human being. From these observations much is also learned about the functioning of the intact immune system. The cellular and molecular basis for these observed functions is the subject of much of this book.

Related to Part V

2-28   Protective immunity can be assessed by challenge with infectious agents.

An adaptive immune response against a pathogen often confers long-lasting immunity against infection with that pathogen; this is the basis of successful vaccination. The very first experiment in immunology, Jenner's successful vaccination against smallpox, is still the model for assessing the presence of such protective immunity. The assessment of protective immunity conferred by vaccination has three essential steps. First, an immune response is elicited by immunization with a candidate vaccine. Second, the immunized individuals, along with unimmunized controls, are challenged with the infectious agent. Finally, the prevalence and severity of infection in the immunized individual is compared with the course of the disease in the unimmunized controls (Fig. 2.49, left panel). For obvious reasons, such experiments are usually carried out first in animals, if a suitable animal model for the infection exists. However, eventually a trial must be carried out in humans. In this case, the infectious challenge is usually provided naturally by carrying out the trial in a region in which the disease is prevalent. The efficacy of the vaccine is determined by assessing the prevalence and severity of new

Fig. 2.49 *In vivo* **assay for the presence and nature of protective immunity after vaccination in animals.** Mice are injected with the test vaccine or a control such as saline solution. Different groups are then challenged with lethal or pathogenic doses of the test pathogen or with an unrelated pathogen as a specificity control (not shown). Unimmunized animals die or become severely infected. Successful vaccination is seen as specific protection of immunized mice against infection with the test pathogen. This is called active immunity and the process is called active immunization. If immunity can be transferred to a normal syngeneic recipient with serum from an immune donor, then immunity is mediated by antibodies, such immunity is called humoral immunity and the process is called passive immunization. If immunity can only be transferred by infusing lymphoid cells from the immune donor into a normal syngeneic recipient, then the immunity is called cell-mediated immunity and the transfer process is called adoptive transfer or adoptive immunization. Passive immunity is short-lived, as antibody is eventually catabolized, but adoptively transferred immunity is mediated by immune cells, which can survive and provide longer-lasting protection.

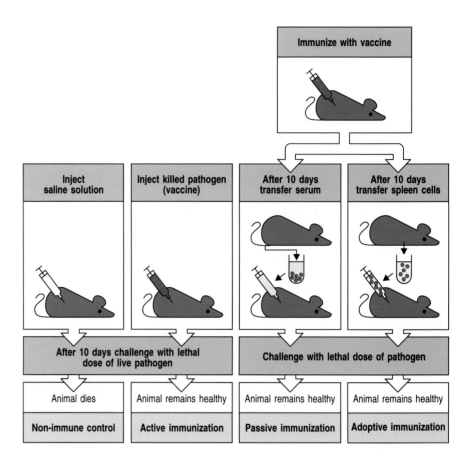

Related to Part V

infections in the immunized and control populations. Such studies necessarily give less precise results than a direct experiment but, for most diseases, they are the only way of assessing a vaccine's ability to induce protective immunity in humans.

2-29   Immunity can be transferred by antibodies or by lymphocytes.

The tests described in the previous section show that protective immunity has been established but cannot tell whether it involves humoral immunity, cell-mediated immunity, or both. When these studies are carried out in immunized or previously infected inbred mice, the nature of protective immunity can be determined by transferring serum or lymphoid cells from an immunized donor to an unimmunized syngeneic recipient (that is, a genetically identical animal of the same inbred strain) (Fig. 2.49). If protection against infection can be conferred by the transfer of serum, the immunity is due to circulating antibodies and is called **humoral immunity**. Transfer of immunity by antiserum or purified antibodies provides immediate protection against many pathogens and against toxins such as those of tetanus and snake venom. However, although protection is immediate, it is temporary, lasting only as long as the transferred antibodies remain active in the recipient's body. This type of transfer is therefore called **passive immunization**. Only **active immunization** with antigen can provide lasting immunity.

Protection against many diseases cannot be transferred by serum but can be transferred by lymphoid cells from immunized donors. The transfer of lymphoid cells from an immune donor to a normal syngeneic recipient is called **adoptive transfer** or **adoptive immunization**, and the immunity transferred is called **adoptive immunity**. Immunity that can be transferred with lymphoid cells only is called **cell-mediated immunity**. Such cell transfers must be between genetically identical donors and recipients, such as members of the same inbred strain of mice, so that the donor lymphocytes are not rejected by the recipient and do not attack the recipient's tissues. Irradiation of the recipient is frequently used to eliminate its own immune response, so that the effect of the adoptively transferred cells can be studied in isolation (see Section 2-32). The relatively low doses of radiation used are not lethal to the recipient but kill all their mature lymphocytes, which are particularly sensitive to radiation. James Gowans originally used this technique to prove the role of the lymphocyte in immune responses. He showed that all active immune responses could be transferred to irradiated recipients by small lymphocytes from immunized donors. This technique can be refined by transferring only certain lymphocyte subpopulations, such as B cells, CD4 T cells, and so on, and even cloned T-cell lines can confer adoptive immunity to their specific antigen. Adoptive transfer of immunity is not used clinically in humans except in experimental approaches to cancer therapy.

2-30 | Local responses to antigen can indicate the presence of active immunity.

Active immunity is often studied *in vivo*, especially in humans, by injecting antigens locally in the skin. If a reaction appears, this indicates the presence of antibodies or immune lymphocytes specific for that antigen; the **tuberculin test** is an example of this. When people have had tuberculosis they develop cell-mediated immunity that can be detected as a local response when their skin is injected with a small amount of tuberculin, an extract of *Mycobacterium tuberculosis*, the pathogen that causes tuberculosis. The response typically appears a day or two after the injection and consists of a raised, red, and hard (or indurated) area in the skin, which then disappears as the antigen is degraded.

Related to Part V

The immune system can also make less desirable responses, such as the hypersensitivity reactions responsible for allergies (see Chapter 11). Local intracutaneous injections of minute doses the antigens that cause allergies are used to determine what antigen triggers a patient's allergic reactions. Local responses that happen in the first few minutes after antigen injection in immune recipients are called **immediate hypersensitivity reactions**, and they can be of several forms, one of which is the wheal and flare response described in Chapter 11. Immediate hypersensitivity reactions are mediated by specific antibodies formed as a result of earlier exposures to the antigen. Responses that take hours to days to develop, such as the tuberculin test, are referred to as **delayed-type hypersensitivity** responses and are caused by pre-existing immune T cells. This latter type of response was observed by Jenner when he tested vaccinated individuals with a local injection of vaccinia virus.

These tests work because the local deposit of antigen remains concentrated in the initial site of injection, eliciting responses in local tissues. They do not cause generalized reactions if sufficiently small doses of antigen are used. However, local tests carry a risk of systemic allergic reactions, and they should be used with caution in people with a history of hypersensitivity.

Related
to Part V

| 2-31 | The assessment of immune responses and immunological competence in humans. |

The methods used for testing immune function in humans are necessarily more limited than those used in experimental animals, but many different tests are available, some of which have been mentioned already. They fall into several groups depending on the reason the patient is being studied.

Assessment of protective immunity in humans generally relies on tests conducted *in vitro*. To assess humoral immunity, specific antibody levels in the patient's serum are assayed using the test microorganism or a purified microbial product as antigen. To test for immunity against viruses, antibody production is often measured by the ability of serum to neutralize the infectivity of live virus for tissue culture cells. In addition to providing information about protective immunity, the presence of antibody to a particular pathogen indicates that the patient has been exposed to it, making such tests of crucial importance in epidemiology. At present, testing for antibody to HIV is the main screening test for infection, critical both for the patient and in blood banking, where blood from infected donors must be removed from the supply. Essentially similar tests are used in investigating allergy, where allergens are used as the antigens in tests for specific IgE antibody by ELISA or radioimmunoassay (see Section 2-7), which may be used to confirm the results of skin tests.

Cell-mediated immunity to infectious agents can be tested either by skin test with extracts of the pathogen, as in the tuberculin test (see Section 2-30), or by the ability of the pathogen or an extract from it to stimulate T-cell proliferative responses *in vitro* (Section 2-18). These tests provide information about the exposure of the patient to the disease and also about their ability to mount an adaptive immune response to it.

Patients with immune deficiency (see Chapter 10) are usually detected clinically by a history of recurrent infection. To determine the competence of the immune system in such patients, a battery of tests is usually conducted (Fig. 2.50); these focus with increasing precision as the nature of the defect is narrowed down to a single element. The presence of the various cell types in blood is determined by routine hematology often followed by FACS analysis (see Section 2-17) for the presence of lymphocyte subsets, and levels of the various serum immunoglobulins are determined. The competence of phagocytic cells is tested on freshly isolated polymorphonuclear leukocytes and monocytes, and the efficiency of the complement system (see Chapter 8) is determined by testing the dilution of serum required for lysis of 50% of antibody-coated red blood cells (CH_{50}) as a screening assay.

In general, if such tests reveal a defect in one of these broad compartments of immune function, more specialized testing is then needed to determine the precise nature of the defect. Tests of lymphocyte function are often valuable, starting with the ability of polyclonal mitogens to induce T-cell proliferation and B-cell secretion of immunoglobulin in tissue culture (see Section 2-18). These tests eventually pinpoint the cellular defect in immunodeficiency.

In patients with autoimmune diseases (see Chapter 11), the same parameters are usually analyzed to determine whether there is a gross abnormality in the immune system. However, most patients with such diseases show few abnormalities in general immune function. To determine whether a patient is producing antibody against their own cellular antigens, the most informative test is to react their serum with tissue sections, which are then examined for bound antibody by indirect

Evaluation of the cellular components of the human immune system		
	B cells	**T cells**	**Phagocytes**
Normal numbers (x10^9 per liter of blood)	Approximately 0.3	Total 1.0–2.5 CD4 0.5–1.6 CD8 0.3–0.9	Monocytes 0.15–0.6 Polymorphonuclear leukocytes Neutrophils 3.00–5.5 Eosinophils 0.05–0.25 Basophils 0.02
Measurement of function *in vivo*	Serum Ig levels, Specific antibody levels	Skin test	—
Measurement of function *in vitro*	Induced antibody production in response to pokeweed mitogen	T-cell proliferation in response to phytohemagglutinin or to tetanus toxoid	Phagocytosis, Nitro blue tetrazolium uptake, Intracellular killing of bacteria
Specific defects	See Fig. 10.7	See Fig. 10.7	See Fig. 10.7

Evaluation of the humoral components of the human immune system				
	Immunoglobulins				**Complement**
Component	IgG	IgM	IgA	IgE	
Normal levels	600–1400 mg dl^{-1}	40–345 mg dl^{-1}	60–380 mg dl^{-1}	0–200 IU ml^{-1}	CH$_{50}$ of 125–300 units ml^{-1}

Fig. 2.50 The assessment of immunological competence in humans. Both humoral and cell-mediated aspects of host defense can be checked, usually in a prescribed sequence, to identify the presence of an immune response or the causes of immunological incompetence. The initial screen consists of measuring levels of immunoglobulin and complement, and counting lymphocytes and phagocytic cells. This usually indicates if a defect in humoral or T-cell mediated immunity is present, and whether it affects the induction or mediation of a response. In Chapter 10, defects in host defense known as immunodeficiency diseases are described in detail.

Related to Part V

immunofluorescence using fluorescent-labeled anti-human immuno-globulin (see Section 2-13). Most autoimmune diseases are associated with the production of characteristic patterns of autoantibodies directed at self tissues. These patterns aid in the diagnosis of the disease and help to distinguish autoimmunity from tissue inflammation due to infectious causes.

Summary.

The measurement of immune function in intact organisms is essential to a full understanding of the immune system in health and disease. The ability of an immunized individual to resist infection is still the standard assay for protective immunity conferred by infection or vaccination. Local reactions to antigens injected into the skin can provide inform-ation about antibody and T-cell responses to the antigen, a procedure that is particularly important in testing for allergic reactions. Finally, many *in vitro* assays such as the analysis of specific antibody in serum and the proliferative responses of T cells to specific antigen are used to assess immune function in human patients. These tests, of necessity, lack the precision and rigor of most cellular and molecular biological assays. However, they provide the very subject matter of immunology. If we cannot relate *in vitro* studies to the behavior of the intact immune system, so that we can efficiently induce protective immunity or inhibit the unwanted responses in allergy, autoimmunity, and graft rejection, then we shall fail to achieve our most important goals.

Related
to Part III

The manipulation of the immune system.

To determine the role of the tissues, cells, and individual molecules of the immune system in intact organisms, immunologists have hitherto relied mainly on naturally occurring mutations and on techniques for generating abnormal immune systems. Much of our current understanding of how the immune system works *in vivo*, and especially of how the system develops, has come from this type of analysis. However, this area is being transformed by new technologies, in particular the ability to generate specific mutations in selected genes and to produce stable strains of mutant or transgenic mice. These approaches, allied to more traditional manipulations of lymphoid cells and tissues, should allow the development and *in vivo* functioning of the intact immune system to be analyzed with the detail and precision of current *in vitro* assays, thus greatly expanding our understanding of immunity. We shall begin by looking at the ways the immune system has been manipulated to produce our current understanding, and then look at novel ways of making genetic alterations *in vivo*. These techniques are already providing much detailed information about the role of certain genes and their products in host defense.

2-32   **Irradiation kills lymphoid cells allowing adoptive transfer of immune function.**

Ionizing radiation from X-ray or γ-ray sources kills lymphoid cells at doses that spare the other tissues of the body. By irradiating a recipient animal with an appropriate dose, the ability of different cell populations from syngeneic donor mice to transfer immune function can be tested. Such adoptive transfer studies are a cornerstone in the study of the intact immune system, as they can be carried out rapidly, simply, and in any strain of mouse.

Somewhat higher doses of irradiation eliminate all cells of hematopoietic origin, allowing replacement of the entire hematopoietic system, including lymphocytes, from donor bone marrow stem cells. The resulting animals are called **radiation bone marrow chimeras** from the Greek word *chimera*, a mythical animal that had the head of a lion, the tail of a serpent and the body of a goat. This technique is used to examine the development of lymphocytes as opposed to their effector functioning, and it has been particularly important in studying T-cell development, as we shall see in Chapter 6. Essentially the same technique is used in humans to replace bone marrow when it fails, as in aplastic anemia or after nuclear accidents, or to eradicate the bone marrow and replace it with normal marrow in the treatment of certain cancers.

2-33   **The *scid* mutation in mice prevents the development of all lymphocytes and homozygous *scid* mice can support a human immune system.**

There are several human immunodeficiencies that are described as severe combined immune deficiency, or SCID. Patients with these disorders are remarkably susceptible to infection with a wide range of agents, and most can survive only if completely isolated from their surroundings. Some SCID patients can be treated by bone marrow transplantation, which shows that the abnormality in these various syndromes is expressed exclusively in hematopoietic cells. SCID individuals are a dramatic illustration of the importance of lymphocytes in host defense and of the origin of all lymphocytes from a bone marrow progenitor.

In the mouse, a recessive mutation called *scid* prevents lymphocyte differentiation (see Chapter 10). Such mice have normal microenvironments for both B- and T-lymphocyte differentiation from stem cells, so grafting normal bone marrow into homozygous *scid/scid* mice can generate an intact immune system. Individual components of the mature immune system can also be transferred to *scid/scid* mice to generate animals expressing only the functions of particular subpopulations of lymphocytes. These mice are useful for distinguishing those immune functions that are innate (see Chapter 9) as opposed to those that require adaptive immunity mediated by specific lymphocytes. A more recent development of this technique uses mice mutant in the *RAG-1* and *RAG-2* genes, which also have no functional T and B cells, instead of *scid* mice, which produce some lymphocytes as they age.

Recently, homozygous *scid/scid* mice have been used to support an immune system derived from humans, a development that, for the first time, allows one to carry out experimental manipulation of the human immune response *in vivo* (Fig. 2.51). It is hoped that such manipulated mice may allow diseases such as AIDS to be studied under defined conditions, permitting vaccination and treatment protocols to be assessed rapidly, in the appropriate conditions, and at no risk to humans.

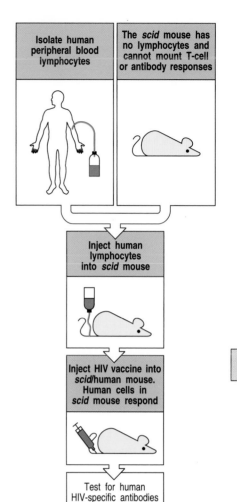

Related to Part III

Fig. 2.51 The use of the *scid*/human mouse to analyze human immune responses. The mouse strain C.B17 (*scid/scid*) or *scid* has an inherited severe combined immune deficiency; it lacks T and B lymphocytes but has normal hematopoietic cells. When these mice are injected with peripheral blood lymphocytes from a normal human donor, the human lymphocytes survive and function for several months in the mouse, producing antibodies and immune T cells when challenged. This human immune system can be tested for its ability to mount a response to a trial vaccine, for instance against HIV.

| 2-34 | **T cells can be selectively eliminated by removal of the thymus or by the *nude* mutation.** |

The importance of T-cell function *in vivo* can be ascertained in mice with no T cells of their own. Under these conditions, the effect of a lack of T cells can be studied, and T-cell subpopulations can be selectively restored to analyze their specialized functions. T lymphocytes originate in the thymus, and **thymectomy**, the surgical removal of the thymus, of a mouse at birth prevents T-cell development from occurring. Alternatively, adult mice can be thymectomized and then irradiated and reconstituted with bone marrow; such mice will develop all hematopoietic cell types except mature T cells.

The recessive *nude* mutation in mice, which in homozygous form causes hairlessness and absence of the thymus, is also associated with failure to develop T cells from bone marrow progenitors. Grafting thymectomized or *nude/nude* mice with thymic epithelial elements depleted of lymphocytes allows the graft recipients to develop normal mature T cells. This procedure allows the role of the non-lymphoid thymic stroma to be examined; it has been crucial in determining the role of thymic stromal cells in T-cell development (see Chapter 6).

| 2-35 | **B cells can be selectively depleted by treatment with anti-μ chain antibody or by genetic manipulation of immunoglobulin genes.** |

There is no single site of B-cell development in mice, so techniques such as thymectomy cannot be applied to the study of B-cell function and development in rodents. Nor are there mutations equivalent to *nude* that provide one with mice that have T cells but no B cells. However, such mutations exist in humans, leading to a failure to mount humoral immune responses or make antibody. The diseases produced by such mutations are called **agammaglobulinemias**, as they were originally detected as the absence of gamma globulins (see Section 2-9). The genetic basis for one form of this disease in humans has now been established (see Chapter 10), and the disease can be reproduced in mice by targeted disruption of the corresponding gene (see Section 2-38). Several different mutations in crucial regions of immunoglobulin genes have already been produced by gene targeting and have provided mice lacking B cells.

Before such mice became available, B-cell depletion could be achieved only by chronic administration of antibody against the μ heavy chains of IgM. This procedure is thought to mimic the process of self tolerance in B cells, signaling the early developing B cells by engaging their receptors and thus leading to their elimination (see Section 5-9). These treatments have to be maintained so that the new B cells emerging each day are eliminated, making this a difficult and costly procedure. Thus, while some information has been obtained about the role of B cells in various infectious diseases using this approach, it is clear that the new mutations that inhibit B-cell development will allow rapid clarification of the unique roles played by B cells in adaptive immunity.

2-36   Antibody treatment *in vivo* can deplete cells or inhibit cellular function.

Antibodies to cell-surface molecules on lymphocytes can inhibit cellular interactions in tissue culture, as we have already seen in the case of antibodies against MHC molecules (Section 2-25). Injection of mice or humans with monoclonal antibodies against particular cell-surface molecules can lead either to the elimination of the cell type bearing them or to inhibition of that cell's function. The outcome depends on whether the antibody is a 'depleting' or 'non-depleting' antibody, a distinction that depends mainly on its isotype, which also determines its effector functions. Antibodies that cause the death of the cells to which they bind are said to be depleting. Knocking out a particular cell type or inhibiting the function of a specific molecule can provide information about their probable function and importance. Monoclonal antibodies have also been used in this way for therapeutic purposes in humans as we shall see in Chapter 12.

Related to Part V

Chronic treatment with monoclonal antibodies is usually required to sustain the effects observed, and this creates problems in humans, who normally make antibodies against the mouse immunoglobulins used for this purpose. This problem has been approached by 'humanizing' mouse monoclonal antibodies, substituting human immunoglobulin sequences for mouse sequences in all but the antigen-binding site, so that the molecule is not recognized as foreign. As we shall see in Chapter 12, treatment of graft rejection, autoimmune disease, and cancer with monoclonal antibodies has demonstrated the therapeutic potential and lack of toxicity of this approach. However, better antibodies are needed before this becomes a major mode of treatment.

2-37   The role of individual genes can be studied in cultured cells by mutagenesis and by transfection.

The function of a gene has traditionally been studied by observing the effect of mutations in that gene in whole organisms and, more recently, in cultured cells. The advent of gene cloning, *in vitro* mutagenesis, and techniques for expressing genes in heterologous cells has revolutionized genetic analysis in immunology, as elsewhere in biology.

In cultured cells, a mutation in a gene encoding a known protein product can be obtained in two ways. In the classical approach, cells in which the gene is known to be expressed are treated with a mutagen and mutant cells are isolated by selecting against expression of the gene product. For cell-surface molecules, this is often done by killing cells expressing the product using a specific antibody and complement, leaving only mutant cells that lack the product. This approach is not always successful, mainly because such recessive or loss-of-function mutations can only be detected if both copies of the gene in the diploid cell are mutated, which is rare using conventional mutagenesis techniques. Moreover, such cells may accumulate several other mutations for which they have not been selected and which confound the analysis.

A more recent way of obtaining homozygous mutant cells is to use the technique of **homologous recombination**. Cloned copies of the target gene are altered to make them non-functional and are then introduced into the cell where they recombine with the homologous gene in the cell's genome, replacing the normal gene with a non-functional copy. Homologous recombination is a rare event in mammalian cells, and thus a powerful selective strategy is required to detect those cells in which it has occurred. Most commonly, the introduced gene construct has its sequence disrupted by an inserted antibiotic-resistance gene such as that for neomycin resistance. If this construct undergoes homologous recombination with the endogenous copy of the gene, the endogenous gene is disrupted but the antibiotic-resistance gene remains functional, allowing cells that have incorporated the gene to be selected in culture for resistance to the neomycin-like drug G418. Antibiotic resistance on its own shows only that the cells have taken up and integrated the neomycin-resistance gene. To select for those cells in which homologous recombination has occurred, the ends of the construct usually carry the thymidine kinase gene from the herpes simplex virus (HSV-tk). Cells that incorporate DNA randomly usually retain the entire DNA construct including HSV-tk, whereas homologous recombination between the construct and cellular DNA, the desired result, involves the exchange of homologous DNA sequences so that the non-homologous HSV-tk genes at the ends of the construct are eliminated. Cells carrying HSV-tk become sensitive to the anti-viral drug gancyclovir, and so cells with homologous recombinations have the unique feature of being resistant to both neomycin and gancyclovir, allowing them to be selected efficiently when these drugs are added to the cultures (Fig. 2.52). The high frequency of homologous recombination obtained with this technique means that both copies of the gene in a diploid cell can be mutated, resulting in a homozygous mutant cell. The same approach applied to embryonic stem cells has allowed the destruction of genes in intact mice, as we shall see in the next section (see Fig. 2.54).

Having obtained a mutant cell with a functional defect, the defect can be ascribed definitively to the mutated gene if the mutant phenotype can be reverted by a copy of the wild-type gene transferred into the mutant cell by **transfection**. Restoration of function means that the defect in the mutant gene has been complemented by the wild-type gene's function. This technique is very powerful, since it allows the gene that is being transferred to be mutated in precise ways to determine which parts of the protein are required for function.

Transfection can also be used to express proteins in cells that normally do not make them. This has been used to isolate genes, as we learned in Section 2-15, and is also useful in many other types of analysis. Some cell-surface molecules are expressed only as parts of multichain complexes: the receptors on T and B lymphocytes are very complex, consisting of products of at least six genes in the case of the T-cell receptor. Transfection of all six genes is required to achieve T-cell receptor

Related to Part V

Fig. 2.52 The deletion of specific genes can be accomplished by homologous recombination. When pieces of DNA are introduced into cells, they can integrate into cellular DNA in two different ways. If they randomly insert into sites of DNA breaks, the whole piece is usually integrated, often in several copies. However, extra-chromosomal DNA can also undergo homologous recombination with the cellular copy of the gene, in which case only the central, homologous region is incorporated into cellular DNA. Inserting a selectable marker gene such as resistance to neomycin (neo^r) into the coding region of a gene does not prevent homologous recombination, and it achieves two goals. First, it protects any cell that has integrated the DNA from the neomycin-like antibiotic G418. Second, when the gene does recombine with homologous cellular DNA, the neo^r gene disrupts the coding sequence of the modified cellular gene. Homologous recombinants can be discriminated from random insertions if the gene for herpes simplex virus thymidine kinase (HSV-tk) is placed at one or both ends of the DNA construct, which is often known as a 'targeting construct' because it targets the cellular gene. In random DNA integrations, HSV-tk is retained. HSV-tk renders the cell sensitive to the anti-viral agent gancyclovir. However, as HSV-tk is not homologous to the target DNA, it is lost from homologous integrants. Thus, cells that have undergone homologous recombination are uniquely both neo^r- and gancyclovir- resistant, and survive in a mixture of the two antibiotics. The presence of the disrupted gene has to be confirmed by Southern blotting or by the polymerase chain reaction (PCR) using primers in the neo^r gene and in cellular DNA lying outside the region used in the targeting construct. By using two different resistance genes one can disrupt the two cellular copies of a gene, making a deletion mutant (not shown).

Related to Part V

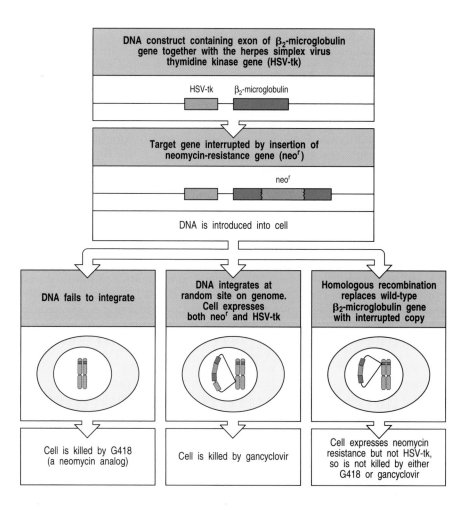

expression in cells that do not express any of these genes. Likewise, MHC class II molecules can be expressed only if genes encoding their two chains are transfected together into the same cell. This type of transfection analysis has provided much information on the subunit structure of complex protein arrays, the role of individual components of the complex, and the forces that hold the complex together. Thus, the combination of mutant phenotypes, created by mutagenesis or gene deletion, with the restoration of function via transfection, teaches us a great deal about detailed structure–function relationships in proteins important in immune system function.

2-38   The role of individual genes can be studied *in vivo* by transgenesis and gene knock-out.

Mice with extra copies or altered copies of a gene in their genome can be generated by **transgenesis**, which is now a well established procedure. There are various ways of introducing new DNA into the mouse genome. One way is by microinjection of a fertilized ovum. The required DNA is injected into the male pronucleus of a fertilized ovum, which is then implanted into the uterus of a pseudopregnant female mouse. In some of the eggs, the injected DNA becomes integrated randomly into the genome, giving rise to a mouse that has an extra genetic element of known structure, the **transgene** (Fig. 2.53). This technique allows one to study the impact of a new gene on development,

Fig. 2.53 The function and expression of genes can be studied *in vivo* using transgenic mice. DNA encoding a gene of interest, here the mouse MHC class II gene Eα, is purified and microinjected into the male pronucleus of fertilized ova or oocytes obtained from mice that lack Eα, which are then implanted into pseudo-pregnant female mice. The resulting offspring are screened for the presence of the transgene in their cells, and positive mice are used as founders that transmit the transgene to their offspring, establishing a line of transgenic mice that carry one or more extra genes. The function of the Eα gene used here is tested by breeding the transgene into C57BL/6 mice that lack an endogenous Eα gene.

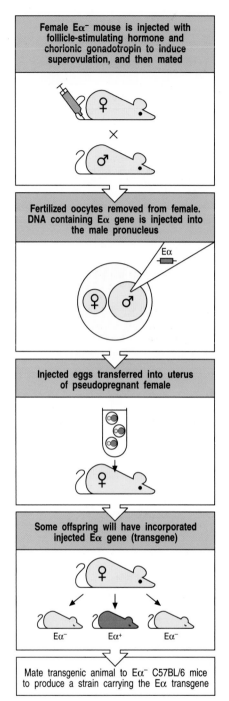

Female Eα⁻ mouse is injected with folllicle-stimulating hormone and chorionic gonadotropin to induce superovulation, and then mated

Fertilized oocytes removed from female. DNA containing Eα gene is injected into the male pronucleus

Injected eggs transferred into uterus of pseudopregnant female

Some offspring will have incorporated injected Eα gene (transgene)

Mate transgenic animal to Eα⁻ C57BL/6 mice to produce a strain carrying the Eα transgene

Related to Part V

to identify the regulatory regions of a gene required for its normal tissue-specific expression, to determine the effects of its overexpression or expression in inappropriate tissues, and to find out the impact of mutations on gene function. Transgenic mice have been particularly useful in studying the role of T-cell and B-cell receptors in lymphocyte development, as will be described in Chapters 5 and 6.

In many cases, the functions of a particular gene can only be fully understood if a mutant animal that does not express the gene can be obtained. While genes used to be discovered through identification of mutant phenotypes, it is now more common to discover and isolate the normal gene and then determine its function by replacing it *in vivo* with a defective copy, using the technique of homologous recombination followed by transgenesis (Fig. 2.54). This strategy is known as **gene knock-out**, and has been made possible by the development of continuously growing lines of pluripotent **embryonic stem cells (ES cells)**. These cells can be maintained in culture in an undifferentiated state but can give rise to all cell lineages when injected into a mouse blastocyst, which is then reimplanted into the uterus. To knock out a gene *in vivo*, embryonic stem cells in culture are first transfected with a copy of the gene that has been altered so that, when it recombines with the homologous cellular DNA, a mutation is created in the cellular gene The mutant cells are selected using essentially the same technique described in Section 2-37, except that only one copy of the cellular gene needs to be disrupted, as the first generation of heterozygous transgenic mice can be interbred to produce homozygous progeny.

When embryonic stem cells carrying the mutant gene are injected into the blastocyst, they become incorporated into the developing embryo, contributing to all tissues of the resulting chimeric offspring including the germline. The mutated gene can therefore be transmitted to some of the offspring of the original chimera, and further breeding of the mutant gene to homozygosity produces mice that completely lack the expression of that particular gene product. The effects of the absence of the gene's function can then be studied. In addition, the parts of the gene that are essential for its function can be identified by determining whether function can be restored by introducing a copy of the gene mutated in various ways into the genome by transgenesis. The manipulation of the mouse genome by gene knock-out and transgenesis is revolutionizing our understanding of the role of individual genes in lymphocyte development and function, as we shall see throughout this book.

A problem with gene knock-outs arises when the function of the gene is essential for the survival of the animal; in such cases, homozygous animals cannot be produced. However, means have been developed to allow the function of recessive lethal genes to be analyzed. In the case of immune system genes that are active in lymphocytes, it is sometimes possible to study the phenotype of lethal loss-of-function mutants by injecting the mutated ES cells in blastocysts of RAG-deficient mice (mice

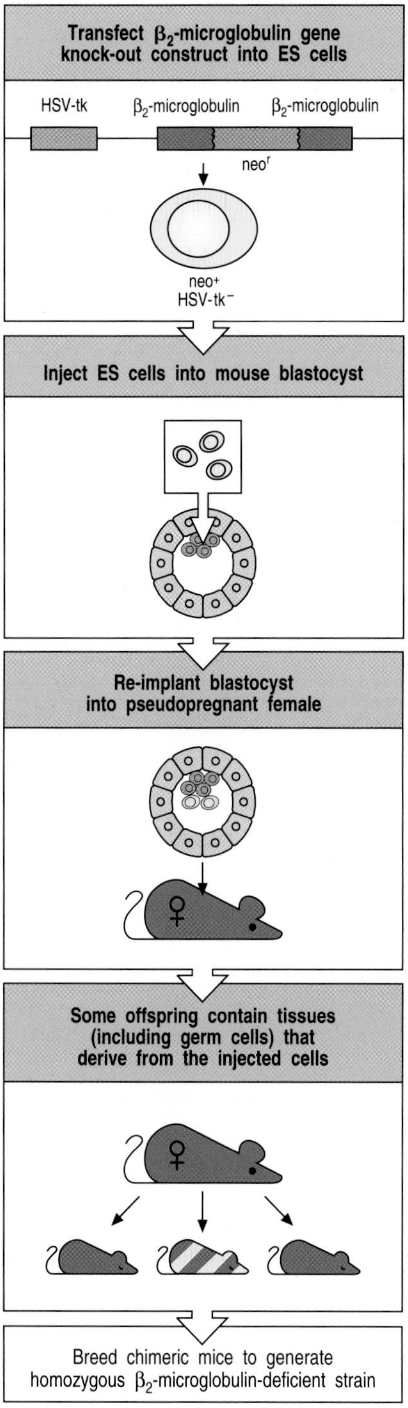

Transfect β$_2$-microglobulin gene knock-out construct into ES cells

HSV-tk   β$_2$-microglobulin   β$_2$-microglobulin

neo^r

neo$^+$
HSV-tk$^-$

Inject ES cells into mouse blastocyst

Re-implant blastocyst into pseudopregnant female

Some offspring contain tissues (including germ cells) that derive from the injected cells

Breed chimeric mice to generate homozygous β$_2$-microglobulin-deficient strain

Fig. 2.54 Gene knock-out in embryonic stem cells (ES cells) enables mutant mice to be produced. Specific genes can be deleted using homologous recombination in tissue cultures of cells known as embryonic stem cells because they can give rise to all cell lineages in a chimeric mouse. The technique of homologous recombination is carried out as described in Fig. 2.52. In this example, the gene for β$_2$-microglobulin is disrupted by homogous recombination of a targeting construct in ES cells. Only a single copy of the gene needs to be disrupted. ES cells in which homologous recombination has taken place are injected into mouse blastocysts. If the mutant ES cells give rise to germ cells in the resulting chimeric mice (striped in the figure), then the mutant gene can be transferred to their offspring. By breeding the mutant gene to homozygosity, a mutant phenotype is generated. In this case, the homozygous mutant mice lack MHC class I molecules on their cells, as MHC class I molecules have to pair with β$_2$-microglobulin for surface expression. The β$_2$-microglobulin-deficient mice can then be bred with mice transgenic for subtler mutants of the deleted gene, allowing the effect of such mutants to be tested *in vivo*.

lacking the ability to rearrange their antigen receptor genes), which themselves fail to make B or T cells. The RAG- cells can compensate for any developmental failure resulting from the gene knock-out in the ES cells. As long as the mutated ES cells can develop in hematopoietic progenitors in the bone marrow, all the lymphocytes in the resulting chimeric mouse will be derived from the ES cells (Fig. 2.55).

A second, and more powerful, technique makes use of the DNA sequences and enzymes used by bacteriophage P1 to excise itself from a host cell's genome. The integrated phage DNA is flanked by recombination signal sequences, called *loxP* sites. A recombinase, Cre, recognizes these sites, cuts the DNA and joins the two ends, thus excising the intervening DNA in the form of a circle. This mechanism can be adapted to allow the deletion of specific genes in a transgenic animal only in certain tissues or at certain times in development. First, *loxP* sites flanking a gene, or perhaps just a single exon, are introduced by homologous recombination (Fig. 2.56). Usually, the introduction of these sequences into flanking or intron DNA does not disrupt the normal function of the gene. Mice containing such *loxP* mutant genes are then mated with mice made transgenic for the Cre recombinase, under the control of a tissue-specific or inducible promoter. When the Cre recombinase is active, either in the appropriate tissue or when induced, it excises the DNA between the inserted *loxP* sites, thus inactivating the gene or exon. Thus, using a T-cell specific promoter to drive expression of the Cre recombinase, a gene can be deleted only in T cells, while remaining functional in all other cells of the animal. This is an extremely powerful genetic technique that is still in its infancy and is certain to yield exciting results in the future.

Summary.

Manipulation of the immune system *in vivo* reveals the need for each of its components. Using irradiation or mutation to eliminate lymphocytes or particular lymphocyte lineages, and then adoptively transferring mature lymphocytes, isolated subpopulations, cloned T-cell lines, or bone marrow stem cells allows one to study the functions and development of individual normal or immune cell types in an *in vivo* setting. The role of individual genes in lymphocyte development and function can be studied *in vivo* by manipulating the mouse genome, adding genes by transgenesis or eliminating them through gene knock-out. These two techniques can be combined to give detailed information

Fig. 2.55 The role of recessive lethal genes in lymphocyte function can be studied using RAG-deficient chimeric mice. Embryonic stem (ES) cells carrying the lethal mutation are injected into a RAG-deficient blastocyst (top panel). The RAG-deficient cells can give rise to all the tissues of a normal mouse except lymphocytes, and so can compensate for any deficiency in the developmental potential of the mutant ES cells (middle panel). If the mutant ES cells are capable of differentiating into hematopoietic stem cells, that is, if the gene function that has been deleted is not essential for this developmental pathway, then all the lymphocytes in the chimeric mouse will be derived from the ES cells (bottom panel), as RAG-deficient mice cannot make lymphocytes of their own.

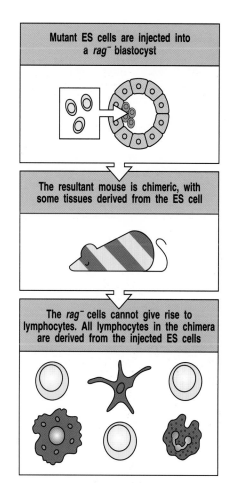

about structure–function relationships in genes and their protein products, either in cultured cells or *in vivo*. These powerful techniques are increasing our understanding of immunobiology at an astonishing rate. The use of mutant mice in the study of host defense should rapidly alter our understanding of these highly complex processes.

Summary to Chapter 2.

The immune system is very complex. To analyze it properly, it must be broken down into its individual components, which can then be assayed in isolation. In this chapter we have described how immune responses are induced and measured, and how the immune system can be manipulated experimentally. An appreciation of the methodologies and findings described in this chapter is essential for a full understanding of immunobiology, and many of the techniques included here are used routinely in the experiments described in subsequent chapters. Some, especially the use of monoclonal antibodies for identifying molecules in cells and tissues, also have general applications in biology.

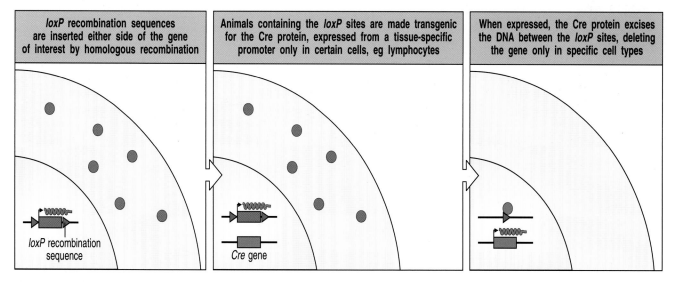

Fig. 2.56 The P1 bacteriophage recombination system can be used to eliminate genes in particular cell lineages. The P1 bacteriophage protein Cre will excise DNA that is bounded by recombination signal sequences called *loxP* sequences. These sequences can be introduced at either end of a gene by homologous recombination (left panel). Animals carrying *loxP*-flanked genes can also be made transgenic for the gene for the Cre protein, which is placed under the control of a tissue-specific promoter so that it is only expressed in certain cells or at certain times during development (middle panel). In the cells in which the Cre protein is expressed, it recognizes the *loxP* sequences and excises the DNA lying between them (right panel). Thus, individual genes can be deleted only in certain cell types or only at certain times. In this way, genes that are essential for the normal development of a mouse may be deleted from, for example, T cells, and the role of such genes in T-cell function studied.

General methods references.

Weir, D. (ed): *The Handbook of Experimental Immunology, vol 1.*, 5th edn. Oxford, Blackwell Scientific Publications, 1996.

Coligan, J.E.: *Current Protocols in Immunology*, 1st edn. New York, Greene Publishing Associates and Wiley Interscience, 1991. Continuous updates added.

Ausubel, M.: *Current Protocols in Molecular Biology*, 1st edn. New York, Greene Publishing Associates and Wiley Interscience, 1987. Continuous updates added.

Sambrook, J., Fritsch, E.F., Maniatis, T.: *Molecular Cloning: A Laboratory Manual*, 2nd edn. Cold Spring Harbor, NY, Cold Spring Harbor Laboratory Press, 1989.

Harlow, E. and Lane, D.: *Antibodies: a Laboratory Manual.* Cold Spring Harbor, NY, Cold Spring Harbor Laboratory Press, 1988.

Green, M.C. (ed): *Genetic Variant and Strains of the Laboratory Mouse*, 1st edn. New York, Gustav Fischer Verlag, 1981.

Rose, N.R., Conway de Macario, E., Fahey, J.L., Friedman, H., Penn, G.M. (eds): *Manual of Clinical Laboratory Immunology*, 4th edn. Washington DC, American Society of Microbiology, 1992.

Journals and Series:

Journal of Immunological Methods

Cytometry

Methods in Enzymology

PART II   THE RECOGNITION OF ANTIGEN

Structure of the Antibody Molecule and Immunoglobulin Genes

3

Antibodies are the antigen-specific products of B cells, and the production of antibody in response to infection is the main contribution of B cells to adaptive immunity. Antibodies were the first of the molecules that participate in specific immune recognition to be characterized and are still the best understood. Antibodies collectively form a family of plasma proteins known as the immunoglobulins, whose basic building block, the immunoglobulin fold or domain, is used in various forms in many molecules of both the immune system and other biological recognition systems.

The antibody molecule itself has two separable functions. One is to bind specifically to molecules from the pathogen that elicited the immune response; the other is to recruit other cells and molecules to destroy the pathogen once the antibody is bound to it. These functions are structurally separated in the antibody molecule, one part of which specifically recognizes antigen, while the other engages the effector mechanisms that will dispose of it. The antigen-binding region varies extensively between antibody molecules and is thus known as the **variable region** or **V region**. The variability of antibody molecules allows each molecule to recognize a particular antigen, and the sum total of all antibodies can bind to virtually any structure. The region of the antibody molecule that engages the effector functions of the immune system does not vary in the same way and is thus known as the **constant region** or **C region**, although it has in fact five main forms, or isotypes, which are specialized for activating different immune effector mechanism.

The remarkable diversity of antibody molecules is the consequence of a highly specialized mechanism by which the antibody genes expressed in any given cell are assembled by DNA rearrangements that join together two or three different gene segments to form a variable-region gene during the development of the B cell. Subsequent DNA rearrangement can attach the assembled variable-region gene to any constant-region gene and thus produce antibodies of any of the five isotypes.

B cells do not secrete antibody until they have been stimulated by specific antigen, which they recognize by means of membrane-bound immunoglobulin molecules, which serve as antigen receptors. Antigen binding to these surface receptors is a crucial step in inducing the B cell to proliferate and differentiate into an antibody-secreting cell.

In this chapter, we will describe the structural and functional properties of antibody molecules and explain the special genetic processes that generate antibody diversity and produce functional versatility, ending with an account of the mechanisms whereby antigen binding to surface immunoglobulin molecules on B cell transmits signals to the cell's interior.

The structure of a typical antibody molecule.

All antibodies are constructed in the same way from four polypeptide chains, and the generic term **immunoglobulin (Ig)** is used for all such proteins. Within this general class of immunoglobulins, however, five **classes** of antibodies — IgM, IgD, IgG, IgA, and IgE — can be distinguished biochemically as well as functionally, while more subtle differences confined to the variable region account for the specificity of antigen binding. In this section, we shall describe the general structural features of immunoglobulin molecules using the IgG molecule as an example. In later sections, the DNA rearrangements underlying antibody diversity and functional versatility will be described, once the basic features of the antibody molecule are understood.

3-1   IgG antibodies consist of four polypeptide chains.

IgG antibodies are large molecules with a molecular weight of approximately 150 kDa. When they are treated with agents that cleave disulfide bonds, two subunits can be distinguished. One, a polypeptide chain of approximately 50 kDa, is termed the **heavy** or **H chain**, and the other, of 25 kDa, is termed the **light** or **L chain** (Fig. 3.1). The two chains are present in an equimolar ratio, and each intact IgG molecule contains two heavy chains and two light chains [(2 x 50) + (2 x 25) = 150)]. The two heavy chains are linked to each other by disulfide bonds and each heavy chain is linked to a light chain by a disulfide bond. In any one immunoglobulin molecule, the two heavy chains and the two light chains are identical, so the molecule has a two-fold axis of symmetry.

There are only two types of light chain, which are termed lambda (λ) and kappa (κ) chains. No functional difference has been found between antibodies having λ or κ light chains. The ratio of the two types of light chain varies from species to species. In mice, the κ:λ ratio is 20:1, whereas in humans it is 2:1, and in cattle it is 1:20. It is likely that these differences reflect variation in the numbers of κ and λ V region genes in each species. Distortions in this ratio can sometimes be used to detect immune system abnormalities: for example, an excess of λ light chains in a human might indicate the presence of a λ chain-producing B-cell tumor.

By contrast, there are five main **heavy-chain classes** or **isotypes,** and these determine the functional activity of an antibody molecule. The five functional classes of immunoglobulin are **immunoglobulin M (IgM), immunoglobulin D (IgD), immunoglobulin G (IgG), immunoglobulin A (IgA)**, and **immunoglobulin E (IgE)**, and their heavy chains are denoted by the corresponding lower case Greek letter (μ, δ, γ, α, and ϵ, respectively). Each isotype has a particular function in immune responses and their distinctive functional properties are conferred by the carboxy-terminal part of the heavy chain, where it is not associated with the light chain. These carboxy-terminal regions differ in their detailed structure from isotype to isotype. We shall describe the distinct heavy-chain isotypes in more detail later. IgG is the most abundant immunoglobulin isotype in blood plasma, being produced at high levels in both primary and secondary immune responses. As the general structural characteristics of all the isotypes are similar, we shall therefore describe the structure of IgG here as a typical antibody molecule.

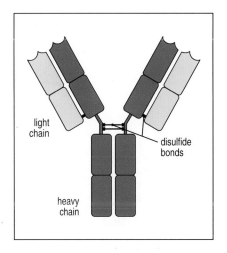

Fig. 3.1 The immunoglobulin molecule has two different polypeptide chains called the heavy chain and the light chain. Each immunoglobulin molecule is made up of two heavy chains (green) and two light chains (yellow) joined by disulfide bridges such that each heavy chain is linked to a light chain and the two heavy chains are linked together.

| 3-2 | **The heavy and light chains are composed of constant and variable regions.** |

The amino acid sequences of many immunoglobulin heavy and light chains have been determined and show that each chain contains distinct sequence domains, each about 110 amino acids in length. The light chains have two domains, while the heavy chain of the IgG antibody has four. All the domains have similarities in amino acid sequence, suggesting that the immunoglobulin chains have evolved by repeated duplication of an ancestral gene corresponding to one domain. As we shall see, these sequence-defined domains correspond to separate structural domains in the folded protein.

Comparison of amino acid sequences of individual antibody molecules reveals that the amino-terminal sequences of both the heavy and light chains vary greatly between different antibodies. The variability in sequence is limited to the first 110 amino acids, corresponding to the first domain, while the carboxy-terminal sequences are constant between immunoglobulin chains, either light or heavy, of the same isotype (Fig. 3.2). The variable domains (**V domains**) make up the variable regions of the antibody, and the constant domains (**C domains**) make up the constant region.

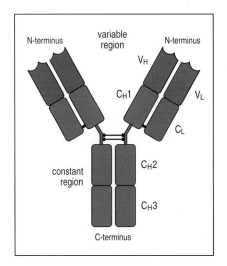

Fig. 3.2 The heavy and light chains of an immunoglobulin can be divided into domains on the basis of sequence similarity. The amino-terminal domain (N-terminus; red) of each chain is variable in sequence when several antibodies are compared; the remaining domains are constant (blue). The two domains of the light chains are termed V_L and C_L. IgG has four domains in the heavy chain, which are termed V_H, C_H1, C_H2, and C_H3.

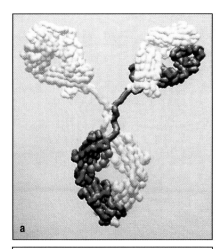

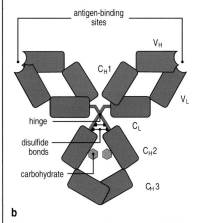

Fig. 3.3 Structure of the antibody molecule. Panel a : A model of an IgG antibody based on structures determined by X-ray crystallography. Light chains are white; the two heavy chains are pink and red, respectively. Carbohydrate side chains are blue and gray. Panel b: Schematic representation of antibody structure showing the different domains and how they interact. The antigen-binding site is formed from the V_L and V_H domains. Panel a courtesy of R S H Pumphrey.

3-3 | **The structure of the antibody molecule has been determined by X-ray crystallography.**

The structure of the antibody molecule has been determined by electron microscopy and X-ray crystallography and is shown in Fig. 3.3 (panel a). The molecule comprises three equal-sized globular portions joined by a flexible stretch of polypeptide chain known as the **hinge region**; the overall shape is roughly that of a Y. Each arm of the Y is formed by the association of a light chain with the amino-terminal half of a heavy chain, while the leg of the Y is formed by the pairing of the carboxy-terminal halves of the two heavy chains. Each of the chains is folded into separate structural domains that correspond to the domains identified by amino acid sequencing. The association of the heavy and light chains is such that the V_H and V_L domains are paired, as are the C_H1 and C_L domains. The two C_H3 domains pair with each other but the C_H2 domains do not interact; carbohydrate side chains attached to the C_H2 domains lie between the two heavy chains. The two antigen-binding sites of the IgG antibody are formed by the paired V_H and V_L domains at the end of the two arms of the Y (Fig. 3.3, panel b).

Proteolytic enzymes (proteases) that cleave polypeptide sequences at particular amino acids have been used to probe the structure of antibody molecules. Limited digestion with the protease papain cleaves antibody molecules into three fragments (Fig. 3.4). Two fragments are identical and contain the antigen-binding activity, and these are termed the **Fab fragments**, for Fragment antigen binding. The other fragment contains no antigen-binding activity but was originally observed to crystallize readily, and for this reason was named the **Fc fragment**, for Fragment crystallizable. The Fab fragments correspond to the arms of the antibody molecule that contain the complete light chains paired with the V_H and C_H1 domains of the heavy chains, whereas the Fc fragment corresponds to the paired C_H2 and C_H3 domains. The disulfide bridges between the heavy chains lie in a hinge region between the C_H1 and C_H2 domains. As illustrated in Fig. 3.4, papain cleaves the antibody molecule on the amino-terminal side of the disulfide bridges, releasing the two arms of the antibody as separate Fab fragments, while the carboxy-terminal halves of the heavy chains remain linked, forming the Fc fragment. Another protease, pepsin, cleaves in the same region of the antibody molecule but on the carboxy-terminal side of the disulfide bridges (see Fig. 3.4), producing a fragment, the F(ab')2 fragment, in which the two arms of the antibody molecule remain linked. These can easily be reduced to form Fab' fragments.

Electron microscopy of antibody complexes with a bivalent hapten capable of crosslinking two antigen-binding sites demonstrates that the hinge region is flexible and that the angle between the two Fab arms can vary (Fig. 3.5). Such flexibility is required to allow the binding of both arms of the antibody molecule to sites that are different distances apart, for instance with sites on bacterial cell wall polysaccharides. It is thought that flexibility of the hinge is also required for the interaction of antibodies with the antibody-binding proteins that mediate immune effector mechanisms, as will be described in Chapter 8. Some flexibility is also found at the junction between the V and C domains, allowing bending and rotation of the V domain relative to the C domain. This range of motion has led to the junction between the two domains being referred to as a 'molecular ball and socket joint'.

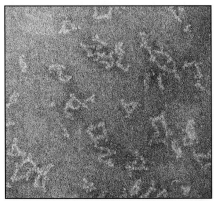

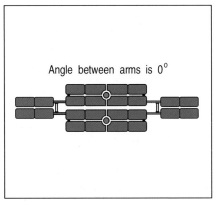

Fig. 3.4 The Y-shaped immunoglobulin molecule can be dissected by partial digestion with proteases. Papain cleaves the immunoglobulin molecule into three pieces, two Fab fragments and one Fc fragment (upper panels). Pepsin cleaves an immunoglobulin to yield one $F(ab')_2$ fragment and many small pieces of the Fc fragment, the largest of which is called the pFc' fragment (lower panels).

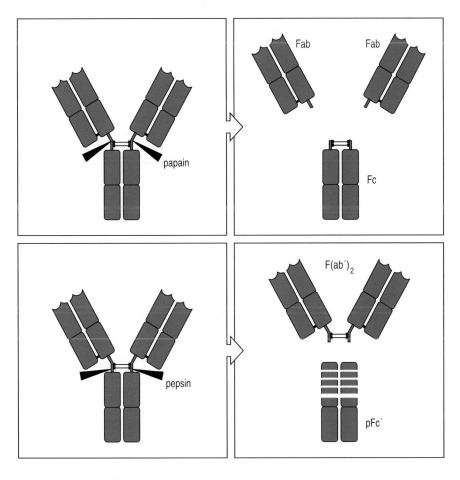

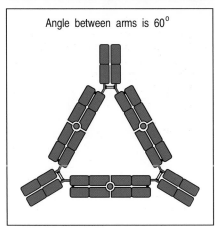

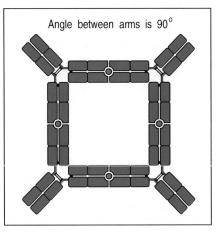

Fig. 3.5 Antibody arms are joined by a flexible hinge. The overall shape of antibodies and the flexibility of the hinge can be seen in the electron micrograph of antibody complexes. A small bifunctional hapten, depicted as a red ball, capable of crosslinking two antigen-binding sites, is used to create antigen:antibody complexes. The complexes can be seen to form linear, triangular and square forms, with short projections or spikes. Limited pepsin digestion removes these spikes, which therefore correspond to the Fc portion of the antibody; the $F(ab')_2$ pieces remain crosslinked by antigen. The interpretation of the complexes is shown in the remaining three panels. The angle between the arms of the antibody molecule varies from 0° in the antibody dimers to 60° in the triangular forms, showing that the connections between the arms in the connection between the arms is flexible. Photograph (x 300 000) courtesy of N M Green.

| 3-4 | **Each domain of an immunoglobulin molecule has a similar structure.** |

The discrete globular domains into which immunoglobulin chains fold fall into two distinct structural classes, corresponding to the domains of the variable and the constant regions, each of about 110 amino acids. The similarities and differences between these two domains can be seen in the diagram of a light chain in Fig. 3.6. The basic structure of an **immunoglobulin domain** consists of two layers of polypeptide chain, linked by a disulfide bridge, that pack together to form a roughly cylindrical shape. Each layer is formed from a number of stretches of polypeptide chain that have a conformation known as a **β strand**. For this reason the layers are termed **β sheets**. The order of the β strands in each sheet is characteristic of immunoglobulin domains, as is the disulfide bond that links the central β strands of each sheet. This characteristic three-dimensional structure is known as the **immunoglobulin fold**. Both the essential similarity of the V and C domains and the critical difference between them are most clearly seen in the bottom panels of Fig. 3.6,

Fig. 3.6 The structure of immunoglobulin variable and constant domains. The upper panels show the folding pattern of the variable and constant domains of an immunoglobulin light chain. Each domain is a globular structure in which a number of strands of polypeptide chain come together to form two antiparallel β sheets that are held together by a disulfide bond. The strands in each sheet are shown in separate colors in the folded structure but their arrangement can be seen more clearly when the sheets are opened out, as shown in the lower panels. The β strands are lettered sequentially with respect to their occurrence in the amino acid sequence of the domains; the order in each β sheet is characteristic of immunoglobulin domains. The β strands found in the variable domains but not in the constant domains are indicated by the shaded background.

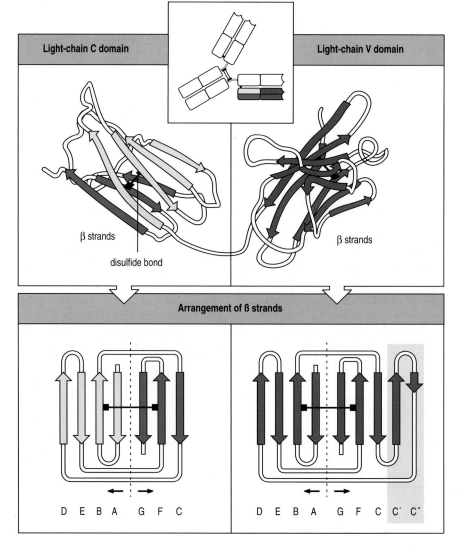

where the cylindrical domains are opened out to reveal the individual β strands that make up each β sheet. The main difference between the V and C domain structures is that the V domain has two more β strands than the C domain, forming an extra loop of polypeptide chain.

Many of the amino acids that are common to all the domains of the heavy and light chains lie in the core of the immunoglobulin fold and are critical to the stability of the structure, including an invariant trypto-phan. For that reason, other proteins having sequences homologous to those of immunoglobulins are believed to have domains with a similar structure. These immunoglobulin domains are found in many proteins of the immune and nervous systems, as well as in other proteins thought to be involved in cell–cell recognition.

| 3-5 | **Localized regions of hypervariable sequence form the antigen-binding site.** |

Sequence variability is not distributed evenly throughout the variable regions. Many amino acids are conserved, particularly those important in determining the structure of the V domain. The distribution of vari-able residues can be seen clearly using what is termed a **variability** or **Wu and Kabat plot** (Fig. 3.7), where the sequences of many different antibody variable regions are compared. Three regions of particular variability can be identified, roughly from residues 28 to 35, from 49 to 59 and from 92 to 103. These were designated **hypervariable regions** and are denoted HV1, HV2, and HV3. The most variable part of the domain is in the HV3 region. The rest of the V domain shows less variability, and the segments between the hypervariable regions, which are relatively invariant, are termed the **framework regions**. There are four such regions, designated FR1, FR2, FR3, and FR4.

The framework regions form the β sheets that provide the structural framework of the domain, with the hypervariable sequences corre-sponding to three loops at one edge of each sheet that are juxtaposed in the folded protein (Fig. 3.8). Thus, not only is sequence diversity focused on particular parts of the variable regions but it is localized to a particular part of the surface of the molecule. Moreover, when the V_H and V_L domains pair in the antibody molecule, the hypervariable loops from each domain are brought together, creating a single hypervariable site at the tip of the Fab fragment, which forms the binding site for anti-gens — the **antigen-binding site**. As the three hypervariable loops constitute the binding site for antigen and determine specificity by form-ing a surface complementary to the antigen, they are more commonly termed the **complementarity determining regions,** or **CDRs,** and denoted **CDR1, CDR2** and **CDR3.** One consequence of the contribu-tion of CDRs from both V_H and V_L domains to the antigen-binding site is that it is the combination of the heavy and the light chain that deter-mines the final antigen specificity. Thus, one way in which the immune system is able to generate antibodies of different specificities is by generating different combinations of heavy- and light-chain variable re-gions. This means of producing variability is known as **combinatorial diversity**; we will encounter a second form of combinatorial diver-sity when we come to consider how the genes encoding the heavy and light chain V regions are created from smaller segments of DNA (see Section 3.11).

Because it is the CDRs that determine the specificity of an antibody, it is possible to manipulate the antigen specificity of an antibody molecule

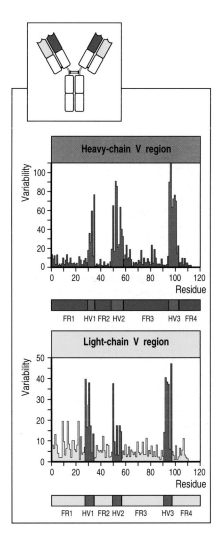

Fig. 3.7 There are discrete regions of hypervariability in variable domains. The degree of variability is the ratio of the number of different amino acids and the frequency of the most common amino acid and is shown for each amino acid position in the variable region of the heavy and light chains. Three hyper-variable regions (HV1, HV2, and HV3) can be discerned (red), flanked by less variable framework regions (FR1, FR2, FR3, and FR4).

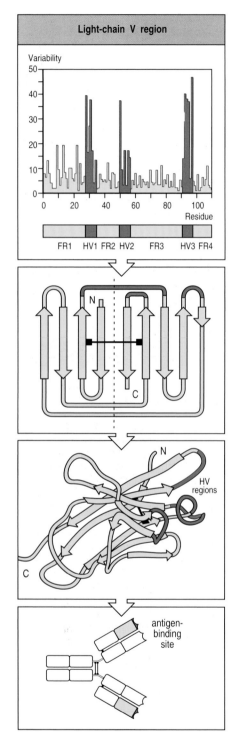

Light-chain V region

Variability

FR1   HV1 FR2 HV2   FR3   HV3 FR4

N

C

N

HV
regions

C

antigen-
binding
site

Fig. 3.8 The hypervariable regions lie in discrete loops of the folded structure.
When the positions of the hypervariable regions are plotted on the structure of a variable domain it can be seen that they lie in loops that are brought together in the folded structure. In the antibody molecule, the pairing of the heavy and light chains brings together the hypervariable loops from each chain to create a single hypervariable surface, which forms the antigen-binding site at each tip of the Fab arms.

solely by replacing the CDRs using genetic engineering. This is of particular value in the case of mouse monoclonal antibodies used clinically in transplantation or cancer therapy (see Chapter 12).

Summary.

IgG antibodies are made up of four polypeptide chains, comprising two identical light chains and two identical heavy chains and can be thought of as forming a flexible Y-shaped structure. Each of the four chains has a variable region at its amino terminus that contributes to the antigen-binding site, and a constant region, which, in the case of the heavy chain, determines isotype and hence the functional properties of the antibody. The light chains are bonded to the heavy chains with disulfide links and the variable regions of the heavy and light chains pair to generate two identical antigen-binding sites, which lie at the tips of the arms of the Y. This allows antibody molecules to crosslink antigens. The leg of the Y, or Fc fragment, is composed of the two carboxy-terminal domains of the two heavy chains. Joining the arms of the Y to the leg are the flexible hinge regions. The amino-terminal domains of each antibody chain have different sequences in antibodies with different specificities, with three distinct regions of hypervariability in each chain. These complementarity determining regions (CDRs) of the heavy and light chains are juxtaposed to create the antigen-binding site at the tip of the Fab fragment. The Fc fragment and hinge regions differ in antibodies of different isotypes, determining their functional properties. However, the overall plan of all isotypes is similar.

The interaction of the antibody molecule with specific antigen.

In the previous section we described the structure of the antibody molecule and how the variable regions of heavy and light chains fold and pair to form the antigen-binding site. In this section we will discuss the different ways in which antigens can bind to antibody and will address the question of how variation in the sequences of the antibody complementarity-determining loops influences the specificity for antigen.

3-6   Small molecules bind between the heavy- and light-chain variable domains.

In the early investigations of antigen binding, the only available sources of single species of antibody molecules were tumors of antibody-secreting cells, which produce homogeneous antibody molecules. The specificities of the tumor-derived antibodies were unknown, so that large numbers of compounds had to be screened to identify ligands that could be used in the analysis of antigen binding. In general, the substances found to bind to the antibodies were small chemical compounds, or haptens, such as phosphorylcholine or vitamin K1. Structural analysis of antigen:antibody complexes between antibodies and their hapten ligands provided the first direct evidence that the hypervariable regions form the antigen-binding site, and established the structural basis for antigen specificity. The antigens were found to lie in a cleft formed by the interface between the heavy- and light-chain variable domains. The sides of the cleft, which provide the amino acids that interact with the antigen and thereby determine the specificity of the antibody, are formed by the CDRs of the heavy and light chains. For these small antigens, not all of the CDRs contribute to antigen binding in any one antibody. Where the antibody is bound to phosphorylcholine, the light-chain variable region contributes only CDR3 to the binding site, whereas all three CDRs of the heavy-chain variable region are involved.

This mode of binding also seems to apply to antibodies binding carbohydrate antigens. Antibodies binding polysaccharides can be classified as **end-binders** or **middle-binders** depending on whether they bind to one end of the polysaccharide chain or to a stretch of sugar units, usually six, in the middle of the chain. The two types of antibodies are thought to represent either those with a deep pocket to bind one end of the molecule, or those with a longer and shallower cleft in which the polysaccharide chain lies lengthwise.

Antibodies can bind peptides in the same way (Fig. 3.9). In the case of a monoclonal antibody binding a synthetic peptide of 19 amino acids, seven amino acids of the peptide are bound into a cleft created by the three heavy-chain CDRs and the CDR1 and CDR3 of the light chain. In a second example, where the ligand is a short stretch of peptide from the HIV gp120 molecule, the peptide is seen to lie along an open-ended groove formed between the V_H and V_L domains (Fig. 3.9, panel b). More extensive contacts, however, are made by antibodies binding intact proteins, as we shall see shortly; in these cases there may be no discrete pocket or cleft. Even for some small molecules it may be difficult to define a discrete pocket or cleft; in the case of an antibody specific for a steroid molecule, the steroid fits into a shallow depression formed by both the heavy and light chain.

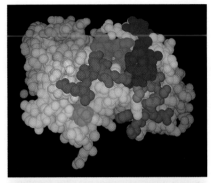

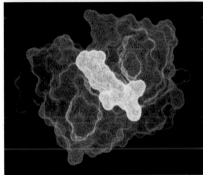

Fig. 3.9 Peptide antigen in pocket- and cleft-type binding sites of antibody Fab fragments. Top panel: Space-filling representation of the interaction of a peptide antigen with the complementarity-determining regions (CDRs) of the Fab fragment as viewed looking into the antigen-binding site. Seven amino acid residues of the antigen, shown in red, are bound in the antigen-binding pocket. Five of the six CDRs (H1, H2, H3, L1, and L3) interact with the peptide, whereas L2 does not make contact with the peptide. The CDR loops are colored as follows: L1, dark blue; L2, magenta; L3, green; H1, cyan; H2, pale magenta; H3, yellow. Bottom panel: In a complex of an antibody with a peptide from the human immuno- deficiency virus, the peptide (yellow) binds along a cleft formed between the heavy- and light-chain variable domains (green). Photographs courtesy of I A Wilson and R L Stanfield.

| 3-7 | Antibodies bind to sites on the surfaces of native protein antigens. |

The biological function of antibodies is to bind to pathogens and their products and facilitate their removal from the body. Although some of the most important pathogens have polysaccharide coats, in many cases the antigens that provoke an immune response are proteins. For example, protective antibodies against viruses recognize viral coat proteins. In such cases, the antibody binds to the native conformation of the protein and the determinants recognized are therefore areas on the surface of proteins (Fig. 3.10). Regions of a molecule that are specifically recognized by antibodies are called **antigenic determinants** or **epitopes**. Such sites on protein surfaces are likely to be composed of amino acids from different parts of the sequence that have been brought together by protein folding. Epitopes of this kind are known as **conformational** or **discontinuous epitopes**, since the site is composed of segments of the protein that are discontinuous in the primary sequence but are contiguous in the three-dimensional structure (Fig. 3.10). In contrast, an epitope composed of a single segment of polypeptide chain is termed a **continuous** or **linear epitope**. Antibodies raised against native

Fig. 3.10 Antibodies bind to the surface of proteins. Known antibody-binding sites are shown on the surface of a polio virus as white patches. At the bottom of the figure are the viral coat proteins VP1 (blue), VP2 (yellow) and VP3 (red). The antigenic sites on each of these proteins are shown in white. In the whole virus, the three proteins come together to create a pentameric structure, shown on the upper left, which is then used to build the complete icosahedral virus (upper right). Not only are the individual antigenic sites located on the surface of each coat protein but, as can be seen from the pentameric subunit and the whole virus, the antigenic sites also lie on the outer surface of the viral particle. Photograph courtesy of D Filman and J M Hogle.

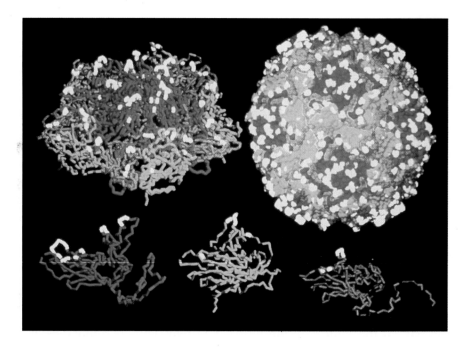

proteins usually recognize discontinuous epitopes, but some can be found to bind peptide fragments of the protein. Conversely, antibodies raised against peptide fragments of a protein or synthetic peptides corresponding to part of its sequence are occasionally found to bind to the native protein. This makes it possible, in some cases, to use synthetic peptides in vaccines aimed at raising antibodies against an intact protein of a pathogen. We shall discuss the design of such vaccines in Section 12-15.

| 3-8 | **The interaction of antibody with protein antigens occurs over a surface involving most or all CDRs.** |

Antibodies binding to native protein antigens make contacts with a larger area of the protein than can be accommodated within a cleft

Fig. 3.11 Antibody binding to protein antigens involves contact between two extended surfaces. In the structure of a complex between hen egg-white lysozyme and the Fab fragment of an antibody to lysozyme, HyHel5, the two surfaces that come into contact are complementary, as can be seen from this computer-generated image, where the surface contour of the lysozyme molecule (yellow dots) is superimposed on the antigen-binding site of the antibody. Residues in the antibody that make contact with lysozyme are shown in full (red) while for the rest of the Fab fragment only the peptide backbone is shown (blue). All six CDRs of the antibody are involved in the binding. Photograph courtesy of S Sherriff.

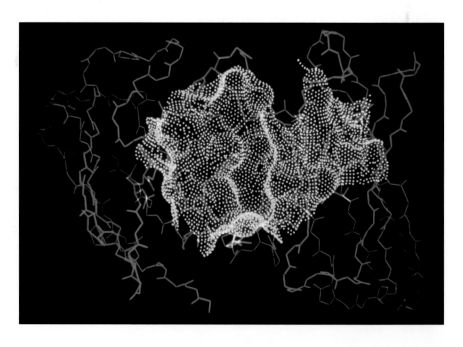

between the V_H and V_L domains. The detailed molecular interactions between antibody and protein antigens have also been studied by the X-ray crystallographic analysis of antibody complexes with protein antigens such as lysozyme (Fig. 3.11) or the influenza virus neuraminidase. Antibodies that bind protein antigens often have no groove between the two variable domains, and the interaction of antibody with antigen extends over the surface of the antibody in the region of the hypervariable loops. Several complexes between antibody Fab fragments and native protein antigens have been analyzed and the surface area involved has been relatively constant, at about 700–900 Å^2, involving most or all of the six CDRs. In some cases, residues lying outside of the hypervariable loops can also contribute to binding.

| 3-9 | **Antigen:antibody interactions involve a variety of forces.** |

The interaction between an antibody and its antigen can be disrupted by high salt concentrations, extremes of pH, and detergents. The binding is therefore a non-covalent interaction. The forces, or bonds, involved in non-covalent interactions are outlined in Fig. 3.12. All are used, to a greater or lesser extent, by antibodies.

Non-covalent forces	Origin	
Electrostatic forces	Attraction between opposite charges	$-NH_3^{\oplus}$ $^{\ominus}OOC-$
Hydrogen bonds	Hydrogen shared between electronegative atoms (N,O)	$-N-H--O=C$ δ^- δ^+ δ^-
Van der Waals forces	Fluctuations in electron clouds around molecules oppositely polarize neighboring atoms	
Hydrophobic forces	Hydrophobic groups interact unfavorably with water and tend to pack together to exclude water molecules. The attraction also involves van der Waals forces	

Fig. 3.12 The non-covalent forces that hold together the antigen–antibody complex. Partial charges found in electric dipoles are shown as δ^+ or δ^-.

The non-covalent forces in antigen:antibody binding mostly, but not always, involve electrostatic interactions, either between charged amino acid side chains as in salt bridges, or between electric dipoles as in hydrogen bonds and van der Waals forces. High salt concentrations and extremes of pH will weaken electrostatic interactions; hence they can disrupt antigen:antibody binding.

Hydrophobic interactions occur when two hydrophobic surfaces come together to exclude water. The strength of hydrophobic interactions is proportional to the surface area that is hidden from water. Thus for very small antigens, the buried surface area may be small and most of the binding energy usually comes from electrostatic interactions and hydrogen bonds. For large antigens, such as native proteins, the surface area buried can account for over half of the binding energy.

The importance of each of the forces to the interaction between antigen and antibody will depend on the specific antibody and antigen involved.

A striking difference from other protein–protein interactions is that anti-bodies possess many aromatic residues in their antigen-binding sites, which participate in many van der Waals and hydrophobic interactions, as well as sometimes forming hydrogen bonds. In general terms, the hydrophobic and van der Waals forces relate to the interaction of two surfaces that must be complementary for good binding to occur; hills on one surface must fit into valleys on the other. On the other hand, the electrostatic and hydrogen-bonding interactions relate to specific features that must interact over and above the general surface complementarity. For example, in the complex of hen egg-white lysozyme with the antibody D1.3, strong hydrogen bonds are formed between the antibody and a specific glutamine residue in the lysozyme molecule that protrudes between the V_H and V_L domains (Fig. 3.13). Lysozymes from partridge and turkey have another amino acid in place of the glutamine and do not bind to the antibody. In the complex of hen egg-white lysozyme with another antibody, HyHel5 (see Fig. 3.11), important inter-actions are two salt bridges formed between two arginine residues from the lysozyme interacting with two glutamic acid residues, one each from the V_H CDR1 and CDR2 loops. Again, lysozymes from different avian species lack one of the two arginine residues, resulting in a 1000-fold decrease in affinity. Thus, overall surface complementarity, together with specific electrostatic and hydrophobic interactions, appear to be the determining features of antibody specificity.

Fig. 3.13 The complex of lysozyme with the antibody D1.3. The interaction of the Fab fragment of D1.3 with hen egg-white lysozyme is shown, with the lysozyme in green, the heavy chain in blue and the light chain in yellow. A glutamine residue of lysozyme, shown in red, protrudes between the two variable domains of the antigen-binding site and makes hydrogen bonds important to the antigen:antibody binding. Photograph courtesy of R J Poljak.

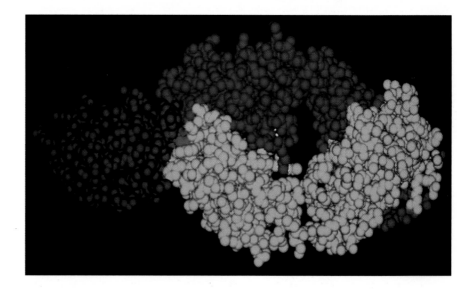

Summary.

X-ray crystallographic analysis of antigen:antibody complexes has dem-onstrated that the hypervariable loops of immunoglobulin variable regions determine the specificity of antibodies; in the case of protein antigens, the antibody molecule contacts the antigen over a broad area of its surface that is complementary to the surface recognized on the antigen. Electrostatic interactions, hydrogen bonds, and van der Waals forces can all contribute to binding. Amino acid side chains in most or all of the hypervariable loops make contact with antigen and determine both the specificity and the affinity of the interaction. Other parts of the variable region play little role in direct contact with the antigen but pro-vide a stable structural framework for the hypervariable loops and help determine their positioning. Antibodies raised against native proteins usually bind to the surface of the protein and make contact with resi-dues that are discontinuous in the primary structure of the molecule but they may occasionally bind peptide fragments of the protein, while antibodies raised against peptides derived from a protein can sometimes be used to detect the native protein molecule. Peptides binding to antibodies usually bind in the cleft between the variable regions of the heavy and light chains, where they make specific contact with some, but not necessarily all, of the hypervariable loops. This is also the usual mode of binding carbohydrate antigens and small molecules, or haptens.

The generation of diversity in the humoral immune response.

Virtually any substance can elicit an antibody response. Furthermore, the response even to a simple antigen is diverse, comprising many different antibody molecules each with a unique affinity and fine specificity. The complete collection of antibody specificities available within an individual is known as the antibody repertoire and in humans consists of as many as 10^{11} different antibody molecules. Before it was posssible to examine the immunoglobulin genes directly, there were two main hypotheses for the origin of this diversity. According to one, the **germline theory**, there is a separate gene for each antibody molecule and the antibody repertoire is largely inherited. By contrast, **somatic mutation theories** were based on the idea that a limited number of inherited antibody genes undergo mutation in B cells during the lifetime of an individual to generate the observed repertoire. The cloning of the genes that encode immunoglobulins showed that the antibody repertoire is, in fact, generated from a relatively small group of variable-region sequences at each locus by DNA rearrangement, and that diversity is further enhanced by a process of somatic hypermutation in B cells. Thus, both theories explain part of antibody diversity.

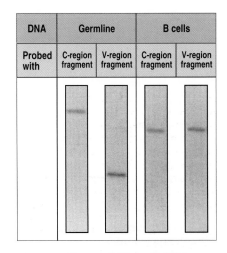

DNA	Germline		B cells	
Probed with	C-region fragment	V-region fragment	C-region fragment	V-region fragment

Fig. 3.14 **The arrangement of the immunoglobulin genes is not the same in B cells as it is in other cells of the body.** The left two photographs ('germline') show agarose gel electrophoresis of a restriction enzyme digest of DNA from peripheral blood granulocytes of a normal person. The location of immunoglobulin DNA sequences are identified by hybridization with V- and C-region probes. The V and C regions are found in quite separate DNA fragments. The right two photographs ('B cells') are of a similar restriction digest of DNA from peripheral blood lymphocytes from a patient with chronic lymphatic leukemia (see Chapter 5), in which a particular clone of B cells is greatly expanded. For this reason, a unique rearrangement is visible. Normal B lymphocytes have many millions of rearranged genes, so they yield only a smear of DNA, normally not visible as a band. In this DNA, the V and C regions are found in the same fragment. Photograph courtesy of S Wagner and L Luzzatto.

3-10	Immunoglobulin genes are rearranged in antibody-producing cells.

The DNA sequences encoding the variable and constant regions of immunoglobulin chains are separated by a great distance in all the cells of the body except for lymphocytes of the B lineage. This was originally discovered 20 years ago in the mouse when it first became possible to study the arrangement of the antibody genes in the chromosomes using restriction enzyme analysis. After cutting DNA with a restriction enzyme, DNA fragments containing V- and C-region sequences were detected by hybridization with two radiolabeled mRNA probes, one of which contained a λ light-chain V sequence and the other the C sequence only. It was found that the location of V- and C-region sequences relative to each other was quite different in germline DNA and in B cells. In the germ line, represented by whole mouse embryo DNA, the V- and C-region sequences were on separate DNA fragments. Owing to the size of the fragments, which were each much larger than the total length of the antibody mRNA, the V and C sequences must have been located some distance apart in the genome. However, in the B cells, represented by a mouse B-cell tumor (a plasmacytoma) from which the mRNA probes had been isolated, both probes hybridized to a single DNA fragment, showing that the V- and C-region sequences were now close together in the DNA. A modern presentation of a similar experiment using human DNA is shown in Fig. 3.14.

This simple experiment first proved that genomic DNA had become rearranged in somatic cells of the B lymphocyte lineage. The process by which the rearrangement occurs is known as **somatic recombination**, to distinguish it from the meiotic recombination that takes place during the production of gametes. Recombination of immunoglobulin genes is a prerequisite for their expression; expressed genes are always **rearranged**, whereas the same genes in tissues not expressing immunoglobulins are in the **germline configuration**.

| 3-11 | Complete variable regions are generated by the somatic recombination of separate gene segments. |

Detailed analysis of rearranged and germline genes for immunoglobulin light chains revealed that each variable domain is encoded in two separate segments of DNA that are brought together in B cells by DNA rearrangement. The first segment encodes the first 95–101 amino acids of the light chain; since this makes up most of the variable domain it is termed a **V gene segment**. A second segment of DNA encodes the remainder of the variable domain (up to 13 amino acids) and is termed a **joining** or **J gene segment**.

The process of rearrangement that leads to the production of an immunoglobulin light-chain gene is shown in Fig. 3.15. The joining of a V and a J gene segment creates a contiguous piece of DNA encoding the whole of the light-chain variable region. The J gene segments are located close to the constant region (C) gene segments, to which they are joined by RNA splicing after transcription, and not by DNA recombination. In the experiment shown in Fig. 3.14 therefore, the germline DNA identified by the 'V-region fragment' contains the V gene segment, and that identified by the 'C-region fragment' actually contains the J and C gene segments.

Fig. 3.15 Light-chain variable regions are constructed from two gene segments. A complete light-chain variable-region gene is constructed by somatic recombination of a variable (V) and a joining (J) gene segment. The constant region is encoded in a separate exon and is joined to the variable-region gene by RNA splicing of the light-chain gene RNA transcript. Immunoglobulin chains are extracellular proteins and the V gene segment is preceded by an exon encoding a leader peptide (L), which directs the protein into the cell's secretory pathways and is then cleaved.

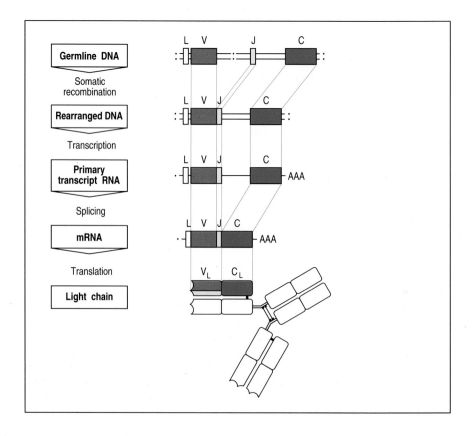

The heavy-chain variable regions are encoded in three gene segments. In addition to the V and J gene segments (denoted V_H and J_H to distinguish them from the light-chain gene segments), a third gene segment called the **diversity** or **D gene segment** lies between the V_H and J_H gene segments. The process of recombination that generates a complete heavy-chain variable region is shown in Fig. 3.16 and occurs in two separate stages. In the first, a D gene segment is joined to a V_H gene segment; this is followed by the rearrangement of a V_H gene segment to DJ_H to complete the variable-region coding region. As with the light chains, the variable-region coding sequence is joined to the constant-region coding sequence by RNA splicing.

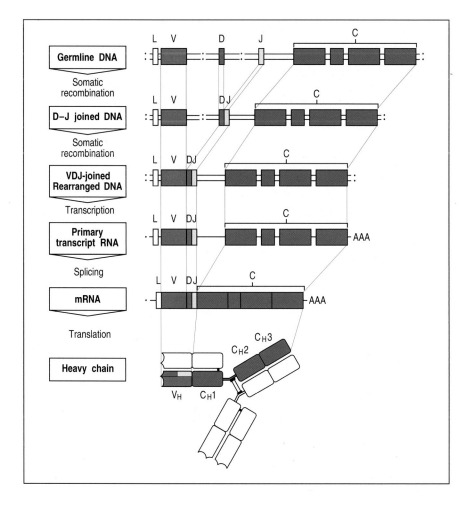

Fig. 3.16 Heavy-chain variable regions are constructed from three gene segments. A complete heavy-chain variable-region gene is constructed by somatic recombination that first joins the diversity (D) and J gene segments, then joins the V gene segment to the combined DJ sequence. The heavy-chain constant-region sequences are encoded in several exons and, together with the leader (L) sequence, are spliced to the variable domain sequence during processing of the heavy-chain gene RNA transcript.

3-12 Variable-region gene segments are present in multiple copies.

For simplicity, we have discussed the formation of a complete immunoglobulin variable-region genes as though there were only single copies of each gene segment. In fact, there are multiple copies of all of the gene segments in germline DNA. The number of the gene segments in humans has been determined by gene cloning and sequencing. Some of these are expressed and some are pseudogenes. The number of functional segments of each type is given in Fig. 3.17. The precise number of functional segments in each person can differ due to the presence or absence of particular segments (known as insertion/deletion polymorphism) or to changes that transform a functional gene into a pseudogene (allelic polymorphism).

Number of segments in human immunoglobulin genes			
Segment	**Light chains**		**Heavy chain**
	κ	λ	H
Variable (V)	40	~29	51
Diversity (D)	0	0	~27
Joining (J)	5	4	6

Fig. 3.17 The numbers of functional gene segments for the variable region of heavy- and light-chain genes in human DNA.

The organization of the variable-region gene segments differs in detail for each of the immunoglobulin chains and is shown in Fig. 3.18. For the λ light chains, located on chromosome 22, there is a cluster of Vλ gene segments, followed by pairs of Jλ gene segments and Cλ genes. In the case of the κ light chains, on chromosome 2, the cluster of Vκ gene segments is followed by a cluster of Jκ gene segments, then by a single Cκ gene. Finally, the organisation of the heavy chains, on chromosome 14, resembles that of the κ genes, with separate clusters of VH, D, and JH gene segments and of CH genes.

The human V gene segments can be grouped into families on the basis of similarity of DNA sequence; both the VH and Vκ gene segments fall into seven families whose members are more than 80% homologous, while there are eight familes of Vλ gene segments. The families can be further grouped into 'clans', whose members are more similar to each other than to families in other clans. Human VH gene segments fall into three such clans. All of the VH gene segments identified from other species also fall into the same three clans, suggesting that all may have evolved by gene duplication from three ancestral V gene segments.

The numbers of V gene segments shown above are fewer than past estimates suggested. The number of VH gene segments had been estimated at more than 100, whereas we know now that there are 95 VH gene segments in the VH gene cluster, of which only 51 are functional. The difference between the estimated and true numbers is partly due to the presence of what are called 'orphon' genes, V segment sequences that have become translocated from their original locations and can no longer contribute to immunoglobulin variable regions.

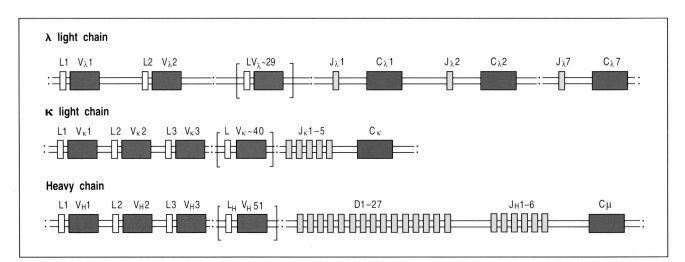

Fig. 3.18 The genomic organization of the heavy- and light-chain gene segments in humans. The upper row shows the gene locus for the λ light chain which has about 29 functional Vλ gene segments and four pairs of functional Jλ segments and Cλ genes. The single κ locus (middle row) is organized similarly, with about 40 functional Vκ gene segments accompanied by a cluster of five Jκ segments and a single Cκ gene. The heavy-chain gene locus (bottom row) has about 50 functional VH gene segments but, in addition, there is a cluster of around 27 D segments lying between the 51 V gene segments and the six JH gene segments. The heavy-chain locus also contains a large cluster of CH genes that will be described in a later section. For simplicity we have shown only a single CH gene in this diagram, and have omitted pseudogenes. L = leader sequence.

3-13 **Rearrangement of V, D, and J gene segments is guided by flanking sequences in DNA.**

When the non-coding regions flanking the different heavy and light chain V gene segments are compared, conserved sequences are found on the 3′ side of V gene segments, the 5′ side of J gene segments, and both sides of D gene segments. These sequences consist of a conserved block of seven nucleotides (**heptamer**), followed by a spacer of roughly 12 or 23 base pairs, followed by a second conserved block of nine nucleotides (**nonamer**) (Fig. 3.19). The heptamer sequence is CACAGTG or, when inverted, CACTGTG, while the nonamer sequence is ACAAAAACC or, inverted, GGTTTTTGT. The spacer is not conserved in sequence but is always either 12 or 23 base pairs, corresponding to one or two turns of the DNA double helix. This would bring the heptamer and nonamer sequences to the same side of the DNA helix, presumably where they can be recognized by the enzymes that carry out the gene rearrangement. The heptamer-spacer nonamer is often called the **recombination signal sequence**.

Although the mechanism of recombination is not known in detail, the process does follow a strict rule (the **12/23 rule**) that recombination can only occur between a gene segment flanked by a heptamer and nonamer separated by a 12mer spacer and one where the heptamer and nonamer are separated by a 23mer spacer. Thus, for the heavy chain, recombination can only join a V gene segment to a D gene segment and a D gene segment to a J gene segment , as both V and J gene segments are flanked by 23 base pair spacers and the D gene segments have 12 base pair spacers on both sides.

The mechanism of gene rearrangement is similar for heavy and light chains, although to construct the light-chain variable gene only one joining event need take place, between the V and the J gene segments, while for heavy chains there are separate rearrangements to join the D and J gene segments and to join the V and DJ gene segments. In the most common type of rearrangement (Fig. 3.20, left-hand panels), the two gene segments to be joined have the same transcriptional orientation. The heptamer and nonamer recombination signal sequences are brought together, most probably by interactions between proteins that bind to them rather than by interactions between the two DNA molecules themselves. Such proteins must also recognize the length of spacer between the heptamer and nonamer signals in order to enforce the 12/23 rule for recombination. The two DNA molecules are then broken and rejoined so that the ends of the heptamer sequences are joined precisely in a head-to-head fashion, forming what is called the **signal joint**. In this process, the pair of recombination signal sequences and the intervening DNA are removed from the genome as a circular molecule. The joining of the V and J gene segments, forming what is called the **coding joint**, is not precise, as we will describe shortly, and generates a large amount of variability.

In a few cases the two gene segments to be joined have opposite transcriptional orientation (Fig. 3.20, right-hand panels). Rearrangement of these gene segments can still take place and differs from the more common case only in the fate of the DNA that lies between the two gene segments. When the recombination signals are brought together and recombination takes place, the intervening DNA is not lost from the chromosome but is inverted.

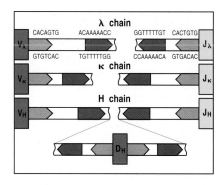

Fig. 3.19 Conserved heptamer and nonamer sequences flank the gene segments encoding the variable regions of heavy and light chains. The spacing between the heptamer and nonamer sequences is always either approximately 12 or approximately 23 base pairs, and joining always involves a 12 base pair and a 23 base pair recombination signal.

3-14 | **There are four main processes by which antibody diversity is generated.**

Antibody diversity is generated in four main ways, three of which are consequences of the process of recombination used to create complete

Fig. 3.20 Variable-region gene segments are joined by recombination. In every variable region recombination event, the signals flanking the gene segments are brought together to allow recombination to take place. For simplicity, the recombination of light chains is illustrated; for heavy chains, two separate recombination events are required to generate a functional variable region. In many cases, as shown in the left-hand panels, the V and J gene segments have the same transcriptional orientation as shown by the arrows. Juxtaposition of the recombination signal sequences results in the looping out of the intervening DNA. Heptamers are shown in orange, nonamers in purple. Recombination occurs at the ends of the heptamer sequences, creating a signal joint and releasing the intervening DNA in the form of a closed circle. Subsequently, the joining of the V and J gene segments creates the coding joint. In some cases, illustrated in the right-hand panels, the V and J gene segments are oriented in opposite directions. Bringing together the signal sequences in this case requires a more complex looping of the DNA. Joining the ends of the two heptamer sequences now results in the inversion of the intervening DNA. Again, the joining of the V and J segments creates a functional variable region gene.

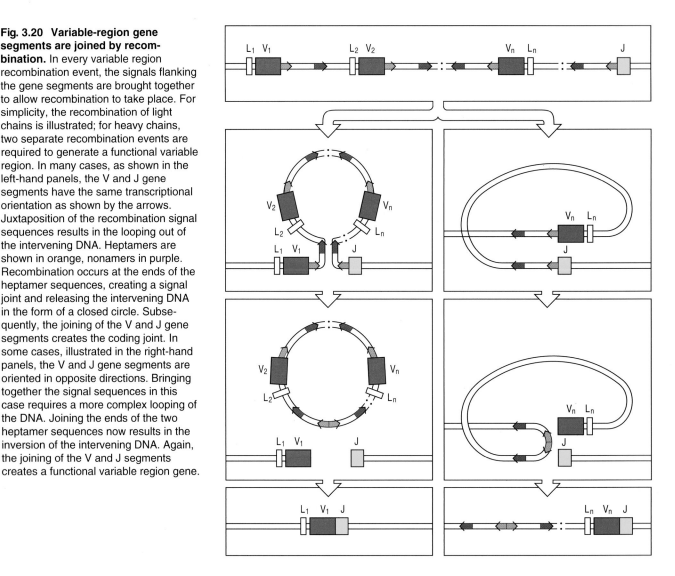

immunoglobulin variable regions, while the fourth is a mutational process that acts only on the rearranged DNA encoding the variable regions.

First, there are multiple copies of each of the gene segments that go to make up an immunoglobulin variable region, and different combinations of segments can be used in different rearrangement events. This is one form of combinatorial diversity. The ability of the heavy and light chains to pair appears, in most cases, to be independent of the variable regions involved and thus a second form of combinatorial diversity arises from the pairing of the heavy and light chains to form a complete antigen binding site. These two processes of combinatiorial diversity alone can generate around 3×10^6 possible antibody molecules (see Section 3-15). Third, as part of the recombination process itself, diversity can be introduced at the joints between the different gene segments. Finally, there is somatic hypermutation. This process introduces point mutations into the rearranged heavy and light chain genes and thus it is the only means by which the specificity of an immunoglobulin can be altered after a complete variable-region gene has been created by recombination. We will discuss these four mechanisms at greater length in the following sections.

3-15   Repertoires of human immunoglobulin genes account for some parts of diversity.

There are multiple copies of the V, D, and J gene segments, each of which is capable of contributing to an immunoglobulin variable region.

The factors that determine which gene segments are used in any particular gene rearrangement are unknown. However, it is clear that many different variable regions can be made by selecting different combinations of V and J gene segments, in the case of light chains, or V, D, and J gene segments in the case of heavy chains. For human κ light chains, there are approximately 40 functional V_κ gene segments and 5 J_κ gene segments, giving the capacity to make 200 different V_κ regions. For λ light chains there are approximately 35 functional V_λ gene segments and 4 J_λ gene segments, yielding 140 V_λ regions. So in all, 340 different light chains can be made: (35 x 4) + (40 x 5) = 340. For the heavy chains of humans, there are 51 functional V_H gene segments , approximately 30 D gene segments and 6 J_H gene segments, giving the capacity to make around 9000 different V_H regions: 51 x 30 x 6 = 9180. As both the heavy- and the light-chain variable regions contribute to antibody specificity, each of the 340 different light chains could be combined with each of the 9000 heavy chains to give approximately 3×10^6 different antibody specificities. The ability to create a large number of different specificities by making many different combinations of a small number of gene segments (40 + 5 + 35 + 4 + 51 + 30 + 6 = 171) is known as combinatorial diversity. For each of these loci, we have given the number of V regions in terms of the number of functional gene segments; the total number of V regions is larger but these additional gene segments do not appear to be used, and many have defects that render them pseudogenes.

The true repertoire of variable regions is likely to be less than the number calculated from the theoretical extent of combinatorial diversity. Not all V gene segments are used at the same frequency; some are common, while others are found only rarely. However, this ignores two processes that greatly add to repertoire diversity, imprecise joining of V, D, and J gene segments and somatic hypermutation.

3-16   Joining of variable gene segments is imprecise.

Although the details of the recombination process still need to be worked out, we know that several steps are required in the joining of V, D, and J gene segments, and that some of these steps create diversity in the variable regions by inserting or deleting nucleotides at the joints between gene segments (Fig. 3.21). This is known as **junctional diversity**. First, the recombinases, enzymes that mediate gene rearrangement, must recognize the recombination signal sequences and bring them together. Second, they must catalyze formation of a double-stranded break, so that a signal joint can form, either by head-to-head joining or by inversion. Third, the double-stranded breaks of the two coding ends, D and J or V and DJ, apparently form a hairpin loop. The hairpin loop is presently inferred from the presence of additional nucleotides found at the joints between V (D) and J gene segments in both heavy- and light-chain joints. These additional nucleotides are called **P-nucleotides** because they tend to be palindromic. In addition, it has been found that the ends of coding joints in *scid* mice, which have a defect in recombination and which make no antibodies, are always hairpin in nature. The resolution of hairpins creates P-nucleotides in many cases, as shown in Fig. 3.21.

Fig. 3.21 Enzymatic steps in the rearrangement of immunoglobulin gene segments. The process is illustrated for a D to J rearrangement, showing the full sequence of the heptamer signal sequence and the first two nucleotides of the gene segments to be joined; however, the same steps occur in V to D and in V to J rearrangements. Rearrangement commences with the action of an exonuclease, which recognizes the recombination signal sequences and cuts one strand of the DNA precisely at the end of the heptamer sequences (top panel). Subsequently, the 5′ end of the DNA strand generated by the cleavage undergoes a chemical reaction with the opposite, uncut strand of DNA, breaking that strand to generate on one side a double-stranded break in the DNA precisely at the end of the heptamer sequence, and on the other side a DNA hairpin (second panel). Subsequently, the two heptamer sequences are ligated together to form the signal joint, although the exact time at which this occurs is unknown, while an endonuclease cleaves the DNA hairpin at a random site (third panel) to yield a single-stranded DNA end (fourth panel). Depending on the site of cleavage, this single-stranded DNA may contain nucleotides that were originally complementary in the double-stranded DNA and which therefore form short DNA palindromes, as indicated by the shaded box in the fourth panel. Such stretches of nucleotides that originate from the complementary strand are known as P-nucleotides. For example, the sequence GA at the end of the D segment shown is complementary to the preceding sequence TC. The subsequent sequence of events differs between light-chain and heavy-chain variable genes, since at the time of heavy-chain gene rearrangement the enzyme terminal deoxynucleotidyl transferase (TdT) is expressed and can add nucleotides to the ends of these single-stranded segments of DNA. Where TdT is present, nucleotides are added at random to the ends of the single-stranded segments before pairing of the strands (fifth panel), indicated by the shaded box surrounding these non-templated, or N, nucleotides. The two single-stranded ends then pair (sixth panel). Exonuclease trimming of unpaired nucleotides and repair of the coding joint by DNA synthesis and ligation leaves both the P- and N-nucleotides present in the final coding joint (indicated by shading).

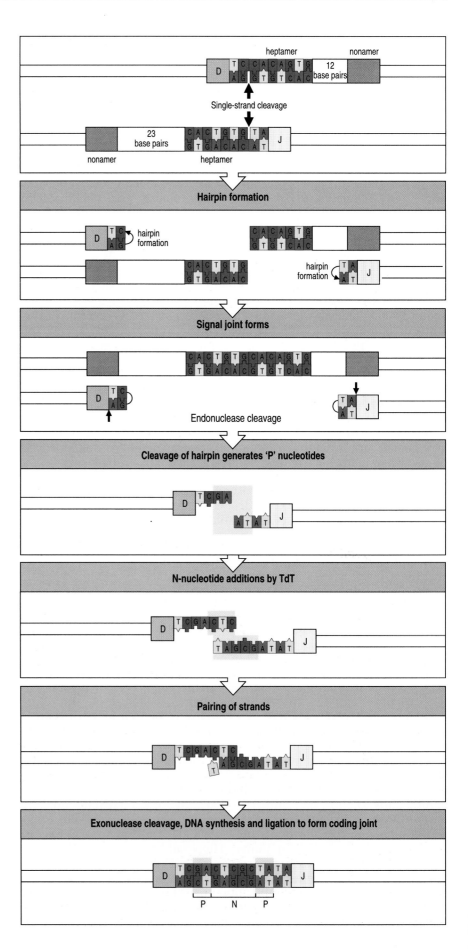

A second process that generates diversity in immunoglobulin molecules is the addition of **N-nucleotides**, so-called because they are non-template encoded but are added to the free 3′ end of a DNA strand by the enzyme **terminal deoxynucleotidyl transferase (TdT)**. Thus in mice whose TdT has been inactivated by homologous recombination (see Section 2-38), N-nucleotides are absent from coding joints. As shown in Fig. 3.21, TdT adds between 1 and 20 nucleotides to the free ends of coding joints, after the hairpins have been cleaved. The two DNA strands then pair, and other enzymes (remaining to be categorized) then fill in and repair the ends.

In mice, N-nucleotides are found only in the heavy chains. During the development of B cells, the heavy-chain genes undergo rearrangement before the light-chain genes (see Chapter 5). TdT is active early in mouse B-cell development, while the heavy chains are being rearranged but is no longer expressed at the time of light-chain gene rearrangement. Hence, the light chains lack N-nucleotides because the necessary enzymatic machinery is not present at the time they are rearranged. In humans, both heavy and some light chains contain N-nucleotides.

Little is known of the other enzymes that participate in gene rearrangement, although the details of the joining of V, D, and J gene segments are rapidly being worked out thanks to studies with *scid* (*severe combined immunodeficient*) mice, which have a genetic defect that makes them deficient in DNA recombination and repair. They make no antibodies or T-cell receptors and are consequently severely immunodeficient. Cells derived from these mice make normal numbers of signal joints but cannot make coding joints. Coding joints are formed by the ligation of two pieces of DNA, each of which has been broken across the two strands. Some of the proteins involved in repairing double-stranded breaks in DNA have now been identified and include a very large protein known as **DNA-dependent protein kinase**. It is the DNA-dependent protein kinase that is defective in *scid* mice, which suggests that in normal cells it is involved in forming the coding joints.

Two other genes have been identified that are likely to be involved in DNA rearrangment as they enable introduced unrearranged antibody gene constructs to become rearranged in cell types that do not normally make antibodies. They are called **RAG-1** and **RAG-2**, for **recombination activating genes.** The *RAG-1* gene has similarities to the yeast gene *HRP-1*, which is involved in recombination. Both *RAG-1* and *HRP-1* gene products have similarities to bacterial enzymes called **topoisomerases**, which catalyze the breakage and rejoining of DNA. Mice defective in either *RAG-1* or *RAG-2* cannot make immunoglobulin, strongly implicating these genes in somatic recombination. Thus, it appears that the joining process is soon going to yield a molecular mechanism.

The result of N- and P-nucleotide addition and of exonuclease trimming, is that extra diversity is created at the junction between gene segments. The exact position of the junction between segments is variable, and the extra nucleotides inserted can encode additional amino acids. In addition, the frame in which the D and J segments will be read depends on the number of bases inserted or deleted at the junction.

| 3-17 | **Rearrangement of immunoglobulin genes is regulated so that each B cell makes antibody of a single specificity.** |

The rearrangement of immunoglobulin genes is tightly regulated during B-cell development, so that only one rearranged heavy-chain gene and one rearranged light-chain gene are finally expressed in each individual developing B cell. This generates B cells that bear a single type of antigen receptor, with two identical light chains and two identical heavy chains and thus two identical antigen-binding sites. So, although there are two chromosomes encoding heavy chains, and a total of four chromosomes encoding light chains (the κ and λ loci are on different chromosomes), only one heavy chain and one light chain are finally expressed. This restriction is known as allelic exclusion. In allelic exclusion, only one of the two chromosomes is allowed to make a productive rearrangement; the other chromosome is either not rearranged or carries an out-of-frame joint. We discuss the mechanism of allelic exclusion in Chapter 5.

As we learned in Chapter 1, the clonal selection theory requires that each lymphocyte has just one receptor specificity. This **monospecificity** is important because it means that cells respond to a particular antigen by making antibodies that bind that antigen, and not the irrelevant antibodies that could be made if the cell had multiple specificities.

3-18	**Rearranged V genes are further diversified by somatic hypermutation.**

The mechanisms for generating diversity that we have described in the previous sections all take place during the rearrangement of gene segments in developing B cells to produce a functional antibody molecule. This tends to focus diversity into the CDR3 region of the variable region. However, there is an additional mechanism that generates diversity throughout the variable region and which operates after functional antibody genes have been assembled. This process is known as **somatic hypermutation** and involves the introduction of point mutations into the variable regions of the expressed heavy- and light-chain genes at a very high rate (Fig. 3.22). Other genes expressed in the B cells do not undergo mutagenesis at the elevated rate and, in particular, the immunoglobulin constant-region genes are not affected. The mechanism by which mutations are introduced into the expressed variable-region genes is unknown.

Somatic hypermutation occurs when B cells respond to antigen and acts randomly on rearranged variable-region genes whether they are expressed, productively rearranged genes or non-expressed, non-productive genes. However, the pattern of mutation is different in these two types of rearranged genes. Base changes that alter amino acid sequences are clustered in the three CDRs that make contact with antigen in the expressed variable-region genes, while silent base changes that preserve amino acid sequences are distributed throughout the framework regions. No such focusing of silent or productive mutations is seen in the non-productive variable-region genes in the same cell.

The pattern of mutation shows that antigen selects those B cells having mutated receptors that bind antigen better; this enhanced binding favors stimulation of such B cells and their secretion of antibody. The process of mutation followed by antigen selection will be discussed in detail in Chapters 8 and 9, where we shall see that it leads to better antigen binding over the course of an antibody response, a process called **affinity maturation**.

The existence of many copies of the variable-region gene segments, all differing in sequence, allows diversity to be distributed throughout the variable regions and thus makes an important contribution to the development of the antibody repertoire. The number of variable-region gene segments represents a heritable contribution to immunoglobulin diversity. However, the inherited component is only the template from

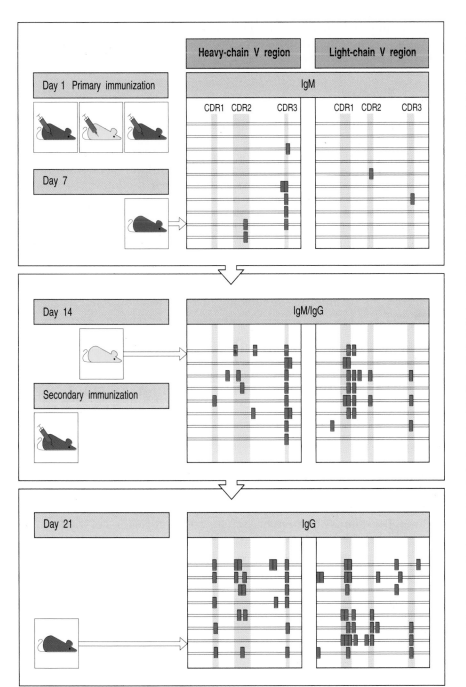

Fig. 3.22 Somatic hypermutation introduces diversity into expressed immunoglobulin genes. This figure illustrates an experiment in which somatic hypermutation in immuno-globulin variable regions was demonstrated by sequencing of heavy- and light-chain variable regions of immuno-globulins specific for the same antigen at different times after immunization. Three groups of mice were immunized, in this case with a small hapten, oxazolone, for which the majority of antibodies produced use a single V_H and V_L. Seven days after immunization, B cells were taken from the first group of animals and oxazolone-specific hybridomas were produced from them. The hybridomas secreted predominantly IgM antibodies and showed little sequence variation in the V regions. Amino acid positions that differ from the prototypic variable region sequences are shown as bars on the lines representing the sequences. At seven days most of the differences lie in the junctional regions, that is, in CDR3. After a further seven days the oxazolone-specific antibodies from the second group of mice were analyzed. At this time, both IgG and IgM antibodies were present and a number of sequence changes were found affecting all six CDRs. A third group of mice were given a secondary immunization and were analyzed after a further seven days. In this last group most of the antibodies were of the IgG type and all showed extensive changes in the V regions. Both productive and silent changes were seen throughout the variable region but productive changes were concentrated in CDRs. Thus, the concentration of mutations in CDRs is a consequence of selection of the mutant B cells for antigen binding, and not of the specific focusing of the mutagenic process.

which random processes of combinatorial diversity, junctional diversity, and somatic hypermutation fashion the final repertoire. Most of the diversity seen in antibodies derives from such random processes and is therefore acquired during the life of the organism. The diversification that occurs during gene rearrangement tends to focus variability into the CDR3 region of the variable region and may not be sufficient by itself to generate the broad spectrum of antibody specificities required to protect the organism from infectious agents. Somatic hypermutation affects diversity in all CDRs, and thus further enhances antibody specificity. The compromise between the heritable and acquired components of diversity that we have described has been found in several mammalian immune systems. Some species have chosen strategies to generate diversity that rely more on one component than another. It seems likely that the important factor is the generation of sufficient diversity in the immune system to protect the organism from common pathogens, rather than how that diversity is generated.

Summary.

Diversity in antibody molecules arises from several sources. Inherited variability arises from the presence of many variable-region gene segments in the genome. Additional diversity results from the formation of a complete variable-region gene by the random recombination of separate V, D, and J gene segments. Furthermore, the joining process is itself a source of diversity as a consequence of imprecise joining of the gene segments and the introduction of P- and N-nucleotides. A third source of diversity is the association of variable regions of the heavy and light chains to form the antigen-binding site. Finally, after an antibody has been expressed, the coding sequence of its varaible region is further diversified by somatic hypermutation upon stimulation of the B cell by antigen. The combination of all these sources of diversity creates a vast repertoire of antibody specificities from a relatively limited number of genes.

Structural variation in immunoglobulin constant regions.

When we described the structure of an antibody molecule earlier in this chapter, we used the example of the most abundant type of antibody in plasma, IgG. IgG is one of the five major classes, or **isotypes**, of antibody molecules, defined by the structure of the heavy-chain constant regions. Differences in the heavy-chain constant regions of the five isotypes confer different functional properties on each class. In this section, we will describe the different isotypes and their functions, and the mechanism by which a given variable region may be expressed with any of the different constant regions.

3-19 | Immunoglobulin constant regions confer functional specificity.

The five main isotypes of immunoglobulin are IgM, IgD, IgG, IgE, and IgA. The heavy chains that define these different isotypes are designated by the lower case Greek letters μ, δ, γ, ε and α, as shown in Fig. 3.23, which also lists the major physical properties of the different human isotypes.

IgG was the first isotype discovered, as it is the most abundant in normal serum. Subsequently, IgM antibodies were distinguished from IgG when they were found in the **macroglobulin** (hence IgM) fraction of serum that sediments more rapidly than IgG during ultracentrifugation. IgA antibodies were first identified as a separate entity by electrophoresis of serum proteins and the IgD isotype was found as a product of a myeloma, an antibody-producing tumor. Finally, IgE was identified as the pathogenic antibody, or **reagin**, in the serum of patients suffering severe allergies. In addition to the five major classes, there are four subclasses of IgG in humans (IgG1, IgG2, IgG3, and IgG4) and in mice (IgG1, IgG2a, IgG2b, and IgG3) and two subclasses of IgA in humans (IgA1 and IgA2).

Immunoglobulin								
IgG1	IgG2	IgG3	IgG4	IgM	IgA1	IgA2	IgD	IgE
Heavy chain γ_1	γ_2	γ_3	γ_4	μ	α_1	α_2	δ	ε
Molecular weight (kDa) 146	146	165	146	970	160	160	184	188
Serum level (mean adult mg ml^{-1}) 9	3	1	0.5	1.5	3.0	0.5	0.03	0.00005
Half-life (days) 21	20	7	21	10	6	6	3	2

Fig. 3.23 The physical properties of the human immunoglobulin isotypes.

The various isotypes and subclasses are functionally distinct, binding to different receptors and carrying out separate functions in the immune response (Fig. 3.24). The effector functions of the immunoglobulin isotypes are carried out by the Fc part of the molecule, consisting of the paired C_H2 and C_H3 domains in IgG and IgA, and of paired C_H2, C_H3, and C_H4 domains in IgM and IgE. Sites on the Fc portion that are involved in some of the effector functions have been identified by studies of mutant immunoglobulins.

Immunoglobulin								
IgG1	IgG2	IgG3	IgG4	IgM	IgA1	IgA2	IgD	IgE
Classical pathway of complement activation ++	+	+++	–	+++	–	–	–	–
Alternative pathway of complement activation –	–	–	–	–	+	–	–	–
Placental transfer	+		+	–	–	–	–	–
Binding to macrophages and other phagocytes +	–	+	–	–	–	–	–	+
High-affinity binding to mast cells and basophils –	–	–	–	–	–	–	–	+++
Reactivity with staphylococcal Protein A +	+	–	+	–	–	–	–	–

Fig. 3.24 The biological functions of the various human immunoglobulin isotypes.

One very important function of immunoglobulins is the binding of complement to initiate the complement cascade, which helps to recruit and activate phagocytes and can also directly destroy pathogens (see Chapter 8). The initial component of the complement cascade is a protein called C1q, which binds to IgM on a region of charged residues on the side of C_H3 and to IgG at a similar region of the C_H2 domain; C1q binding is also affected by the glycosylation of the C_H2 domain. The site at which C1q binds on IgG is shown on the structure of the Fc fragment in Fig. 3.25, which also shows the binding of a fragment of Protein A, an immunoglobulin-binding protein synthesized by the bacterium *Staphylococcus aureus* (see Section 2-9).

A second critical function of antibodies, as we shall see in Chapter 8, is to enable macrophages and other phagocytic cells to engulf microorganisms and other foreign antigens they cannot recognize directly. Such antigens, when coated with antibodies, can be bound by receptors on the surface of phagocytes that recognize the Fc portion of the antibodies

Fig. 3.25 The complement component C1q binds to the C$_H$2 domain of the Fc fragment. The structure of the Fc fragment of a single IgG heavy chain is shown, complexed with a fragment of the immunoglobulin- binding protein from *Staphylococcus aureus*, Protein A (see Section 2-9). The Fc fragment has two domains, C$_H$2 and C$_H$3, shown in purple. A carbohydrate chain is attached to an asparagine residue in the C$_H$2 domain; all the atoms are shown and the surface is outlined in green. The fragment of Protein A (white), is shown binding to the Fc fragment between the two domains. Amino acid residues involved in the binding of the complement component, C1q, are shown on the structure in red and lie in the C$_H$2 domain. The binding site for the Fcγ receptor lies in the hinge region that links the Fc fragment to the Fab arms and is not shown in this structure. Photograph courtesy of C Thorpe.

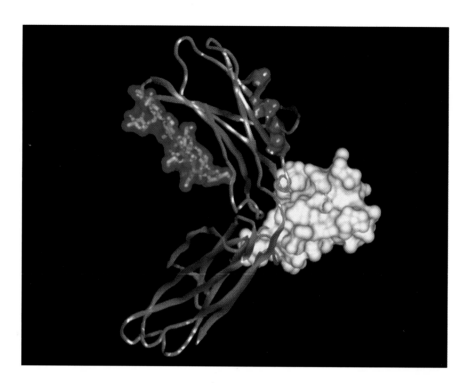

and are thereby stimulated to internalize the antigen. Coating with antibodies in this way is known as opsonization (see Chapter 8), and the opsonizing antibody isotype is IgG; IgM antibodies can also act as opsonins but only when the phagocytes have been activated. The receptors on the surface of phagocytes that recognize the antibody's Fc region are therefore known as Fcγ receptors. These receptors bind to the hinge region of most immunoglobulins. Flexibility of the hinge region is important for C1q binding, perhaps because it enables the Fab arms to move from positions in which they obscure the C1q-binding site.

3-20 | Isotypes are distinguished by the structure of their heavy-chain constant regions.

Comparing the structural organization of the different immunoglobulin heavy chains (Fig. 3.26), it is clear that the various isotypes differ in the number and location of interchain disulfide bonds and in the number of oligosaccharide moieties attached to the heavy chain. In addition, IgM

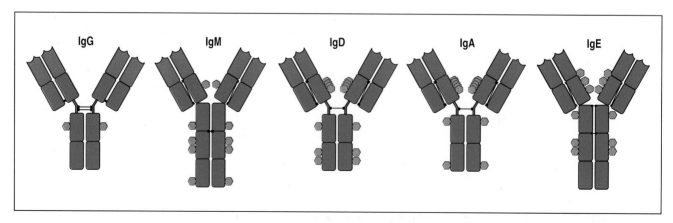

Fig. 3.26 The structural organization of the main human immunoglobulin isotypes. In particular, note the differences in the numbers and location of the disulfide bonds linking the chains and that both IgM and IgE lack a hinge region. The isotypes also differ in the distribution of N-linked carbohydrate groups, as shown in green.

and IgE heavy chains contain an extra constant-region domain that replaces the hinge region found in γ, δ, and α chains. The absence of the hinge region does not imply that the IgM and IgE molecules lack flexibility; electron micrographs of IgM molecules binding to ligands clearly show that the Fab arms can bend relative to the Fc portion. However, such a difference in structure may have functional consequences that are not yet characterized.

The domain structure of the different constant regions of the proteins corresponds exactly to the exon structure of the genes encoding them. Each of the different immunoglobulin heavy-chain isotypes is encoded by a separate gene, and these genes form a large cluster that lies to the 3' side of the J_H gene segments (Fig. 3.27). The cluster spans a large amount of DNA, covering some 200 kilobases (kb) in the mouse. Each constant-region gene is split into three or four exons, each encoding a separate domain within the protein structure (Fig. 3.28).

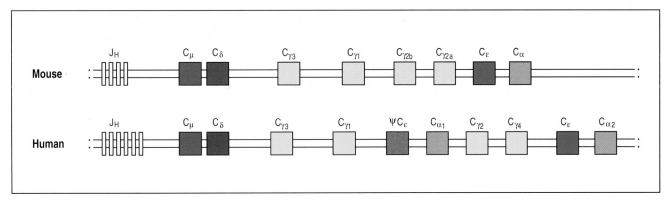

Fig. 3.27 The organization of the immunoglobulin heavy-chain constant-region genes in humans and mice. In the mouse the complex spans some 200 kilobases. In humans, the cluster shows evidence of evolutionary duplication of a unit consisting of two γ genes, an ε and an α gene. One of the ε genes has become inactivated and is now a pseudogene (ψ), hence only one subtype of IgE is expressed. For simplicity, other pseudogenes are not illustrated.

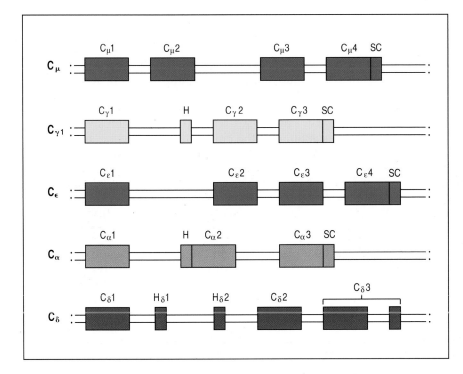

Fig. 3.28 The structure of the genes encoding the main immunoglobulin isotypes in humans. The structure of the genes encoding the secreted form of the immunoglobulin is shown; SC stands for the carboxy terminus utilized in secreted immunoglobulin. A different exon (not shown) encodes a trans-membrane domain used for cell-surface receptors on B cells (see Section 3-26). H stands for hinge. The δ gene differs from the others in having its secreted carboxy terminus encoded on an exon that is separate from the last constant-gene exon. In the mouse, the δ hinge region is contained in a single exon.

| 3-21 | **The same V$_H$ region can associate with different C$_H$ regions.** |

For the heavy chain, there is only one set of variable-region gene segments associated with the cluster of constant-region genes. Therefore, heavy chains of antibodies of all isotypes can share variable regions, and antibody molecules of different isotypes can contain exactly the same variable region.

The association of a variable region with different constant regions occurs during the maturation of a B cell after stimulation with antigen. All B cells initially produce a μ heavy chain and therefore make IgM antibodies. The C$_μ$ gene lies closest to the rearranged V$_H$ gene (see Fig. 3.27) and a complete immunoglobulin mRNA is constructed by splicing from the rearranged variable-region gene to the start of the C$_μ$ gene. After antigen stimulation, the B cells proliferate and can differentiate to produce other isotypes. The particular V$_H$ gene that is expressed is determined by the irreversible recombination process that must occur before the expression of immunoglobulin by the B cell, and it is thus fixed in all progeny of that B cell. The association of a variable region with different constant regions enables antibodies of a given specificity to change their function and is known as **isotype switching** or **class switching**. Although no further variable-region gene rearrangement occurs after the assembly of a functional variable-region gene, somatic hypermutation can and often does occur in the assembled V$_H$ gene after isotype switching. No class switching occurs in light chains as κ and λ are encoded on different chromosomes and cannot therefore interchange.

| 3-22 | **Isotype switching involves site-specific recombination.** |

When B cells switch from producing μ heavy chains to the production of other isotypes, most of the DNA between the V$_H$ region and the desired C$_H$ region is deleted by a site-specific recombination process. In the intron between the rearranged V$_H$ gene and the C$_μ$ gene lies a stretch of repetitive DNA known as a **switch region**, and there are sequences homologous to this switch region 5′ to each of the γ, α, and ε genes (Fig. 3.29. Here we show the switch regions indicated upstream of the mouse constant-region genes; switch regions are also found upstream of the human constant-region genes, again with the exception of the δ gene.) The μ switch region consists of about 150 repeats of the sequence [(GAGCT)n GGGGGT], where n is usually 3 but can be as many as 7. The sequences of the other switch regions differ in detail but all contain repeats of the GAGCT and GGGGGT sequences. Each switch region is given the same designation as the corresponding C gene, hence the μ gene switch region is called S$_μ$ and the γ3 switch region is called Sγ3. To produce an IgG3 antibody, recombination takes place between the S$_μ$ and Sγ3 switch regions, as shown in Fig. 3.29, with the deletion of the intervening constant-region genes. Transcription now proceeds from the VH to the C$_γ3$ gene, allowing a functional immunoglobulin mRNA to be constructed by splicing.

Recombination can take place between the μ switch region and any of the other switch regions to allow production of any isotype, with the exception of IgD, which is always co-expressed with IgM by differential transcription and splicing of the exons of the μ and δ constant-region genes, as we discuss later. The right-hand part of Fig. 3.29 shows the recombination event that allows switching from IgM to IgA production. Switching events can also take place sequentially, allowing a B cell that has already switched to, say IgG3 (left panel), to switch again to produce

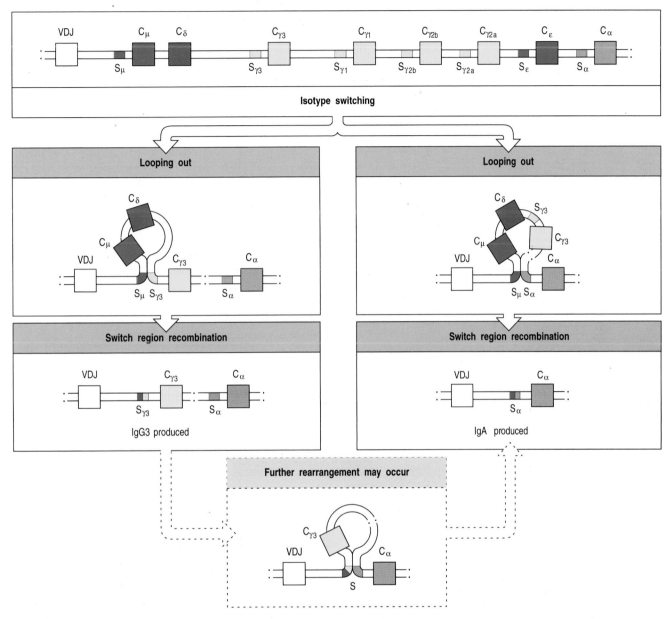

Fig. 3.29 Isotype switching involves recombination between specific signals. Repetitive DNA sequences are found in front of each of the immunoglobulin constant-region genes, with the exception of the δ gene. Switching occurs by recombination between the switch signals, with deletion of the intervening DNA. The initial switching event takes place from the μ switch region; switching to other isotypes can take place subse-

IgA, as shown at the bottom of the figure. Because the switch sequences lie in an intron, all switch recombination events produce genes that can encode a functional protein. Hence, switch recombination is unlike variable-gene segment recombination as all isotype switch recombination is productive.

Isotype switching occurs in activated B cells that have been stimulated by antigen to divide and differentiate. It ensures that the same variable region, and hence the same antigen specificity, can be expressed with different constant-region isotypes, which direct different effector functions. The switching process is not random but is regulated by proteins secreted by T cells, as will be discussed in Section 8-4. Thus the immune system can alter the effects of an antibody response to particular antigens by regulating the isotype of antibody produced.

3-23 | **Expression of IgD depends on RNA processing and not on DNA rearrangement.**

Expression of the IgD isotype differs from the expression of the other isotypes in two important details. First, IgD is co-expressed with IgM on the surface of mature naive B cells, the only case in which two different antibody isotypes are expressed by the same cell. Second, the C_δ gene is not preceded by a switch region. The C_μ and C_δ genes lie close together in the DNA (see Fig. 3.23). B cells expressing IgM and IgD produce two different primary RNA transcripts: in one, the transcript is terminated after the C_μ gene; in the other, both C_μ and C_δ genes are transcribed, and the transcript is terminated after the C_δ gene (Fig. 3.30). The transcripts

Fig. 3.30 IgD expression is regulated by RNA processing. Transcription of the μ and δ genes can terminate at one of two sites, either after the μ gene segments (pA1) or after the δ gene segments (pA2), where pA stands for polyadenylation site. For simplicity we have not shown all the individual constant-region exons. Transcripts that terminate at pA2 are spliced to remove the μ constant-region exons, giving an mRNA encoding a δ heavy chain. The relative amounts of IgM and IgD produced can be varied by regulating either RNA termination or the splicing of the μ–δ transcript.

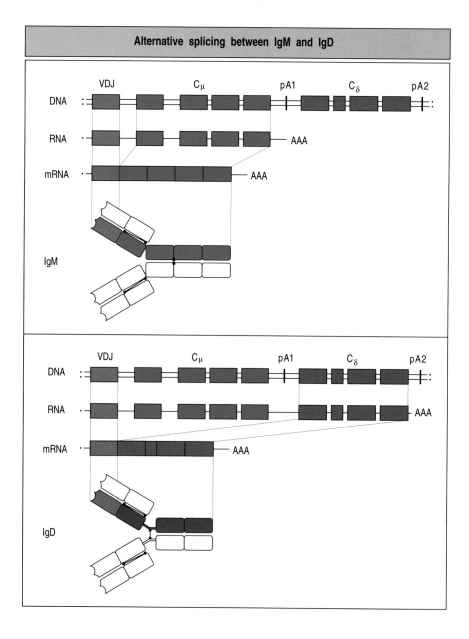

terminating after the C_μ gene are spliced to yield a μ chain mRNA: in those terminating after the C_δ gene, the C_μ exons are removed during RNA processing to yield a δ chain mRNA.

By regulating the sites at which the primary transcripts end, the B cell can express either IgM alone or can co-express IgM with IgD. Moreover, the decision to express IgD is reversible, as the DNA encoding the transcripts is not affected. The function of IgD is not known but the level of IgM and IgD expression in developing B cells correlates with the elimination of B cells expressing self-reactive antibodies (see Section 5-9), and recent data from transgenic mice suggest that mice that lack IgD in the transgene can break B-cell self tolerance. If this is so, then the importance of IgD will turn out to be in shutting off autoreactive B cells during development. The expression of IgM and IgD can also be regulated by post-translational events. As we will describe in more detail in Chapter 5, when B cells capable of recognizing self-antigens develop, they are rendered unresponsive (anergic). In this state they express IgD at the cell surface but not IgM. IgM is still synthesized, but is retained within the cell and never reaches the cell surface. The means by which this selective expression of IgD is achieved is not known.

| 3-24 | IgM and IgA can form polymers. |

Although all immunoglobulin molecules consist of a basic unit of two heavy and two light chains, both IgM and IgA can form higher order polymers. IgM molecules mainly form pentamers while IgA mainly forms dimers (Fig. 3.31). Polymerization is aided by a separate 15 kDa polypeptide chain called the J chain; the IgM pentamer and the IgA dimer both contain one molecule of the J chain.

The polymerization of immunoglobulin molecules is thought to be important in antibody binding to repetitive epitopes. The rate at which an antigen dissociates from the binding site is dependent on the strength of binding, or **affinity** of that site (see Section 2-12). However, antibodies have two or more identical antigen-binding sites and if both bind to epitopes on a single moiety (such as a bacterium) the molecule will only dissociate when both sites are empty. The dissociation rate of the whole antibody will therefore be much slower than the rate for the individual binding sites, giving a greater effective binding strength, or **avidity**. This consideration is particularly relevant for pentameric IgM, which has 10 antigen-binding sites. IgM antibodies frequently recognize repetitive epitopes such as those expressed by bacterial cell wall polysaccharides but the binding of individual sites is often of low affinity. The increase in avidity as a consequence of polymerization may be important for IgM antibodies to be able to bind antigens effectively.

Pentameric IgM antibody is also highly efficient in enlisting the activity of the complement cascade once it binds a pathogen (see Chapter 8). The initiating event of the complement cascade involves the binding of the plasma protein, C1q, to the Fc portion of immunoglobulin. The C1q molecule has six immunoglobulin-binding sites of which at least two must be occupied before the complement cascade is activated. The pentameric IgM molecule has five C1q-binding sites and is very efficient at stimulating complement activity as just one molecule of the pentamer is sufficient to activate the cascade. IgA does not bind to C1q and so the benefits of IgA dimerization must lie elsewhere. The polymerization of IgA is required for transport of IgA through epithelia, as discussed in Chapter 8.

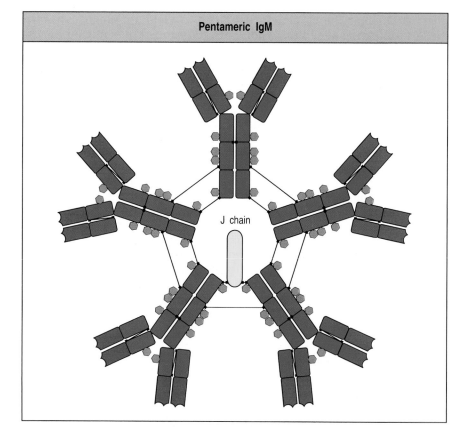

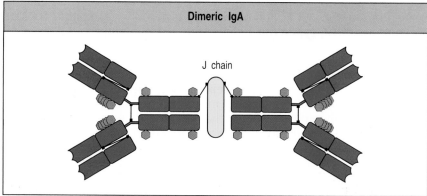

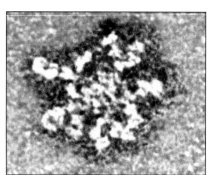

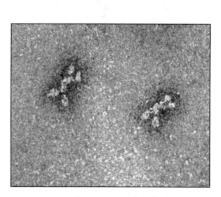

Fig. 3.31 The IgM and IgA molecules can form multimers.
IgM and IgA are usually synthesized as multimers in association with an additional polypeptide chain, the J chain. In the pentameric IgM, the monomers are crosslinked by disulfide bonds to each other and to the J chain. The panel to the left shows an electron micrograph of an IgM pentamer, showing the arrangement of the monomers in a flat disc. IgM can also form hexamers which lack a J chain but are more efficient in complement activation. In dimeric IgA, the monomers have disulfide bonds to the J chain and not to each other. The bottom left panel shows an electron micrograph of dimeric IgA. Photographs (x 900 000) courtesy of K H Roux and J M Schiff.

3-25	Antibodies can recognize amino acid differences in immunoglobulins.

When an immunoglobulin is used as an antigen, it will be treated like any other foreign protein and will elicit an antibody response. Anti-immunoglobulin antibodies can be made that recognize the amino acids that characterize the isotype of the injected antibody (see Section 2-9).

Such anti-isotypic antibodies recognize all immunoglobulins of the same isotype in all members of the species from which the injected antibody came.

It is also possible to raise antibodies that recognize differences in antibodies from members of the same species that are due to genetic variation or **polymorphism**. Such allelic variants are called **allotypes** and represent polymorphic differences at the loci encoding heavy- and light-chain constant regions. In contrast to anti-isotypic antibodies, anti-allotypic antibodies will recognize immunoglobulins of a particular isotype only in some members of a species. Finally, as individual antibodies differ in their variable regions, one can raise antibodies agaist unique sequence variants, which are called **idiotypes**. Anti-idiotypic antibodies have been used widely to manipulate a particular response via an **idiotypic network**, which we shall consider in Chapter 12.

A schematic picture of the differences between idiotypes, allotypes, and isotypes is shown in Fig. 3.32. Historically, the main features of immunoglobulins were defined using isotypic and allotypic markers. The independent segregation of allotypic markers revealed the existence of separate heavy-chain, κ, and λ chain genes. Rabbits, which are unique in having heavy-chain variable-region allotypes, provided the earliest evidence that the variable and constant regions were encoded by distinct gene segments. The finding that variable-region allotypes could be associated with different isotypes of immunoglobulin confounded the dogma that one gene encoded one polypeptide chain and presaged the discovery of somatic recombination.

Isotypic differences	Allotypic differences	Idiotypic differences
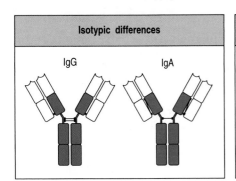	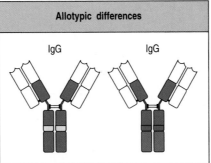	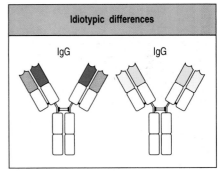

Fig. 3.32 Amino acid variation in immunoglobulin chains can be recognized by other immunoglobulins. Differences between constant-region genes are called isotypes, those between two alleles of the same constant genes are called allotypes and amino acid changes specific to a particular rearranged V_H and V_L gene are called idiotypes.

Summary.

The isotypes of immunoglobulins are defined by their heavy-chain constant regions, each isotype being encoded by a separate constant-region gene. The heavy-chain constant-region genes lie in a cluster 3′ to the variable-region genes. The same rearranged variable-region gene can be expressed with each isotype by the process of isotype switching in which recombination juxtaposes the rearranged variable region just 5′ to the expressed constant-region gene. Unlike VDJ recombination, isotype switching occurs only in specifically activated B cells and is always productive. The immunological functions of the various isotypes differ; thus isotype switching allows the immune system to vary the response to the same antigen at different times or under different conditions.

> # The B-cell antigen receptor and B-cell activation.

Antibodies were originally discovered in their secreted form as proteins that appeared in the plasma following immunization or infection. However, before antibody can be produced, an immunoglobulin molecule encoded by exactly the same rearranged heavy- and light-chain genes must function as the cell-surface antigen receptor for the B cell. We shall use the terms **cell-surface immunoglobulin** and **B-cell antigen receptor (B-cell receptor)** interchangeably in this book. Antigen binding to these transmembrane immunoglobulin molecules initiates the clonal expansion and differentiation of B cells into antibody-secreting plasma cells. This is known as B-cell activation. Although some antigens can activate B cells just by binding surface immunoglobulin, B-cell responses to most antigens require specialized interactions with other cells that provide additional signals. These cell–cell interactions, which we mention only briefly here, will be discussed in detail in Chapters 7 and 8. In the following sections, we shall be concerned chiefly with the mechanism whereby B cells switch from the production of membrane immunoglobulin to the secreted molecule, and with the complex of associated chains that enables the surface immunoglobulin to signal to the interior of the cell on antigen binding.

3-26   Transmembrane and secreted forms of immunoglobulin are generated from alternative heavy-chain transcripts.

Antibodies of all heavy-chain isotypes can be produced either in secreted form or as a membrane-bound receptor. In its membrane-bound form, the immunoglobulin molecule has a hydrophobic transmembrane domain that anchors it to the surface of the B lymphocyte; this domain is absent from the secreted form. In the case of IgM and IgA, the transmembrane form is always monomeric (in other words it is a single immunoglobulin molecule containing two heavy and two light chains) and lacks the cysteine residues necessary for polymer formation (see Fig. 3.31). In the case of IgM, the carboxy terminus of the secreted form has an additional glycosylation site that may increase the solubility of the secreted pentameric molecule.

The two different carboxy termini of the transmembrane and secreted forms of immunoglobulin heavy chains are encoded in separate exons. As with the regulation of IgM and IgD expression (see Section 3-23), the regulation of transmembrane versus secreted immunoglobulin is determined by the point at which the initial RNA transcript ends (Fig. 3.33). The last exon of the constant-region gene contains the sequence encoding the carboxy-terminal end of the transmembrane form of immunoglobulin, and if the primary transcript includes this exon, the sequence encoding the secreted form is removed during RNA splicing and the cell-surface form of immunoglobulin is produced. If the transcript terminates before reaching the transmembrane exon, only the secreted form can be produced.

The mechanism of expression of the transmembrane versus secreted forms of immunoglobulins is the same for all isotypes. Although all B cells initially express the transmembrane form of IgM, after isotype switching memory B cells express transmembrane immunoglobulins of the new isotype. These convert to secretory immunoglobulin of that isotype upon suitable stimulation.

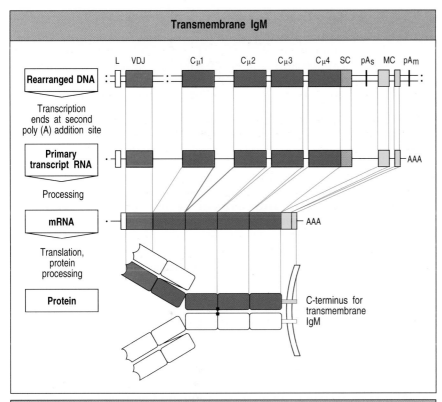

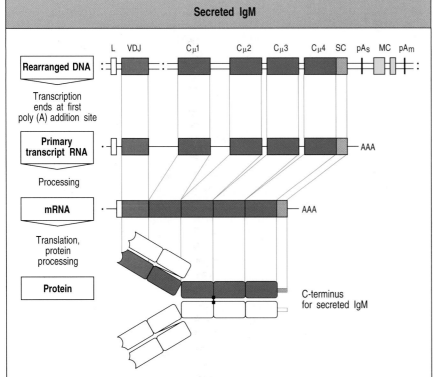

Fig. 3.33 Transmembrane and secreted forms of immunoglobulins are derived from the same gene by alternative RNA processing. Each immunoglobulin gene has two exons (MC; yellow) that encode the transmembrane region and cytoplasmic tail of the transmembrane form and an SC sequence (orange) encoding the carboxy terminus of the secreted form. In the case of IgD the SC sequence is present on a separate exon but for the other isotypes, including IgM shown here, the SC sequences are contiguous with the last constant-domain exon. The events that dictate whether an immunoglobulin RNA will encode a secreted or transmembrane immunoglobulin occur during the processing of the initial transcript. Each immunoglobulin gene has two potential transcription termination sites (shown as pAs and pAm). In the upper panel, the transcript terminates at the second site (pAm). The transcript is spliced to a cryptic splice donor site in the last constant-region exon to remove the SC sequences and to join the MC exons, generating the transmembrane form of immunoglobulin. In the lower panel, the transcript terminates at the first site (pAs), excluding the transmembrane exons and giving rise to the secreted variant.

| 3-27 | Transmembrane immunoglobulin is associated with a complex of invariant proteins. |

The cytoplasmic tail of transmembrane immunoglobulins consists of only a few amino acids and is presumed to be too short to interact with

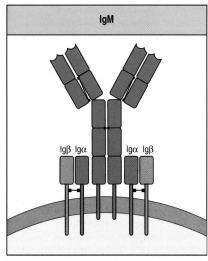

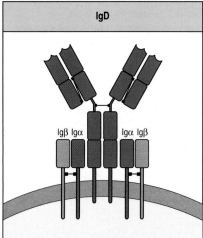

Fig. 3.34 Transmembrane immunoglobulins are found in a complex with two other proteins, Igα and Igβ. Igα and Igβ are disulfide-linked but the exact stoichiometry is unknown, nor is it known which chain binds to the heavy chain. Igα varies in its glycosylation depending on which heavy chain it associates with.

the proteins required for intracellular signaling. Transmission of signals depends instead on at least two other chains associated with immunoglobulin in the membranes of B cells. These proteins are called Igα and Igβ (Fig. 3.34). The Igα and Igβ chains are also required for the expression of immunoglobulin at the cell surface; in the absence of these chains the immunoglobulin stays in an intracellular compartment.

The cytoplasmic tails of the Igα and β chains contain sequences that can be phosphorylated by intracellular Src-family tyrosine kinases and that can subsequently bind other tyrosine kinases. Similar short sequences can be found in the cytoplasmic domains of other immune system signaling molecules such as the T-cell receptor (see Section 4.26) and Fc receptors (see Section 8.16) and have been called **Immunoreceptor Tyrosine-based Activation Motifs,** or **ITAMs** (these were previously known as antigen receptor homologies — ARHs — or antigen-receptor activation motifs — ARAMs). The ITAMs associated with the Igα and β chains allow surface immunoglobulin to associate with cytosolic enzymes that provide the means of intracellular signaling when B cells bind antigen.

3-28 | **B-cell antigen receptor crosslinking can activate B cells.**

Most of what is known about the mechanism of signaling through the B-cell receptor has come from experiments *in vitro* in which the surface immunoglobulin molecules are crosslinked by anti-immunoglobulin antibodies, causing their aggregation in the membrane. Natural antigens can activate B cells in this way only if they have multiple identical epitopes; however, as such antigens include bacterial cell-surface polysaccharides, virions, cell-bound antigens and other complexes, B-cell activation by receptor crosslinking plays an important part in protective immunity.

The B-cell receptor is associated through the cytoplasmic tails of Igα and Igβ with several intracellular **protein tyrosine kinases** of the Src family — Blk, Lck, Fyn, and Lyn. These phosphorylate specific tyrosine residues on other proteins, including those within the ITAMs of Igα and Igβ, activating them in their turn.

Signaling in B cells occurs by a rapid sequence of phosphorylation steps. On receptor crosslinking, the tyrosine kinases are activated to phosphorylate the Igα and Igβ chains, causing the binding of an additional tyrosine kinase, called Syk, to the receptor. Syk contains two protein domains, called SH2 domains, which bind to the conserved tyrosine residues in the ITAMs only when these have been phosphorylated. Once bound, Syk is also activated and this augments transmission of the signal (see legend to Fig. 3.35). The activity of the receptor-associated kinases is positively regulated by another cell-surface protein, CD45, which is a tyrosine-specific phosphatase found on all hematopoietic cells, and which removes a specific inhibitory phosphate from these kinases. CD45 is also called the **leukocyte common antigen**, as it is found on all white blood cells.

One of the most important of the proteins activated by the receptor-associated kinases is the enzyme **phospholipase C-γ**, which cleaves the membrane phospholipid phosphatidylinositol-4,5-bisphosphate (PIP$_2$) into **inositol trisphosphate**, which releases calcium ions from intracellular stores, and **diacylglycerol**, an activator of protein kinase C, which leads to further protein phosphorylation reactions (Fig. 3.35). The cascade of intracellular reactions that follows the activation of the receptor-associated tyrosine kinases leads ultimately to changes in gene expression, which results in the proliferation and differentiation of the

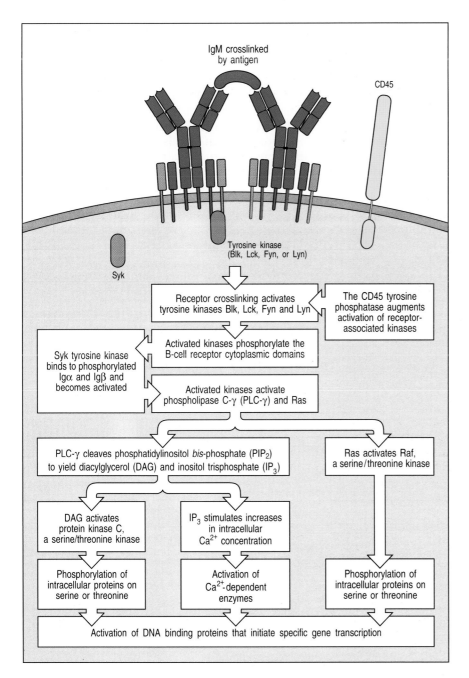

IgM crosslinked by antigen

CD45

Tyrosine kinase
(Blk, Lck, Fyn, or Lyn)

Syk

Receiver crosslinking activates tyrosine kinases Blk, Lck, Fyn and Lyn	The CD45 tyrosine phosphatase augments activation of receptor-associated kinases

Syk tyrosine kinase binds to phosphorylated Igα and Igβ and becomes activated

Activated kinases phosphorylate the B-cell receptor cytoplasmic domains

Activated kinases activate phospholipase C-γ (PLC-γ) and Ras

PLC-γ cleaves phosphatidylinositol *bis*-phosphate (PIP$_2$) to yield diacylglycerol (DAG) and inositol trisphosphate (IP$_3$)

Ras activates Raf, a serine/threonine kinase

DAG activates protein kinase C, a serine/threonine kinase

IP$_3$ stimulates increases in intracellular Ca^{2+} concentration

Phosphorylation of intracellular proteins on serine or threonine

Activation of Ca^{2+}-dependent enzymes

Phosphorylation of intracellular proteins on serine or threonine

Activation of DNA binding proteins that initiate specific gene transcription

Fig. 3.35 Crosslinking of cell-surface immunoglobulin molecules initiates an intracellular signaling cascade. Antigens that bind and crosslink surface immunoglobulin molecules activate the Src-family protein tyrosine kinases Blk, Lck, Fyn, and Lyn, which become associated with the receptor complex. The CD45 phosphatase, which can remove a specific inhibitory phosphate from these kinases, is probably also involved. Activation of the receptor-associated kinases results in a signaling cascade involving several reaction pathways. First, the receptor-associated kinases phosphorylate the proteins of the receptor complex itself, which then bind and activate another kinase, Syk. Syk then initiates the phosphorylation of phospholipase C-γ, which cleaves the membrane phospholipid phosph-atidylinositol-4,5-bisphosphate (PIP$_2$) into inositol trisphosphate and diacylglycerol. Inositol trisphosphate releases calcium ions from intracellular stores, increasing intracellular calcium concentrations, while diacyglycerol activates the serine/threonine protein kinase C. Finally, the GTP-binding protein Ras is activated, and in turn activates an associated protein kinase, Raf, which in turn activates protein kinases that phosphorylate gene transcription regulatory proteins.

B cell. This intracellular signaling cascade, which in B cells links antigen receptor binding to the activation of specific transcriptional regulators, serves in many different cell types to link a specific signal at the cell surface to changes in gene expression, which vary depending upon the cell type involved. T-cell activation, as we shall see in Chapter 4, depends upon a similar cascade.

Although crosslinking of surface immunoglobulin can initiate the bio-chemical signaling pathway we have just described, this is not normally sufficient on its own to activate the proliferation and differentiation of the B cell, which also requires signals from growth factors released by other cells such as helper T cells and macrophages. For antigens that do not crosslink the B-cell receptor, other activation signals as well as those from growth factors are required.

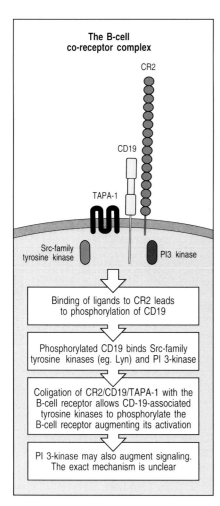

The B-cell co-receptor complex

CR2

CD19

TAPA-1

Src-family tyrosine kinase

PI3 kinase

Binding of ligands to CR2 leads to phosphorylation of CD19

Phosphorylated CD19 binds Src-family tyrosine kinases (eg. Lyn) and PI 3-kinase

Coligation of CR2/CD19/TAPA-1 with the B-cell receptor allows CD-19-associated tyrosine kinases to phosphorylate the B-cell receptor augmenting its activation

PI 3-kinase may also augment signaling. The exact mechanism is unclear

Fig. 3.36 The B-cell co-receptor is a complex of three cell-surface molecules, CD19, TAPA-1, and CR2.
Binding of ligands to the CR2 component of the co-receptor results in the phosphorylation of tyrosine residues in the cytoplasmic domain of CD19; it is not known which tyrosine kinases(s) are involved. Once CD19 is phosphorylated it can bind the Src-family tyrosine kinase Lyn and a second enzyme, phosphatidylinositol 3-kinase. Coligation of the B-cell receptor with the co-receptor brings the bound Lyn in close proximity to the Igα and Igβ cytoplasmic domains, and Lyn may be able to phosphorylate these and augment the signaling through the receptor. In addition, phosphatidylinositol 3-kinase bound to the co-receptor may also augment signaling, possibly by activating a distinct isoform of protein kinase C or by activating other enzymes in the signaling pathway. The exact role of phosphatidylinositol 3-kinase is thus not clear.

3-29   Helper T cells are required for most B-cell responses to antigen.

Most antigens are not able to activate B cells simply by crosslinking their receptors; although they may contain repeated epitopes, as do virions for example, the density of these may not be sufficient to stimulate the B cell. B-cell responses to these antigens are driven by interactions with a specialized subset of T cells, the **helper T cells (T_H2)**, which recognize antigen presented on the surface of B cells and deliver signals that appear to be sufficient on their own to activate the B cell. The role of antigen binding in signaling during this interaction is unclear. The crucial function of the B-cell antigen receptor is to capture antigen for presentation to antigen-specific helper T cells. The signaling function of the antigen receptor is not required for antigen internalization, although it can initiate cell-surface changes in the B cell that promote this interaction; we shall return to this topic in Chapters 4 and 8.

Once a B cell has been activated by a helper T cell, its antigen receptor may once again play a crucial role. The amplification of the antibody response is thought to depend upon a second specialized cell–cell interaction that occurs in the lymphoid follicles (see Chapter 1). Lymphoid follicles contain cells called follicular dendritic cells that are specialized to hold antigen on their surface, to which activated B cells bind through multiple antigen receptor molecules. This crosslinks the receptor molecules, presumably inducing the biochemical changes seen when anti-immunoglobulin is used to crosslink the receptor.

However, even activated B cells whose surface immunoglobulin molecules are effectively crosslinked make very limited amounts of antibody in the absence of other signals. Follicular dendritic cells are thought to increase the sensitivity of the B cells to antigen through the retention of antigen:antibody:complement complexes on their surfaces. While the antigen in the complex binds to the B-cell antigen receptor, complement component C3d binds to complement receptor 2 (CR2), part of a B-cell surface complex known as a co-receptor. Stimulation of the B-cell antigen receptor and CR2 at the same time greatly potentiates signaling via the antigen receptor although binding of ligand to CR2 by itself does not induce any response from the B cell. This means that the B cell homes in on molecules previously tagged by pre-existing antibodies or by the alternative complement pathway.

The **B-cell co-receptor** is a complex of three proteins (Fig. 3.36). The first of these is a receptor, CR2, which binds an activated complement component, C3d. The second component is called CD19, and the third component is TAPA-1, a protein that spans the membrane four times.

One way that co-receptors may enhance signaling of antigen receptors is by bringing more Src-family tyrosine kinases to the receptor. For example, when CR2 is ligated, CD19 becomes phosphorylated and binds phosphatidylinositol 3-kinase (PI 3-kinase) and Src-family tyrosine kinases such as Lyn, a component of the signaling pathway shown in Fig. 3.35. These then become activated, generating intracellular signals that augment the signal transduced via the B-cell receptor itself. Thus, when the co-receptor is triggered at the same time as the B-cell antigen receptor, a much lower level of antigen is needed to generate an activating signal.

Many details of the signaling events that activate B cells remain to be elucidated. We shall discuss B-cell activation by signals from T cells in Chapter 8, after we have described the activation of the T cells themselves but, at present, our understanding of the interplay between the different cell-surface signaling molecules that contribute to activation is incomplete.

Summary.

Immunoglobulin is not simply a serum protein but is also found on the surface of all B cells where it acts as the receptor for antigen. The transmembrane and secreted forms of immunoglobulin produced by one B cell share the same antibody specificity and the difference between the two forms results from alternative heavy-chain termination of transcription and RNA processing. Thus one principle of the clonal selection hypothesis, that the antigen specificity of the secreted antibody should be identical to that of the cellular antigen receptor, is upheld. Expression of transmembrane immunoglobulins at the cell surface and signal transduction by immunoglobulins require the association of the heavy chains with two other membrane proteins, Igα and Igβ, to form a complex in the cell membrane. Crosslinking of the complex by antigen is required to activate enzymes within the cell that initiate a series of biochemical processes leading to the activation of several different protein kinases and raised intracellular calcium ion concentrations. Antigens that do not strongly crosslink surface immunoglobulin molecules cannot activate B cells in the absence of helper T cells. However, after the B cell has been activated in this way it can be stimulated further through crosslinking of its receptors by antigen arrayed on the surface of follicular dendritic cells, which present antigen in the form of antigen:antibody:complement complexes. The complement forms a ligand for the B-cell co-receptor complex, thereby amplifying the effect of the antigen.

Summary to Chapter 3.

This chapter has provided an overview of the antibody molecule. In Chapter 1 we introduced the clonal selection hypothesis and suggested that the principles of clonal selection provide a framework for understanding the immune system. The clonal selection hypothesis requires that there be a broad repertoire of antibody specificities and that these specificities should be distributed clonally. The organization of the antibody molecule and of the genes encoding the antibody molecule allows diversity to be generated within the antigen-binding site. Moreover, the mechanisms that create this diversity ensure that the specificity of each receptor is unique to the B cell in which it occurs, and hence is distributed clonally. A second principle of the clonal selection hypothesis requires that the effector antibody molecules secreted by a B cell have the same specificity as the cellular receptor. Alternative splicing of heavy-chain RNA transcripts, varying the carboxy-terminal sequences of the heavy chains, allows the same gene to make both transmembrane and secreted immunoglobulins, ensuring that the antigen specificity remains the same. The existence of different heavy-chain constant-region genes provides for the diversification of effector functions in different antibody isotypes. The mechanism of isotype switching by moving an active heavy-chain variable-region gene to a new expression site upstream of various constant-region genes ensures that the same antigen specificity is retained in antibodies of different functional properties. The transmembrane form of immunoglobulin exists in association with at least two other proteins, forming a complex that functions as an antigen receptor able to signal to the interior of the cell that antigen has bound. This can activate B cells when the receptors are crosslinked by multivalent antigens in the presence of growth factors but a second signal is required for other antigens and this is provided by signaling molecules expressed by helper T cells.

General references.

Kindt, T.J., and Capra, J.D.: *The antibody enigma*. New York, Plenum Press, 1984.

Honjo, T., Alt., F.W., and Rabbits, T.H. *Immunoglobulin genes*. London, Academic Press, 1989.

Schatz, D.G., Oettinger, M.A., and Schlissel, M.S.: **V(D)J recombination: Molecular biology and regulation**. *Ann. Rev. Immunol.* 1992, **10**:359.

Reth, M.: **Antigen receptors on B lymphocytes**. *Ann. Rev. Immunol.* 1992, **10**:97.

Reth, M. **B-cell antigen receptors**. *Curr. Opin. Immunol.* 1994, **6**:3.

Section references.

3-1   IgG antibodies consist of four polypeptide chains.

Edelman, G.M., Cunningham, B.A., Gall, W.E., Gottlieb, P.D., Rutihauser, U., and Waxdal, M.J.: **The covalent structure of an entire gamma G immunoglobulin molecule**. *Proc. Natl. Acad. Sci. USA* 1969, **63**:78-85.

Fleischman, J.B., Pain, R.H., and Porter, R.R.: **Reduction of gammaglobulins**. *Arch. Biochem. Biophys. Suppl.* 1962, **1**:174.

3-2   The heavy and light chains are composed of constant and variable regions.

Hilschman, N., and Craig, L.C.: **Amino acid sequence studies with Bence-Jones proteins**. *Proc. Natl. Acad. Sci. USA* 1969, **53**:1403-1409.

Dreyer, W.J., and Bennett, J.C.: **The molecular basis of antibody formation: a paradox**. *Proc. Natl. Acad. Sci. USA* 1965, **54**:864-869.

3-3   The structure of the antibody molecule has been determined by X-ray crystallography.

Valentine, R.C., and Green, N.M.: **Electron microscopy of an antibody-hapten complex**. *J. Mol. Biol.* 1967, **27**:615-617.

Porter, R.R.: **The hydrolysis of rabbit gammaglobulin and antibodies by crystalline papain**. *Biochem. J.* 1959, **73**:119.

Alzari, P.M., Lascombe, M., and Poljak, R.J.: **Three-dimensional structure of antibodies**. *Ann Rev. Immunol.* 1988, **6**:555-580.

Poljak, R.J.: **X-ray diffraction studies of immunoglobulins**. *Adv. Immunol.* 1975, **21**:1-33.

Lesk, A.M. and Chothia, C. **Elbow motion in the immunoglobulins involves a molecular ball-and-socket joint**. *Nature* 1988, **335**:188-190.

3-4   Each domain of an immunoglobulin molecule has a similar structure.

Amzel, L.M., and Poljak, R.J.: **Three-dimensional structure of immunoglobulins**. *Ann. Rev. Biochem.* 1979, **48**:961.

Williams, A.F.: **A year in the life of the immunoglobulin superfamily**. *Immunol. Today* 1987, **8**:298.

3-5   Localized regions of hypervariable sequence form the antigen-binding site.

Wu, T.T., and Kabat, E.A.: **An analysis of the sequences of the variable regions of the Bence-Jones proteins and myeloma light chains and their implications for antibody complementarity**. *J. Exper. Med.* 1970, **132**:211-250.

Kabat, E.A., Wu, T.T., Reid-Miller, M., Perry, H.M., and Gottesman, K.S.: *Sequences of Proteins of Immunologic Interest*, 4th edn. US Dept of Health and Human Services, 1991.

3-6   Small molecules bind between the heavy- and light-chain variable domains.

Davies, D.R., Padian, E.A., and Sheriff, S.: **Antigen:antibody complexes**. *Ann. Rev. Biochem.* 1990, **59**:439-473.

Wilson, I.A., Ghiara, J.B., and Stanfield, R.L.: **Structure of anti-peptide antibody complexes**. *Res. Immunol.* 1994, **145**:73.

Arevalo, J.H., Hassig, C.A., Stura, E.A., Sims, M.J., Taussig, M.J., and Wilson, I.A.: **Structural analysis of antibody specificity. Detailed comparison of five Fab′-steroid complexes**. *J. Mol. Biol.* 1994, **241**:663-690.

3-7   Antibodies bind to sites on the surfaces of native protein antigens.

Sheriff, S., Silverton, E.W., Padian, E.A., Cohen, G.H., Smith-Gill, S.J., Finxel, B.C., and Davies, D.R.: **Three-dimensional structure of an antigen:antibody complex**. *Proc. Natl. Acad. Sci. USA* 1987, **84**:8075-8079.

3-8   The interaction of antibody with protein antigens occurs over a surface involving most or all CDRs.

Amit, A.G., Mariuzza, R.A., Phillips, S.E.V., and Poljak, R.J.: **Three-dimensional structure of an antigen-antibody complex at 2.8Å resolution**. *Science* 1986, **233**:747-753.

Tulip, W.R., Varghese, J.N., Laver, W.G., Webster, R.G., and Colman, P.M.: **Refined crystal structure of the influenza virus N9 neuraminidase-NC41 Fab complex**. *J. Mol. Biol.* 1992, **227**:122-148.

Wison, I.A., and Stanfield, R.L.: **Antibody-antigen interactions: New structures and new conformational changes**. *Curr. Opin. Struct. Biol.* 1994, **4**:857-867.

3-9   Antigen:antibody interactions involve a variety of forces.

Novotny, J., and Sharp, K.: **Electrostatic fields in antibodies and antibody/antigen complexes**. *Prog. Biophys. Mol. Biol.* 1992, **58**:203-224.

3-10   Immunoglobulin genes are rearranged in antibody-producing cells.

Tonegawa, S., Hozumi, N., Matthyssens, G., and Schuller, R.: **Somatic changes in the content and context of immunoglobulin genes**. *Cold Spring Harbor Symposium on Quantitative Biology* 1975, **41**:877-888.

Tonegawa, S.: **Somatic generation of antibody diversity**. *Nature* 1983, **302**:575.

3-11   Complete variable regions are generated by the somatic recombination of separate gene segments.

Seidman, J.G., Max, E.E., and Leder, P.: **A κ immunoglobulin gene is formed by site-specific recombination without further somatic hypermutation**. *Nature* 1979, **280**:370.

Early, P., Huang, H., Davis, M., Calame, K., and Hood, L.: **An immunoglobulin heavy-chain variable region gene is generated from three segments of DNA: VH, D and JH.** *Cell* 1980, **19**:981-992.

Bernard, O., Hozumi, N., and Tonegawa, S.: **Sequences of mouse immunoglobulin light chain genes before and after somatic changes.** *Cell* 1978, **15**:1133-1144.

Sakano, H., Maki, R., Kurosawa, Y., Roeder, W., and Tonegawa, S.: **Two types of somatic recombination are necessary for the generation of complete immunoglobulin heavy-chain genes.** *Nature* 1980, **286**:676-683.

Sakano, H., Kurosawa, Y., Weigert, M., and Tonegawa, S.: **Identification and nucleotide sequence of a diversity DNA segment (D) of immunoglobulin heavy-chain genes.** *Nature* 1981, **290**:562-565.

| 3-12 | Variable-region gene segments are present in multiple copies. |

Seidman, J.G., Leder, A., Edgell, M.H., Polsky, F., Tilghman, S.M., Tiemeier, D.C., and Leder, P.: **Multiple related immunoglobulin variable region genes identified by cloning and sequence analysis.** *Proc. Natl. Acad. Sci. USA* 1978, **75**:3881-3885.

Seidman, J.G., and Leder, P.: **The arrangement and rearrangement of antibody genes.** *Nature* 1978, **276**:790-795.

Tomlinson, I.M., Cook, G.P., Carter, N.P., Elaswarapu, R., Smith,S., Walter, G., Buluwela, L., Rabbitts, T.H., and Winter, G.: **Human immunoglobulin V(H) and D segments on chromosomes 15q11.2 and 16p11.2.** *Molec. Genet.* 1994, **3**:853-860.

Cook, G.P., Tomlinson, I.M., Walter, G.,Riethman, H., Carter, N.P., Buluwela, L., Winter, G., and Rabbitts, T.H.: **A map of the human immunoglobulin V(H) locus completed by analysis of the telomeric region of chromosome 14q.** *Nature Genet.* 1994, **7**:162-168.

Cox, J., Tomlinson, I.M., and Winter, G.: **A directory of human germ-line V (kappa) segments reveals a strong bias in their usage.** *Eur. J. Immunol.* 1994, **24**:827-836.

| 3-16 | Joining of variable gene segments is imprecise. |

Lafaille, J.J., DeCloux, A., Bonneville, M., Takagari, Y., and Tonegawa, S: **Functional sequences of T cell receptor γ:δ T cell lineages and for a novel intermediate of V-(D)-J Joining.** *Cell* 1989, **59**:859-870.

Leiber, M.R.: **Site-specific recombination in the immune system.** *FASEB J,* 1991, **5**:2934-2944.

| 3-18 | Rearranged V genes are further diversified by somatic hypermutation. |

Berek, C., and Milstein, C.: **Mutation drift and repertoire shift in the maturation of the immune response.** *Immunol. Rev.* 1987, **96**:23-41.

Kim, S., Davis, M., Sinn, E., Patten, P., and Hood, L.: **Antibody diversity: Somatic hypermutation of rearranged Vh genes.** *Cell* 1981, **27**:573-581.

Gorski, J., Rollini, P., and Mach, B.: **Somatic mutations of immunoglobulin variable genes are restricted to the rearranged V gene.** *Science* 1983, **220**:1179-1181.

Sablitzsky, F., Weisbaum, D., and Rajewsky, K.: **Sequence analysis of non-expressed immunoglobulin heavy-chain loci in clonally related, somatically mutated hybridoma cells.** *EMBO J.* 1985, **4**:3435-3437.

| 3-19 | Immunoglobulin constant regions confer functional specificity. |

Davies, D.R., and Metzger, H.: **Structural basis of antibody function.** *Ann. Rev. Immunol.* 1983, **1**:87-117.

| 3-20 | Isotypes are distinguished by the structure of their heavy-chain constant regions. |

Natvig, J.B., and Kunkel, H.G.: **Human immunoglobulin: Classes, subclasses, genetic variants, and idiotypes.** *Adv. Immunol.* 1973, **16**:1-59.

Pumphrey, R.S.: **Computer models of the human immunoglobulins.** *Immunol. Today* 1986, **7**:206-211.

| 3-21 | The same V_H region can associate with different C_H regions. |

Wabe, M.R., Forn,i L. and Loor, F.: **Switch in immunoglobulin class production observed in single clones of committed lymphocytes.** *Science* 1978, **199**: 1078-1080.

| 3-22 | Isotype switching involves site-specific recombination. |

Kataoka, T., Kawakami, T., Takahashi, N., and Honjo, T.: **Rearrangement of immunoglobulin γ1-chain gene and mechanism for heavy-chain class switch.** *Proc. Natl. Acad. Sci. USA* 1980, **77**:919-923.

Honjo, T., and Kataoka, T.: **Organization of immunoglobulin heavy-chain genes and allelic deletion model.** *Proc. Natl. Acad. Sci. USA* 1978, **75**:2140-2144.

Cory, S., and Adams, J.M.: **Deletions are associated with somatic rearrangement of immunoglobulin heavy-chain genes.** *Cell* 1980, **19**:37-51.

| 3-23 | Expression of IgD depends on RNA processing and not on DNA rearrangement. |

Cheung, H.-L., Blattner, F.R., Fitzmaurice, L., Mushinski, J.F., and Tucker, P.W.: **Structure of genes for membrane and secreted murine IgD heavy-chains.** *Nature* 1982, **296**:410-415.

| 3-24 | IgM and IgA can form polymers. |

Cann, G.M., Zaritsky, A., and Koshland, M.E.: **Primary structure of the immunoglobulin J chain from the mouse.** *Proc. Natl. Acad. Sci. USA* 1982, **79**:6656.

Chapus, R.M., and Koshland, M.E.: **Mechanisms of IgM polymerization.** *Proc. Natl. Acad. Sci. USA* 1974, **71**:657-661.

| 3-25 | Antibodies can recognize amino acid differences in immunoglobulins. |

Bentley, G., Boulot, G., Riottot, M.M., and Poljak, R.J.: **Three-dimensional structure of an idiotype-anti-idiotype complex.** *Nature* 1990, **348**:254-257.

| 3-27 | Transmembrane immunoglobulin is associated with a complex of invariant proteins. |

Venkitaraman, A.R., Williams, G.T., Dariavich, P., and Neuberger, M.S.: **The B-cell antigen receptor of the five immunoglobulin classes.** *Nature* 1991, **352**:777-781.

Hombach, J., Tsubata, T., Leclerq, L., Stappert, H., and Reth, M.: **Molecular components of the B-cell antigen receptor complex of the IgM class.** *Nature* 1990, **343**:760-762.

Campbell, K.S., and Cambier, J.C.: **B-lymphocyte antigen receptors (mig) are non-covalently associated with a disulfide-linked, inducibly phosphorylated glycoprotein complex.** *EMBO J.* 1990, **9**:441-448.

Pleiman, C.M., Dambrosio, D., and Cambier, J.C.: **The B-cell antigen receptor complex: Structure and signal transducttion.** *Immunol. Today* 1994, **15**:393-399.

Sefton, B. M., and Taddie, T.A.: **Role of tyrosine kinases in lymphocyte activation.** *Curr. Opin. Immunol.* 1994, **6**:372-379.

Peaker, C.: **Transmembrane signaling by the B-cell antigen receptor.** *Curr. Opin. Immunol.* 1994, **6**:359-363.

3-28   B-cell antigen receptor crosslinking can activate B cells.

Abbas, A.K.: **A reassessment of the mechanisms of antigen-specific T-cell dependent B-cell activation.** *Immunol. Today* 1988, **9**:89-94.

Burkhardt, A.L., Brunswick, M., Bolen, J.B., and Mond, J.J.: **Anti-immunoglobulin stimulation of B lymphocytes activates src-related protein-tyrosine kinases.** *Proc. Natl. Acad. Sci. USA* 1991, **88**:7410-7414.

Early, P., Rogers, J., Davis, M., Calame, K., Bond, M., Wall, R., and Hood, L.: **Two mRNAs can be produced from a single immunoglobulin μ gene by alternative RNA processing pathways.** *Cell* 1980, **20**:313-319.

Alt, F., Bothwell, A.L., Knapp, M., Siden, E., Mather, E., Koshland, M., and Baltimore, D.: **Synthesis of secreted and membrane-bound immunoglobulin μ heavy chains is directed by mRNAs that differ at their 3′ ends.** *Cell* 1980, **20**:293-301.

Rogers, J., Early, P., Carter, C., Calame, K., Bond, M., Hood, L., and Wall, R.: **Two mRNAs with different 3′ ends encode membrane-bound and secreted forms of immunoglobulin μ chain.** *Cell* 1980, **20**:303-312.

Yamanishi, Y., Kakiuchi, T., Mizuguchi, J., Yamamoto, T., and Toyoshima, K.: **Association of B-cell antigen receptor with protein tyrosine kinase Lyn.** *Science* 1991, **251**:192-194.

3-29   Helper T cells are required for most B-cell responses to antigen.

Yamanishi, Y., Fukui, Y., Wongsasant, B., Kinishita, Y., Ichimori, Y., Toyoshima, K., and Yamamoto, T.: **Activation of Src-like protein-tyrosine kinase Lyn and its association with phospatidylinositol 3-kinase upon B-cell antigen receptor-mediated signaling.** *Proc. Natl. Acad. Sci. USA* 1992, **89**:1118-1122.

Cambier, J.C.: **Signal transduction by T- and B-cell antigen receptors: converging structures and concepts.** *Curr. Opin. Immunol.* 1992, **4**:257-264.

Fearon, D.T.: **The CD19-CR2-TAPA-1 complex, CD45 and signaling by the antigen receptor of B lymphocytes.** *Curr. Opin. Immunol.* 1993, **5**:341-348.

Carter, R.H., Fearon, D.T.: **Lowering the threshold for antigen receptor stimulation of B lymphocytes.** *Science* 1992, **256**:105-107.

Lankester, A.C., Van, S.G., Rood, P., Verhoeven, A.J., and Van, L.R.: **B-cell antigen receptor crosslinking induces tyrosine phosphorylation and membrane translocation of a multimeric Shc complex that is augmented by CD19 co-ligation.** *Eur. J. Immunol.* 1994, **24**:2818-2825.

Tedder, T.F., Zhou, L.J. and Engel, P.: **The CD19/CD21 signal transduction complex of B lymphocytes.** *Immunol. Today* 1994, **15**:437-442.

Antigen Recognition by T Lymphocytes

4

In an adaptive immune response, antigen is recognized by two distinct sets of highly variable receptor molecules — the immunoglobulins that serve as antigen receptors on B cells, and the antigen-specific receptors of T cells. As we saw in Chapter 3, immunoglobulins are secreted as antibodies by activated B cells, and bind pathogens or their toxic products in the extracellular spaces of the body. Binding by antibody neutralizes viruses, and marks pathogens for destruction by phagocytes and complement, mechanisms that will be the topic of Chapter 8. T cells, by contrast, recognize only antigens that have been generated inside the cells of the body and that are displayed on cell surfaces. These antigens may derive from pathogens, such as viruses or intracellular bacteria, that replicate within cells, or from pathogens or their products that cells internalize by endocytosis from the extracellular fluid.

T cells can detect cells infected with intracellular pathogens because such cells display on their surface peptide fragments derived from the pathogens' proteins. These foreign peptides are delivered to the cell surface by specialized cellular glycoproteins, which are encoded in a large cluster of genes first identified by their potent effects on the immune response to transplanted tissues. For that reason, the gene complex was termed the **major histocompatibility complex (MHC)**, and the peptide-binding glycoproteins are still called **MHC molecules**. The recognition of antigen as a small peptide fragment bound to an MHC molecule and displayed at the cell surface is one of the most distinctive features of T cells, and will be the central focus of this chapter.

We shall begin by discussing the mechanisms of antigen processing and presentation, whereby protein antigens are degraded into peptides inside cells and the peptides then carried to the cell surface by MHC molecules. We shall see that there are two different classes of MHC molecules, known as MHC class I and MHC class II, each of which deliver peptides from a different cellular compartment to the surface of the infected cell. Having reached the surface, peptides bound to MHC class I and MHC class II molecules activate the two major classes of T cells — CD8 and CD4 T cells respectively. The two functional subsets of T cells are activated to destroy pathogens resident in different cellular compartments. The activation of another subset of CD4 T cells by peptide:MHC class II complexes provides activated helper T cells required to stimulate antibody production by B cells.

In the second part of this chapter, we shall see that there are several genes for each class of MHC molecule, that is, the MHC is polygenic. Each of these genes has many alleles, that is, the MHC is also polymorphic. Indeed, the most remarkable feature of MHC genes is their genetic variability. MHC polymorphism has a profound effect on antigen recognition by T cells, and the combination of polygeny and polymorphism greatly extends the range of peptides that can be presented to T cells by one individual.

Finally, we will describe the **T-cell receptors** themselves. As might be expected from their function as highly variable antigen recognition structures, T-cell receptors are closely related to antibody molecules in structure and, like immunoglobulins, are encoded in V, D, and J gene segments that rearrange to form a complete variable-region exon. T-cell receptors are complexes of proteins very similar to B-cell receptors; they signal the cell when they bind antigen, using analogous biochemical pathways. There are, however, important differences between T-cell receptors and immunoglobulins, which reflect the unique features of antigen recognition by the T-cell receptor.

The generation of T-cell ligands.

The actions of T cells depend on their ability to recognize cells that are harboring pathogens or have internalized pathogens or their products. T cells do this by recognizing peptide fragments of proteins derived from the pathogen that are bound to MHC molecules on the surface of these cells. In this section, we shall see how the structure and intracellular transport of the two classes of MHC molecules enables them to bind to a wide range of peptides derived from pathogens and their antigens in each of the two main intracellular compartments of cells, and to present them for recognition by the appropriate functional type of T cell.

4-1   T cells with different functions recognize peptides produced in two distinct intracellular compartments.

Infectious agents can replicate in either of two distinct compartments within cells (Fig. 4.1). Viruses and some bacteria replicate in the cytosol or in the contiguous nuclear spaces, while some important pathogenic bacteria and some eukaryotic parasites replicate in the endosomes and lysosomes that form part of the vesicular system of cells (Fig. 4.2, left and center panels). The immune system has different strategies for eliminating infections from these two sites. Cells infected with viruses or with bacteria that live in the cytosol are eliminated by **cytotoxic T cells,** which are distinguished by the cell-surface molecule **CD8.** The function of CD8 T cells is to kill infected cells; this is an important means of eliminating sources of new viral particles and cytosolic bacteria and thus freeing the host of infection. Pathogens and their products in the vesicular compartments of cells are detected by a different class of T cell, distinguished by surface expression of the molecule **CD4.** CD4 T cells are specialized to activate other cells and fall into two functional classes: **T$_H$1 cells** (sometimes known as inflammatory T cells), which activate macrophages to kill the intravesicular bacteria they harbor, and **T$_H$2 cells** or helper T cells, which activate B cells to make antibody.

Microbial antigens may enter the vesicular compartment in either of two ways. Some bacteria, including the mycobacteria that cause tuberculosis and leprosy, invade macrophages and flourish in intracellular vesicles. Other bacteria, which normally proliferate outside cells, secrete toxins and other proteins, and these and bacterial degradation products can be internalized by cells by endocytosis and enter intracellular vesicles in that way. In particular, B cells take up and internalize specific antigen by receptor-mediated endocytosis of antigen bound to their surface immunoglobulin receptor (Fig. 4.2, right panel).

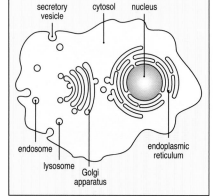

Fig. 4.1 There are two major compartments within cells, separated by membranes. The first is the cytosol, which is continuous with the nucleus via the nuclear pores in the nuclear membrane. The second is the vesicular system, which comprises the endoplasmic reticulum, Golgi apparatus, endosomes, lysosomes and other intracellular vesicles. The vesicular system can be thought of as contiguous with the extracellular fluid, as secretory vesicles bud off from the endoplasmic reticulum and are transported via the Golgi membranes to deliver vesicular contents out of the cell, while endosomes take up extracellular material into the vesicular system. All cell-surface proteins, including the MHC class I and MHC class II molecules, are synthesized on ribosomes attached to the cytoplasmic face of the endoplasmic reticulum and co-translationally transported into the lumen, where they are modified and folded.

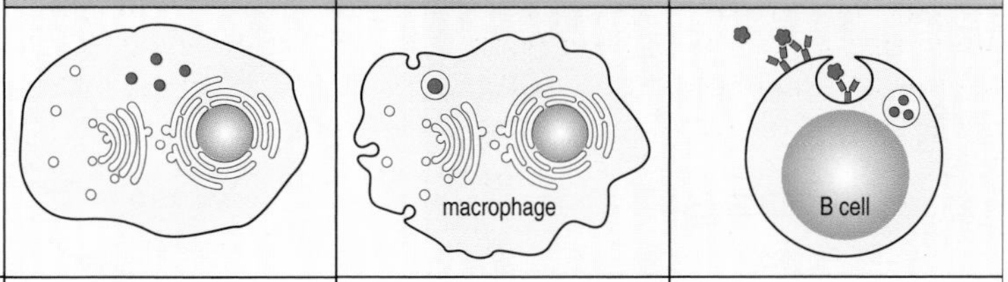

Cytosolic pathogens	Intravesicular pathogens	Extracellular pathogens and toxins
	macrophage	B cell

	Cytosolic pathogens	Intravesicular pathogens	Extracellular pathogens and toxins
Degraded in	Cytoplasm	Acidified vesicles	Acidified vesicles
Peptides bind to	MHC class I	MHC class II	MHC class II
Presented to	CD8 T cells	CD4 T cells	CD4 T cells
Effect on presenting cell	Cell death	Activation to kill intravesicular bacteria and parasites	Activation of B cells to secrete Ig to eliminate extracellular bacteria/toxins

Fig. 4.2 Pathogens and their products can be found in either the cytoplasmic or the vesicular compartment of cells. Left panel: all viruses and some bacteria replicate in the cytosolic compartment. Center panel: other bacteria and some parasites are engulfed into endosomes, usually by phagocytic cells such as macrophages, and are able to proliferate within the vesicles themselves. Right panel: proteins derived from extracellular pathogens may enter the vesicular system of cells by binding to surface molecules followed by endocytosis. This is illustrated for proteins bound by surface immunoglobulin of B cells, which thereby present antigens to CD4 helper T cells; this stimulates them to produce soluble antibody. (The endoplasmic reticulum and Golgi apparatus have been omitted for simplicity.) Other types of cells may also internalize antigens in this way and be able to activate T cells.

To produce an appropriate response to infectious microorganisms, T cells must be able to distinguish between foreign material coming from the cytosolic and vesicular compartments. This is achieved through delivery of peptides to the cell surface from different intracellular compartments by the two distinct classes of MHC molecule (Fig. 4.2). MHC class I molecules deliver peptides originating in the cytosol to the cell surface, where the peptide:MHC complex is recognized by CD8 T cells. MHC class II molecules deliver peptides originating in the vesicular system to the cell surface, where they are recognized by CD4 T cells. Because the generation of peptides involves modifications of the native protein, it is commonly referred to as **antigen processing**, while the display of the peptide at the cell surface by the MHC molecule is referred to as **antigen presentation**.

One difficulty encountered by MHC molecules in effecting this separation of effort is that both MHC class I and MHC class II molecules are synthesized in the endoplasmic reticulum and transported to the cell surface through the Golgi apparatus. We shall see that this separation of function requires adaptations both in the MHC molecules themselves and in the molecules with which they associate during their passage through the system, thus allowing each MHC class to bind and deliver only peptides originating from the appropriate site. Later, when we discuss the recognition of MHC molecules by the T-cell receptor, we will also see how the molecules CD4 and CD8, which characterize the two major subsets of T cells, help in the differential recognition of MHC class I and MHC class II molecules by the T-cell receptor.

4-2 The two classes of MHC molecule have a distinct subunit structure but a similar three-dimensional structure.

The **MHC class I** and **MHC class II molecules** are cell-surface glycoproteins closely related in overall structure and function, although they have readily distinguishable subunit structures. The structures of both MHC class I and MHC class II glycoproteins have been determined by X-ray crystallography. MHC class I structure is outlined in Fig. 4.3.

Fig. 4.3 The structure of an MHC class I molecule, determined by X-ray crystallography. Panel a shows a computer graphics representation of a human MHC class I molecule, HLA-A2, which has been cleaved from the cell surface by the enzyme papain. Panel b shows a ribbon diagram of that structure. Shown schematically in panel d, the MHC class I molecule is a heterodimer of a membrane-spanning α chain (43 000 kDa), non-covalently associated with β2-microglobulin (12 000 kDa), which does not span the membrane. The α chain folds into three domains, α1, α2, and α3. The α3 domain and β2-microglobulin show similarities in amino-acid sequence to immunoglobulin constant domains and have a similar folded structure, while the α1 and α2 domains fold together into a single structure consisting of two segmented α helices lying on a sheet of eight antiparallel β-strands. The folding of the α1 and α2 domains creates a long cleft or groove, which is the site at which peptide antigens bind to the MHC molecules. The transmembrane region and the short stretch of peptide that connects the external domains to the cell surface are not seen in panels a and b as they have been removed by the papain digestion. As can be seen in panel c, looking down on the molecule from above, the sides of the cleft are formed from the inner faces of the two α helices, while the β-pleated sheet formed by the pairing of the α1 and α2 domains creates the floor of the cleft. We shall use the schematic representation in panel d throughout this text. Photograph courtesy of C Thorpe.

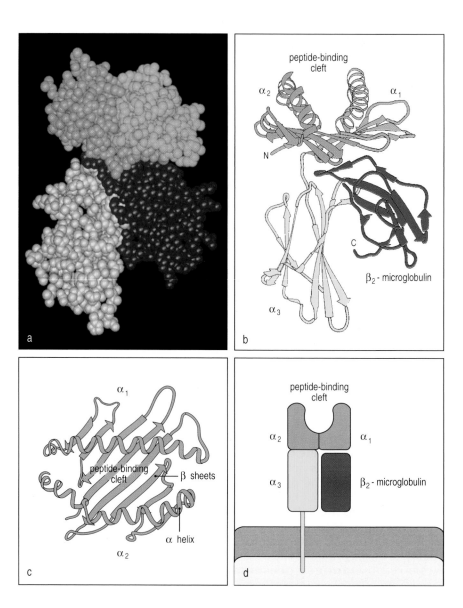

MHC class I molecules consist of two polypeptide chains, an α or heavy chain encoded in the MHC, and a smaller non-covalently associated chain, **β2-microglobulin**, which is not encoded in the MHC. Only the class I α chain spans the membrane. The molecule has four domains, three formed from the MHC-encoded α chain, and one contributed by β2-microglobulin. The α3 domain and β2-microglobulin have a folded structure that closely resembles that of an immunoglobulin domain (see Section 3-4). The most remarkable feature of MHC molecules is the structure of the α1 and α2 domains, which pair to generate a cleft on the surface of the molecule that is the site of peptide binding.

MHC class II molecules consist of a non-covalent complex of two chains, α and β, both of which span the membrane (Fig. 4.4). The crystal structure of the MHC class II molecule shows that it has a folded structure very similar to that of the MHC class I molecule. The major differences in the folded structures of the two molecules lie at the ends of the peptide-binding cleft, which are more open in MHC class II molecules. The main consequence of these differences is that the ends of a peptide bound to an MHC class I molecule are substantially buried within the molecule, while the ends of peptides bound to MHC class II molecules are not.

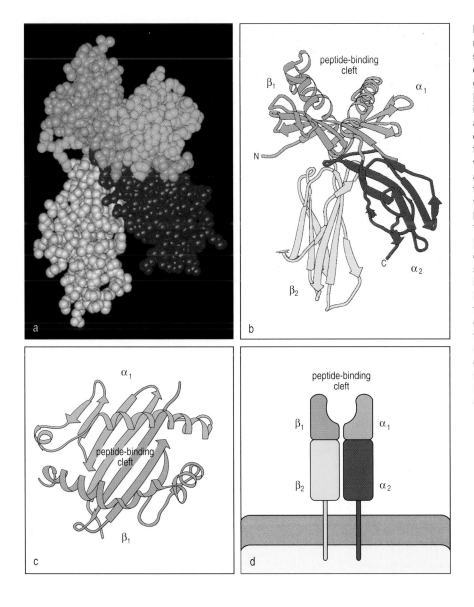

Fig. 4.4 MHC class II molecules resemble MHC class I molecules in structure. The MHC class II molecule is composed of two transmembrane glycoprotein chains, α (34 000 kDa) and β (29 000 kDa), as shown schematically in panel d. Each chain has two domains, and the two chains together form a compact four-domain structure similar to that of the class I molecule (compare with panel d of Fig. 4.3). Panel a shows a computer graphics representation of the MHC class II molecule, in this case, the human protein HLA-DR1, and panel b shows the equivalent ribbon diagram. The $α_2$ and $β_2$ domains, like the $α_3$ and $β_2$-microglobulin domains of the MHC class I molecule, have amino acid sequence and structural similarities to immunoglobulin constant domains; in the MHC class II molecule, the two domains forming the peptide-binding cleft are contributed by different chains, and are therefore not joined by a covalent bond (see panels c and d). Another important difference, not apparent in this diagram, is that the peptide-binding groove of the MHC class II molecule is open at both ends. Photograph courtesy of C Thorpe.

4-3   A T cell recognizes a complex of a peptide fragment bound to an MHC molecule.

The recognition of protein antigens by B-cell receptors and their secreted counterpart, antibody molecules, involves direct binding to the native protein structure. It can be shown by X-ray crystallography that, typically, antibodies bind to the protein surface, contacting amino acids that are discontinuous in the primary structure but are brought together in the folded protein.

Such a direct approach to analyzing antigen recognition has not been possible with T cells, which do not secrete their receptors; as a consequence it has been difficult to obtain sufficient amounts of purified receptors to allow a detailed physical and structural analysis. However, the use of protein engineering techniques to produce soluble T-cell receptors is soon likely to yield a description of T-cell receptor:MHC:peptide interactions comparable to that obtained for antibody:antigen interactions. Until such data is available, the features of antigen recognition by T cells have to be deduced from the functional assays described

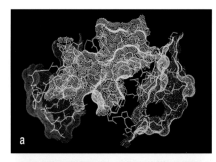

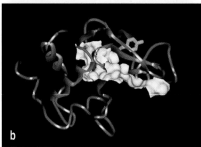

Fig. 4.5 The epitopes recognized by antibodies and by T cells are distinct. B-cell receptors and their secreted counterparts, immunoglobulins, can be shown by X-ray crystallography to bind epitopes on the surface of proteins, as shown in panel a, where the epitopes of three antibodies are shown on the surface of hen egg-white lysozyme. (The interaction between one of these antibodies and hen egg-white lysozyme has already been shown in Fig. 3.13). In contrast, the epitopes recognized by T-cell receptors need not lie on the surface of the molecule, as the T-cell receptor recognizes not the antigenic protein itself but a peptide fragment of the protein. The peptide corresponding to a T-cell epitope of lysozyme is shown in panel b, where that portion of the protein is shown in white. A tyrosine residue (green) known to be recognized by the T-cell receptor protrudes into the core of the protein and is inaccessible in the folded protein. For this residue to be accessible to the T-cell receptor the protein must be unfolded and processed. Panel a courtesy of S Sheriff. Panel b courtesy of C Thorpe.

in Chapter 2. T cells always respond to contiguous short sequences in proteins that often lie internal in their structure. This is illustrated clearly in Fig. 4.5, which compares the parts of the lysozyme molecule bound by antibody (see also Fig. 3.13) and those recognized by T cells. The peptides that stimulate T cells are recognized only when bound to the appropriate MHC molecule. This can be shown conclusively by stimulating T cells with purified peptide:MHC complexes.

Purified peptide:MHC complexes have been characterized structurally (Fig. 4.6). The peptide binds to the cleft on the outer face of the MHC molecule so that, viewed from above as a T-cell receptor would see the complex, the peptide occupies the center of this site and, in an MHC class I molecule, is surrounded by the two α helices from the α_1 and α_2 domains. Similarly, in the MHC class II molecule, the peptide is held between the α helices of the α_1 and β_1 domains. Assuming that a T-cell receptor interacts with this ligand much as an antibody does with a protein, then ~700–900 Å^2 of surface area will be in contact with the T-cell receptor, with the periphery consisting of contacts with the MHC molecule and the center of contacts with the peptide fragment of antigen. As we shall see in the last part of this chapter, the most variable part of the T-cell receptor are the central CDR3 loops that are believed to make contact with the peptide.

4-4   Peptides are stably bound to MHC molecules.

Cells make only a few distinct MHC class I molecules but an individual may be infected by a wide variety of different pathogens whose proteins will not necessarily have peptide sequences in common. For example, if T cells are to be alerted to all possible intracellular infections, the MHC class I molecules on each cell must be able to bind stably to many different peptides. This behavior is quite distinct from that of peptide-binding receptors, such as those for peptide hormones, which bind only a single peptide with great specificity. Rather, it resembles the specificity of some proteases where, although the binding site encompasses some six amino acids, only a single amino acid of the substrate determines its ability to bind.

One major difference between MHC molecules and other peptide-binding proteins, however, is that the peptide ligand appears to be an integral part of the structure of the MHC molecule, which is unstable when peptides are not bound. The crystal structures of peptide:MHC complexes have helped to show how a single binding site can bind peptides with high affinity while retaining the ability to bind a wide variety of different peptides.

When MHC class I molecules are purified from cells, their bound peptides co-purify with them, illustrating the tight association between the MHC molecules and their peptide ligands. The peptides can then be eluted from the MHC class I molecules by denaturing the complex in acid, releasing the bound low molecular weight peptides, which can be purified and sequenced.

Pure synthetic versions of these peptides can then be co-crystallized with previously empty MHC class I molecules and the structure of the complex determined, revealing details of the contacts between the MHC molecule and the peptide. Peptides that bind to MHC class I molecules are usually eight to ten amino acids long. The binding of the peptide is stabilized at its two ends by contacts between atoms in the free termini common to most short peptides and invariant sites in the peptide-binding groove of all MHC class I molecules. The terminal amino group of the

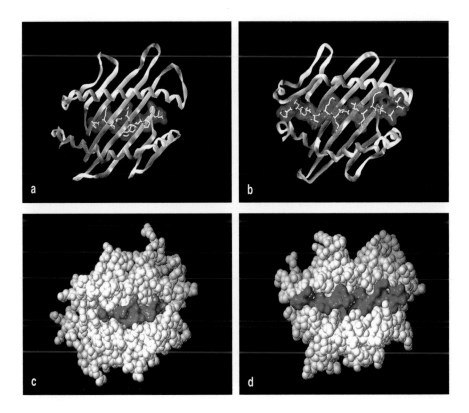

Fig. 4.6 MHC molecules bind peptides tightly within the cleft. The original crystal structure of an MHC class I molecule contained a mixture of naturally occurring peptide antigens and details of the peptide:MHC interaction could not be discerned. When MHC molecules are crystallized with a single synthetic peptide antigen bound to their cleft, the details of peptide binding are revealed. In MHC class I molecules (panel a) the peptide is bound in an elongated conformation with both ends tightly bound at either end of the cleft. In the case of MHC class II molecules (panel b), the peptide is also bound in an elongated conformation but the ends of the peptide are not tightly bound and the peptide extends beyond the cleft. The upper surface of the MHC molecules, the surface recognized by T cells, is composed of residues of the MHC molecule (shown in white for MHC class I molecules in panel c and for MHC class II molecules in panel d) and of the peptide (shown in red in panels c and d).

peptide makes contact with an invariant site at one end of the peptide-binding groove, and the terminal carboxyl group binds to an invariant site at the other end of the groove. The binding of the carboxy terminus may not be an absolute requirement for peptide binding as there is one known example of a peptide binding to a class I molecule where the carboxy-terminal amino acid protrudes from the peptide-binding cleft. The peptide lies in an elongated conformation along the groove; variations in peptide length appear to be accommodated by a kinking in the peptide backbone, although the single case where the peptide is able to extend out of the groove at the carboxy terminus suggests that some length variation may also be accommodated in this way.

In addition to the broad binding specificity provided by these interactions between common structural features, the preference for binding one peptide rather than another arises from interactions of side chains on peptides and MHC molecules. MHC molecules are highly polymorphic and this has consequences for their peptide-binding specificity. The sequences of peptides bound by many different MHC alleles have been determined; peptides binding to a given allelic variant of an MHC molecule have the same or very similar amino acid residues at two or three specific positions along the peptide sequence (Fig. 4.7).

These amino acid side chains insert into pockets in the MHC molecule that are lined by amino acids that vary between the different MHC alleles. Because the binding of these peptide side chains into the pockets anchors the peptide to the MHC molecule, the peptide residues involved have been called **anchor residues**. Most peptides that bind to MHC class I molecules have an anchor residue at the carboxy terminus, and this residue is frequently a hydrophobic or a basic residue. Changing any anchor residue can prevent the peptide from binding, and conversely, most, but not all, synthetic peptides of correct length that contain these anchor residues will bind the appropriate MHC class I

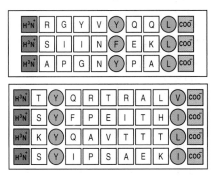

Fig. 4.7 Peptides bind to MHC molecules through relatively invariant anchor residues. Peptides eluted from two different MHC class I molecules are shown. The anchor residues (green) differ for peptides binding different MHC molecules but are similar for all peptides binding to the same MHC molecule. The upper and lower panels show peptides that bind to two different MHC class I molecules respectively. The anchor residues binding a particular MHC molecule need not be identical but are always related (for example, phenylalanine (F) and tyrosine (Y) are both aromatic amino acids, whereas valine (V), leucine (L) and isoleucine (I) are all hydrophobic amino acids). Peptides also bind to MHC class I molecules through their amino (blue) and carboxy termini (red).

molecule, irrespective of the sequence of the peptide at other positions (Fig. 4.7). Thus, the characteristics of peptide binding allow MHC class I molecules to bind a wide variety of different peptides of suitable length. Moreover, because the peptides can kink in the middle where they protrude above the groove and contact the T-cell receptor, the anchor residues are not always at precisely the same position in the linear sequence of peptides that bind to a given MHC class I molecule.

Although only a few residues of the peptide may protrude above the peptide-binding cleft and be available for recognition by the T-cell receptor, T cells are clearly able to discriminate efficiently between different peptide:MHC complexes. From a comparison of the structures of different peptides bound by the same MHC class I molecule, it is clear that even for peptides of the same length, the conformation of the peptide backbone can vary. Finally, when different peptides are bound by the same MHC class I molecule, there can be small changes in the conformation of the class I molecule itself, which could also influence the binding of the T-cell receptor.

Peptide binding to MHC class II molecules has also been analyzed, both by elution of bound peptides and by X-ray crystallography, and they are different in several ways from peptides binding to MHC class I molecules. Peptides that bind to MHC class II molecules are at least 13 amino acids in length and can be much longer; they lie in an extended conformation along the MHC class II peptide-binding groove. The ends of the peptide are not bound by MHC class II molecules, and the clusters of residues in MHC class I molecules that bind the two ends of peptides are not found in MHC class II molecules. Instead, the peptide backbone is held by interactions both with side chains of conserved residues that line the peptide-binding groove and with backbone atoms of the MHC molecule. This way of binding the peptide backbone, together with the more open ends of the MHC class II peptide-binding groove, allows peptides bound to class II molecules to extend beyond the groove at both ends.

Although there are clear differences in specificity of peptide binding between allelic variants of MHC class II molecules, their molecular basis is not yet well established. The sole crystal structure of an MHC class II:peptide complex so far determined indicates that, as for the class I molecules, as well as peptide backbone binding to conserved residues, side chains of the peptide bind into pockets in the MHC molecule composed of polymorphic residues. Patterns of anchor residues in peptides binding to several MHC class II alleles have been defined (Fig. 4.8), and it is possible to see how the differences in sequence of the different alleles could alter the pockets in the class II molecule to give rise to the observed peptide specificities. However, to determine whether these interpretations are correct will require more crystal structures of class II:peptide complexes.

MHC molecules differ from other known peptide-binding proteins in that the binding of peptide appears to be essential for the correct folding and stabilization of the MHC molecule. For both MHC class I and MHC class II molecules, failure to bind peptide results in a molecule that is unstable, and that dissociates readily into its constituent chains. For MHC class I molecules, the important interactions made by the peptide appear to be those involving the amino- and carboxy-termini of the peptide; synthetic peptide analogs lacking terminal amino and carboxyl groups fail to stabilize the class I molecule. For MHC class II molecules the critical interactions are not yet known. Removing a peptide from an MHC molecule requires the partial unfolding of the molecule, which accounts for the extreme stability of most MHC:peptide complexes — the peptides are essentially bound irreversibly.

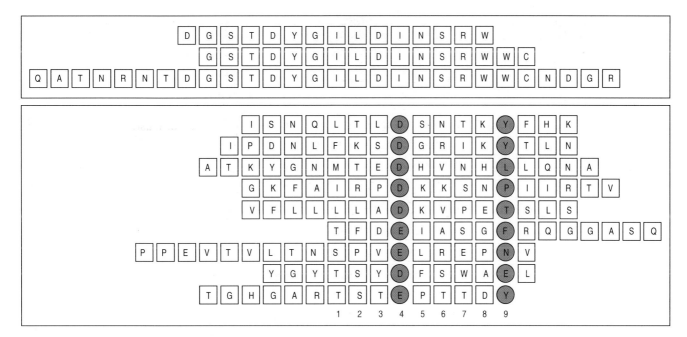

Fig. 4.8 Peptides that bind MHC class II molecules are variable in length and their anchor residues lie at various distances from the ends of the peptide. The sequences of several peptides that bind to the mouse MHC class II allele IA^k are shown in the upper panel. All contain the same core sequence but differ in length. In the lower panel, different peptides binding to the human class II allele HLA-DR3 are shown. The lengths of these peptides can vary, and so by convention the first anchor residue is denoted the P1 residue. Note that all of the peptides share a negatively charged residue (aspartic acid (D) or glutamic acid (E)) in the P4 position (blue) and tend to have a hydrophobic residue (eg tyrosine (Y), leucine (L), proline (P), phenylalanine (F)) in the P9 position (green).

4-5   The two classes of MHC molecule are expressed differentially on cells.

We have seen (in Section 4-1) that the two classes of MHC molecule deliver peptides from different intracellular compartments to the cell surface, where they are recognized by two major functional classes of T cells that can be distinguished on the basis of the cell-surface molecules CD4 and CD8. We shall now see that MHC class I and MHC class II molecules have a distinct distribution among cells that directly reflects the different effector functions of the T cells that recognize them.

As described earlier, MHC class I molecules present peptides from pathogens in the cytosol, commonly viruses, to CD8 cytotoxic T cells, which, once activated, generally kill any cell that they specifically recognize. Because viruses can infect any nucleated cell, almost all such cells express MHC class I molecules, although the level of expression varies from one cell type to the next (Fig. 4.9). Cells of the immune system express abundant MHC class I on their surface, while liver cells (hepatocytes) express relatively low levels. As might be expected, the level of MHC molecule expression influences T-cell activation; cells that express few MHC class I molecules may not be easily killed by cytotoxic T cells.

Non-nucleated cells such as mammalian red blood cells express little or no MHC class I, and thus the interior of red blood cells is a site in which an infection can go undetected by cytotoxic T cells. As red blood cells cannot support viral replication, this is of no great consequence for viral infection, but it may be the absence of MHC class I that allows the *Plasmodium* species that cause malaria to live in this privileged site.

The main function of CD4 T cells by contrast is to activate other cells of the immune system. Thus MHC class II molecules are normally found on B lymphocytes and macrophages — cells that participate in immune

Fig. 4.9 The expression of MHC molecules differs between tissues.
MHC class I molecules are expressed on all nucleated cells, although they are most highly expressed in hematopoetic cells. MHC class II molecules are only expressed by a subset of hematopoietic cells and by thymic stromal cells.
* In humans, activated T cells express MHC class II molecules.
† In the brain, most cell types are MHC class II negative but microglia, which are related to macrophages, are MHC class II positive.

Tissue	MHC class I	MHC class II
Lymphoid tissues		
T cells	+++	– *
B cells	+++	+++
Macrophages	+++	++
Other antigen-presenting cells (eg Langerhans' cells)	+++	+++
Epithelial cells of the thymus	+	+++
Other nucleated cells		
Neutrophils	+++	–
Hepatocytes	+	–
Kidney	+	–
Brain	+	– †
Non-nucleated cells		
Red blood cells	–	–

responses — but not on other tissue cells (see Fig. 4.9). When **helper CD4 T cells** (T$_H$2) recognize peptides bound to MHC class II molecules on B cells, they stimulate the B cells to produce antibody. Likewise, **inflammatory CD4 T cells** (T$_H$1) recognizing peptides bound to MHC class II molecules on macrophages activate these cells to destroy the pathogens in their vesicles. We shall see in Chapter 7 that MHC class II molecules are also expressed on specialized antigen-presenting cells in lymphoid tissues where encounter with antigen first primes naive T cells to become effector T cells and induces CD4 T cells to differentiate into effector T$_H$1 or T$_H$2 cells. Many other cell types can be induced to express MHC class II molecules by cytokines released during immune responses. This may be very important both in normal immune functioning and in autoimmunity.

4-6   Peptides that bind to MHC class I molecules are actively transported from cytosol to the endoplasmic reticulum.

Typically, the antigen fragments that bind to MHC class I molecules for presentation to CD8 T cells are derived from viruses that take over the cell's biosynthetic machinery to make their own proteins in the cytosol or nucleus. Proteins destined for the cell surface, including both classes of MHC molecule, are translocated during synthesis from the cytosol into the lumen of the endoplasmic reticulum, where they must fold correctly before they can be transported to the cell surface. Since the peptide-binding site of the MHC class I molecule is first formed in the lumen of the endoplasmic reticulum, how are peptides derived from viral proteins in the cytosol able to bind to MHC class I molecules for delivery to the cell surface?

The answer to this question was first suggested by mutant cells with a defect in antigen presentation by MHC class I molecules. Although both chains of MHC class I molecules are synthesized normally in these cells, the MHC class I proteins are expressed only at very low levels on the cell surface. This defect in class I expression could be corrected by the addition of synthetic peptides, suggesting that the mutation affects the supply of peptides to MHC class I molecules, and that peptide is required for their normal cell-surface expression.

Analysis of the affected DNA in the mutant cells supported this view: two genes encoding members of the ATP-binding cassette, or ABC, family of proteins were mutant or absent in several cells with this phenotype. These two genes map within the MHC itself (see Section 4-13). ATP-binding cassette proteins are found associated with membranes in many cells, including bacterial cells, and they are always involved in ATP-dependent transport, whether of ions, sugars, amino acids, or peptides, across these membranes. The two ATP-binding cassette proteins deleted in the mutant cells are associated with the endoplasmic reticulum membrane, and transfection of the mutant cells with both genes restores the ability of the cell's MHC class I molecules to present peptides of cytosolic proteins. These proteins are now called **Transporters associated with Antigen Processing-1** and **-2 (TAP-1** and **TAP-2)**. The two TAP proteins form a heterodimer (Fig. 4.10) and mutations in either *TAP* gene prevent antigen presentation by MHC class I molecules.

In assays *in vitro* using microsomal vesicles that mimic the endoplasmic reticulum, vesicles from normal cells will internalize peptides, which then bind to MHC class I molecules already present in the microsomal lumen. Vesicles from TAP-1 or TAP-2 mutant cells do not transport peptides. Peptide transport into the normal microsomes requires ATP hydrolysis, proving that the TAP-1:TAP-2 complex is an ATP-dependent peptide transporter that selectively loads peptides into the lumen of the endoplasmic reticulum. Such experiments have also shown that the TAP transporter has some specificity for the peptides it will transport. The TAP-1:TAP-2 transporter prefers peptides of eight or more amino acids with hydrophobic or basic residues at the carboxy terminus, the exact features of peptides that bind MHC class I molecules. In the rat, there are two allelic variants of the TAP-2 transporter that differ in their capacity to transport peptides. One variant (TAP-2^a) transports peptides with either basic or hydrophobic carboxy-terminal residues, while the other (TAP-2^u) transports only those peptides with hydrophobic carboxy-terminal residues. Genetic variation in the TAP proteins can thus affect the repertoire of peptides available for binding by MHC class I molecules; hence the original description of the *TAP-2* locus in the rat as the class I modifier, or *cim*, locus.

4-7   Newly synthesized MHC class I molecules are retained in the endoplasmic reticulum by binding to TAP-1 until they bind peptide.

The discovery of the TAP-1:TAP-2 heterodimer explained how peptides get from the cytosol to the lumen of the endoplasmic reticulum, and its ability to restore antigen presentation in mutant cells suggested that peptide binding is necessary for the cell-surface expression of newly synthesized MHC class I molecules. We shall now see that newly synthesized MHC class I molecules are held in the endoplasmic reticulum in a

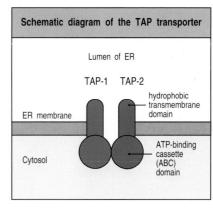

Schematic diagram of the TAP transporter

Lumen of ER

TAP-1   TAP-2

hydrophobic transmembrane domain

ER membrane

Cytosol

ATP-binding cassette (ABC) domain

Fig. 4.10 The TAP-1 and TAP-2 transporter molecules form a heterodimer in the endoplasmic reticulum membrane. All protein molecules that belong to the ATP-binding casette (ABC) transporter family have four domains, two transmembrane domains and two ATP-binding domains. Both TAP-1 and TAP-2 encode one hydrophobic and one ATP-binding domain and assemble into a heterodimer to form a four-domain transporter. On the basis of similarities between the TAP molecules and other members of the ABC-transporter family it is believed that the ATP-binding domains lie within the cytoplasm of the cell, while the hydrophobic domains project through the membrane into the lumen of the endoplasmic reticulum (ER).

partially folded state until they bind peptide, and that without bound peptide the MHC class I molecule is unstable. This explains why cells with mutations in *TAP-1* or *TAP-2* fail to express MHC class I molecules at the cell surface.

In humans, newly synthesized MHC class I α chains rapidly bind an 88 kDa membrane-bound protein known as **calnexin**, which retains the MHC class I molecule in a partially folded state in the endoplasmic reticulum. Calnexin also associates with partially folded T-cell receptors, immunoglobulins, and MHC class II molecules, and so has a central role in the assembly of many molecules important in immunology. When β_2-microglobulin binds to the α chain, the α:β_2-microglobulin complex dissociates from calnexin and now binds to the TAP-1 subunit of the transporter, awaiting the transport of a suitable peptide from the cytosol. Finally, the binding of a peptide to the partially folded MHC class I molecule releases it from TAP and allows the now fully folded class I molecule to leave the endoplasmic reticulum and be transported to the cell surface (Fig. 4.11). Most of the peptides transported by TAP will not bind to the MHC molecules in that cell and are cleared out of the endoplasmic reticulum rapidly; there is evidence that they are transported back into the cytosol by an ATP-dependent transport mechanism distinct from the TAP transporter.

It is not yet clear whether the TAP transporter plays a direct role in loading class I molecules with peptide or whether binding to the TAP transporter merely allows the class I molecule to see a high local concentration of peptide before the peptides diffuse through the lumen of the endoplasmic reticulum and are transported back into the cytosol. One consequence of the binding of class I molecules to the TAP

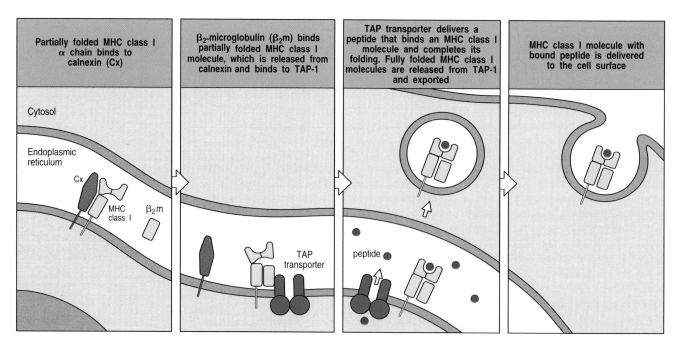

Fig. 4.11 MHC class I molecules do not leave the endoplasmic reticulum unless they bind peptides. Peptides generated by degradation of proteins in the cytoplasm are transported into the lumen of the endoplasmic reticulum. MHC class I α chains assemble in the endoplasmic reticulum with a membrane-bound protein, calnexin (Cx). When this complex binds β_2-microglobulin (β_2m) it is released from calnexin and the partially folded MHC class I molecule then binds to the TAP-1 subunit of the TAP transporter and is retained within the endoplasmic reticulum. Release of the MHC class I molecule from TAP-1 is dependent on the binding of a peptide, which completes the folding of the MHC class I molecule. The peptide:MHC complex is then transported through the Golgi complex to the cell surface.

transporter is that it effectively allows class I molecules to scan every peptide transported into the endoplasmic reticulum and to select those that will bind for transport to the cell surface.

In cells with mutant *TAP* genes, the MHC class I molecules are unstable and appear to be degraded within the endoplasmic reticulum, indicating that it is the binding of peptide to the MHC class I molecule that allows it to complete its folding and releases it from the endoplasmic reticulum. Even in normal cells, MHC class I molecules are retained in the endoplasmic reticulum for some time, suggesting that MHC class I molecules are usually present in excess of peptide. This is very important for the function of MHC class I molecules because they must be immediately available to transport viral peptides to the cell surface at any time the cell becomes infected. In uninfected cells, peptides derived from self proteins fill the peptide-binding cleft of mature MHC class I molecules present at the cell surface. When a cell is infected by a virus, the presence of excess MHC class I molecules in the endoplasmic reticulum allows the rapid presentation at the infected cell's surface of peptides derived from the pathogen.

4-8	**Peptides of cytosolic proteins are generated in the cytosol prior to transport into the endoplasmic reticulum.**

Proteins in cells are degraded continuously and replaced with newly synthesized proteins. A major part in cytosolic protein degradation is played by a large, multicatalytic protease complex of 28 subunits, each between 20 to 30 kDa, called the **proteasome** (Fig. 4.12). Various lines of evidence implicate the proteasome in the production of peptide ligands for MHC class I molecules. For example, the proteasome takes part in the ubiquitin-dependent degradation pathway for cytosolic proteins; experimentally tagging proteins with ubiquitin also results in the more efficient presentation of their peptides by MHC class I molecules. Moreover, inhibitors of the proteolytic activity of the proteasome also inhibit antigen presentation by class I molecules. Thus it is likely that the proteasome can generate peptides for transport into the endoplasmic reticulum, although whether it is the only cytosolic protease capable of so doing is not known.

Two subunits of the proteasome, called LMP2 and LMP7, first identified as low molecular weight polypeptides by immunoprecipitation with anti-MHC antisera (see Section 2-13), are encoded within the MHC near the *TAP-1* and *TAP-2* genes (see Section 4-13) and, like the MHC class I and TAP molecules, their expression is induced by interferons. Expression of the LMP2 and LMP7 subunits displaces two constitutive subunits from the proteasome. A third subunit, MECL-1, which is not encoded within the MHC, is also induced by interferon treatment and also displaces a constitutive proteasome subunit. Comparison of proteasome components with those of archebacterial proteasomes, whose structure is known, suggests that only these three inducible subunits and their constitutive counterparts are likely to be active proteases. The replacement of the constitutive components by their interferon-inducible counterparts is thus likely to change the activity of the proteasome; experimental evidence suggests that, in interferon-treated cells, the specificity of the proteasome is changed to increase cleavage of polypeptides after hydrophobic and basic residues and to inhibit cleavage after acidic residues. This produces peptides with carboxy-terminal residues that are the preferred anchor residues for peptide binding to most MHC class I molecules and are also the preferred structures for transport by TAP. The MHC thus encodes molecules essential for the production and translocation of cytosolic peptides and their presentation at the cell surface.

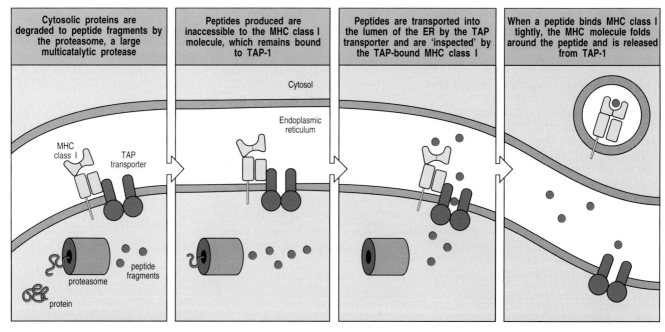

| Cytosolic proteins are degraded to peptide fragments by the proteasome, a large multicatalytic protease | Peptides produced are inaccessible to the MHC class I molecule, which remains bound to TAP-1 | Peptides are transported into the lumen of the ER by the TAP transporter and are 'inspected' by the TAP-bound MHC class I | When a peptide binds MHC class I tightly, the MHC molecule folds around the peptide and is released from TAP-1 |

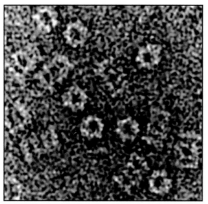

Fig. 4.12 Degradation and transport of antigens that bind MHC class I molecules. The source of peptides for MHC class I molecules is the degradation of proteins in the cytosol. It is believed that the digestion of cytosolic proteins is carried out by a large protease complex, the proteasome. The proteasome contains 28 subunits arranged, as shown in the electron micrograph, to form a cylindrical structure composed of four rings, each of seven subunits. It is not known how the proteasome degrades cytosolic proteins. Here we show a protein unfolding and passing through the center of the cylindrical structure but there is no evidence that this is what really happens. Peptide fragments generated by the proteasome are transported into the lumen of the endoplasmic reticulum (ER) by the TAP transporter. There, the peptides bind to the complex of the partially folded MHC molecule and TAP-1, liberating the MHC class I molecule and allowing the peptide:MHC complex to be delivered to the cell surface. Photograph (x 667 000) courtesy of W Baumeister.

If the peptides that bind to MHC class I molecules are produced in the cytosol of the cell, how can MHC class I molecules present peptide fragments of membrane or secreted proteins, which are normally translocated into the lumen of the endoplasmic reticulum during their synthesis? Probably, a small fraction of such proteins fails to be synthesized and translocated correctly into the endoplasmic reticulum and, instead, remains within the cytosol where it is degraded into peptides. Certain amino-terminal amino acids that protect cell-surface and secreted proteins from degradation in the endoplasmic reticulum are associated with rapid degradation in the cytosol (and vice versa); thus, any misdirected cell-surface or secreted proteins that end up in the cytosol will be targeted for rapid degradation, providing a source of peptides that can be transported across the endoplasmic reticulum membrane to interact with MHC class I molecules. This mechanism may explain, for example, how viral envelope glycoproteins produce peptides that are presented by MHC class I molecules.

4-9   Peptides presented by MHC class II molecules are generated in acidified intracellular vesicles.

Whereas viruses and some bacteria replicate in the cytosol, several classes of pathogens, including *Leishmania* species and the mycobacteria that cause leprosy and tuberculosis, replicate in intracellular vesicles in macrophages. As they reside in membrane-enclosed vesicles, the proteins of these pathogens are not accessible to proteasomes. Instead, proteins in these sites are degraded by vesicular proteases into peptides that bind to MHC class II molecules, which deliver them to the cell surface (Fig. 4.13). Here they are recognized by CD4 T cells. CD4 T cells also recognize peptide fragments derived from extracellular pathogens and proteins that are internalized into similar intracellular vesicles.

Most of what we know about the processing of proteins in vesicles has come from experiments in which simple proteins are added to MHC class II positive antigen-presenting cells because, in this way, processing of added antigen can be quantified. This pathway is also crucial in the processing of proteins that bind to surface immunoglobulin on B cells and are internalized by endocytosis.

Internalized protein antigens enter cells through endocytosis and become enclosed in vesicles — endosomes — in which they are eventually degraded. The vesicles on the endosomal pathway become increasingly acidic with progress down the pathway, and contain proteases, known as acid proteases, that are activated at low pH.

Drugs that raise the pH of vesicles inhibit the processing of proteins that enter the cell in this way, suggesting that acid proteases are important in antigen processing in these vesicles. Among these acid proteases are cathepsins B and D, and cathepsin L, which is the most active enzyme in this family of related proteases. Antigen processing can be mimicked to some extent by digestion of proteins with these enzymes *in vitro* at acid pH. Proteins of pathogens growing in intracellular vesicles are also handled by this pathway of antigen processing.

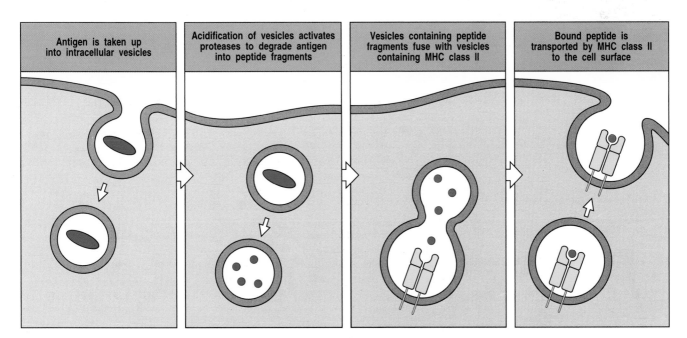

| Antigen is taken up into intracellular vesicles | Acidification of vesicles activates proteases to degrade antigen into peptide fragments | Vesicles containing peptide fragments fuse with vesicles containing MHC class II | Bound peptide is transported by MHC class II to the cell surface |

Fig. 4.13 Antigens that bind to MHC class II molecules are degraded in acidified endosomes. In some cases, the source of the peptides may be bacteria or parasites that have invaded the cell and replicate in intracellular vesicles. In other cases, as illustrated here, microorganisms or foreign proteins may be engulfed by phagocytic cells and routed to lysosomes for degradation. En route to the lysosomes, the pH of the vesicles (endosomes) containing the engulfed pathogens progressively decreases, activating proteases that reside within the endosome to degrade the engulfed material. At some point on their pathway to the cell surface, newly synthesized MHC class II molecules pass through such acidified endosomes and bind peptide fragments of the pathogens, transporting the peptides to the cell surface.

| 4-10 | **The invariant chain directs newly synthesized MHC class II molecules to acidified intracellular vesicles.** |

The function of MHC class II molecules is to present peptides generated in the intracellular vesicles of B cells, macrophages, and other antigen-presenting cells to CD4 T cells. However, the biosynthetic pathway for MHC class II molecules, like that of other cell-surface glycoproteins, starts with their translocation into the endoplasmic reticulum, and they must therefore be prevented from binding prematurely to peptides transported into the endoplasmic reticulum lumen by the TAP transporter. It may be even more important to avoid binding to the cell's own nascent polypeptides, given the ability of MHC class II molecules to bind such structures owing to the open ends of the peptide-binding groove. As the endoplasmic reticulum is richly endowed with unfolded and partially folded proteins, one needs a general mechanism to avoid MHC class II binding to peptides or proteins.

This is achieved by the assembly of newly synthesized MHC class II molecules, with a specialized protein known as the MHC class II-associated **invariant chain (Ii)**. The invariant chain forms trimers, with each subunit binding non-covalently to a class II α:β heterodimer (Fig. 4.14; for convenience, we show the MHC class II:invariant chain complex as only a single α:β:Ii complex). While this complex is being assembled in the endoplasmic reticulum, its component parts are associated with calnexin. Only when assembly is completed to produce a nine-chain complex is it released from calnexin for transport onward from the endoplasmic reticulum. In this nine-chain complex, the MHC class II molecule cannot bind peptides or unfolded proteins, so that peptides present in the endoplasmic reticulum are not usually presented by

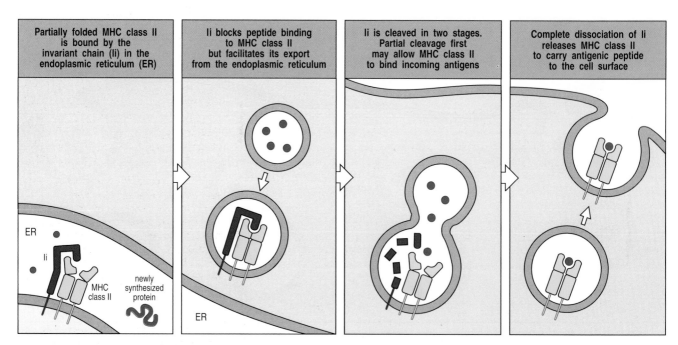

| Partially folded MHC class II is bound by the invariant chain (Ii) in the endoplasmic reticulum (ER) | Ii blocks peptide binding to MHC class II but facilitates its export from the endoplasmic reticulum | Ii is cleaved in two stages. Partial cleavage first may allow MHC class II to bind incoming antigens | Complete dissociation of Ii releases MHC class II to carry antigenic peptide to the cell surface |

Fig. 4.14　The MHC class II-associated invariant chain delays peptide binding and targets MHC class II molecules to the endosomes. The invariant chain (Ii) assembles with newly synthesized MHC class II molecules in the endoplasmic reticulum where it prevents the MHC class II molecule from binding intracellular peptides and partially folded proteins present in the lumen, and directs its export through the Golgi apparatus, to acidified endosomes containing peptides of resident bacteria or engulfed extracellular proteins. Here the invariant chain is cleaved, freeing the MHC class II molecule to bind peptide and be transported to the cell surface.

MHC class II molecules. Moreover, in the absence of invariant chains there is evidence that many MHC class II molecules are retained in the endoplasmic reticulum as complexes with misfolded proteins.

The invariant chain has a second function, which is to target delivery of the MHC class II molecules from the endoplasmic reticulum to an appropriate low pH endosomal compartment. The complex of MHC class II $\alpha{:}\beta$ heterodimers with invariant chain is retained for two to four hours in this compartment. During this time, the invariant chain is cleaved by proteases such as cathepsin L at several sites (see Fig. 4.14). The cleavage is ordered, so that the initial cleavage events generate a truncated form of the invariant chain that remains bound to the MHC class II molecule and retains it within the proteolytic compartment. A subsequent cleavage releases the MHC class II molecule, bound to a short fragment of Ii, called CLIP (for class II-associated invariant-chain peptide). MHC class II molecules that have CLIP associated with them are still prevented from binding other peptides and CLIP must either dissociate or be displaced in order for the MHC class II molecule to bind processed peptide and deliver it to the cell surface.

The intracellular location at which invariant chain is cleaved and MHC class II molecules encounter peptides is not clearly defined. Most newly synthesized MHC class II molecules are thought to travel to the cell surface in vesicles, which, at some point after leaving the trans-Golgi network, fuse with the incoming endosomes. However, there is also evidence that some class II:Ii complexes are transported first to the cell surface and then re-internalized into endosomes. Nevertheless, in either case, MHC class II:Ii complexes enter the endosomal pathway and are there exposed to an acidic, proteolytic environment in which both the invariant chain is cleaved and pathogens and their proteins are broken down into peptides available for binding to the class II molecule. Electron microscopic studies using antibodies tagged with gold particles to reveal the intracellular location of MHC class II molecules and invariant chain suggest that there is a specialized vesicular compartment, called the MIIC (MHC class II compartment), where the final cleavage of the invariant chain and the interaction of the class II molecule with peptide occur (Fig. 4.15). Parallel experiments, using density-gradient centrifugation or free-flow electrophoresis to separate intracellular vesicles, also suggest the presence of a specialized intracellular vesicle, in this case called the CIIV (class II vesicle), in which MHC class II molecules accumulate before encounter with peptide antigens.

It is likely that both the MIIC and the CIIV are descriptions of the same vesicular compartment, although this is yet to be proven. The MIIC/CIIV compartment lies late in the endosomal pathway, shortly before endocytosed pathogens and proteins would enter the lysosome, and bears some similarities to an intracellular compartment called the multivesicular body, where it is believed that endosomal vesicles are sorted into those that progress to the lysosome and those that return to the cell surface. This compartment is an attractive candidate for the site at which MHC class II molecules interact with peptide fragments and from which the MHC class II:peptide complexes are transported to the cell surface.

As with MHC class I molecules, MHC class II molecules in uninfected cells bind peptides derived from self proteins. MHC class II molecules that do not bind peptide after dissociation from the invariant chain aggregate and are rapidly degraded at the acidic pH of the endosomal compartment. It is therefore not surprising that peptides derived from the MHC class II molecules themselves form a large proportion of the peptides presented by MHC class II molecules in normal cells. This suggests that, as for MHC class I molecules, excess MHC class II molecules are generated. Thus, when a cell is infected by mycobacteria or other

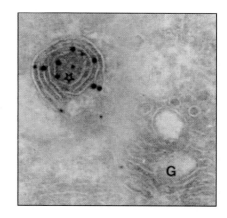

Fig. 4.15 The electron micrograph shows the site where the two pathways, containing internalized proteins and MHC class II molecules, meet, the protein being degraded into peptides and binding to the empty MHC class II molecules. The specialized vesicle in which MHC class II interact with antigen is indicated by a star, and the presence of MHC class II molecules in this compartment is revealed by immunogold staining (see Section 2-13) with 5 nm gold particles (small dots). The presence of the MHC class II-like molecule, DM, in the same compartment is also shown by staining with 10 nm gold particles (larger dots). The Golgi apparatus is also shown (G). Photograph courtesy of F Sanderson.

engulfs a pathogen or a B cell binds antigen to its immunoglobulin receptor, the peptides generated from them find plentiful empty MHC class II molecules to bind. These MHC class II:foreign peptide complexes can then be presented at the cell surface. There, they are recognized by the two subsets of CD4 T cells whose functions are to activate macrophages or B cells.

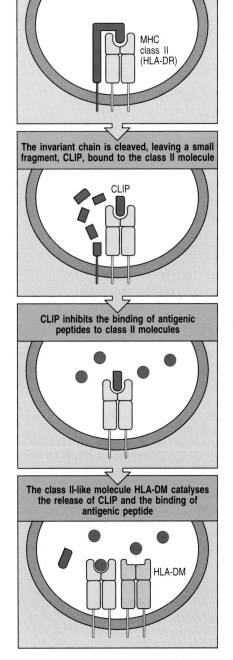

Class II molecules are transported to the MHC in association with the invariant chain

MHC class II (HLA-DR)

The invariant chain is cleaved, leaving a small fragment, CLIP, bound to the class II molecule

CLIP

CLIP inhibits the binding of antigenic peptides to class II molecules

The class II-like molecule HLA-DM catalyses the release of CLIP and the binding of antigenic peptide

HLA-DM

Fig. 4.16 HLA-DM facilitates the loading of antigenic peptides onto MHC class II molecules. As a result of the proteolysis of the invariant chain, a small fragment, called the class II-associated invariant chain peptide, or CLIP, remains bound to the MHC class II molecule, in this example HLA-DR (top panel). Under normal circumstances the CLIP peptide is replacd by antigenic peptides but, in the absence of HLA-DM, this does not occur. The HLA-DM molecule must therefore play some part in removal of the CLIP peptide and in the loading of antigenic peptides. It appears to act catalytically, since it can function at sub-stoichiometric levels.

4-11 **A specialized MHC class II-like molecule catalyzes loading of MHC class II molecules with endogenously processed peptides.**

While many steps in the assembly and export of MHC class II molecules are known, the details of how the MHC class II molecule meets up with a peptide fragment of antigen and binds to it remain obscure. This has been highlighted by experimental observations in mutant human B cell lines in which the correct interaction of MHC class II molecules with peptide antigens does not occur. As with the MHC class I molecule, binding of peptide to the MHC class II molecule is required to create a stable dimer and, in these mutant cells, the class II molecule dissociates readily into its component α and β chains. For this reason the mutation in these cells was called the 'falling-apart' mutation. Further analysis of MHC class II molecules in these mutant cell lines has shown that they assemble correctly with the invariant chain, and seem to be transported to a compartment where the invariant chain is cleaved. However, peptides derived from proteins that have been internalized and degraded within the endosomal pathway do not bind to the MHC class II molecules in the mutant cells and the CLIP peptide remains associated with many class II molecules.

The defect in these 'falling-apart' cells lies in a class II-like molecule, called **HLA-DM** (H2-M in mice), which is encoded near the *TAP* and LMP genes in the class II region of the MHC (see Fig. 4.17). The HLA-DM locus encodes an α chain and a β chain that closely resemble those of other MHC class II molecules, although, unlike other class II molecules, it does not appear to require peptide in order to generate a stable dimeric molecule. The DM molecule also differs from other MHC class II molecules in that it is not expressed at the cell surface but rather is found predominantly in the MIIC/CIIV compartment within the cell. From experiments that involved mixing HLA-DR:CLIP complexes from the cells with the 'falling apart' mutation either with DM alone or with both DM and antigenic peptides, it has recently been shown how the HLA-DM molecule is able to direct the loading of peptides onto other MHC class II molecules. With the addition of DM alone, the stability of HLA-DR is not restored; but it is restored if antigenic peptides are also added. This suggests that HLA-DM is needed for the exchange of CLIP with antigenic peptides. Moreover, the work suggests that DM molecules catalyze HLA-DR peptide loading since they stabilize HLA-DR molecules purified from DM negative cells, when added at sub-stoichiometric amounts together with peptide.

The role of the DM molecule in facilitating the binding of peptides to MHC class II molecules appears to parallel the role of the TAP molecules in facilitating the binding of peptides to class I molecules. Thus it seems likely that both classes of molecule interact inefficiently with peptides free in solution and that a specialized mechanism to deliver peptides efficiently has co-evolved with the MHC molecules themselves.

| 4-12 | **The characteristics of peptide binding by MHC molecules allow effective antigen presentation at the cell surface.** |

The ability of MHC molecules to bind a wide range of different peptides is essential for detection of intracellular pathogens by T cells. It is important that the peptide:MHC complex should be stable at the cell surface. If the complex were to dissociate too readily, the pathogen in the infected cell could escape detection. Also, MHC molecules on uninfected cells could pick up peptides released by dissociated MHC molecules on infected cells; this could falsely signal to cytotoxic T cells that a healthy cell is infected, resulting in its unwanted destruction. The stable binding of peptide by MHC molecules makes both these undesirable outcomes unlikely.

It can be seen from the peptide:MHC complexes shown in Fig. 4.6 that the peptide is actually enclosed within the three-dimensional structure of the MHC molecule. Moreover, it can be shown that peptide:MHC complexes expressed on live cells are lost at the same rate as the MHC molecule itself, indicating that the binding of peptide is essentially irreversible. This stability of binding permits even rare peptides to be transported efficiently to the cell surface by MHC molecules, and allows long-term display of these complexes on the surface of the infected cell, thus fulfilling the first of the requirements for effective antigen presentation.

The second criterion for effective antigen presentation is that if dissociation of a peptide from an MHC molecule should occur, new peptides would not be able to bind to the now empty peptide-binding groove. Indeed, if one were to remove the peptide from the binding cleft shown in Fig. 4.6, then structural considerations would predict that this MHC class I molecule would be unstable. In fact, removal of the peptide from a purified MHC class I molecule denatures the molecule. When peptide dissociates at the cell surface, the MHC class I molecule changes conformation, the β_2-microglobulin moiety dissociates, and the α chain is internalized and rapidly degraded. Thus, empty MHC class I molecules are quickly lost from the cell surface.

At neutral pH, empty MHC class II molecules are more stable than empty MHC class I molecules, yet empty class II molecules are also removed from the cell surface. Peptide loss from MHC class II molecules is most likely when the class II molecules are recycled through acidified intracellular vesicles. At the acidic pH of these endocytic vesicles, MHC class II molecules that are not associated with peptides aggregate and are rapidly degraded. Thus loss of peptide again leads to the rapid loss of the empty MHC molecule. This feature of peptide binding is important in the antigen presentation function of MHC molecules as it helps to prevent the MHC molecules on a cell surface from acquiring peptides from the surrounding extracellular fluid. This ensures that T cells act selectively on infected cells that efficiently display foreign peptides bound to MHC molecules on their surfaces, while sparing surrounding healthy cells.

Summary.

The most distinctive feature of antigen recognition by T cells is the form of the ligand recognized by the T-cell receptor. This comprises a peptide derived from the foreign antigen bound to an MHC molecule. MHC molecules are cell-surface glycoproteins whose non-cytoplasmic face has a peptide-binding groove that can bind a wide variety of different peptides. The MHC molecule binds the peptide in an intracellular location and delivers it to the cell surface, where the combined ligand can be recognized by a T cell. There are two classes of MHC molecule, MHC class I and MHC class II, which deliver peptides from proteins degraded in different intracellular sites. MHC class II molecules, which present peptides to CD4 T cells, bind peptides from proteins that are degraded in acidified intracellular vesicles. Typically, macrophages infected with mycobacteria, or a B cell that has bound and internalized a specific protein antigen, will present peptides from these foreign proteins bound to MHC class II molecules to CD4 T cells, which then activate the macrophage or B cell. MHC class I molecules, which present peptides to CD8 T cells, bind peptides from proteins degraded in the cytosol. Typically, foreign peptides presented by MHC class I molecules come from viral proteins, and the CD8 T cell kills the infected cell upon recognizing the foreign peptide:MHC class I complex on the cell surface. Thus, the two classes of MHC molecule deliver peptides from different cellular compartments to the cell surface where they are recognized by T cells mediating distinct and appropriate effector functions.

The major histocompatibility complex of genes: organization and polymorphism.

As we have seen, the function of the MHC molecules is to bind peptide fragments derived from pathogens by degradation inside the cell and to display those fragments on the cell surface where the complex is recognized by the appropriate T cells. The consequences of such presentation are almost always deleterious to the pathogen; virus-infected cells are killed, macrophages are activated to kill bacteria in intracellular vesicles, and B cells are activated to produce antibody molecules capable of eliminating or neutralizing extracellular pathogens. Thus, there is strong selective pressure in favor of any pathogen that can mutate its structural genes to escape presentation by an MHC molecule, allowing it to survive undetected by the host immune system.

Two separate mechanisms counter this means of evading immune responses: first, the MHC is **polygenic** — there are several MHC class I and MHC class II genes, encoding proteins with different ranges of peptide-binding specificities; second, the MHC is highly **polymorphic** — there are multiple alleles of each gene. The MHC genes are, in fact, the most polymorphic genes known. In this section, we shall describe the organization of the genes in the MHC and discuss how the allelic variation in MHC molecules arises. We shall also see how the effect of polygeny and polymorphism on the range of peptides bound contributes to the ability of the immune system to respond to a multitude of different and rapidly evolving pathogens. Finally, we shall see that the polymorphism of MHC molecules places unique constraints on the T-cell receptor repertoire, such that T cells can only recognize peptides bound to the MHC molecules present at the time of T-cell **priming** (see Chapter 7). This property is called MHC restriction of the T-cell response.

4-13 | The proteins involved in antigen processing and presentation are encoded by genes in the major histocompatibility complex.

The major histocompatibility complex extends over 2–3 centimorgans of DNA, or about 4×10^6 base pairs, and contains at least 50 genes in humans. The genes encoding the α chains of MHC class I molecules and the α and β chains of MHC class II molecules are linked within the complex; the genes for β_2-microglobulin and the invariant chain lie on separate chromosomes. Fig. 4.17 shows the general organization of these genes in the MHC of humans and of the mouse. Separate regions contain the genes encoding the MHC class I and MHC class II molecules, and within these regions there are several genes for each chain.

In humans, there are three class I α-chain genes, called HLA-A, -B, and -C. There are also three pairs of MHC class II α- and β-chain genes, called HLA-DR, -DP, and -DQ. However, the HLA-DR cluster contains an extra β-chain gene, whose product can pair with the DRα chain. This means that the three sets of genes give rise to four types of MHC class II molecule. All the MHC class I and class II molecules are capable of presenting antigens to T cells and, as each protein binds a different range of peptides, the presence of several loci means that any one individual is equipped to present a much broader range of different peptides than if only one MHC protein of each class were expressed at the cell surface.

The two *TAP* genes lie in the MHC class II region, in close association with the *LMP* genes that encode components of the proteasome. The genetic linkage of the MHC class I molecules, which deliver cytosolic peptides to the cell surface, with the *TAP* and proteasome genes, which encode the molecules that generate these peptides in the cytosol and transport them into the endoplasmic reticulum, suggests that the entire major histocompatibility gene complex has been selected during evolution for antigen processing and presentation.

Moreover, when cells are treated with the cytokines interferon-α, -β or -γ, transcription of MHC class I α chain, β_2-microglobulin, and the MHC-linked proteasome and *TAP* genes are all markedly increased.

Fig. 4.17 The genetic organization of the major histocompatibility complex in humans and the mouse. The organization of the principal MHC genes is shown for both human (where the MHC is called HLA and is on chromosome 6) and mouse (in which the MHC is called H-2 and is on chromosome 17). The organization of the MHC genes is similar in both species. There are separate regions of class I and of class II genes, although in the mouse a class I gene appears to have translocated relative to the human MHC so that, in mice, the class I region is split in two. In both species there are three main class I genes, which are called HLA-A, -B, and -C in humans and H2-K, -D, and -L in the mouse. The gene for β_2-microglobulin, although it encodes part of the MHC class I molecule, is located on a different chromosome, chromosome 15 in humans and chromosome 2 in the mouse. The genes for the TAP-1:TAP-2 peptide transporter, the LMP genes that encode proteasome subunits, and the DMA and DMB genes (encoding DMα and DMβ chains) are all in the MHC class II region as well. The so-called class III genes encode various other proteins with functions in immunity (see Fig. 4.18).

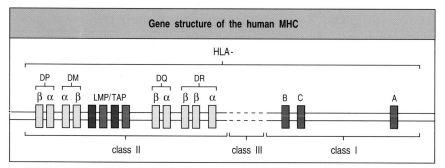

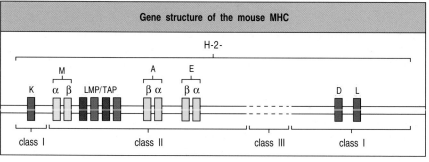

Interferon-γ is produced early in viral infections as part of the innate immune response, as described in more detail in Chapter 9, and this effect of interferon-γ, which increases the ability of cells to process viral proteins and present the resulting peptides at the cell surface, can help to activate T cells and initiate the later phases of the immune response. The coordinated regulation of the genes encoding these components may be facilitated by the linkage of many of them in the MHC.

The DM genes, whose function is to catalyze peptide binding to MHC class II molecules, are clearly related to the class II genes, and no particular conclusions can be drawn from their placement in the MHC class II region. There is also coordinate regulation of the DM genes with those encoding other class II molecules and the invariant chain; the expression of all is induced by interferon-γ (but not by interferon-α or -β), and expression of all results from the action of an **MHC class II transactivator (CIITA)** whose production is stimulated by interferon-γ. The absence of CIITA in patients with the bare lymphocyte syndrome causes severe immunodeficiency as described later in Chapter 10.

| 4-14 | **A variety of genes with specialized functions in immunity are also encoded in the MHC.** |

While the most important known function of the gene products of the MHC is the processing and presentation of antigens to T cells, many other genes map within this region and, although some of these are known to have other roles in the immune system, many have yet to be characterized functionally. Fig. 4.18 shows the detailed organization of the human MHC.

In addition to the highly polymorphic MHC class I and class II genes, there are several MHC class I genes encoding variants of these proteins that show little polymorphism, most of which have no known function. Many genes linked to the class I region of the major histocompatibility complex encode class I-like α chains; the exact number of genes varies greatly between species and even between members of the same species. These genes have been termed **class IB** genes, and like MHC class I genes, they encode β2-microglobulin-associated cell-surface molecules. Their expression on cells is variable, both in terms of the amount expressed at the cell surface and the tissue distribution.

In mice, one of these molecules, H2-M3, can present peptides with N-formylated amino-termini, which is interesting because all prokaryotes initiate protein synthesis with N-formylmethionine, and cells infected with cytosolic bacteria can be killed by CD8 T cells that recognize N-formylated bacterial peptides bound to this MHC class IB molecule. Whether an equivalent class IB molecule exists in humans is not known. The function of most other class IB genes and their products is unclear.

The large number of MHC class IB genes (50 or more in the mouse) means that many different class IB molecules can exist in a single animal. These may, like the protein that presents N-formylmethionyl peptides, have specialized roles in antigen presentation. Some class IB genes appear to be under a different regulatory control from the classical MHC class I genes, and are induced in response to cellular stress (such as heat shock). These class IB genes may play a part in innate immunity, or in the induction of immune responses in circumstances where interferons are not produced.

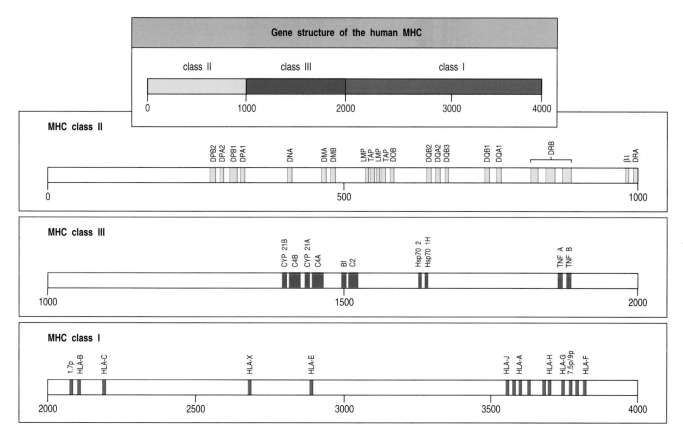

Fig. 4.18 Detailed map of the human MHC region. The organization of the class I, class II and class III regions of the MHC are shown, with approximate genetic distances given in thousands of base pairs (kb). Most of the genes in the class I and class II region are mentioned in the text; the additional genes indicated in the class I region (for example HLA-E, -F, -G, -H, -J, and -X) are class I-like genes, encoding class IB molecules, while the additional class II genes are pseudogenes. The genes shown in the class III region encode the complement proteins C4 (two genes, shown as C4A and C4B), C2 and Factor B (shown as Bf) as well as genes that encode the cytokines tumor necrosis factor (TNF) α and β. Closely linked to the C4 genes are the genes encoding 21-hydroxylase (shown as CYP 21A and CYP 21B), an enzyme involved in steroid synthesis. Deficiencies in 21-hydroxylase cause congenital adrenal hyperplasia and salt-wasting syndrome. Finally, the position of two heat-shock protein genes (Hsp70 1H and Hsp70 2) are shown. It is not known if these have any role in the immune system.

A second MHC class II-like molecule, in addition to the DM molecule discussed previously (see Section 4-13), is encoded within the MHC class II region. The DO molecule is formed from the pairing of the DNα and DOβ chains; these genes appear to be expressed only in the thymus and on B cells. The role of the DO gene products in the immune system is unknown.

Of the other genes that map within the MHC, some have products such as the complement components C2, Factor B and C4 or the **cytokines** tumor necrosis factor α and β (lymphotoxin), that have important functions in immunity. These have been termed MHC class III genes, and are shown in Fig. 4.18. The functions of these genes will be discussed in Chapters 8 and 9.

Some MHC class I-like genes map outside the MHC region. One family of such genes, called CD1, also functions in antigen presentation to T cells, although it does not present a peptide antigen. In cells infected with mycobacteria, the CD1 molecule is able to bind and present a mycobacterial membrane component, mycolic acid. Whether CD1 molecules can also present peptide antigens remains to be determined.

As we shall see in Chapter 11, many studies have established associations between susceptibility to certain diseases and particular allelic variants of genes in the MHC. While most of these diseases are known or suspected to have an immune etiology, this is not true of all of them, and it is important to remember that there are many genes lying in the MHC class II region that have no known or suspected immunological function. One of these is the enzyme 21-hydroxylase, deficiencies of which cause congenital adrenal hyperplasia and salt-wasting syndrome. Disease associations mapping to the MHC must therefore be interpreted with caution, based on a detailed understanding of its structure. Much remains to be learned about the functions of individual molecules, and the significance of their localization within the MHC. For instance, the C4 genes are highly polymorphic, and this genetic variability may have adaptive significance in resistance to disease, like that of the MHC class I and class II proteins to which we now turn.

4-15 The protein products of MHC class I and class II genes are highly polymorphic.

Because there are three genes encoding MHC class I molecules and four possible sets of MHC class II genes, every individual will express at least three different MHC class I proteins and four MHC class II proteins on his or her cells. In fact, the number of different MHC proteins expressed on the cells of most individuals is greater because of the extreme polymorphism of the MHC and the co-dominant expression of MHC genes.

The term polymorphism comes from the Greek *poly*, meaning many, and *morph*, meaning shape or structure. As used here, it means variation at a single genetic locus and its product within a species; the individual variant genes are termed **alleles**. There are more than 100 alleles of some MHC class I and class II loci (Fig. 4.19), each allele being present at a relatively high frequency in the population. For these reasons, the chance that the corresponding MHC locus on both chromosomes of an individual will encode the same allele is small; most individuals will be **heterozygous** at these loci. The products of both alleles are expressed on the same cell, so expression is said to be **co-dominant**, and both function in presenting antigens to T cells (Fig. 4.20). The extensive polymorphism at each locus has the potential to double the number of distinct MHC molecules expressed by each cell in an individual and thereby increases the diversity already available through polygeny, the existence of multiple functionally equivalent loci (Fig. 4.21).

Thus, with three MHC class I genes and four potential sets of MHC class II genes on each chromosome, a typical human will express six different MHC class I molecules and eight different MHC class II molecules on his or her cells. For the MHC class II genes the number of different products may be increased still further by the combination of α and β chains from different chromosomes (so that two α chains and two β chains can give rise to four different products). In mice, it has been shown that not all combinations of α and β chains can pair to form stable dimers and so, in practice, the exact number of different MHC class II molecules expressed will depend on which alleles are present on each chromosome.

Pairing between a class II α chain of one sort and a β chain of another can occur (for example, human DRβ pairing with DQα, or mouse Eα pairing with Aβ) but it is only seen when the correct partner fails to be expressed and even then is found only at a very low level. It is unlikely that such combinations have any significant role *in vivo*.

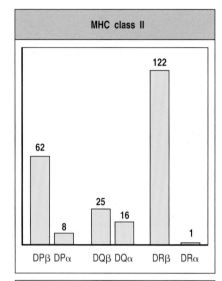

MHC class II

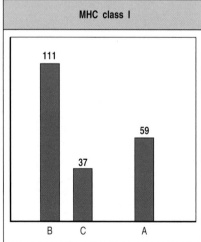

MHC class I

Fig. 4.19 Human MHC genes are highly polymorphic. With the notable exception of the DRα locus, which is monomorphic, each locus has many alleles. The number of different alleles is shown in this figure by the height of the bars and is obtained from studies mainly of Caucasoid populations. In other populations, such as Amerindian or Oriental populations, new alleles are found, so that the total diversity in these loci is greater than represented here. In fact, it is impossible to determine the total amount of variability at these loci without detailed worldwide studies.

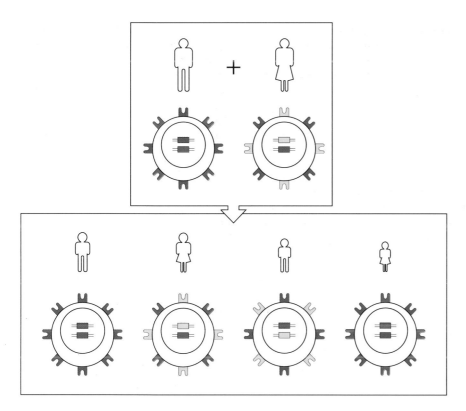

Fig. 4.20 Expression of MHC alleles is co-dominant. The MHC is so polymorphic that most individuals are likely to be heterozygous at each locus. Both alleles are expressed and the products of both alleles are found on all expressing cells. In any mating, there are four possible combinations of alleles that can be found in the offspring; thus siblings are also likely to differ in the MHC alleles they express, there being one chance in four that an individual will share both alleles with a sibling. One consequence of this is the difficulty in finding suitable donors for tissue transplantation.

All MHC products are polymorphic to a greater or lesser extent, with the exception of the DRα chain and its homolog in mouse, Eα. These chains do not vary in sequence between different individuals and are said to be **monomorphic**. This might indicate a functional constraint that prevents variation in the DR and Eα proteins but no such special function has yet been found. Many mice, both domestic and wild, have a mutation in the Eα gene that prevents synthesis of the Eα protein, and thus lack cell-surface E molecules; so if E molecules have a special function it is unlikely to be an essential one. All other MHC class I and class II genes are polymorphic.

Polymorphism

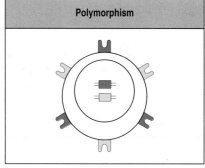

| 4-16 | **MHC polymorphism affects antigen recognition indirectly by controlling peptide binding.** |

The products of individual MHC alleles can differ from one another by up to 20 amino acids, making each allele quite distinct. Most of these differences are localized to exposed surfaces of the outer domain of the molecule, and to the peptide-binding groove in particular (Fig. 4.22). The polymorphic residues that line the peptide-binding groove determine the peptide-binding properties of the different MHC molecules.

Polygenism

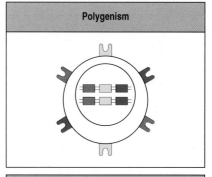

Fig. 4.21 Polymorphism and polygenism contribute to the diversity of MHC molecules expressed by an individual. The MHC genes are highly polymorphic, so that each individual is likely to be heterozygous, that is, to express two different, allelic MHC molecules from each locus. However, no matter how polymorphic the genes, no individual can express more than two alleles of a given gene. The duplication of the MHC genes, leading to polygenism, overcomes this limitation. Polymorphism and polygenism combine to produce the diversity in MHC molecules seen both within an individual, and in the population at large.

Polymorphism and polygenism

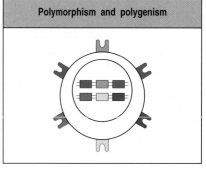

We have seen that peptides bind to MHC class I molecules through specific anchor residues (see Section 4-4) — peptide amino-acid side chains that are held in pockets lining the peptide-binding groove. Polymorphism in MHC class I molecules affects the amino acids lining these pockets and thus their binding specificity. In consequence, the anchor residues of peptides that bind to each allelic variant are different. The set of anchor residues that allows binding to a given MHC class I molecule is called a **sequence motif**. These sequence motifs make it possible to identify peptides within a protein that can potentially bind the appropriate MHC molecule, which may be very important in designing peptide vaccines (see Chapter 12). Different allelic variants of MHC class II molecules also bind different peptides but the more open structure of the MHC class II peptide-binding groove, and the greater length of the peptides bound in it, allow greater flexibility in peptide binding, so that it is more difficult to predict which peptides will bind to MHC class II molecules.

Because different MHC molecules bind different peptides, the T cells responding to a given protein antigen presented by several different MHC molecules will usually have to recognize different peptides. In rare cases, a protein will have no peptides with a suitable motif for binding to any of the MHC molecules expressed on the cells of an individual. When this happens, the individual fails to respond to the antigen. Such failures in responsiveness were first reported in inbred animals, where they were called **immune response (Ir) gene** defects, long before the function of MHC molecules was understood. These defects could be mapped to genes within the MHC, and were the first clue to the

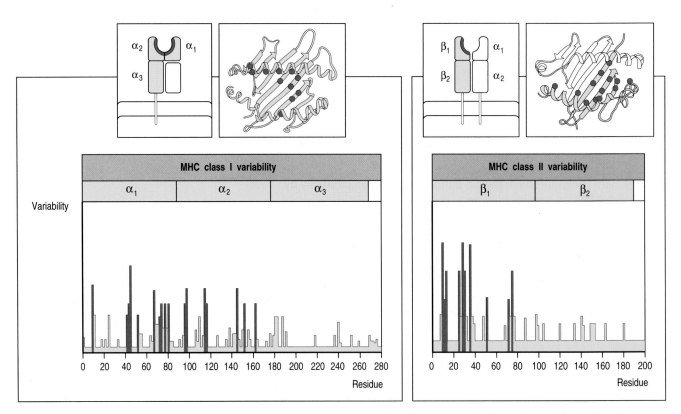

Fig. 4.22 Allelic variation occurs at specific sites within the MHC molecules. Variability plots of the MHC molecules show that the variation due to polymorphism in the MHC molecules is restricted to the amino-terminal domains (α_1 and α_2 domains of class I and predominantly the β_1 domain of MHC class II molecules), the domains that form the peptide-binding cleft. Moreover, allelic variability is clustered in specific sites within the amino-terminal domains, lying in positions that line the peptide-binding cleft, either on the floor of the groove or directed inwards from the walls.

antigen-presenting function of MHC molecules; however, it was only much later that the Ir genes were shown to encode MHC class II molecules. Ir gene defects are common in inbred strains of mice because the mice are homozygous for all their MHC genes and thus express only one allelic variant from each gene locus. Ordinarily, the polymorphism of MHC molecules guarantees a sufficient number of different MHC molecules in a single individual to make this type of non-responsiveness unlikely. This has obvious importance for host defense.

4-17   MHC polymorphism directly affects antigen recognition by T cells.

Ir gene defects were identified in experimental animals (guinea pigs and subsequently mice) through the failure to mount an immune response to specific foreign antigens, and initially the only evidence linking the defect to the MHC was genetic — mice of one MHC genotype could make antibody in response to a particular antigen, while mice of a different MHC genotype but otherwise genetically identical could not. MHC molecules were somehow controlling the ability of the immune system to detect or respond to specific antigens but it was not clear at that time that direct recognition of MHC molecules was involved. This emerged from later experiments.

The immune responses that led to the discovery of the Ir genes were known to be dependent upon T cells, and this led to a series of experiments aimed at ascertaining how MHC polymorphism might control the responses of T cells. The earliest of these experiments showed that T cells could be activated only by macrophages or B cells that shared MHC alleles with the mouse in which the T cells originated; this provided the first evidence for the direct recognition by T cells of MHC molecules themselves. The clearest example of this recognition, however, came from studies of virus-specific cytotoxic T cells.

When mice are infected with a virus, they generate cytotoxic T cells that kill self cells infected with the virus, while sparing uninfected cells or cells infected with unrelated viruses. The cytotoxic T cells are thus virus-specific. A particularly striking outcome of these experiments, however, was that the specificity of the cytotoxic T cells was also affected by allelic polymorphism in MHC molecules: cytotoxic T cells induced by viral infection in mice of MHC genotype a (MHC^a) would kill any cell of MHC genotype a infected with that virus, but would not kill cells of MHC type b, or c, and so on, even if they were infected with the same virus. Because the MHC genotype restricts the antigen specificity of T cells, this effect is called **MHC restriction**. Together with the earlier studies on both B cells and macrophages, this showed that MHC restriction is a critical feature of antigen recognition by all functional classes of T cells.

Because different MHC molecules bind different peptides, MHC restriction in responses to viruses and other complex antigens could be explained solely on this indirect basis. However, it can be seen from Fig. 4.22 that some of the polymorphic amino acids on MHC molecules are located on the α helices flanking the peptide-binding cleft in such a way that they would be exposed on the outer surface of the peptide:MHC complex. It is therefore not surprising that when T cells are tested for their ability to recognize the same peptide bound to different MHC molecules, they readily discriminate between peptide bound to MHC^a and the same peptide bound to MHC^b. Thus, specificity in a T-cell receptor is defined both by the peptide and by the MHC molecule binding it (Fig. 4.23). This restricted recognition is sometimes due to differences in the conformation of the bound peptide imposed by the different MHC molecules, and sometimes by the conformational changes that occur in the MHC

Fig. 4.23 T-cell recognition of antigens is MHC-restricted. The antigen-specific receptor of T cells (TCR) recognizes a complex of antigenic peptide and MHC. One consequence of this is that a T cell specific for peptide X and a particular MHC allele, MHC^a (left panel), will not recognize the complex of peptide X with a different MHC allele, MHC^b (center panel), or the complex of antigen Y with MHC^a (right panel). The co-recognition of peptide and MHC molecule is known as MHC restriction, because the MHC molecule is said to restrict the ability of the T cell to recognize antigen. This restriction may result either from direct contact between MHC molecule and T-cell receptor, or be an indirect effect of MHC polymorphism on the peptides that bind or their bound conformation.

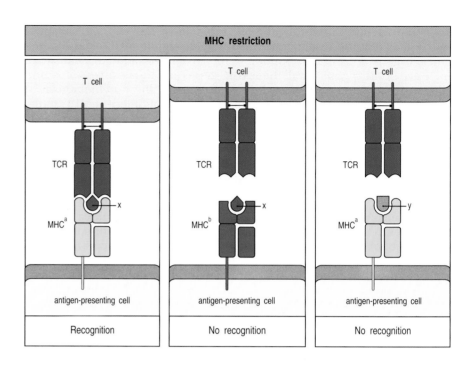

molecule on binding different peptides, rather than by direct recognition of polymorphic amino acids on the MHC molecule itself. However, it can be shown by other means that direct contact of the T-cell receptor with polymorphic residues on the MHC molecule affects antigen recognition, and thus MHC restriction in antigen recognition reflects the combined effect of differences in peptide binding and of direct contact between the MHC molecule and the T-cell receptor.

The discovery of MHC restriction, in revealing the physiological function of the MHC molecules, also led to the explanation of the otherwise puzzling phenomenon of non-self MHC recognition in graft rejection, to which we shall turn briefly before discussing other implications of MHC polymorphism.

4-18   Non-self MHC molecules are recognized by 1–10% of T cells.

Transplanted tissues or organs from donors bearing MHC molecules that differ from those of the recipient are reliably rejected. Tissue grafts can be rejected on the basis of MHC molecules that differ by as little as one amino acid. This rapid and very potent **cell-mediated immune response** results from the presence of large numbers of T cells in any individual that are specifically reactive to particular non-self or **allogeneic** MHC molecules. Studies on T-cell responses to allogeneic MHC molecules using the mixed lymphocyte reaction (see Section 2-24) have shown that roughly 1–10% of all T cells in an individual will respond to stimulation by cells from any allogeneic individual. This type of T-cell response is called **alloreactivity**, because it represents recognition of allelic polymorphism on allogeneic MHC molecules.

Before the role of the MHC molecules in antigen presentation was understood, it was a mystery why so many T cells should recognize non-self MHC molecules, as there is no reason why the immune system should have evolved a defense against tissue transplants. It is now thought that this alloreactivity reflects cross-reactivity of T-cell receptors normally specific for a variety of foreign peptides bound by self MHC molecules. This cross-reactivity results in part from the many peptides bound by non-self MHC molecules on the transplanted tissues but not by the host's own MHC molecules, which form complexes to which the host T cells are not tolerant. Other alloreactive T cells respond because of direct binding of the T-cell receptor to distinctive features of the non-self MHC molecule (Fig. 4.24). In the former case (peptide-dominant binding), the peptide bound by the non-self MHC molecule must interact strongly with a T-cell receptor normally specific for a self MHC molecule binding a different antigenic peptide. In the latter case (MHC-dominant binding), the recognition is independent of the type of peptide bound. T-cell receptor binding to unique features of the non-self MHC molecule generates a strong signal because of the high concentration of the non-self MHC molecule on the surface of the presenting cell. Both these mechanisms contribute to the high frequency of T cells responding to the non-self MHC molecules on the transplanted tissue, which clearly reflects the commitment of the T-cell receptor to the recognition of MHC molecules in general.

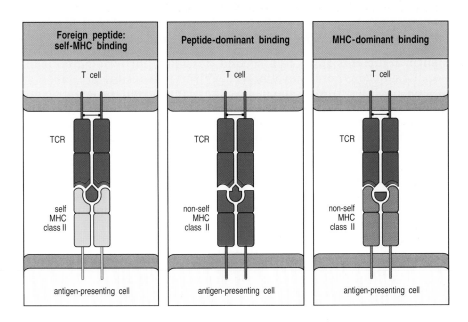

Foreign peptide: self-MHC binding	Peptide-dominant binding	MHC-dominant binding
T cell	T cell	T cell
TCR	TCR	TCR
self MHC class II	non-self MHC class II	non-self MHC class II
antigen-presenting cell	antigen-presenting cell	antigen-presenting cell

Fig. 4.24 Two modes of cross-reactive recognition that may explain alloreactivity. A T cell that is specific for one peptide:MHC combination (left panel) may cross-react with peptides presented by other (allogeneic) MHC molecules. This may come about in either of two ways. The peptides bound to the allogeneic MHC molecule might fit well to the T-cell receptor (TCR), allowing binding even though there is not a good fit with the MHC molecule (center panel). Alternatively, and apparently less frequently, the allogeneic MHC molecule may provide a better fit to the T-cell receptor, giving a tight binding that is independent of the peptide bound to the MHC molecule (right panel).

4-19 MHC polymorphism extends the range of antigens to which the immune system can respond.

Most polymorphic genes encode proteins that vary by only one or a few amino acids. As we have seen, the different allelic variants of MHC proteins differ by up to 20 amino acids. Because the role of the immune system is to protect against infection, it is here we must look for the nature of the selective advantage conferred by the extensive polymorphism of the MHC proteins.

Pathogens have several possible strategies for avoiding an immune response either by evading detection or by suppressing the ensuing response. The requirement that pathogen antigens must be presented by an MHC molecule provides two possible means of evading detection. Although MHC molecules have a broad specificity of peptide binding, only certain peptides will bind to a given MHC molecule, and those that do not bind are not immunogenic. A pathogen could therefore escape detection by mutations that eliminated from its proteins all peptides able to bind MHC molecules. An example of this type of strategy can be seen in regions of South East China and in Papua New Guinea, where about 60% of the population carry the HLA-A11 allele. Many isolates of the Epstein-Barr virus obtained in this population have mutated a dominant epitope presented by HLA-A11, so that the mutant peptides no longer bind to HLA-A11 and cannot be recognized by HLA-A11-restricted T cells. This strategy is plainly much more difficult to follow if there are many different MHC molecules, and the presence of different loci encoding functionally related proteins may have been an evolutionary adaptation by hosts to this strategy by pathogens.

Polymorphism at each locus can potentially double the number of different MHC molecules expressed by an individual, as most individuals will be heterozygotes. Polymorphism has the additional advantage that different individuals in a population will differ in the combinations of MHC molecules they express, and will therefore present different sets of peptides from each pathogen. This makes it unlikely that all individuals in a population will be equally susceptible to a given pathogen. Its spread will therefore be limited. That exposure to pathogens over an evolutionary timescale can select for expression of particular MHC alleles is strongly indicated by the strong association of the HLA-B53 allele with recovery from a potentially lethal form of malaria; this allele is very common in individuals from West Africa where malaria is endemic.

Similar arguments apply to a second possibility for evading recognition. If pathogens could develop mechanisms to block the presentation of their peptides by MHC molecules, they could avoid the adaptive immune response. Adenoviruses encode a protein that binds to MHC class I molecules in the endoplasmic reticulum and prevents their transport to the cell surface, thus preventing recognition of viral peptides by CD8 cytotoxic T cells. This MHC-binding protein must interact with a polymorphic region of the MHC class I molecule, as some alleles are retained while others are not. Increasing the variety of MHC molecules expressed therefore reduces the likelihood that a pathogen will be able to block presentation by all of them, and so completely evade an immune response.

These arguments raise a question: if having three MHC class I molecules is advantageous, and six even more so, why are there not far more MHC class I loci? A full answer to this question must await a discussion of the mechanisms by which the repertoire of T-cell receptors is selected in the thymus, which will be the topic of Chapter 6. Briefly, the probable explanation is that each time a distinct MHC molecule is added to the MHC repertoire, all T cells that can recognize self peptides bound to that molecule must be removed in order to maintain self tolerance. It seems that the number of MHC loci present in humans and mice is about optimal to balance out the advantages of presenting an increased range of foreign peptides and the disadvantages of increased presentation of self peptides and the loss of T cells that accompanies it.

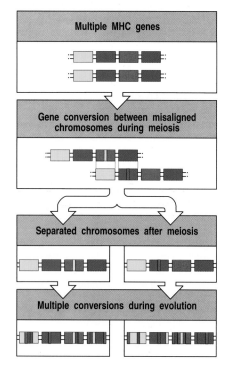

Fig. 4.25 Gene conversion can create polymorphisms by transferring sequences from one MHC gene to another. Sequences can be transferred from one gene to a similar gene by a process known as gene conversion. In this process, which can occur between two alleles or, as shown here, between two closely related genes generated by gene duplication during evolution, the two genes are apposed during meiosis. This can occur as a consequence of the misalignment of the two chromosomes when there are many copies of similar genes arrayed in tandem — somewhat like buttoning in the wrong buttonhole. The DNA sequence from one chromosome can then be copied to the other, giving rise to a new gene sequence. In this way a number of nucleotide changes can be inserted all at once into a gene and can cause several amino-acid changes between the new gene and the original gene. The process of gene conversion has occurred many times in the evolution of MHC alleles.

Labels within the figure:
- Multiple MHC genes
- Gene conversion between misaligned chromosomes during meiosis
- Separated chromosomes after meiosis
- Multiple conversions during evolution

4-20   **Multiple genetic processes generate MHC polymorphism.**

MHC polymorphism appears to have been strongly selected by evolutionary pressures. However, for selection to work efficiently in slowly reproducing organisms like humans, there must also be powerful mechanisms that generate variability in MHC alleles on which selection can act. The generation of polymorphism in MHC molecules is an evolutionary problem not readily analyzed in the laboratory but it is clear that several genetic mechanisms contribute to the generation of new alleles. Some new alleles are the result of point mutations but many arise from combining sequences from different alleles either by genetic recombination or by **gene conversion**, in which one sequence is replaced in part by another from a homologous gene (Fig. 4.25).

Evidence for gene conversion comes from studies of the sequences of different MHC alleles, which reveal that some changes involve clusters of several amino acids in the MHC molecule and require multiple nucleotide changes in a contiguous stretch of the gene. Even more significantly, the same sequences are found within other MHC genes on the same chromosome, a prerequisite for gene conversion.

Recombination between alleles at the same locus may, however, have been more important than gene conversion in generating MHC polymorphism. A comparison of sequences of MHC alleles shows that many different alleles could represent recombination events between a set of hypothetical ancestral alleles. If one postulates a small number of ancestral alleles, most present-day alleles could have been generated by one or more recombination events (Fig. 4.26).

The effects of selective pressure in favor of polymorphism can be seen clearly in the pattern of point mutations in the MHC genes. Point mutations can be classified as replacement substitutions, which change an amino acid, or silent substitutions, which simply change the codon but leave the amino acid the same. Replacement substitutions occur within the MHC at a higher frequency relative to silent substitutions than would be expected, providing evidence that polymorphism has been actively selected for in the evolution of the MHC.

Summary.

The major histocompatibility complex (MHC) of genes consists of a linked set of genetic loci encoding many of the proteins involved in antigen presentation to T cells, most notably the MHC glycoproteins that present peptides to the T-cell receptor. The most outstanding feature of MHC genes is their extensive polymorphism. This polymorphism is of critical importance in antigen recognition by T cells. A T cell recognizes antigen as a peptide bound by a particular allelic variant of an MHC molecule, and will not recognize the same peptide bound to other MHC molecules. This behavior of T cells is called MHC restriction. Most MHC alleles differ from one another by multiple amino-acid substitutions, and these differences are focused on the peptide-binding site and adjacent regions that make direct contact with the T-cell receptor. At least three properties of MHC molecules are affected by MHC polymorphism: the range of peptides bound; the conformation of the bound peptide; and the interaction of the MHC molecule directly with the T-cell receptor. The central role of the MHC in immune responses and the highly polymorphic nature of the MHC strongly suggest that polymorphism is critical to the function of the MHC molecules. Powerful genetic mechanisms generate this polymorphism, and an argument can be made that selective pressure to maintain a wide variety of MHC molecules in the population comes from infectious agents.

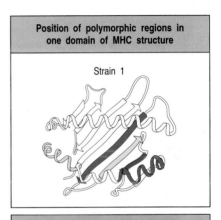

Position of polymorphic regions in one domain of MHC structure

Strain 1

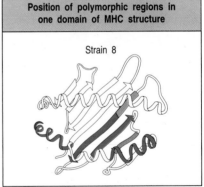

Position of polymorphic regions in one domain of MHC structure

Strain 8

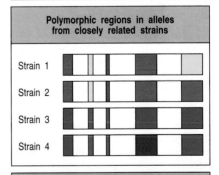

Polymorphic regions in alleles from closely related strains

Strain 1
Strain 2
Strain 3
Strain 4

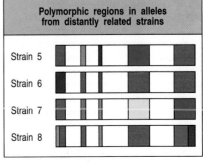

Polymorphic regions in alleles from distantly related strains

Strain 5
Strain 6
Strain 7
Strain 8

Fig. 4.26 Recombination can create new alleles by reassorting discrete polymorphic regions. Recombination differs from gene conversion in that the DNA segments are exchanged between different chromosomes rather than, as in gene conversion, being copied so that one sequence replaces sequences in another gene. Analysis of many MHC allele sequences has shown that the swapping of segments of DNA has occurred many times in the evolution of MHC alleles. The variable parts of MHC domains correspond to segments of the structure, such as β strands or parts of the α helix, as shown in the upper two panels. Closely related strains of mice have MHC genes where only one or two segments have been swapped between alleles (third panel), while more distantly related strains show a patchwork effect that results from the accumulation of many such recombination events (bottom panel).

The T-cell receptor complex.

The mechanisms by which a diverse set of B-cell antigen receptors are generated through recombination of a limited set of gene segments are so powerful that it is not surprising that the antigen receptor of T cells uses the same mechanisms operating on homologous genes. The T-cell antigen receptor resembles a membrane-bound Fab fragment of immunoglobulin and, like the immunoglobulin antigen receptor of B cells (see Section 3-27), is found on the cell surface in association with a complex of invariant proteins that are required for the cell-surface expression of the receptor and also play a part in signal transduction. In this section, we shall describe the structure of the T-cell receptor proteins and the organization of the T-cell receptor genes. We shall also see how, despite their overall similarity, T-cell receptors differ from immunoglobulins in important ways, and how the MHC-binding co-receptor molecules CD4 and CD8 contribute to antigen recognition.

4-21   The T-cell receptor resembles a membrane-associated Fab fragment of immunoglobulin.

T-cell receptors were first identified by making monoclonal antibodies against individual cloned T-cell lines (see Section 2-20). Some of these antibodies reacted only with the immunizing clone, suggesting that they might be detecting a unique receptor on the T-cell surface. Moreover, such **clonotypic** antibodies could specifically inhibit antigen recognition, consistent with the notion that these antibodies recognized the T-cell receptor for antigen. The clonotypic antibodies were then used to show that each T cell bears about 30 000 T-cell receptor molecules on its surface, each receptor consisting of two different polypeptide chains, termed the **T-cell receptor α and β chains**, bound to one another by a disulfide bond in a structure that is very similar to a Fab fragment of an immunoglobulin (Fig. 4.27). These α:β heterodimers account for antigen recognition by all the functional classes of T cells we have described so far. There is an alternative type of T-cell receptor made up of different polypeptides designated γ and δ but its discovery was unexpected and its functional significance is not yet clear, as we shall see later (see Section 4-30).

Although the use of clonotypic antibodies enabled some characteristic features of the α:β T-cell receptor to be determined, most of what we now know about its structure and function came from studies of cloned DNA encoding the receptor chains. The genes encoding the T-cell receptor α and β chains were first identified as cDNAs that were isolated on the basis of their expression in T cells but not B cells. As T and B cells are closely related, there are relatively few such cDNAs. Those encoding the T-cell receptor were sought on the basis of two criteria. First, it was expected that they would be encoded by gene segments that had undergone rearrangement only in T cells. The second criterion was sequence homology to immunoglobulin. Using these approaches, the first cDNAs encoding T-cell receptor α and β chains were identified.

Preliminary peptide fragmenation studies of T-cell receptors isolated using clonotypic antibodies indicated that, like antibodies, they contain variable and constant peptides. However, it was the predicted amino-acid sequence from T-cell receptor cDNAs that demonstrated clearly that both chains of the T-cell receptor have an amino-terminal variable region with homology to an immunoglobulin V domain, a constant

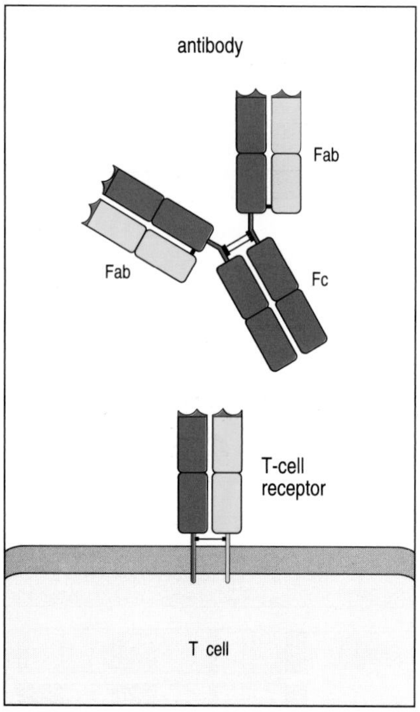

Fig. 4.27 The T-cell receptor resembles a membrane-bound Fab fragment. The Fab fragment of antibody molecules is a disulfide-linked heterodimer, each chain of which contains one immunoglobulin constant domain and one variable domain; the juxtaposition of the variable domains forms the antigen-binding site (see Chapter 3). The T-cell receptor is also a disulfide-linked heterodimer, with each chain containing an immunoglobulin constant-like domain and an immuno-globulin variable-like domain. Finally, as in the Fab fragment, the juxtaposition of the variable regions forms the antigen recognition site.

region with homology to an immunoglobulin C domain, and a short hinge region with a cysteine residue that forms the interchain disulfide bond (Fig. 4.28). Each chain spans the lipid bilayer by a hydrophobic transmembrane domain whose notable feature is the presence of positively charged amino acids. The presence of such charged residues in transmembrane domains is unusual and would normally tend to destabilize them. We will see later that these charged residues play an important part in the interaction of the T-cell receptor chains with appropriately charged polypeptides known as CD3 γ, δ, and ε, which are homologous to the Igα and Igβ proteins of the B-cell receptor. Finally, each chain ends with a short cytoplasmic domain.

The V-like domains comprise V-, D- and J-like elements in the β chain and V- and J-like elements in the α chain. It is these close similarities of T-cell receptor chains to the heavy and light immunoglobulin chains that lead to the conclusion that T-cell receptor proteins must closely resemble a Fab fragment of immunoglobulin. The structure of the T-cell receptor has not yet been determined directly, but many groups are actively pursuing this structure and its solution is close. The structure of the T-cell receptor β chain has been determined and, as expected, closely resembles that of an immunoglobulin light chain.

Some differences do exist, most notably in the interface between the V and C domains, that suggest that the T-cell receptor may be a more rigid structure than a Fab fragment, and this may have some effect on the ability of the receptor to transmit to the interior of the cell a signal that it has bound an MHC:peptide complex. T-cell receptors differ from B-cell receptors in that the T-cell receptor is monovalent, while immunoglobulin is bivalent, and in that the T-cell receptor is not secreted, while immunoglobulin is adapted to be secreted upon B-cell activation (see Fig. 3.33).

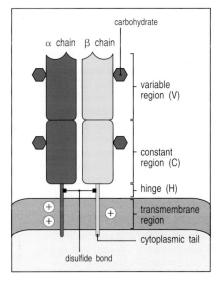

Fig. 4.28 Structure of the T-cell receptor. The T-cell receptor heterodimer is composed of two transmembrane glycoprotein chains, α and β. The external portion of each chain consists of two domains, resembling immunoglobulin variable and constant domains, respectively. Both chains have carbohydrate side chains attached to each domain. A short segment, analogous to an immunoglobulin hinge region, connects the immunoglobulin-like domains to the membrane and contains the cysteine that forms the interchain disulfide bond. The transmembrane helices of both chains are unusual in containing positively charged (basic) residues within the hydrophobic transmembrane segment. The α chains carry two such residues, while the β chains have one.

| 4-22 | **The T-cell receptor genes resemble immunoglobulin genes.** |

The organization of the gene segments encoding T-cell receptor α and β chains (Fig. 4.29) is generally homologous to that of the immunoglobulin gene segments (see Sections 3-11 and 3-12 for comparison). The α chains, like immunoglobulin light chains, are assembled from V and J gene segments, although the T-cell receptor α-chain genes have many more J gene segments. 61 J_α gene segments are distributed over about 80 kb of DNA, while immunoglobulin light-chain genes have only five J gene segments. We shall see later that this has important consequences for the recognition of antigen by the T-cell receptor. The β-chain genes, like those of immunoglobulin heavy chains, have D gene segments in addition to V and J gene segments.

Like immunoglobulin genes in B cells, the T-cell receptor gene segments rearrange in thymocytes to form complete V-domain exons (Fig. 4.30). (The process of rearrangement is dealt with in more detail in Chapter 6.) The T-cell receptor gene segments are flanked by heptamer and nonamer recombination signals homologous to those found in immunoglobulin genes (see Section 3-14) and are recognized by the same enzymes: defects in three distinct genes that control gene segment rearrangement affect T- and B-cell receptor genes equally, and animals with these genetic defects lack functional lymphocytes altogether.

A further shared feature of immunoglobulin and T-cell receptor gene rearrangement is the presence of P- and N-nucleotides in the junctions between the V, D, and J gene segments of the β chain, although in T cells P- and N-nucleotides are also added between the V and J gene segments

Fig. 4.29 The organization of the human T-cell receptor α- and β-chain genes. The arrangement of the gene segments resembles that of the immunoglobulins with separate variable (V), diversity (D), joining (J) and constant (C) gene segments. The α-chain gene consists of 70–80 variable segments, each containing an exon encoding a variable region (V) preceded by an exon encoding the leader sequence (L) that targets the protein to the endoplasmic reticulum for transport to the cell surface. How many of these are functional is not known exactly. A cluster of about 60 J segments is located a considerable distance from the V segments. The J segments are followed by a single constant-domain segment, which contains separate exons for the constant and hinge domains and a single exon encoding the transmembrane and cytoplasmic regions. The β-chain gene has a different organization with a cluster of about 50 functional V segments located distantly from two separate clusters each containing a single D segment, together with six or seven J segments and a single constant segment. Each β-chain constant segment has separate exons encoding the constant, hinge, transmembrane, and cytoplasmic regions. The α-chain locus is interrupted between the J and V segments by another TCR locus — the δ-chain locus (not shown here; see Fig. 4.38).

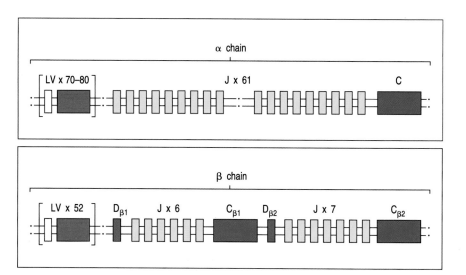

of all α chains, while V to J gene segment joints in immunoglobulin light-chain genes are only modified in some instances.

The main differences between the immunoglobulin genes and those encoding the T-cell receptor reflect the fact that all the effector functions of B cells depend upon secreted antibodies whose distinct constant-region isotypes trigger distinct effector mechanisms. The effector functions of T cells, on the other hand, depend upon cell–cell contact and are not mediated directly by the T-cell receptor, which serves only for antigen recognition. Thus, the constant-region genes of the T-cell receptor are much simpler than those of antibodies: there is only one C_α gene and, although there are two C_β genes, there is no known functional distinction between their products. The T-cell receptor constant-region genes encode only transmembrane polypeptides: there are no exons encoding an alternative secreted form.

Fig. 4.30 T-cell receptor α- and β-chain gene rearrangement and expression. The T-cell receptor α- and β-chain genes are composed of discrete segments that are joined by somatic recombination during development of the T cell. For the α chain, a V_α gene segment rearranges to a J_α gene segment to create a functional exon. Transcription and splicing of the VJ_α exon to C_α generates the mRNA that is translated to yield the TCR α-chain protein. For the β chains, like the immunoglobulin heavy chains (see Chapter 3), the variable domain is encoded in three gene segments, V_β, D_β, and J_β. Rearrangement of these gene segments generates a functional exon that is transcribed, spliced to join VDJ_β to C_β and the resulting mRNA translated to yield the T-cell receptor β-chain protein. The α and β chains pair soon after their biosynthesis to yield the α:β T-cell receptor heterodimer. Not all J segments are shown.

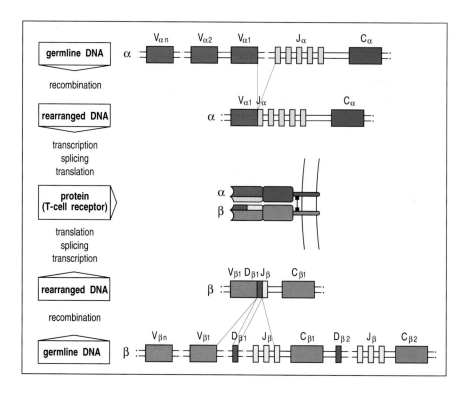

4-23	**T-cell receptor diversity is focused in CDR3.**

Just as the absence of a secreted form of the T-cell receptor reflects the need for recognition by T cells to focus on antigens presented on the cell surface, so the extent and pattern of diversity of T-cell receptors and immunoglobulins should reflect the distinct nature of their ligands. While antibodies must conform to the surfaces of an almost infinite variety of different antigens, the ligand for the T-cell receptor is always an MHC molecule; the T-cell receptors will therefore have a relatively invariant shape with most of the variability focused on the bound antigenic peptide occupying the center of the surface in contact with the receptor.

The three-dimensional structure of a complete T-cell receptor is not yet known, although that of the β chain alone has been obtained, but it will almost certainly look much like an antibody molecule because of its similarity in sequence, function, and gene structure.

In an antibody, the center of the antigen-binding site is formed by the third complementarity determining regions (CDR3) of the heavy and light chains. The CDR3 loops of the T-cell receptor α and β chains, to which the D and J gene segments contribute, are therefore expected to form the center of the antigen-binding site on T-cell receptors, while the periphery of the site will consist of the equivalent of the CDR1 and CDR2 loops, which are encoded within the germline V gene segments for the α and β chains. By comparing the origins of diversity in immunoglobulin and T-cell receptor genes, we can determine whether the distribution of variability in the two receptor types conforms to these predictions.

T-cell receptor genes have roughly the same number of V gene segments as immunoglobulins (Fig. 4.31) but only immunoglobulins show extensive diversification of expressed rearranged variable-region genes by somatic hypermutation. (However, somatic mutations of

Element	Immunoglobulin		αβ receptors	
	H	κ+λ	β	α
Variable segments (V)	51	69	52	~70
Diversity segments (D)	~30	0	2	0
D segments read in 3 frames	rarely	–	often	–
Joining segments (J)	5	5	13	61
Joints with N and P nucleotides	2	(1)	2	1
Number of V gene pairs	3519		3640	
Junctional diversity	~10^{13}		~10^{13}	
Total diversity	~10^{16}		~10^{16}	

Fig. 4.31 The numbers of T-cell receptor gene segments and the sources of T-cell receptor diversity compared with those of immunoglobulin. The table shows human gene numbers. The number of κ chain joints with N and P regions is shown in brackets as only about half of human κ chains contain N and P regions. Adapted from Davis, M. M., and Bjorkman, P. J. *Nature* 1988, **334**:395–402.

unknown significance have recently been described in the α chains of T cells within germinal centers). Thus, diversity in the periphery of the antigen-binding site of an antibody molecule comprising the CDR1 and CDR2 loops will be far greater than it is in a T-cell receptor. By contrast, T-cell receptor genes have many more J segments, and although there are only two Dβ gene segments, they can be read in all three reading frames, unlike those of immunoglobulin heavy chains where at least one frame contains a premature termination codon. The large number of J gene segments increases diversity only in CDR3 loops. Perhaps an even greater contributor to diversity in the CDR3 loops of the T-cell receptor is the presence of N-nucleotides, which are introduced at the junctions between gene segments on both α and β chains, whereas only immunoglobulin heavy chains and some light chains have N-nucleotides.

Comparing the origins of diversity in T-cell receptors and immunoglobulins, it can be seen that most of the variability in T-cell receptors occurs within the junctional region encoded by D, J, and N-nucleotides. This region encodes the CDR3 loops in immunoglobulins that form the center of the antigen-binding site. Assuming that the structure of the T-cell receptor is similar, the center of the T-cell receptor will be highly variable, while the periphery will be subject to relatively little variation. So, when one superimposes the proposed structure of a T-cell receptor on its ligand, the most variable part of the receptor lies over the most variable part of the ligand, the bound foreign peptide (Fig. 4.32). The periphery of the receptor, formed mainly from the CDR1 and CDR2 loops of the α and β variable domains, will contact the periphery of the ligand, comprising mainly amino acids contributed by the α helices of the two outer MHC domains.

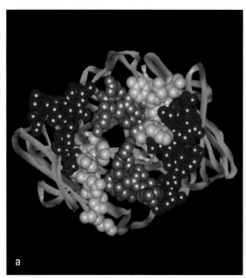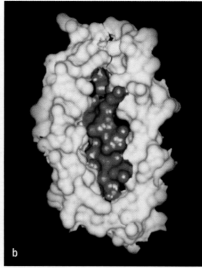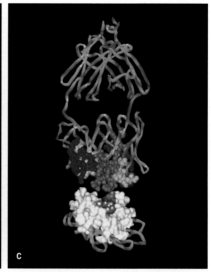

Fig. 4.32 The variability of the T-cell receptor complements the variability in the peptide:MHC complex. The proposed conformation of the antigen-binding site of the T-cell receptor (panel a) is based on the assumption that the variable domains of the T-cell receptor resemble immunoglobulin variable domains. The antigen-binding site is composed of the CDR1 (yellow), CDR2 (dark blue) and CDR3 (pink) loops of both the α and β chains of the T-cell receptor, and extends over a broad surface at one end of the molecule. The diversity in T-cell receptors is concentrated in the CDR3 loops, which lie in the center of the antigen-binding site. The CDR1 and CDR2 loops, which form the periphery of the binding site, show less variability than the CDR3 loops. The most variable part of a peptide antigen:MHC complex (panel b) is the peptide, shown in red, which binds into the cleft between the α helices of the MHC molecule, shown in white. It is likely that the T-cell receptor binds to the antigen peptide:MHC complex in the manner shown in panel c, such that the least variable parts of the T-cell receptor binding site, the CDR1 and CDR2 loops, make contact with the α helices of the MHC molecule while the CDR3 loops make contact with the peptide antigen. Adapted from Davis, M. M., and Bjorkman, P.J. *Nature* 1988, **334**:395–402.

4-24   **Diversity in T-cell receptors is not extended by somatic hypermutation.**

When we discussed the generation of antibody diversity in Section 3-18, we saw that somatic hypermutation increases the diversity of all three complementarity determining regions of both immunoglobulin chains. As a general principle, somatic hypermutation does not occur in T-cell receptor genes, so that variability of the CDR1 and CDR2 regions is limited to that of the germline V gene segments. Somatic mutation has been reported for the α chain V regions expressed by T cells isolated from germinal centers, but it is not known whether these mutated α chains contribute to a cell-surface T-cell receptor and so generate an altered specificity. At present, therefore, it appears as though the bulk of diversity in T-cell receptors is generated during rearrangement and is consequently focused on the CDR3 regions.

Why T-cell and B-cell receptors differ in their ability to undergo somatic hypermutation is not clear, but several explanations can be suggested on the basis of the functional differences between T and B cells. Because the central role of T cells is to stimulate both humoral and cellular immune responses, it is crucially important that T cells do not react with self proteins. T cells that recognize self antigens are rigorously purged during development (see Chapter 6), and the absence of somatic hypermutation helps to ensure that somatic mutants recognizing self proteins do not arise later in the course of immune responses. This constraint does not apply with the same force to B-cell receptors, as B cells usually require T-cell help in order to secrete antibodies. A B cell whose receptor mutates to become self reactive would, under normal circumstances, fail to make antibody for lack of self-reactive T cells to provide this help. An additional argument might be that T cells already interact with a self component, namely the MHC molecule that makes up part of the ligand for the receptor, and thus might be unusually prone to developing self-recognition capability through somatic hypermutation. In this case, the obverse argument can also be made: because T-cell receptors must be able to recognize self MHC molecules as part of their ligand, it is important to avoid somatic mutation that might result in the loss of recognition and consequent loss of any ability to respond. However, the most likely explanation for this difference between immunoglobulins and T-cell receptors is the simple one that somatic hypermutation is an adaptive specialization for B cells alone, because they must make very high affinity antibodies in order to capture toxin molecules in the extracellular fluids. We shall see in Chapter 9 that they do this through somatic hypermutation followed by selection for antigen binding.

4-25   **Many T cells respond to superantigens.**

Not all antigens that bind to MHC class II molecules are presented as peptides in the peptide-binding groove. A few fall into a distinct class known as **superantigens**, which have a distinctive mode of binding that enables them to stimulate very large numbers of T cells, often with disastrous consequences. Superantigens are produced by many different pathogens, including bacteria, mycoplasmas, and viruses, and bind directly to MHC molecules without being previously processed; indeed, fragmentation of a superantigen destroys its biological activity. Instead of binding in the groove of the MHC molecule, superantigens bind to the upper surface of both the MHC class II molecule and the V_β region of the T-cell receptor (Fig. 4.33). Thus, the α chain V region and the DJ junction of the β chain of the T-cell receptor have little effect on superantigen recognition, which is determined largely by the V gene segment

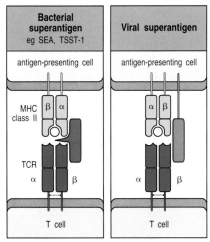

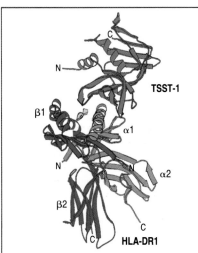

Fig. 4.33 Superantigens bind directly to T-cell receptors (TCR) and to MHC molecules. Superantigens interact with MHC class II molecules and T-cell receptors in a way that is quite distinct from the way that normal peptide antigens bind. Superantigens can bind independently to MHC class II molecules and to T-cell receptors, binding to the β chain of the T-cell receptor, away from the complementarity determining region, and to the outer faces of the MHC class II molecule, outside the peptide-binding site. Two distinct classes of superantigens have been described so far. Bacterial superantigens, like staphlyococcal enterotoxins (SEs) or the toxic shock syndrome toxin (TSST-1) are soluble proteins secreted by bacteria. The so-called endogenous viral superantigens are proteins expressed by some viruses that infect mammalian cells and integrate into the DNA of their host. The best characterized viral superantigens are membrane proteins produced by endogenous viruses of mice, especially the murine mammary tumor virus, MMTV. The crystal structures of complexes of MHC class II molecules with staphylococcal enterotoxin B (SEB) and with TSST-1 have been determined (that of the HLA-DR1:TSST-1 complex is shown in the bottom panel) and show clearly that the superantigens binds to the α chain of the class II molecule. In the case of the TSST-1 superantigen, peptides bound by the class II molecule and parts of the β chain may also contact the superantigen and influence its binding. The viral superantigen MMTV-7 binds to the β chain of MHC class II molecules. Each of these superantigens contacts a separate site on the T-cell receptor Vβ domain. Bottom panel courtesy of J Kim.

that encoded the β chain. Each superantigen can bind one or a few of the different products of Vβ gene segments, of which there are 20–50 in mice and humans, so a superantigen can stimulate 2–20% of all T cells.

This mode of stimulation is not specific for the pathogen and thus does not lead to adaptive immunity. Instead, it causes massive production of cytokines by CD4 T cells, the predominant responding population. These cytokines have two effects on the host, systemic toxicity and suppression of the adaptive immune response. Both of these effects contribute to microbial pathogenicity. Among the bacterial superantigens are the **staphylococcal enterotoxins (SE)** that cause common food poisoning and the **toxic shock syndrome toxin (TSST)**.

The role of viral superantigens is less clear. Endogenous viral superantigens are very common in mice, and we shall see in Chapter 6 that the study of these superantigens has played a critical role in elucidating one of the major mechanisms of self tolerance.

4-26 | The T-cell receptor associates with the invariant proteins of the CD3 complex.

Neither chain of the T-cell receptor heterodimer has a large cytoplasmic domain that might serve to signal the cell that the T-cell receptor has bound antigen. Instead, that function is carried out by a complex of proteins, known as the **CD3 complex**, which is stably associated with the T-cell receptor on the surface of T cells (Fig. 4.34). The complex consists of three distinct proteins with some homology to immunoglobulins, and two other proteins not homologous to immunoglobulins but closely related to each other. Unlike the T-cell receptor heterodimer, the CD3 proteins have cytoplasmic extensions that allow them to interact with signal-transducing proteins. The proteins showing sequence homologies to immunoglobulins are known as CD3γ, CD3δ, and CD3ε. These three proteins, like Igα and Igβ, consist of extracellular domains that bear weak amino acid homology to immunoglobulin domains, a transmembrane region, and modest cytoplasmic domains. The transmembrane domains are characterized by an acidic (negatively charged) residue in the appropriate location to form a salt bridge with the basic (positively charged) amino acids in the transmembrane region of the T-cell receptor. The cytoplasmic domains contain sequences called **immuno-receptor tyrosine-based activation motifs (ITAMs)** (see Section 3-27) that allow them to associate with cytosolic **protein tyrosine kinases** following receptor stimulation, and those of the CD3ε chain are an important target for phosphorylation by tyrosine kinases. The genes encoding CD3γ, δ, and ε are closely linked in the genome, and their expression is coordinately regulated.

Another protein, known as ζ, also forms part of this complex as a disulfide-linked dimer (see Fig. 4.34). In mice, a second form of the ζ chain, the η chain, arises by alternative splicing of the ζ chain RNA transcript to yield a protein with a distinct carboxy-terminal domain. About 80% of T-cell receptors at the cell surface associate with a ζ:ζ homodimer, the rest containing a ζ:η heterodimer. In humans, where the η chain has not been found, the γ chain of the Fcε receptor is also found associated with the T-cell receptor. It is not known if there are functional differences between these various forms. In contrast to the other CD3 chains, neither the ζ, η nor Fcε receptor γ polypeptides extend far outside the cell; the bulk of their polypeptide chains lie in the cytoplasm. The ζ chain contains three sets of ITAM sequences that allow it to interact with cytosolic tyrosine kinases, and it is also a major target for tyrosine phosphorylation.

The CD3 proteins are also required for the cell-surface expression of the T-cell receptor. Mutant cells lacking either of the T-cell receptor chains, or any of the γ, δ, or ε chains of the CD3 complex, fail to express any of the chains of the complex at the cell surface. Sequences lying within the plasma membrane which contain the basic or acidic residues of the α:β heterodimer or of the CD3γ, δ, or ε chains respectively (see Fig. 4.34), seem to be required for the complex to assemble and be transported to the cell surface. Mutant cells lacking ζ chains express much reduced levels of the T-cell receptor at the cell surface, suggesting that the ζ chain plays an important, but not vital, role in transport.

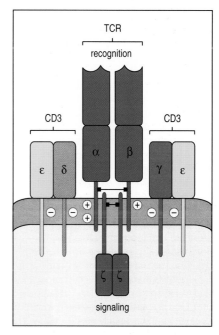

Fig. 4.34 The outline structure of the T-cell receptor:CD3 complex. The receptor for antigens on the surface of T cells is composed of eight polypeptide chains. Two are the disulfide-bonded chains of the T-cell receptor that recognizes antigen (TCR). The other six chains, collectively called CD3, signal to the interior of the cell that antigen binding has occurred. These chains are coordinately expressed at the T-cell surface.

| 4-27 | **The co-receptor molecules CD4 and CD8 cooperate with the T-cell receptor in antigen recognition.** |

We have seen that T cells fall into two major classes that differ in the class of MHC molecule they recognize, have different effector functions, and are distinguished by the cell-surface proteins CD4 and CD8. CD4 and CD8 were known for some time as markers for different functional sets of T cells before it became clear that they play an important part in the differential recognition of MHC class II and class I molecules. It is now known that CD4 binds to invariant parts of the MHC class II molecule and CD8 to invariant parts of the MHC class I molecule. During antigen recognition, CD4 and CD8 molecules associate on the T-cell surface with components of the T-cell receptor. For this reason, they are called **co-receptors**.

CD4 is a single-chain molecule composed of four immunoglobulin-like domains (Fig. 4.35). The first two domains (D_1 and D_2) of the CD4 molecule are packed tightly together to form a rigid rod some 60 Å long, which is believed to be joined by a flexible hinge to a similar rod formed by the third and fourth domains (D_3 and D_4). The cytoplasmic domain interacts strongly with a cytoplasmic tyrosine kinase called Lck, which

Fig. 4.35 The outline structures of the CD4 and CD8 co-receptor molecules. The CD4 molecule exists as a monomer (panel a) and contains four immunoglobulin-like domains. The crystal structure of the first two domains of human CD4 has been obtained and is shown here in panel b. The amino-terminal domain, D_1, in white, is similar in structure to an immunoglobulin variable domain. The second domain, D_2, in purple, although it is clearly related to immunoglobulin domains, is different from both V and C domains and has been termed a C_2 domain. The first two domains of CD4 form a rigid rod-like structure that is linked to the two carboxy-terminal domains by a flexible link. The binding site for MHC class II molecules is thought to involve both the D_1 and D_2 domains of CD4. The CD8 molecule is a heterodimer of an α and a β chain that are covalently associated by a disulfide bond (panel a). The two chains of the dimer have very similar structures, each having a single domain resembling an immunoglobulin variable domain and a stretch of peptide believed to be in a relatively extended conformation that links the variable region-like domain to the cell membrane. The structure shown in panel c is that of a homodimer of CD8α chains, which both resembles and functions like the α:β heterodimer. Photographs courtesy of C Thorpe.

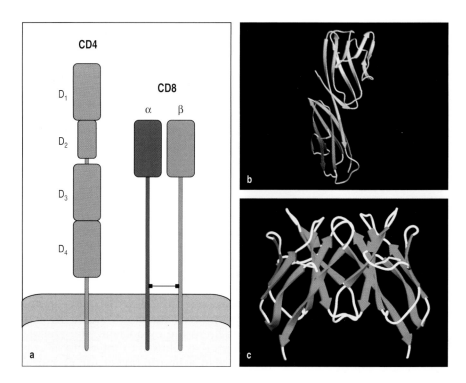

enables the CD4 molecule to participate in signal transduction. CD4 binds MHC class II molecules through a region that lies mainly on a lateral face of the first domain, although it is thought that residues in the second domain may also be involved. CD4 binding to MHC class II is weak on its own, and it is not clear whether this binding is able to transmit any signal to the interior of the T cell. As CD4 binds to a site on the β_2 domain of the MHC class II molecule that is well away from the site where the T-cell receptor binds (Fig. 4.36), the CD4 molecule and the T-cell receptor can bind the same peptide:MHC class II complex. Because they bind independently to the peptide:MHC class II complex, they come together only during antigen recognition when they act synergistically in signaling. The presence of CD4 results in a marked increase in the sensitivity of a T cell to antigen presented by MHC class II molecules, lowering by 100-fold the dose of antigen required for activation, as discussed in the next section.

Although CD4 and CD8 both function as co-receptors, their structures are quite distinct. The CD8 molecule is a disulfide-linked heterodimer comprising α and β chains, each containing a single immunoglobulin-like domain linked to the membrane by a segment of polypeptide chain that is believed to have an extended conformation (see Fig. 4.35). It is not known whether a single domain of the CD8 molecule contacts MHC class I proteins or whether the binding site is formed by the interaction of the CD8α and CD8β chains, although it is known that CD8α homodimers can also bind MHC class I molecules. CD8 binds weakly on its own to the α_3 domain of MHC class I molecules (see Fig. 4.36), allowing it to bind simultaneously with the T-cell receptor to specific peptide:MHC class I complexes. CD8 also binds Lck with its cytoplasmic tail and increases the sensitivity of T cells bearing the CD8 co-receptor to antigen presented by MHC class I molecules by about 100-fold. Thus, the two co-receptor proteins have similar functions, although their structures are only distantly related.

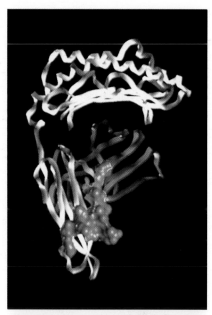

Fig. 4.36 The binding site for CD8 and CD4 on MHC class I and class II molecules lies in the immunoglobulin-like domains. The binding sites for CD8 and CD4 on the MHC class I and class II molecules respectively lie in the membrane proximal, immunoglobulin-like domains, distant from the peptide-binding cleft. CD8 binds to a site, shown as a green surface in the top panel, at the base of the α_3 domain of the MHC class I molecule. The α chain of the class I molecule is shown in white while the β_2-microglobulin is shown in purple. CD4 binds to a site on the β_2 domain that, as shown on the structure of a MHC class II molecule, as a green surface in the bottom panel, is also at the base of the domain and distant from the peptide-binding site. The α chain of the class II molecule is shown in purple while the β chain is in white. Photographs courtesy of C Thorpe.

4-28 Antigen recognition activates protein tyrosine kinases in the T cell.

Signaling through the antigen-specific T-cell receptor requires aggregation of the T-cell receptors themselves by the array of peptide:MHC complexes on the surface of a target cell, just as stimulation of B cells requires crosslinking and clustering of cell-surface immunoglobulin. Optimal signaling through the T-cell receptor requires a clustering with the co-receptors CD4 or CD8, just as CD19 co-aggregation with immunoglobulin enhances B-cell signaling (see Section 3-29). The aggregation of the receptors and co-receptors results in the increased association of the co-receptor-associated tyrosine kinases with the receptor and CD3 cytoplasmic tails; this type of association is a trigger for the activation of many cell types by growth factors or hormones. In addition, some evidence suggests that changes in T-cell receptor conformation induced by ligand binding also contribute to signaling.

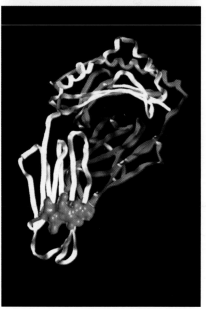

As described earlier (see Section 4-26), the cytoplasmic domains of the CD3 proteins, especially the ζ chains, contain sequences that, when phosphorylated, allow the binding of cytosolic protein tyrosine kinases. The co-receptor molecules, CD4 and CD8, are also associated with a protein tyrosine kinase, Lck. When T cells recognize their specific peptide:MHC complex, the T-cell receptor complex is aggregated together with the appropriate co-receptor, and the tails of the T-cell receptor complex are brought together with those of the co-receptor (Fig. 4.37). About 100 specific peptide:MHC complexes on a target cell are required to trigger a T cell that expresses a suitable co-receptor. In the absence of the co-receptor, 10 000 identical complexes (or about 10% of all the MHC molecules on the cell) would be required. Thus, co-receptors are virtually essential for T-cell activation by peptides bound to MHC molecules.

One substrate phosphorylated by the cytosolic tyrosine kinases that become associated with the CD3 tails are the cytoplasmic domains of CD3ε and ζ. Phosphorylated ζ chains then bind and activate a cytosolic tyrosine kinase of 70 kDa known as zeta-associated protein-70 (ZAP-70). This kinase is related to Syk in B cells, and it probably has a role in sustaining T-cell receptor signaling. Patients lacking ZAP-70 have recently been described, and their CD4 T cells, while maturing normally, fail to respond to signals delivered via their T cell receptors.

T-cell activation through the tyrosine kinases associated with the receptor complex is modulated by another T-cell surface molecule called **CD45**. CD45 is a transmembrane molecule whose cytoplasmic domain has tyrosine-specific phosphatase activity. It is believed that CD45 activates the tyrosine kinases associated with the receptor and co-receptor molecules by removing inhibitory phosphate groups. T cells that lack CD45 are defective in signaling through the T-cell receptor. Like the co-receptors, CD45 is believed to associate physically with the T-cell receptor complex, although in this case the mechanism of association is not known.

Fig. 4.37 Binding of antigen to the T-cell receptor initiates a series of biochemical changes within the T cell. It is believed that protein tyrosine phosphorylation plays an important part in the activation of T cells as both the T-cell receptor complex and the co-receptor (in this example the CD4 molecule) are associated with cytoplasmic tyrosine kinases. Further, the CD45 molecule, a T-cell surface protein known to be required for activation of T cells, has protein tyrosine phosphatase activity in its cytoplasmic domain. It is thought that ligand binding to the T-cell receptor and the co-receptor brings together CD4, the T-cell receptor:CD3 complex and CD45, thus allowing the CD45 tyrosine phosphatase to activate the Lck and Fyn tyrosine kinases associated with the co-receptor and T-cell receptor:CD3 complex. The events occurring after the activation of these tyrosine kinases are not known in detail. One effect is to phosphorylate ζ, which then binds and activates a cytosolic tyrosine kinase called zeta-associated protein-70 (ZAP-70). Activation of these kinases also leads to activation of phospholipase C-γ, which cleaves the phospholipid, phosphatidyl-inositol-4,5-bisphosphate (PIP$_2$), to yield diacylglycerol (DAG) and inositol trisphosphate (IP$_3$). DAG acts within the cell to activate a protein serine/threonine kinase, protein kinase C (PKC) and IP$_3$ acts to release calcium ions (Ca^{2+}) from intracellular stores. In addition, a calcum-specific ion channel is opened in the T-cell membrane to allow the influx of calcium ions from extracellular sources. The activation of protein kinase C and the elevation of calcuim ion concentrations within the cell are common features of the stimulation of cell proliferation in a number of cell types. The combination of these two signals activates intracellular DNA-binding proteins and transcription factors that act upon the chromatin of the T cell, initiating a cascade of events that results in the proliferation and differentiation of the T cell, as will be discussed in more detail in Chapter 7.

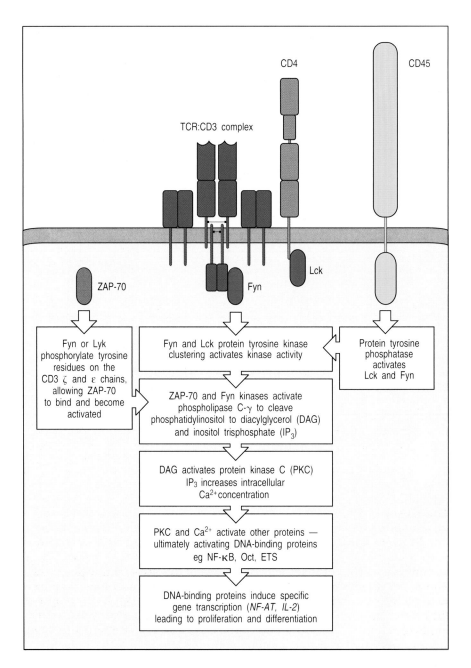

One of the earliest consequences of the activation of T-cell receptor-associated tyrosine kinases is the activation through tyrosine phosphorylation of the enzyme phospholipase C-γ within the T cell. This activated enzyme breaks down phosphatidylinositol-4,5-bisphosphate (PIP$_2$) into inositol trisphosphate (IP$_3$), which releases calcium from intracellular stores, and diacylglycerol, an activator of the enzyme protein kinase C, a serine/threonine kinase. In addition, a channel specific for calcium ions is opened in the T-cell membrane, allowing entry of calcium ions from the surrounding extracellular fluid. Both intracellular calcium ions and protein kinase C subsequently activate a variety of enzymes within the cell, including other protein kinases. The enzymes phosphorylate a variety of proteins within the cell, leading ultimately to a cellular response that requires new gene expression (see Chapter 7).

Signal transduction in T cells is potently inhibited by two drugs called **cyclosporin A** and **FK506** (see Chapter 12). These drugs are widely used to prevent graft rejection, which they do by inhibiting the activation of alloreactive T cells. Cyclosporin A and FK506 both inhibit a ser- ine/threonine-specific protein phosphatase called **calcineurin**. Thus, removal of phosphates from serine and/or threonine residues on an as yet unidentified protein must also be crucial for T-cell activation.

The signaling events described here occur in fully differentiated effector T cells and lead to the release of effector molecules by the activated T cell. These may be the cytotoxins released by cytotoxic T cells, which help cause the death of virus-infected cells, or the cytokines released by helper T cells that help activate antigen-binding B cells to produce anti- bodies. These effector molecules will be discussed in more detail in Chapter 7. The same signals are also crucial earlier in the development of T cells, both for the initiation of maturation to effector status on first encounter with antigen, and for proper differentiation of T cells during their development in the thymus. However, in these latter settings other signals are also required, and these will be discussed in detail in Chapters 6 and 7.

| 4-29 | **Certain variants of antigenic peptides generate partial signals for activation, or can inhibit T-cell responses.** |

So far, we have assumed that any MHC:peptide complex that is recog- nized by a T-cell receptor will activate the T cell bearing that receptor. However, some experiments originally designed to explore the struc- tural basis for antigen recognition by T cells showed unexpectedly that recognition does not necessarily lead to activation. Some MHC:peptide complexes that do not themselves activate a given T cell can actually inhibit its response to the MHC:peptide complex that it normally recog- nizes. These peptides are usually called **antagonist peptides**, or **altered peptides ligands**.

In these experiments, variants of a known peptide ligand were made in which the changes were thought to affect amino acids that contact the T-cell receptor, but not those that direct binding to the MHC molecule. Some of these peptides proved to be unable to stimulate responses in the appropriate T cells, while others (called **partial agonist peptides**) elicited partial responses. More surprisingly, some peptides rendered the T cells unresponsive to stimulation with agonist peptides, whether presented to the T-cell receptor on the same antigen-pre- senting cell or, even more strikingly, when exposed to the activating peptide at a later time.

These effects are unlikely to be significant for most physiological immune responses, although they may contribute to some persistent viral infections. For example, mutant peptides of epitopes on cells in- fected with human immunodeficiency virus can inhibit activation of CD8 T cells at a 1:100 ratio of antagonist to agonist; this allows the infected cells to survive even though virus-specific cytotoxic cells are present. Differential signaling by variants of agonist peptides may also be important for the development of T cells in the thymus, where the immature cells are selected for the ability to recognize foreign peptides antigens in the context of self MHC molecules. This process, which we shall discuss in detail in Chapter 6, would seem to require immature T cells to be signaled by a self-peptide:self-MHC complex that is related to but not identical with the foreign peptide:self MHC complex that the mature T cell will specifically recognize.

It is not known how antagonist peptides work. One possibility is that the affinity of the T-cell receptor for the antagonist peptide:MHC complex is lower than that for the activating complex, and the T-cell receptor dissociates too quickly from its ligand for a full activating signal to be delivered. An alternative possibility is that conformational changes in the T-cell receptor contribute to signaling, and antagonist peptides fail to trigger these conformational changes.

4-30 Some T cells bear an alternative form of T-cell receptor with γ and δ chains.

At the time of the discovery of the T-cell receptor α:β heterodimer, all known specific immune responses could be accounted for by the action of cells bearing these polypeptides. Thus, it was a real surprise when during the search for genes encoding T-cell receptors, a third T cell-specific cDNA was discovered that also encoded a protein with homology to immunoglobulin and that rearranged in T lymphocytes. As this gene clearly did not encode either the α or the β chain of the T-cell receptor, it was termed T-cell receptor γ. The γ polypeptide is found on the cell surface associated with a second polypeptide, called the T-cell receptor δ chain. The **γ:δ heterodimer**, like the homologous α:β heterodimer, is also associated with the CD3 complex on the cell surface and the γ:δ receptor chains should not be confused with the CD3 γ and δ chains.

Similarly, the organization of the γ and δ genes shown in Fig. 4.38 resembles that of the α and β genes, although there are some important differences. The gene complex encoding the δ chain is found entirely within the T-cell receptor α-chain gene complex between the $V_α$ and the $J_α$ gene segments. As a result, any rearrangement of the α-chain genes inactivates the genes encoding δ chains. There are many fewer V gene segments at the γ and δ loci than at either the T-cell receptor α or β loci or for any of the immunoglobulin loci. Increased junctional variability in the δ chains may compensate for the small number of possible variable regions and has the effect of focusing almost all of the variability in the γ:δ receptor in the junctional region. As we have seen, the amino acids encoded in the junctional region lie at the center of the binding site.

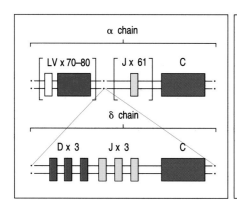

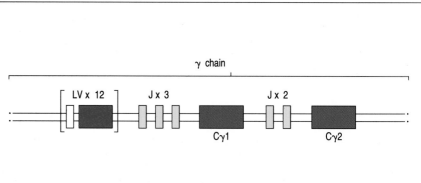

Fig. 4.38 The organization of the T-cell receptor γ and δ chain genes of the human. The γ and δ genes, like the α and β genes, have discrete V, D, J, and C gene segments. Uniquely, the gene encoding the δ chain is located entirely within the gene encoding the α chain, lying between the cluster of $V_α$ segments and the cluster of $J_α$ segments. There are three $D_δ$ segments, three $J_δ$ segments, and a single constant segment. The $V_δ$ gene segments are interspersed among the $V_α$ gene segments; it is not known exactly how many $V_δ$ segments there are but there are at least four. The human γ chain resembles the β chains, with two constant-region gene segments each with its own J segments. The mouse γ genes (not shown) have a more complex organization and there are three functional clusters of γ genes, each containing variable, joining and constant segments. Rearrangement of the γ and δ genes proceeds as for the other T-cell receptor genes, with the exception that during δ-chain rearrangement both D segments can be used in the same gene. Use of two D segments greatly increases the variability, mainly because extra N-region nucleotides can be added at the junction between the two D segments as well as at the VD and DJ junctions.

T cells bearing γ:δ receptors are a distinct lineage of cells of unknown function. The ligand for this receptor is also unknown, although some γ:δ T cells can recognize products of certain class IB genes (see Section 4-14) while others appear to be able to recognize antigen directly, much as antibodies do, without the requirement for presentation by an MHC molecule or processing of the antigen. Detailed analysis of the rearranged variable regions of γ:δ T cell receptors show that they resemble variable regions of antibody molecules more than they resemble the variable regions of α:β T cell receptors. In peripheral lymphoid tissues, only a very small percentage (generally 1–5%) of CD3-positive cells express γ:δ receptors instead of α:β receptors. However, in epithelial tissues, especially in the epidermis and small intestine of the mouse, most T cells express γ:δ receptors. The receptors of these epithelial γ:δ T cells show extremely restricted variability. We shall return to the possible functional significance of these findings in Chapter 9.

Summary.

T-cell receptors are closely similar to immunoglobulins and are encoded by homologous genes. However, diversity is distributed differently in T-cell receptors, which have roughly the same number of V gene segments, but more J and D gene segments and more powerful mechanisms for diversification of junctions between gene segments. Moreover, T-cell receptors are not known to diversify their V genes after rearrangement through somatic hypermutation. This leads to a T-cell receptor structure where the highest diversity is in the central part of the receptor, which contacts the bound peptide fragment of the ligand. The cell-surface T-cell receptor resembles in many ways the cell-surface form of immunoglobulins. Both are associated in the cell membrane with a complex of invariant proteins that are required for transport of the receptors to the cell surface and for signal transduction. Both receptors must not only bind antigen but also become clustered or crosslinked in order to stimulate the cell. The co-receptor molecules CD4 and CD8 bind MHC class II and MHC class I molecules respectively, and act synergistically with the T-cell receptor in signaling, resulting in about a 100-fold increase in the sensitivity of T cells to antigen. The biochemical events that follow from antigen binding to the T-cell receptor share many features with other signaling systems, including that of B cells, in which cell growth or cell activation is regulated by the binding of growth factors or hormones.

Summary to Chapter 4.

The T-cell receptor is very similar to immunoglobulins, both in structure and in the way in which variability is introduced into the antigen-binding site. However, there are also important differences between T-cell receptors and immunoglobulins that are related to the nature of the antigens recognized by T cells. The mechanism of generation of diversity in T-cell receptors focuses the diversity into the CDR3 loops of T-cell receptor variable regions, which lie in the center of the antigen-binding site. This pattern of diversity reflects the form in which antigen is recognized by the T-cell receptor, which is as a complex formed by a peptide antigen bound to an MHC molecule on the target cell surface. There are two classes of MHC molecule: MHC class I molecules, which bind peptides derived from proteins synthesized and degraded in the cytosol; and MHC class II molecules, which bind peptides derived from proteins degraded in cellular vesicles. There are several genes for each class of MHC molecule, arranged in a cluster in the major histocompatibility complex (MHC), together with genes involved in the degradation of protein antigens into peptides and their transport to the cell surface bound to MHC molecules. Because the genes for the MHC class I and class II molecules are highly polymorphic, each cell expresses several different MHC class I and class II proteins, and is thus able to bind many different peptide antigens. The binding site for the peptide on an MHC molecule lies in a cleft between two α helices; thus the T-cell receptor recognizes a ligand that has a region of high variability (the peptide antigen) lying between regions of lesser variability (the α helices of the MHC). The distribution of variability in the T-cell receptor thus correlates with the distribution of variability in the ligand it must recognize. Unlike immunoglobulins, T-cell receptors are not known to use somatic hypermutation as a means of increasing receptor variability. Thus, the features that are unique to the T-cell receptor can all be understood in terms of the unique biology of the T cell.

General references.

Klein, J.: *Natural History of the Major Histocompatibility Complex.* New York: J. Wiley & Sons; 1986.

Haas, W., Pereira P., and Tonegawa S.: **Gamma/delta cells.** *Ann. Rev. Immunol.* 1993, **11**:637-685.

Neefjes, J.J., and Mombourg, F.: **Cell biology of antigen presentation.** *Curr. Opin. Immunol.* 1993, **5**:27-34.

Klein, J., Satta, Y., and OHuigin, C.: **The molecular descent of the major histocompatibility complex.** *Ann. Rev. Immunol.* 1993, **11**:269-295.

Davis, M.M., and Bjorkman, P.J.: **T-cell antigen receptor genes and T-cell recognition.** *Nature* 1988, **334**:395-402.

Monaco, J.J.: **A molecular model of MHC class I-restricted antigen processing.** *Immunol. Today* 1992, **13**:173-179.

Bodmer, J.G., Marsh, S.G.E., Albert, E.D., Bodmer, W.F., DuPont, B., Erlich, H.A., Mach, B., Mayr, W.R., Parham, P., Saszuki, T., *et al.*: **Nomenclature for factors of the HLA system, 1991.** *Tissue Antigens* 1992, **39**:161-173.

Townsend, A., and Bodmer, H.: **Antigen recognition by class I-restricted T lymphocytes.** *Ann Rev. Immunol.* 1989, **7**:601-624.

Bjorkman, P.J., and Parham, P.: **Structure, function and diversity of class I major histocompatibility complex molecules.** *Ann. Rev. Biochem.* 1990, **59**: 253-288.

Rammensee, H.G.: **Chemistry of peptides associated with MHC class I and class II molecules.** *Curr.Op. Immunol.* 1995, **7**:85-96.

Moller, G. (ed): **Origin of major histocompatibility complex diversity.** *Immunol. Rev.* 1995, **143**:5-292.

Germain, R.N.: **MHC-dependent antigen processing and peptide presentation: Providing ligands for T lymphocyte activation.** *Cell.* 1994, **76**:287-299.

Section references.

4-1   **T cells with different functions recognize peptides produced in two distinct intracellular compartments.**

Morrison, L.A., Lukacher, A.E., Braciale, V.L., Fan, D.P., and Braciale, T.J.: **Differences in antigen presentation to MHC class I- and class II-restricted influenza virus-specific cytolytic T-lymphocyte clones**. *J. Exper. Med.* 1986, **163**:903.

4-2   **The two classes of MHC molecule have a distinct subunit structure but a similar three-dimensional structure.**

Bjorkman, P.J., Saper, M.A., Samraoui, B., Bennett, W.S., Strominger, J.L., and Wiley, D.C.: **The foreign antigen-binding site and T-cell recognition regions of class I histocompatibility antigens.** *Nature* 1987, **329**:512-518.

Bjorkman, P.J., Saper, M.A., Samraoui, B., Bennet, W.S., Strominger, J.L., and Wiley, D.C.: **Structure of the human class I histocompatibility antigen HLA-A2.** *Nature* 1987, **329**:506-512.

Brown, J.H., Jardetzky, T.S., Gorga, J.C., Stern, L.J., Urban, R.G., Strominger, J.L., and Wiley, D.C.: **The three-dimensional structure of the human class II histocompatibility antigen HLA-DR1.** *Nature* 1993, **364**:33-39.

4-3   **A T cell recognises a complex of a peptide fragment bound to an MHC molecule.**

Guillet, J.G., Lai, M.Z., Briner, T.J., Smith, J.A., and Gefter, M.L.: **Interaction of peptide antigens and class II major histocompatibility complex antigens.** *Nature* 1986, **324**:260-262.

Watts, T.M., Brian, A.A., Kappler, J.W., Marrack, P., and McConnell, H.M.: **Antigen presentation by supported planar membranes containing I-A**[d]. *Proc. Natl Acad. Sci. USA* 1984, **81**:7564.

4-4   **Peptides are stably bound to MHC molecules.**

Falk, K., Rotzsche, O., Stevanovic, S., Jung, G., Rammensee, H.-G.: **Allele-specific motifs revealed by sequencing of self peptides eluted from MHC molecules.** *Nature* 1991, **351**:290-296.

Hunt, D.F., Henderson, R.A., Shabanowitz, J., Sakaguchi, K., Michel, H., Sevilir, N., Cox, A.L., Appella, E., and Engelhard, V.H.: **Characterization of peptides bound to the class I MHC molecule HLA-A2.1 by mass spectrometry.** *Science* 1992, **255**:1261-1263.

Madden, D.R., Gorga, J.C., Strominger, J.L. and Wiley, D.C.: **The three-dimensional structure of HLA-B27 at 2.1Å resolution suggests a general mechanism for tight peptide binding to MHC.** *Cell* 1992, **70**:1035-1048.

Guo, H-C., Jardetsky, T.S., Lane, W.S., Strominger, J.L. & Wiley, D.C.: **Different length peptides bind to HLA-Aw68 similarly at their ends but bulge out in the middle.** *Nature* 1992, **360**:364-366.

Fremont, D.H., Matsumura, M., Stura, E.A., Peterson, P.A. & Wilson, I.: **Crystal structures of two viral peptides in complex with murine MHC class 1 H-2K**[b]. *Science*, 1992, **257**:919-927.

4-6 Peptides that bind to MHC class I molecules are actively transported from cytosol to the endoplasmic reticulum.

Shepherd, J.C., Schumacher, T.N.M., Ashton-Rickardt, P.G., Imaeda, S., Ploegh, H.L., Janeway, C.A. Jr., and Tonegawa, S.: **TAP1-dependent peptide translocation** *in vitro* **is ATP-dependent and peptide-selective.** *Cell* 1993, **74**:577-584.

Townsend, A., Ohlen, C., Foster, L., Bastin, J., Lunggren, H.-G., and Karre, K.: **A mutant cell in which association of class I heavy and light chains is induced by viral peptides.** *Cold Spring Harbor Symp. Quant. Biol.* 1989, **54**:299-308.

4-7 Newly synthesized MHC class I molecules are retained in the endoplasmic reticulum by binding to TAP-1 until they bind peptide.

Degen, E., and Williams, D.B.: **Participation of a novel 88kD protein in the biogenesis of murine class I histocompatibility molecules.** *J. Cell Biol.* 1991, **112**:1099-1155.

Ortmann, B., Androlewicz, M.J., and Cresswell, P.: **MHC class I Isol β2-microglobulin complexes associate with TAP transporters before peptide binding.** *Nature.* 1994, **368**,864-867.

Williams, D.B. and Watts, T.H.: **Molecular chaperones in antigen presentation.** *Curr. Op. Immunol.* 1995, **7**:77-84.

4-8 Peptides of cytosolic proteins are generated in the cytosol prior to transport into the endoplasmic reticulum.

Van Kaer, L., Ashton-Rickardt, P.G., Eichelberger, M., Gaczynska, M., Nagashima, K., Rock, K.L., Goldberg, A.L., Doherty, P.C., and Tonegawa, S.: **Altered peptides and viral specific T cell responses in LMP2 mutant mice.** *Immunity.* 1994, **1**:533-541.

4-9 Peptides presented by MHC class II molecules are generated in acidified Intracellular vesicles.

Cresswell, P.: **Assembly, transport and function of MHC class II molecules.** *Ann. Rev. Immunol.* 1995, **12**:259-293.

4-10 The invariant chain directs newly synthesized MHC class II molecules to acidified intracellular vesicles.

Roche, P.A., and Cresswell, P.: **Invariant chain association with HLA-DR molecules inhibits immunogenic peptide binding.** *Nature* 1990, **345**:615-618.

Roche, P.A., Marks, M.S., Cresswell, P.: **Formation of a nine subunit complex by HLA class II glycoproteins and the invariant chain.** *Nature* 1991, **354**:392-394.

Peters, P.J., Neefjes, J.J., Orschot, V., Ploegh, H.L., and Geuze, H.J.: **Segregation of MHC class II molecules from MHC class I molecules in the Golgi complex for transport to lysosomal compartments.** *Nature* 1991, **349**:669-676.

Davidson, H.W., Reid, P.A., Lanzavecchia, A., and Watts, C.: **Processed antigen binds to newly synthesized MHC class II molecules in antigen specific B lymphocytes.** *Cell* 1991, **67**:105-116.

Tulip, A., Verwoerd, D., Dobberstein, B., Ploegh, H.L., and Pieters, J.: **Isolation and characterization of the Intracellular MHC Class II compartment.** *Nature* 1994, **369**:120-126.

Amigorena, S., Drake, J.R., Webster, P., and Mellman, I.: **Transient accumulation of new class II MHC molecules in a novel endocytic compartment in B lymphocytes.** *Nature* 1994, **369**:113-120.

4-11 A specialized MHC class II-like molecule catalyzes loading of MHC class II molecules with endogenously processed peptides.

Denzin, L.K., Robbins, N.F., Carboy-Newcomb, C., and Cresswell, P.: **Assembly and intracellular transport of HLA-DM and correction of the class II antigen processing defect in T2 cells.** *Immunity*, 1994, **1**:595-606.

Morris, M., Shaman, J., Attaya, M., Amaya, M., Goodman, S., Bergman, C., Monaco, J., and Mellins, E.: **An essential role for HLA-DM in antigen presentation by class II major histocompatibility molecules.** *Nature* 1994, **368**:551-554.

Fling, S., Arp B., and Pious, D.: **HLA-DMA and -DMB genes are both required for MHC class II/peptide complex formation in antigen presenting cells.** *Nature* 1994 **368**:554-558.

4-12 The characteristics of peptide binding by MHC molecules allow effective antigen presentation at the cell surface.

Lanzavecchia, A., Reid, P.A., and Watts, C.: **Irreversible association of peptides with class II MHC molecules in living cells.** *Nature* 1992, **357**:249-252.

4-13 The proteins involved in antigen processing and presentation are encoded by genes in the major histocompatibility complex.

Trowsdale, J., and Campbell, R.D.: **Complexity in the major histocompatibility complex.** *Eur. J. Immunogenet.* 1992, **19**:45-55.

4-14 A variety of genes with specialized functions in immunity are also encoded in the MHC.

Campbell, R.D. and Trowsdale, J.: **Map of the human MHC.** *Immunol. Today* **14**:349-352.

4-15 The protein products of MHC class I and class II genes are highly polymorphic.

Klein, J., Satta, Y., and O'Huigin, C.: **The molecular descent of the major histocompatibility complex.** *Ann. Rev. Immunol.* 1993, **11**:269-295.

4-16 MHC polymorphism affects antigen recognition indirectly by controlling peptide binding.

Babbitt, B., Allen, P.M., Matsueda, G., Haber, E., and Unuanue, E.R.: **Binding of immunogenic peptides to Ia histocompatibility molecules.** *Nature* 1985, **317**:359.

Buus, S., Sette, A., Colon, S.M., Miles, C., and Grey, H.M.: **The relation between major histocompatibility complex (MHC) restriction and the capacity of Ia to bind immunogenic peptides.** *Science* 1987, **235**:1353.

4-17 MHC polymorphism directly affects antigen recognition by T cells.

Ajitkumar, P., Geier, S.S., Kesari, K.V., Borriello, F., Nakagawa, M., Bluestone, J.A., Saper, M.A., Wiley, D.C., and Nathenson, S.G.: **Evidence that multiple residues on both the alpha helices of the class I MHC molecule are simultaneously recognized by the T-cell receptor.** *Cell* 1989, **54**:47.

Zinkernagel, R.M., and Doherty, P.C.: **Restriction of** *in vivo* **T-cell mediated cytotoxicity in lymphocytic choriomeningitis within a syngeneic or semiallogeneic system.** *Nature* 1974, **248**:701-702.

Rosenthal, A.S., and Shevach, E.M.: **Function of macrophages in antigen recognition by guinea pig T lymphocytes. I. Requirement for histocompatible macrophages and lymphocytes.** *J. Exper. Med.* 1973, **138**:1194.

Katz, D.H., Hamaoka, T., Dorf, M.E., Maurer, P.H., and Benacerraf, B.: **Cell interactions between histoincompatible T and B lymphocytes. IV. Involvement of immune response (Ir) gene control of lymphocyte interaction controlled by the gene.** *J. Exper. Med.* 1973, **138**:734.

4-18   Non-self MHC molecules are recognized by 1–10% of T cells.

Kaye, J., and Janeway, C.A. Jr.: **The Fab fragment of a directly activating monoclonal antibody that precipitates a disulfide-linked heterodimer from a helper T-cell clone blocks activation by either allogeneic Ia or antigen and self-Ia.** *J. Exper. Med.* 1984, **159**:1397-1412.

4-19   MHC polymorphism extends the range of antigens to which the immune system can respond.

Parham, P., Chen, B.P., Clayberger, C., Ennis, P.D., Krensky, A.M., Lawlor, D.A., Littman, D.R., Norment, A.M., Orr, H.T., Salter, R.D., and Zemmour, J.: **Diversity of class I HLA molecules: Functional and evolutionary interactions with T cells.** *Cold Spring Harbor Symp. Quant. Biol.* 1989, **54**:529.

Hill, A.V.,Elvin, J., Willis, A.C., Aidoo, M., Allsopp, C.E.M. Gotch, F.M., Gao, X.M., Takiguchi, M., Greenwood, B.M., Townsend, A.R.M., McMichael, A.J., and Whittle, H.C.: **Molecular analysis of the association of B53 and resistance to severe malaria**, *Nature*, 1992, **360**: 434-440.

4-20   Multiple genetic processes generate MHC polymorphism.

Nathenson, S.G., Geliebter, J., Pfaffenbach, G.M., and Zeff, R.A.: **Murine major histocompatibility complex class I mutants: Molecular analysis and structure:function implications.** *Annu. Rev. Immunol.* 1986, **4**:471.

Begovich, A.B., McClure, G.R., Suraj, V.C., Helmuth, R.C., Fildes, N., Bugawan T.L., Erlich H.A. and Klitz, W.: **Polymorphism, recombination and linkage disequilibrium within the HLA class II region.** *Immunol.*, 1992, **148**: 249-258.

Erlich, H.A. and Gyllensten, U.B.: **Shared epitopes among HLA class II alleles: Gene conversion, common ancestry and balancing selection.** *Immunol. Today*, 1991, **12**: 411-414.

She, J.X., Boehme, S.A., Wang, T.W., Bonhomme F., and Wakeland, E.K.: **Amplification of major histocompatibility complex class II gene diversity by intraexonic recombination.** *Proc. Natl. Acad. Sci. USA* 1991, **88**:453-457.

4-21   The T-cell receptor resembles a membrane-associated Fab fragment of immunoglobulin.

Allison, J.P., McIntyre, B.W., and Bloch, D.: **Tumor-specific antigen of murine T lymphoma defined with monoclonal antibody.** *J. Immunol.* 1982, **129**:2293.

Meuer, S.C., Fitzgerald, K.A., Hussey, R.E., Hodgdon, J.C., Schlossman, S.F., and Reinharz, E.L.: **Clonotypic structures involved in antigen-specific human T-cell function: Relationship to the T3 molecular complex.** *J. Immunol.* 1982, **129**:2293.

4-23   T-cell receptor diversity is focused in CDR3.

Davis, M.M. and Bjorkman, P.J.: **T-cell antigen receptor genes and T cell recognition.** *Nature 1988,* **334**:395-402.

4-24   Diversity in T-cell receptors is not extended by somatic hypermutation.

Zheng, B., Xue, W., and Kelsoe, G.: **Locus-specific somatic hypermutation in germinal centre T cells.** *Nature 1994,* **372**:556-559.

4-25   Many T cells respond to superantigens.

Choi, Y.W., Herman, A., DiGiusto, D., Wade, T., Marrack, P., and Kappler, J.: **Residues of the variable region of the T-cell receptor beta chain that interact with *S. aureus* toxin superantigens.** *Nature* 1990, **346**:471-473.

Janeway, C.A. Jr., Yagi, J., Conrad, P.J., Katz, M.E., Jones, B., Vroegrop, S., and Buxser, S.: **T-cell responses to Mls and to bacterial proteins that mimic its behavior.** *Immunol. Rev.* 1989, **197**:61-88.

Fraser, J.D.: **High-affinity binding of staphylococcal enterotoxins A and B to HLA-DR.** *Nature* 1989, **339**:221-223.

4-26   The T-cell receptor associates with the invariant proteins of the CD3 complex.

Weissman, A.M., Baniyash, M., Hou, D., Samelson, L.E., Burgess, W.H., and Klausner, R.D.: **Molecular cloning of the zeta chain of the T-cell antigen receptor.** *Science* 1988, **239**:1018.

Weiss, A., and Stobo, J.D.: **Requirement for the co-expression of T3 and T-cell antigen on a malignant human T-cell line.** *J. Exper. Med.* 1984, **160**:1284-1299.

4-27   The co-receptor molecules CD4 and CD8 cooperate with the T-cell receptor in antigen recognition.

Janeway, C.A. Jr.: **The T-cell receptor as a multicomponent signaling machine: CD4/CD8 coreceptors and CD45 in T-cell activation.** *Ann. Rev. Immunol.* 1992, **10**:645-674.

4-28   Antigen recognition activates protein tyrosine kinases in the T cell.

Pingel, J.R., and Thomas, M.L.: **Evidence that the leukocyte common antigen is required for antigen-induced T-lymphocyte proliferation.** *Cell* 1989, **58**:1055.

Samelson, L.E., Patel, M.D., Weissman, A.M., Harford, J.B., and Klausner, R.D.: **Antigen activation of murine T cells induces tyrosine phosphorylation of a polypeptide associated with the T-cell antigen receptor.** *Cell* 1986, **46**:1083.

Irving, B.A., and Weiss, A.: **The cytoplasmic domain of the T cell receptor chain is sufficient to couple to receptor-associated signal-transduction pathways.** *Cell* 1991, **64**:891.

4-29   Certain variants of antigenic peptides generate partial signals for activation, or can inhibit T-cell responses.

Sloan-Lancaster, J., and Allen, P.M.: **Significance of T cell stimulation by altered peptide ligand in T cell biology.** *Curr. OP. Immunol.* 1995, **7**:103-109.

De Magistris , M.T., Alexander, J., Coggeshall, M., Altman, A., Gueta, F.C.A., Grey, H.M., Sette, A.: **Antigen analog-major histocompatibility complexes act as antagonists of the T-cell receptor.** *Cell* 1992 **68**:625-634.

4-30   Some T cells bear an alternative form of the T-cell receptor with γ and δ chains.

Haas, W., Pereira, P., and Tonegawa, S.:**γ Isol δ cells.** *Ann. Rev. Immunol.* 1993, **11**:637-685.

PART III

THE DEVELOPMENT OF LYMPHOCYTE REPERTOIRES

The Development of B Lymphocytes

B lymphocytes are generated throughout human life, though in gradually decreasing numbers with age, providing a continuous supply of new B cells to make antibodies against the broad range of possible pathogens that must be recognized and repelled. In birds, B cells originate in a specialized organ called the bursa of Fabricius, while in mammals B-cell development occurs in the bone marrow: hence the term B lymphocyte, or B cell, for these cells. As we saw in Chapter 3, each B cell bears a unique receptor generated through somatic rearrangement of the immunoglobulin genes. In mammals, the separate rearrangement events that lead to the production of the two chains of the immunoglobulin molecule occur during the development of B cells in the bone marrow and are regulated so that each mature B cell produces only one heavy chain and one light chain, and thus bears receptors of a single specificity. In this way, a large and diverse repertoire of B-cell receptors is generated during the early phases of B-cell development.

The expression of antigen receptors on the surface of the B lymphocyte marks a major watershed in its life cycle. The B cell can now detect ligands in its environment and self tolerance must be established before it is allowed to undergo further maturation. The binding of antigen to surface immunoglobulin early in development leads to inactivation or loss of the B cell, guaranteeing tolerance to ubiquitous self antigens. The remaining cells express a broadly distributed repertoire of receptors that provides the raw material for clonal selection.

In this chapter, we shall define the different stages of B-cell development and see how the unselected B-cell receptor repertoire is generated, before discussing what is known of the mechanisms whereby tolerance is ensured while the B cells are still in the bone marrow. Finally, we shall follow the fate of B cells after their maturation in the bone marrow, up to the point at which they disperse to the lymphoid tissues where they may encounter foreign antigen. The main phases of B-cell development are summarized in Fig. 5.1. The activation of B lymphocytes and their subsequent production of antibody, their sole effector function, will be discussed in Chapter 8.

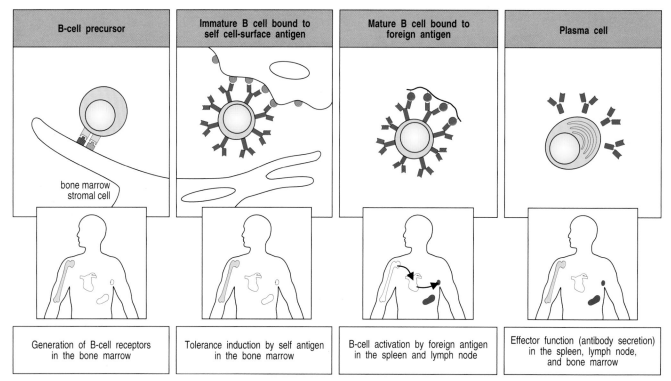

B-cell precursor	Immature B cell bound to self cell-surface antigen	Mature B cell bound to foreign antigen	Plasma cell
bone marrow stromal cell			
Generation of B-cell receptors in the bone marrow	Tolerance induction by self antigen in the bone marrow	B-cell activation by foreign antigen in the spleen and lymph node	Effector function (antibody secretion) in the spleen, lymph node, and bone marrow

Fig. 5.1 The life history of B cells can be divided into four broad phases. First panel: B cells develop from progenitor cells in the bone marrow and rearrange their immunoglobulin genes to produce a receptor with unique antigen specificity. As no surface immunoglobulin can be expressed until gene rearrangement is completed, this process is independent of antigens in the environment; it is, however, dependent on interactions with bone marrow stromal cells. Second panel: immature B cells expressing surface IgM can interact with antigens in their environment; if they encounter antigen at this stage they are either deleted or rendered tolerant. These first two phases occur in the bone marrow, from which the surviving immature B cells emerge into the peripheral lymphocyte pool. Third panel: a newly mature B cell starts to express IgD as well as IgM and can be activated by encounter with antigen in a secondary lymphoid organ. It then responds by proliferating and differentiating into the last phase of the B-cell life span, the antibody-secreting plasma cell, which may remain in the lymphoid organ but more usually migrates to the bone marrow, where it persists.

Generation of B cells.

Perhaps no developmental process is so well characterized as the differentiation of B cells from their progenitor cells. This is partly because the successive stages of B-cell differentiation are marked by the successive steps in the rearrangement of the immunoglobulin genes. In this section, we shall concentrate on the steps leading to the production of mature B cells expressing surface immunoglobulin (see Fig. 5.1, third panel), which entail a series of gene rearrangements each of which seems to be regulated by the protein product of the preceding step.

5-1   **The bone marrow provides an essential microenvironment for B-cell development.**

The differentiation pathway leading from a hematopoietic stem cell to an immature B cell can conveniently be subdivided into four steps. The first step results in the production of an **early pro-B cell.** Early pro-B cells appear before immunoglobulin gene rearrangement has begun, and are identified by cell-surface proteins characteristic of B cells. The subsequent stages are defined by steps in the rearrangement of the immunoglobulin genes, changes in cell-surface molecules, dependence on growth factors, and location within the bone marrow stroma. Thus, at the **late pro-B cell** stage D–J$_H$ joining within the heavy-chain gene has occurred, and at the **pre-B cell** stage intact heavy chains are produced. The light-chain genes then undergo rearrangement, leading to the expression of a complete immunoglobulin M molecule on the cell surface to produce an **immature B cell**, thus completing the first phase of B-cell development (Fig. 5.2).

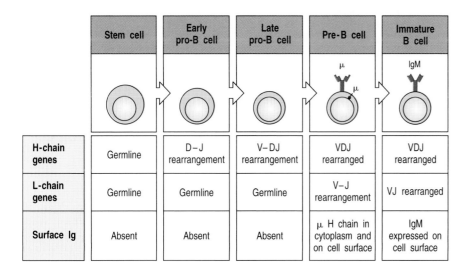

	Stem cell	Early pro-B cell	Late pro-B cell	Pre-B cell	Immature B cell
H-chain genes	Germline	D–J rearrangement	V–DJ rearrangement	VDJ rearranged	VDJ rearranged
L-chain genes	Germline	Germline	Germline	V–J rearrangement	VJ rearranged
Surface Ig	Absent	Absent	Absent	μ H chain in cytoplasm and on cell surface	IgM expressed on cell surface

Fig. 5.2 The development of B cells proceeds through several stages marked by the rearrangement of the immunoglobulin genes. The bone marrow stem cell that gives rise to the B-lymphocyte lineage has not yet begun to rearrange its immunoglobulin genes; they are in germline configuration. The first rearrangements of D gene segments to J$_H$ gene segments, occur in the early pro-B cells, generating late pro-B cells. In the late pro-B cells, a V$_H$ gene segment becomes joined to the rearranged DJ$_H$, producing a pre-B cell that is expressing both low levels of surface and high levels of cytoplasmic μ heavy chain. Finally, the light-chain genes are rearranged and the cell, now an immature B cell, expresses both light chains (L chains) and μ heavy chains (H chains) as surface IgM molecules.

All these stages in B-cell development occur initially in the fetal liver and, after birth, exclusively in the bone marrow. B-cell development is dependent upon the non-lymphoid stromal cells found in these sites: stem cells removed from the bone marrow and grown in culture fail to differentiate into B cells unless fetal liver or bone marrow stromal cells are also present. The contribution of the stromal cells is two-fold. At early stages, the B-cell precursors must be in direct contact with the stromal cells; at later stages, the developing B cells are dependent on growth factors secreted by them (Fig. 5.3).

The earliest B-cell precursors are bound to the stromal cell surface by adhesive interactions involving several **cell adhesion molecules (CAMs)**. (Cell adhesion molecules are discussed in more detail in Section 7-2, and some are also listed under their CD numbers in Appendix I.) Studies of cultured cells directly implicate the integrin VLA-4 (CD49d), on pre-B cells, in binding to its ligand, VCAM-1 (CD106), which is expressed constitutively on stromal cells. Antibodies to either of these molecules cause detachment of lymphocytes from stromal cells and block lymphocyte production in bone marrow cultures. Antibodies to CD44 also block development of both myeloid and lymphoid cells in culture; CD44 has a well-defined ligand, hyaluronan, but it is not yet clear how this pair of molecules functions in bone marrow. These and other cell adhesion molecules could mediate bidirectional communication between B-cell precursors and the microenvironment. Alternatively, they may simply facilitate contact with essential growth and differentiation factors that are produced in small amounts and are possibly immobilized on the surface of stromal cells or on the extracellular

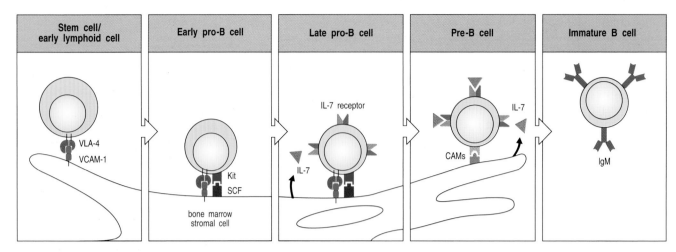

Fig. 5.3 The early stages of B-cell development are dependent on bone marrow stromal cells. Lymphoid progenitor cells and early pro-B cells bind to VCAM-1 through the α4:β1 integrin VLA-4, as well as to other cell adhesion molecules (CAMs) on stromal cells. This promotes the binding of their surface Kit receptor tyrosine kinase to stem-cell factor (SCF) on the stromal cell surface, activating the kinase and inducing proliferation. Late pro-B cells require both stem-cell factor on the surface of stromal cells and soluble interleukin-7 (IL-7) for their growth and maturation, while pre-B cells require only IL-7. At later developmental stages, other CAMs may bind developing B cells to stromal cells.

matrix. **Stem-cell factor (SCF)**, a transmembrane protein on stromal cells, binds to **Kit**, a signaling receptor carried on B cells, which possesses an intracellular tyrosine kinase domain; Kit is activated by binding of stem-cell factor and stimulates proliferation of the early pro-B cell (see Fig. 5.3) but *in vivo* this interaction seems of greater importance for production of non-lymphoid cells than for B-cell precursors.

In later phases of B-cell development, other molecules provide the adhesive and growth-promoting interactions. At the late pro-B cell stage, receptors for the growth factor interleukin-7 (IL-7) appear on the cell surface. Interleukin-7 is secreted in only small amounts by the stromal cells; nevertheless, it is absolutely required to drive proliferation and survival of pre-B cells. At this stage in their development, the lymphocytes lose their dependence on stem-cell factor, cease to express Kit, and become detached from the bone marrow stromal cells. The immature B cells that emerge from this developmental stage are non-dividing cells that do not require interleukin-7 to survive. Other growth factors produced by the bone marrow stromal cells may have a role in B-cell development; this is an active area of research and a full understanding of the factors that regulate B-cell differentiation has yet to be achieved.

One of the earliest markers on developing B cells is an isoform of the transmembrane tyrosine phosphatase CD45, known as CD45R (or B220 in mice). CD45 is expressed in different forms on cells of all hematopoietic lineages and we have already discussed its participation in signaling through the antigen receptors of both B and T cells (see Sections 3-28 and 4-28). CD45 can modulate the activity of tyrosine kinases such as Kit but the precise function of CD45R in B-cell development is unknown. B-cell development is also marked at relatively early stages by the appearance of several other cell-surface proteins known to be important in the activation of mature B cells by helper T cells. These include the B-cell co-receptor protein CD19 (see Section 3-29), MHC class II molecules, and CD40 (Fig. 5.4). The functions of these molecules will be discussed in Chapter 8 when we deal with the interactions between T and B cells. It is likely that the early regulated expression of each of these molecules has important functional consequences for B-cell development; however, most of these functions are still to be discovered.

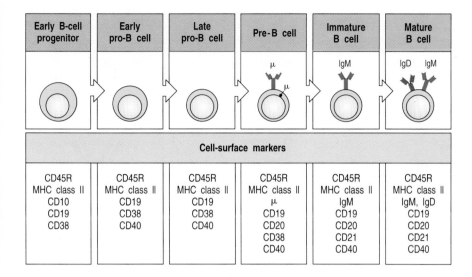

Early B-cell progenitor	Early pro-B cell	Late pro-B cell	Pre-B cell	Immature B cell	Mature B cell
			μ / μ	IgM	IgD IgM

Cell-surface markers

CD45R	CD45R	CD45R	CD45R	CD45R	CD45R
MHC class II	MHC class II	MHC class II	MHC class II	MHC class II	MHC class II
CD10	CD19	CD19	μ	IgM	IgM, IgD
CD19	CD38	CD38	CD19	CD19	CD19
CD38	CD40	CD40	CD20	CD20	CD20
			CD38	CD21	CD21
			CD40	CD40	CD40

Fig. 5.4 Changes in the expression of cell-surface molecules during human B-cell development. Various cell-surface markers are expressed at each stage in human B-cell development and can be used to identify B cells at different stages. Most of these proteins have known functions in mature B cells, though their functional significance during B-cell development is not known. Thus, CD19, CD21 (also called CR2), and CD45 are important in signaling during B-cell activation; MHC class II molecules display antigen to helper T cells, and CD40 participates in the interactions of B cells with T cells. The functions of CD10, CD20, and CD38 are not known but they make useful surface markers for B cells during development. While pre-B cells express some cell-surface μ heavy chains, the presence of intracellular μ chains is characteristic of these cells. Immature B cells express only IgM on their surface. Mature B cells are marked by the additional appearance of IgD on the cell surface.

Immature B cells differentiate within a few days into mature B cells expressing surface IgM and IgD. These two molecules have the same antigen specificity in any given B cell and arise by alternative splicing of heavy-chain mRNA (see Section 3-23). We shall look next at how B-cell development depends on successful rearrangement of the immunoglobulin genes.

5-2 | B-cell development depends on the productive, sequential rearrangement of a heavy- and a light-chain gene.

The developing B cell must make successful rearrangements of a heavy-chain gene and a light-chain gene; cells that fail to do so will be lost. The chances of making an unsuccessful rearrangement are quite high. Each time an immunoglobulin V gene segment undergoes rearrangement to a J or a DJ segment there is a roughly two-in-three chance of generating an out-of-frame sequence, although for heavy chains, the D gene segment can be read in more than one frame and so most DJ joins are potentially useful. In the case of the heavy chains, the cell has only two chances to make a productive rearrangement as, on each chromosome, the rearrangement of one V, D and J gene segment deletes all of the remaining D gene segments and no further rearrangements are possible. For the light-chain genes, partly because of the existence of two different loci and partly because, as we shall see, their gene organization allows repeated rearrangement attempts, there is much more scope for making a productive rearrangement and thus less wastage at later stages when the light chains are rearranging. The sequence of gene rearrangement events during B-cell development is summarized in Fig. 5.5.

Immunoglobulin heavy-chain gene rearrangement begins in early pro-B cells with the rearrangement of D gene segments to J gene segments. This rearrangement occurs on both chromosomes of the diploid set before the cell, now classified as a late pro-B cell, proceeds to the next step, the rearrangement of a V_H gene segment to join the DJ_H complex. The V_H to DJ_H rearrangement occurs first on only one chromosome. There is about a one-in-three chance that this latter rearrangement will generate a V_H exon in a correct translational reading frame, in which case intact μ chains are produced and the cell can be classified as a pre-B cell. If the first V_H to DJ_H rearrangement is not 'in-frame', then rearrangement continues on the other chromosome and a pre-B cell may still be

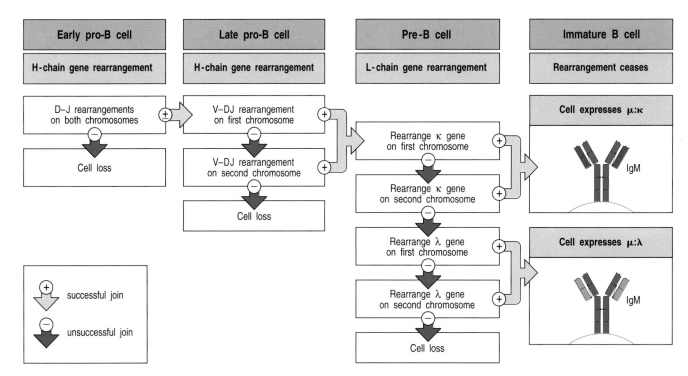

Fig. 5.5 Steps in immunoglobulin gene rearrangement leading to the expression of cell-surface immunoglobulin. The rearrangement events are shown in columns corresponding to the cell type in which they occur. Each rearrangement has about a one-in-three chance of being in the correct reading frame, thus allowing the cell to progress to the next stage in its development. Each cell has more than one chance to achieve a successful rearrangement, and if the first attempt is non-productive it will make further attempts.

generated if this rearrangement is in-frame. However, if both rearrangements are out-of-frame, then the late pro-B cell, which has deleted all the intervening D elements in the course of its abortive attempts at productively joining V_H to DJ_H, can never mature and is lost from the lineage. This is the fate of about 45% of pro-B cells.

Once a productive heavy-chain gene rearrangement has been achieved, the cell is thought to divide several times before reaching the pre-B cell stage, at which light-chain gene rearrangement begins. This means that a cell with a particular rearranged heavy-chain gene can give rise to many progeny, each with different light-chain gene rearrangements; this increases the diversity of the antibody molecules generated. In mice, κ light chains almost always rearrange before λ light chains but it is not clear whether this is developmentally programmed or whether the choice of which light chain locus rearranges first is random, and depends, at least in part, on the number of V gene segments capable of being rearranged at each locus. In the mouse, there are many more $V_κ$ gene segments than $V_λ$ segments and thus it is more likely that rearrangement would start with a κ segment. In humans, where the numbers of $V_κ$ and $V_λ$ gene segments are more equal, light chain rearrangement can begin either with a κ chain or with a λ chain. What is clear is that rearrangement occurs only at one locus at a time; B cells never make simultaneous rearrangements of their κ and λ light chains.

In the following description of gene rearrangement in human immunoglobulin genes, we have assumed that the first light-chain gene rearrangement occurs on one of the two chromosomes encoding the κ light chains. A successful rearrangement leads to the production of a κ chain and to intact IgM (μ:κ) molecules and the termination of further receptor gene rearrangement. Because the human κ locus contains many V and five J gene segments, more than one rearrangement can be attempted on each chromosome (Fig. 5.6). Finally, if κ-chain gene rearrangement does not lead to the production of intact IgM molecules, the λ light-chain locus rearranges. The multiple V and J elements in the λ light-chain locus also allow several attempts at this process as well. A reciprocal pattern is seen where λ chains rearrange first; many attempts to generate a functional λ light chain will be made before the κ chains are rearranged. The result of the redundancy in light-chain genes is that most B-cell precursors that reach the pre-B cell stage eventually generate progeny that bear intact IgM molecules and can be classified as immature B cells.

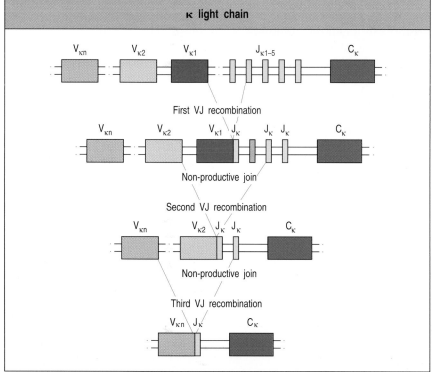

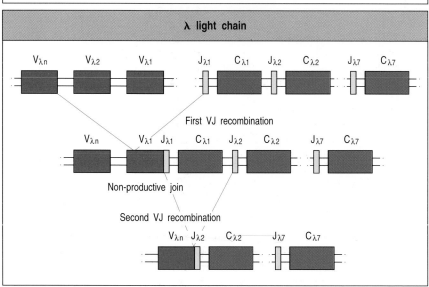

Fig. 5.6 Non-productive light-chain gene rearrangements may be rescued by further gene rearrangement. The organization of the light-chain genes in mice and humans offers many opportunities for rescue of pre-B cells that initially make an out-of-frame light-chain gene rearrangement. Light-chain rescue is illustrated for mice, where it has been demonstrated experimentally. First, a 5′ V_κ gene segment can recombine with a 3′ J_κ gene segment to remove an out-of-frame join and replace it with one that is in-frame (top panel). In principle, this can happen up to four times on each chromosome, since there are four functional J_κ segments in the mouse (the fifth is a pseudogene). In humans, there are five functional J_κ segments. If all rearrangements of κ-chain genes fail to yield a productive light-chain join, λ-chain gene rearrangement may succeed. λ light-chain genes are arranged in four sets of V, J, and C gene segments; although one of these is a pseudogene, this organization nonetheless allows several λ light-chain gene rearrangements to occur on each chromosome. Thus, there is a very high probability of productive light-chain gene rearrangement in developing B cells and most pre-B cells successfully complete their differentiation to immature B cells.

The expression of the enzymes involved in immunoglobulin gene rearrangements is developmentally programmed.

While the sequential steps in immunoglobulin gene rearrangement provide defining markers for the different stages in B-cell development, various intracellular proteins also mark specific stages in differentiation (Fig. 5.7). Thus, *RAG-1* and *RAG-2*, genes that encode proteins required for immunoglobulin gene rearrangement (see Section 3-16), are active in the earliest B lineage cells examined but are not expressed in mature B cells in which gene rearrangement has ceased. Similarly, **terminal deoxynucleotidyl transferase (TdT),** an enzyme involved in N-nucleotide addition (see Section 3-16), ceases to be expressed at the pre-B cell stage, when heavy-chain gene rearrangement is complete and light-chain gene rearrangement has commenced. This is in keeping with the presence of N-nucleotides in the V–D and D–J joints of immunoglobulin heavy-chain genes and their lower frequency in the V–J joints of immunoglobulin light-chain genes. The stage-specific expression of some key proteins in B-cell development is shown in Fig. 5.7. Three of these are DNA-binding proteins, which play a part in the tissue-specific transcriptional regulation of immunoglobulin genes, to which we now turn.

Fig. 5.7 The expression of several important cellular proteins changes during B-cell development. The generation of a cell-surface receptor by B cells involves the precise temporal regulation of several different processes. E32 is a protein involved in the transcription of immunoglobulin heavy chains and is produced early in B-cell development, while NF-κB, which is required for light-chain transcription, is produced at a later stage. Likewise, expression of the *RAG-1* and *RAG-2* genes are required for gene rearrangement, the enzyme terminal deoxynucleotidyl transferase (TdT) is required for the addition of N-nucleotides, and λ5 and VpreB, which are needed for regulating surface μ-chain expression, are all produced only at certain stages of development. λ5 and VpreB are proteins that substitute for immunoglobulin light chains in pre-B cells (see Section 5-6). Finally, Oct-2 is a transcription factor involved in regulating B-cell proliferation. The tight temporal regulation of the expression of these proteins imposes a strict sequence on the events of B-cell differentiation.

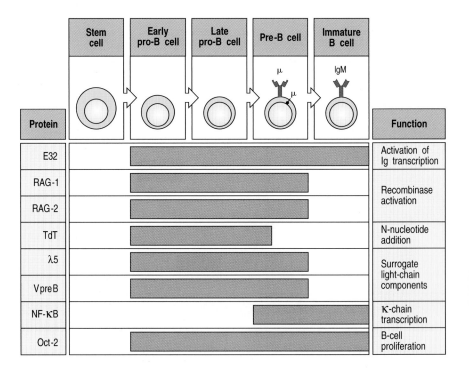

Gene rearrangement in B cells is controlled by proteins that regulate the state of chromatin.

Only genes that contain the conserved recombination signal sequences can be rearranged by the V(D)J recombinase system (see Chapter 3). These recombination signals, which consist of conserved heptamer and nonamer sequences separated by a spacer (see Fig. 3.19), are shared by immunoglobulin heavy- and light-chain genes as well as by T-cell receptor genes, and the same enzymes mediate somatic rearrangement of all these genes. Thus, in mice lacking *RAG-1* or *RAG-2* as a result of gene knock-out by homologous recombination (see Section 2-38), neither T-cell nor B-cell receptor genes undergo somatic recombination. Yet productive rearrangement of T-cell receptor genes does not occur in B cells, and immunoglobulin genes show only some DJ$_H$ rearrangement in T cells. This is because in each cell type, the accessibility of the receptor gene chromatin to the recombination enzymes is controlled by gene-regulatory proteins specific to T cells or to B cells. Variability in chromatin state may also account for the sequential rearrangement of heavy- and light-chain immunoglobulin genes.

Before a gene rearrangement occurs, there is a low level of transcription from the separate immunoglobulin gene segments that are to be joined at that step. This transcription is activated by promoters located upstream of each V gene segment and of the J–C segments. The activity of these promoters is controlled, in turn, by the binding of gene-regulatory proteins to tissue-specific enhancers, which, in the case of the heavy-chain genes and the κ light-chain genes, lie in the intron between the J gene segments and the C-region exons and also 3′ to the C exons (Fig. 5.8).

It is believed that the B-cell specific proteins that bind to the immunoglobulin enhancers are responsible for 'opening' the chromatin in the region of the immunoglobulin genes so that it is accessible not only to transcriptional activation but also to the enzymes that mediate somatic

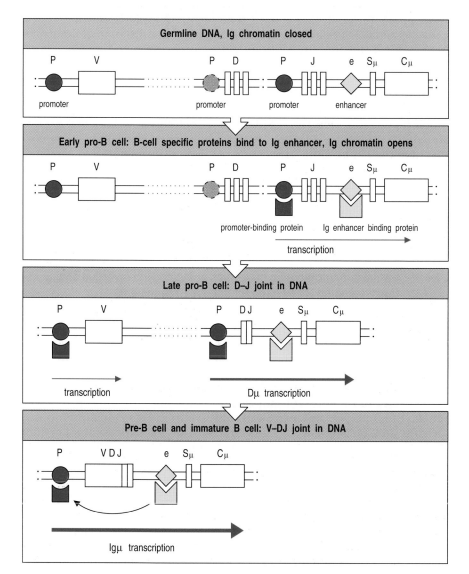

Fig. 5.8 Proteins binding to promoter (P) and enhancer (e) elements contribute to the sequence of gene rearrangement and regulate the level of RNA transcription. Top panel: in germline DNA, or non-lymphoid cells, the chromatin containing the immunoglobulin genes is in a closed conformation. Second panel: in the early pro-B cell, specific proteins bind to the Ig enhancer elements; for the heavy chain, these are in the J–C intron and 3′ to the C exons (not shown). Third panel: this binding opens up the DNA, activating a low level of transcription from promoters located upstream of the J gene and D gene segments and the opening of the DNA also allows DNA rearrangement to occur. Fourth panel: subsequent rearrangement of a V gene segment brings its promoter under the influence of the heavy-chain enhancer (e), leading to the production of mRNA in pre-B and immature B cells at a much higher rate than that of Dμ transcription.

recombination. In mice containing unrearranged immunoglobulin transgenes together with their associated gene-regulatory DNA elements, rearrangement of the transgenes occurs only in B cells, unless the DNA has inserted into regions of chromatin that allow its transcription in T cells. However, because the proteins that bind the immunoglobulin gene-regulatory DNA and open the immunoglobulin chromatin are made in developing B cells but not in developing T cells, full rearrangement of immunoglobulin genes occurs only in B cells. The DJ_H joins found in some T cells may suggest 'leakiness' in the process, or may reflect early events in a common progenitor of B- and T-cell lineages. Similarly, T-cell specific DNA-binding proteins would open the receptor-gene chromatin in T cells. Similar events may also regulate the order of gene rearrangements in B cells, so it is likely that the heavy-chain genes are opened before the light-chain genes.

5-5 Rearrangement of immunoglobulin genes alters the activity of immunoglobulin promoters.

Immunoglobulin gene rearrangement dramatically increases the transcriptional activity of the rearranged gene segments. Before rearrangement, the J and C gene segments are transcribed at a low level from a weak promoter upstream of the J gene segments and transcription of V_H gene segments is variably activated because of the distance of their promoters from the immunoglobulin gene enhancer (see Fig. 5.8, upper two panels). Once rearrangement has occurred, the promoter upstream of the V gene segment is brought into proximity with enhancers in the J–C intron and other enhancers lying 3' to the C exons, with the result that, in mature B cells, the entire rearranged gene is transcribed at a much higher rate (see Fig. 5.8, bottom panel; the 3' enhancers are not shown). Thus, gene rearrangement can be viewed as a powerful mechanism for regulating gene expression, as well as for generating receptor diversity. Several cases of gene rearrangement bringing genes under the control of a new promoter are known from prokaryotes and single-celled eukaryotes but, in vertebrates, only the immunoglobulin and T-cell receptor genes are known to use gene rearrangement to regulate gene expression.

5-6 Partial immunoglobulin molecules combine with invariant chains in the developing B cell to direct gene rearrangement.

The increased transcription of successfully rearranged immunoglobulin genes and the resulting rapid appearance of their protein products plays an important part in the developmental programming that ensures each fully differentiated B cell contains only one successfully rearranged heavy-chain gene and one successfully rearranged light-chain gene. This can be shown dramatically by introducing an already rearranged immunoglobulin heavy-chain gene into the germline of a mouse; virtually all B cells in such a transgenic mouse will express the product of the rearranged heavy-chain transgene and, in these B cells, rearrangement of the endogenous heavy-chain genes is suppressed. The endogenous light-chain genes, however, rearrange normally, thus generating a complete immunoglobulin molecule. A similar suppression, but of light-chain gene rearrangement, occurs in mice transgenic for a rearranged light-chain gene.

The suppression of heavy-chain gene rearrangement depends on the cell-surface expression of the products of the rearranged genes. Because μ heavy chains cannot be expressed on the cell surface on their own, a special mechanism is needed to bring the μ chain to the surface. Pre-B cells produce two immunoglobulin-like proteins, which together make up a surrogate light chain (Fig. 5.9). One of these proteins, called λ5, is similar to a Cλ domain, while the other, called VpreB, resembles a V domain but bears an extra N-terminal protein sequence. Together, these two polypeptides form a cell-surface complex with the μ heavy chain and the attendant constant chains Igα and Igβ (see Section 3-27). This immunoglobulin-like molecule apparently signals to the developing B cell that a complete μ-chain gene has been formed, triggering rapid growth of the cell and inhibiting further heavy-chain gene rearrangement, while triggering the onset of κ light-chain gene rearrangement. Once a light-chain gene has been rearranged successfully, its product combines with the heavy chain to form intact IgM (see Fig. 5.9).

When mice have mutant μ-chain genes that cannot form transmembrane molecules, B-cell development is blocked after heavy-chain gene

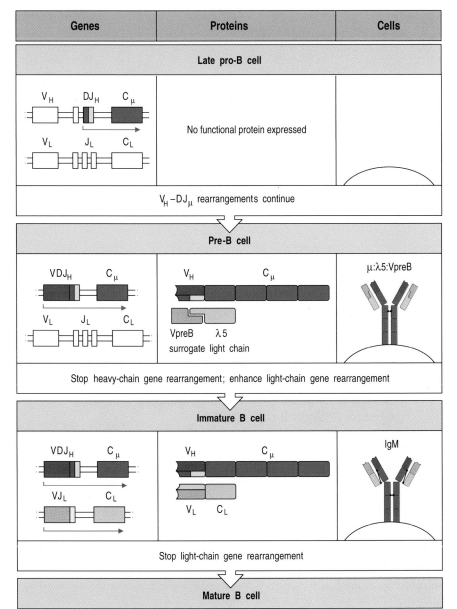

Fig. 5.9 Cell surface μ-chain expression during B-cell development. Top panel: in late pro-B cells, although mRNA is transcribed from the promoter upstream of the D gene segments (see Fig. 5.8), no functional μ protein is expressed at this stage. Second panel: in the pre-B cell, where heavy-chain gene rearrangement has taken place, μ chains can be expressed at the cell surface in an immunoglobulin-like complex with two chains, λ5 and VpreB, which together make up a surrogate light chain. Signaling via this immunoglobulin-like molecule is thought to trigger pre-B-cell proliferation and/or survival, the cessation of heavy-chain gene rearrangement, and the start of light-chain gene rearrangements. Successful light-chain gene rearrangement results in the production of a light-chain protein that binds the μ chain to form a complete IgM molecule at the cell surface (third panel). Signaling via the IgM molecules is thought to trigger the cessation of light-chain gene rearrangement.

rearrangement. Absence of λ5 has a similar effect, although some B cells can be formed in such mutant mice. This suggests that the complex of μ:λ5:VpreB acts as the pre-B-cell receptor and may trigger proliferation and/or survival of pre-B cells prior to light-chain gene rearrangement. Thus, its absence leads to a much reduced output of B cells.

Perhaps as an accidental side effect of this important feedback mechanism, B-cell development is sometimes aborted when partially rearranged heavy chains are expressed on the cell surface. This happens when D–J joining activates heavy-chain transcription from a previously inactive promoter 5′ to D (see Fig. 5.8, top panel), and can allow the production of a truncated heavy chain known as a Dμ protein when the join is in a suitable reading frame (Fig. 5.10). Pre-B cells that express the resulting Dμ:λ5:VpreB complex on the cell surface are lost from the B-cell developmental lineage unless rescued by secondary DJ$_H$ rearrangements, perhaps because further rearrangement of the heavy-chain locus is thereby suppressed, preventing the V to DJ$_H$ joining necessary for the completion of B-cell maturation.

Fig. 5.10 Some DJ$_H$ junctions allow production of a truncated heavy chain known as D$_\mu$ that blocks B-cell development. D$_\mu$ lacks a V$_H$ region and is produced when D–J joining in pro-B cells prematurely activates heavy-chain transcription from a previously inactive promoter 5′ to D. Not all D gene segments give rise to D$_\mu$ proteins, and only one D gene segment reading frame allows protein production. Antibodies with D in this reading frame are not found in mature B cells. This is because the D$_\mu$ protein binds λ5 and VpreB, as well as a possible surrogate V$_H$ domain (designated V$_H$preB in this figure) and goes to the surface. Here, the D$_\mu$ complex is thought to signal for cessation of V$_H$ to DJ$_H$ joining, thus blocking further B-cell maturation. Most developing B cells do not make D$_\mu$ and so can rearrange V$_H$ to DJ$_H$.

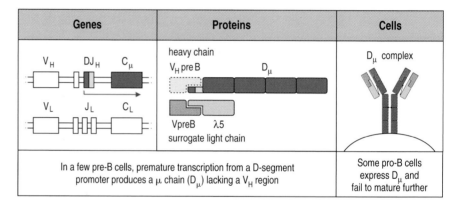

Genes	Proteins	Cells
V$_H$ DJ$_H$ C$_\mu$ V$_L$ J$_L$ C$_L$	heavy chain V$_H$ pre B D$_\mu$ VpreB λ5 surrogate light chain	D$_\mu$ complex
In a few pre-B cells, premature transcription from a D-segment promoter produces a μ chain (D$_\mu$) lacking a V$_H$ region		Some pro-B cells express D$_\mu$ and fail to mature further

The expression of IgM on the B-cell surface, once light-chain rearrangement has been successful, corresponds to the cessation of further light-chain gene rearrangement, although the exact nature of the signals by which the B cell senses the presence of surface IgM is not yet characterized. Thus, each step in the rearrangement of immunoglobulin genes is thought to be regulated by the product of the preceding step, ensuring that each B cell expresses only one type of heavy and one type of light chain.

5-7   The immunoglobulin gene rearrangement program leads to monospecificity of B-cell receptors.

We saw in Chapter 1 that individual B cells must produce only one specificity of antibody to ensure that all the antibodies secreted by an activated B cell are specific only for the antigen that originally triggered its proliferation. This prevents the secretion of antibodies of other specificities that could be wasteful or even harmful. We can now see that the regulated program of immunoglobulin gene rearrangement guarantees monospecificity, and is the explanation for the phenomenon of allelic exclusion (see Section 3-17), whereby only one of the two parental chromosomes produces an immunoglobulin chain from each set of immunoglobulin gene segments. Allelic exclusion is so called for historical reasons that are explained in Fig. 5.11.

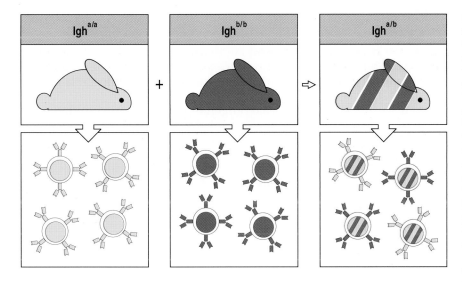

Fig. 5.11 The phenomenon of allelic exclusion of immunoglobulin gene expression in single B cells. Most species have genetic polymorphisms of the constant regions of their immunoglobulin heavy- and light-chain genes known as allotypes. In rabbits, for example, all of the B cells in an individual homozygous for the *a* allele of the immunoglobulin heavy chain (Igh) will express immunoglobulin of type *a*, while in an individual homozygous for the *b* allele all the B cells express immunoglobulin of type *b*. In a heterozygous animal, carrying both *a* and *b* alleles, individual B cells express either type *a* or type *b* immunoglobulin but never both. The expression of only one of the parental alleles in any one B cell reflects productive rearrangement of only one of the two parental chromosomes carrying the Igh locus.

Once a complete immunoglobulin molecule is generated, the mono-specific B cell, now called an **immature B cell**, is exposed to selection by antigens in its environment. Before they leave the bone marrow for the peripheral lymphoid tissues, where they can be stimulated to make antibody, the immature B cells that recognize self antigens must be removed or inactivated to assure self tolerance. We shall describe the mechanisms of B-cell tolerance in subsequent sections, while the activation of B cells in the periphery will be discussed in Chapter 8.

5-8   **Lymphoid organs provide a second essential environment for B cells.**

After B cells leave the bone marrow, they recirculate around the body, passing from the blood into the secondary lymphoid organs — the spleen, lymph nodes and mucosal-associated lymphoid tissues (see Chapter 1) — and returning from these organs to the blood via the lymphatic system. Within the secondary lymphoid organs, the B cells are localized into discrete clusters, called follicles, comprised primarily of B cells and a specialized stromal cell, the follicular dendritic cell. This cell plays an important part in the development of antibody responses and we will return to its properties in Chapter 8. The microenvironment provided by the lymphoid follicle seems to provide signals essential for the survival of B cells, although what these signals are and what cell provides them still remain to be answered. Any B cells that fail to lodge within a follicle die within a matter of days. B cells that do manage to migrate into follicles, and thus receive a survival signal, subsequently migrate from the follicles into the efferent lymphatics and so return to the circulation. However, these cells continue to require survival signals and so must eventually recirculate back to a lymphoid follicle.

New B cells continue to be produced by the bone marrow throughout life, yet the number of follicles is limited; the excess B cells die by being excluded from the follicles. Thus the life of a B cell can be viewed as a continuing Darwinian struggle in which B cells compete with each other for access to lymphoid follicles. As we shall see, this competition plays an important part in the elimination of some self-reactive B cells.

☐   **Summary.**

B cells are generated throughout life in the specialized environment of the human bone marrow and require a second environment, the lymphoid follicle, to maintain their existence. As B cells differentiate from primitive stem cells, they proceed through a series of steps that are marked by the sequential rearrangement of immunoglobulin gene segments to generate a diverse repertoire of antigen receptors. As each intact immunoglobulin chain is generated by somatic gene rearrangement, it signals the developing cell to cease rearrangement of the set of gene segments specifying that chain and to begin rearrangement of the next set. The end product of this process is a B cell with surface immunoglobulin of a single specificity. At this stage in its development, the B cell is ready for selective events driven by antigen binding to these cell-surface receptor molecules.

Selection of B cells.

If B lymphocytes recognize antigen for the first time as immature B cells, they are eliminated or inactivated. Thus, those immature B cells that recognize self antigens while still in the bone marrow are prevented from developing further and going on to make antibodies that bind self cells or tissues. This results in an immature B-cell receptor repertoire that is self tolerant. Only after this screening for potential autoreactivity do the B cells complete their maturation and migrate to the peripheral lymphoid tissues. Here, they may encounter other self antigens that were not present in the bone marrow environment. Mature B cells that can recognize self antigens are inactivated by a variety of mechanisms.

5-9 | Immature B cells can be eliminated or inactivated by contact with self antigens.

The immature B cells generated in the bone marrow express only surface IgM molecules. The completion of B-cell development involves emigration from the bone marrow and the alternative splicing of heavy-chain transcripts to generate mature B cells expressing surface IgM and IgD (see Fig. 3.30). Immature B cells expressing only IgM are eliminated or inactivated if they bind to abundant multivalent ligands in their environment. This can be demonstrated by using anti-μ chain antibodies to crosslink the surface IgM of immature B cells, mimicking the effect of multivalent antigen; such treatment results in the inactivation or death of all immature B cells. This distinguishes immature B cells from mature B cells, which are normally activated by multivalent antigens (see Section 3-28). Thus, the elimination of potentially self-reactive immature B cells must occur during the few days before the cells differentiate into mature B cells bearing IgM and IgD.

Experiments with transgenic mice have shown that two different mechanisms ensure tolerance to self antigens encountered by immature B cells. One of them operates in the case of multivalent antigens, for example cells bearing multiple copies of a cell-surface MHC molecule; the other operates when the antigens are of low valence, for example small soluble proteins. In mice transgenic for the rearranged genes of both chains of an antibody specific for H-2^k MHC class I molecules, all their B cells express the anti-MHC antibody as surface IgM. When the transgenes are introduced into a mouse strain that does not express H-2^k, normal numbers of B cells develop, all bearing anti-H-2^k receptors. However, when the transgenes are introduced into a strain expressing H-2^k, normal numbers of pre-B cells are found but B cells expressing the anti-H-2^k never develop; instead most of these immature B cells die in the bone marrow, probably by apoptosis, and are lost from the B-cell population, a process known as **clonal deletion** (Fig. 5.12, left panels). A similar situation obtains in mice transgenic for a modified form of hen egg-white lysozyme (HEL) and for anti-HEL antibodies, in which the normally soluble lysozyme is expressed as a transmembrane molecule on their bone marrow stromal cells.

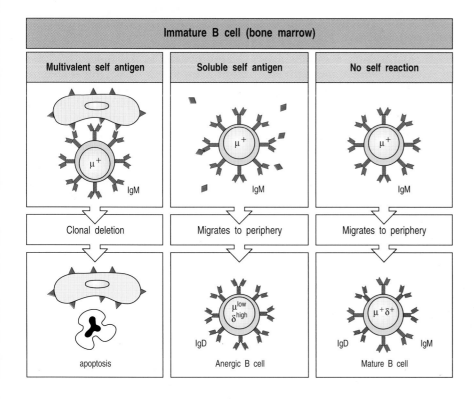

Fig. 5.12 **Self antigens in the bone marrow can lead to deletion or inactivation of immature B cells.** When developing B cells express receptors that recognize ubiquitous self cell-surface antigens, such as those of the MHC, they are deleted from the repertoire. These B cells are believed to undergo programmed cell death or apoptosis (left panels). Immature B cells that bind soluble self antigens are rendered unresponsive or anergic to the antigen and lose surface IgM. They migrate to the periphery where they express IgD but remain anergic (center panels). Only immature B cells that do not encounter antigen in the bone marrow at this early stage of development mature normally, and migrate from the bone marrow to the peripheral lymphoid tissues as B cells bearing both IgM and IgD on their surface (right panels).

In contrast, when the lysozyme transgene is expressed as a soluble secreted protein in mice also transgenic for anti-HEL, the B cells (which all bear anti-HEL receptors) mature but are unable to respond to antigen. The non-responsive cells have lost expression of IgM at the cell surface; instead the IgM is retained within the cell. In addition, they have developed a block in signal transduction so that even though they go on to express normal levels of IgD at the cell surface, the cells cannot be stimulated by crosslinking this receptor. It appears that this blockade in signal transduction lies prior to the phosphorylation of the Igα and Igβ associated with the B-cell receptor (see Section 3-27), although its exact nature is not yet known. This state of non-reactivity is called **anergy**, and such B cells are defined as **anergic** (Fig. 5.12, center panels). B cells that encounter neither form of antigen in bone marrow continue to express IgM, leave the bone marrow for the periphery, express IgD and become mature naive IgM- and IgD-positive B cells (see Fig. 5.12, right panels).

5-10 Some potentially self-reactive B cells may be rescued by further immunoglobulin gene rearrangement.

Although most of the B cells recognizing multivalent self antigens, such as those recognizing self MHC in transgenic mice, are destined to die in the bone marrow, some continue to express *RAG-1* and *RAG-2*, allowing ongoing rearrangement of their endogenous light-chain genes. It is not known why the expression of *RAG-1* and *RAG-2* is sustained in some cells. In the transgenic mice, one possibility is that signaling occurs through the surface immunoglobulin that is prematurely expressed on these cells from an already rearranged transgene. This signaling could substitute for the signaling through the complex of μ heavy chain and surrogate light chain that normally sustains *RAG-1* and *RAG-2* expression at the pre-B cell stage. The rearrangement of the endogenous light-chain genes that then occurs in such transgenic cells can alter the specificity of the receptor by replacing the transgenic light chain that confers autoreactivity with one that does not, a process known as **receptor editing** (Fig. 5.13).

In normal B cells, a similar process could result in the deletion of the previously rearranged light-chain gene (see Fig. 5.6), or the displacement of its product by a new light chain that binds more effectively to the rearranged heavy chain. In either case, the B cell would lose its autoreactivity and be saved from elimination. So far, receptor editing has only been found in mice transgenic for rearranged immunoglobulin genes; however, rare immature B cells with active *RAG-1* and *RAG-2* have been found in the bone marrow of normal mice, and these may represent self-reactive B cells undergoing further receptor gene rearrangement. This process only occurs while B cells are still relatively immature, before they have left the bone marrow.

5-11 In some species, most immunoglobulin gene diversification occurs after gene rearrangement.

In humans and mice, as we have seen, all stages of B-cell development and immunoglobulin gene rearrangement occur in the bone marrow, and a large proportion of receptor diversity is generated at this stage (see Section 3-14). In some other species, B cells develop in a strikingly different fashion. In birds, rabbits, and sheep, there is little or no **germline diversity** in V, D, and J gene segments, and the rearranged

H-2^b mouse made transgenic for rearranged Igμ and κ genes from anti-K^b hybridoma

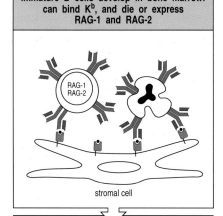

Immature B cells develop in bone marrow: can bind K^b, and die or express RAG-1 and RAG-2

Few peripheral B cells. All express different light chains. None binds K^b

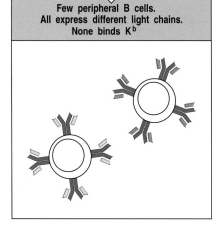

Fig. 5.13 Replacement of light chains by receptor editing can rescue some self-reactive B cells from elimination by changing their antigen specificity. In an H-2^d mouse made transgenic for the heavy- and light-chain genes of an immunoglobulin specific for the MHC class I molecule, H-2K^b, normal numbers of B cells develop. They all express the transgenes and are specific for H-2K^b (not shown). Top panel: if the same rearranged immunoglobulin genes are introduced into an H-2K^b mouse, which expresses the H-2K^b molecule on its tissues, the developing B cells express the immunoglobulin at a very early stage and can bind to the H-2K^b molecule expressed by the bone marrow stromal cells. Center panel: this apparently signals the B cells to express *RAG-1* and *RAG-2* genes, enabling the B cell to make further light-chain gene rearrangements, generating a new receptor specificity. Most of the B cells do not make new rearrangements and are deleted. If the new receptor does not bind self antigens in the bone marrow, the B cell matures and enters the peripheral circulation. Thus, in the transgenic H-2K^b mice, there are many fewer B cells than normal and none expresses the transgenic light chain (bottom panel).

variable-region sequences are identical or very similar in all B cells. As a result, all B cells are initially generated with identical or very similar receptors. These B cells then migrate to a specialized microenvironment, the best known of which is the bursa of Fabricius in chickens. Here, surface immunoglobulin-positive B cells proliferate rapidly, and their already rearranged receptor genes undergo diversification. In birds and rabbits, this occurs by a process of **gene conversion**, in which homologous inactive V gene segments exchange short sequences with the active, rearranged variable-region gene; in sheep, diversification is the result of somatic hypermutation.

It is possible that the B-cell receptor first generated in these animals is specific for a ligand expressed by cells in the bursa of Fabricius or its equivalent, and that recognition of this ligand by the invariant B-cell receptor drives the intense B-cell proliferation found at such sites. The cells can only stop proliferating and emerge from the bursa as mature B cells when their receptors have diversified to such an extent that they no longer recognize this self ligand (Fig. 5.14).

It is not known why this alternative strategy of diversifying an initially homogeneous pool of receptors exists in these species, nor is it clear whether it has any counterpart in mice and humans. The phenomenon would be similar to the continuation of light-chain gene rearrangement

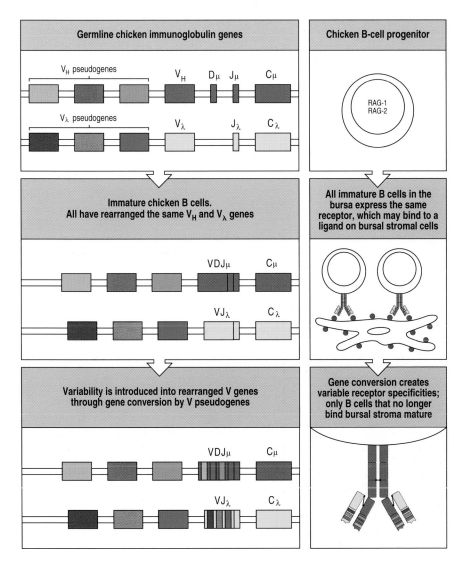

Fig. 5.14 Binding to a self ligand may drive the diversification of chicken immunoglobulins. In chickens, all B cells express the same surface immunoglobulin initially; there is only one active V(D) and J gene segment for both the chicken heavy- and light-chain genes (top panels) and gene rearrangemnt can produce only a single receptor specificity. Immature B cells expressing this receptor migrate to the bursa of Fabricius, where the receptor is thought to bind to a self cell-surface molecule, inducing proliferation. Gene-conversion events introduce sequences from adjacent V pseudogenes into the expressed gene, creating diversity in the receptors. In this scheme, only when a B cell loses reactivity to the bursal antigen does it cease to proliferate and emigrate to the periphery.

that occurs when B cells have receptors specific for self cell-surface molecules. Thus, it may be a general rule that immature B cells that recognize a self ligand can alter their antigen specificity. This could occur if all B cells were programmed to maintain expression of the *RAG* genes for as long as the B-cell receptor is binding a ligand, initially through λ5 and VpreB, and later, for self-reactive cells, via the B-cell receptor itself. We shall see in Chapter 6 that the interaction of receptors on newly formed lymphocytes with self molecules in a specialized microenvironment is also crucial for the development of the other major lymphocyte subset—the T cells.

| 5-12 | **Mature self-reactive B cells can be silenced in the periphery.** |

Not all potentially self-reactive B cells are eliminated or inactivated early in development. Although screening for tolerance to ubiquitous multivalent antigens such as cell-surface MHC class I molecules is usually completed in the bone marrow, B cells recognizing soluble self antigens, such as serum proteins, or proteins expressed only on certain cell types, such as the liver, may survive to mature and migrate to the periphery.

Although such potentially self-reactive B cells mature, they do not necessarily cause disease. Mature B cells exposed to multivalent self antigens in the periphery are deleted from the repertoire. Thus, when mice transgenic for anti-H-2K^b receptors are also made transgenic for H-2K^b expressed under the control of a liver-specific promoter so that it is only expressed on liver cells, immature H-2K^b-specific B cells are found in the bone marrow but all mature B cells are deleted (Fig. 5.15, left panels). In this case there is no evidence that a new receptor is produced by receptor editing, providing support for the idea that receptor editing can only occur in immature B cells. Why the mature B cells are deleted rather than becoming anergic, as is the case for B cells specific for soluble self antigens (see later), is not clear; it may reflect the fact that

Fig. 5.15 Mature B cells may be made tolerant if antigen is presented inappropriately. Potentially self-reactive B cells can mature if the antigens they recognize are not present in the bone marrow. Such cells rarely cause disease. B cells recognizing self cell-surface proteins can be made anergic or deleted when they recognize their antigen in the absence of the necessary additional signals, usually provided by helper T cells (left panels). In addition (center panels), abundant soluble proteins can also induce a state of anergy in mature B cells. Only if the B cell recognizes its antigen and receives the necessary additional signals, delivered in the example shown here by a helper T cell (T$_H$2), does antibody production result (right panels).

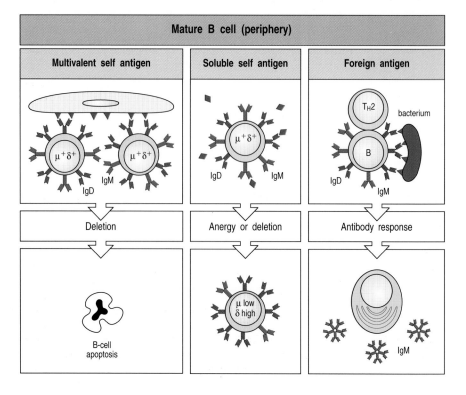

cell-surface antigens can crosslink the B-cell receptor, whereas soluble antigens can not.

In most cases, however, the survival of potentially self-reactive B cells does not matter. This is because most B cells require helper T cells for their activation (Fig. 5.15, right panels) and in the absence of T-cell help they never proliferate or differentiate into antibody-secreting cells. Provided that T-cell tolerance to self antigens has been established, therefore, no B-cell responses can be induced. It appears that B-cell non-responsiveness to many self antigens that are present at low levels is of this type, affecting the helper T cell but not the B cell.

In the case of abundant soluble self proteins, however, B cells do not differentiate to secrete antibodies even if suitable helper T cells are provided. An ingenious extension of the HEL transgenic mouse experiment described in Section 5-9 suggests that this is because binding of abundant soluble antigen to mature B cells also leads to their inactivation. By placing the HEL transgene under an inducible promoter that can be controlled by changes in the diet of the mouse, it is possible to vary the stage of development at which the lysozyme is expressed and thereby study its effects on B cells at different stages of maturation. Experiments along these lines have demonstrated that inactivation occurs whether the B cells are chronically or acutely exposed to the monomeric antigen, and is independent of the developmental stage of the B cell at the time of the encounter (see Fig. 5.15, center panels).

The mature, surface IgM- and IgD-positive B cells that bind soluble self-protein antigens lose surface expression of IgM, which is sequestered in the endoplasmic reticulum. Moreover, even though these cells continue to express normal levels of IgD, they are unable to respond to the antigen through this receptor, as explained in Section 5-9. In a normal animal, in which such anergic cells are in the minority, mature anergic B cells are excluded from the primary follicles and, in the absence of T-cell help, are rapidly lost. However, it appears that the failure to enter the lymphoid follicles is not simply a consequence of the loss of the cell-surface IgM, nor of the inability to respond to antigen stimulation; if the self antigen is removed, B cells regain the ability to enter lymphoid follicles with a matter of hours, whereas they do not re-express IgM and return to antigen responsiveness for several days.

Thus, self tolerance in the B-cell repertoire is achieved in at least four different ways: (1) clonal deletion in the bone marrow and in the periphery; (2) receptor modulation by, and loss of response to, antigen (anergy), which can also occur either in the bone marrow or in the periphery; (3) failure of B cells to enter the primary follicles and subsequent death; and (4), in transgenic mice at least, modification of self-reactive receptors by receptor editing, so that they no longer recognize the self antigen.

5-13 | B cells are produced continuously but only some contribute to a relatively stable peripheral pool.

Many B cells have a short life span once they leave the bone marrow and enter the peripheral B-cell pool and, at least in humans, B cells are continuously replenished throughout life. Labeling studies in mice show that the remaining long-lived B cells have a broad distribution of life spans, with some B cells comprising a non-dividing population that is very long-lived. These may include the memory B cells that differentiate from mature B cells after their first encounter with antigen and persist for long periods after antigenic stimulation (Fig. 5.16). We shall return to B-cell memory in Chapter 9. The rapid production and loss of new B

Fig. 5.16 Proposed population dynamics of conventional B cells. B cells are produced as receptor-positive cells in the bone marrow. Most auto-reactive B cells are removed at this stage. Upon maturation, B cells migrate to the periphery where they enter the re-circulating pool. There appear to be two classes of B cell, long-lived B cells and short-lived B cells. It is estimated that 30–50 million mature B cells are produced in the bone marrow and exported each day in a mouse, and an equal number is lost from the periphery. Most of the turnover of short-lived B cells may result from B cells that fail to enter lymphoid follicles. However, about half of all mature B cells are longer-lived. The long-lived B cells may include memory B cells, which have been activated previously by antigen and T cells. The short-lived B cells are recently formed B cells by definition.

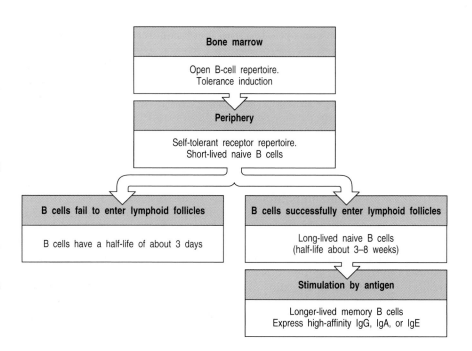

cells ensures that different receptors are produced continuously to meet new antigenic challenges, while the persistence of the clonal progeny of cells that have been activated ensures that those cells proven to recognize pathogens are retained to combat infection.

Summary.

Four different mechanisms remove self-reactive B cells from the repertoire. B cells specific for ubiquitous multivalent ligands such as self MHC molecules are deleted early in development, just after antigen receptor is first expressed. A proportion of self-reactive immature B cells may also be driven by antigen stimulation in the bone marrow to vary their receptors by receptor editing so that they are no longer autoreactive. B cells specific for soluble self antigens are rendered anergic as mature B cells; these cells are excluded from lymphoid follicles, and die in T-cell areas of lymphoid organs. B cells need specific T-cell help to respond to most antigens, so helper T-cell tolerance also ensures that mature B cells will not make antibody even when they can bind self antigens. To maintain a B-cell repertoire that is maximally diverse, new B cells are generated and lost continuously. Once B cells are tested for self tolerance, they are ready to occupy peripheral lymphoid tissues and produce antibody in response to antigenic challenge.

B-cell heterogeneity.

After their maturation in the bone marrow, B cells migrate through the bloodstream to the peripheral lymphoid organs. The B cells in peripheral lymphoid tissues are quite heterogeneous in their morphology and location, and in the cell-surface molecules they express. Part of this heterogeneity results from B-cell maturation in the periphery in response to antigenic stimulation. There is also a population of B cells that may arise from distinct stem cells early in an animal's development and which renews itself by continuing division in the peripheral lymphoid tissues of adult animals. In this section, we will describe these populations of B cells, and some malignant tumors of B-lineage cells that reflect their distinctiveness.

5-14 | CD5 B cells have a distinctive repertoire.

Not all B cells conform to the developmental pathway we have described in previous sections. A significant subset of B cells in mice and humans, and the majority population in rabbits, arises early in ontogeny and has a distinctive receptor repertoire and functional properties (Fig. 5.17). These B cells are identified by surface expression of the protein CD5, and are hence called **CD5 B cells** or **B-1 cells**, and also by the expression of surface IgM with little or no IgD. CD5 can bind to another B-cell surface protein called CD72, which may promote interaction between B cells, but its functional significance is currently unknown since cells with the properties of CD5 B cells develop normally in mice lacking the CD5 gene.

Property	CD5 B cells	Transitional CD5 B cells	Conventional B cells
When first produced	Fetus	Newborn	After birth
Mode of renewal	Self renewing	Self renewing	Replaced from bone marrow
Production of immunoglobulin	High	Intermediate	Low
Specificity	Degenerate	Precise	Precise
Isotypes secreted	IgM >> IgG	IgG = IgM	IgG > IgM
Somatic hypermutation	Low–none	Intermediate	High
Response to carbohydrate antigen	Yes	Maybe	Maybe
Response to protein antigen	Maybe	Yes	Yes

Fig. 5.17 A comparison of the properties of CD5 B cells, transitional B cells, and conventional B cells.

Currently, little is known about the function of CD5 B cells in present-day organisms. Although relatively sparse in lymph nodes or spleen, CD5 B cells are the predominant B-cell population in the peritoneal and pleural cavities. CD5 B cells make little contribution to the adaptive immune response to protein antigens but contribute strongly to some antibody responses that do not require helper T cells, as we shall see in Chapter 8. Moreover, much of the immunoglobulin found in normal serum (see Fig. 3.23) is produced by CD5 B cells and their progeny. These unusual features may reflect an independent origin for CD5 B cells and the unique repertoire of their receptors.

CD5 B cells arise early in ontogeny. In mice, where they have been studied most carefully, most CD5 B cells derive from an immature stem cell that is most active in the prenatal period (Fig. 5.18). The antigen

Fig. 5.18 Stem cells at different stages of development give rise to distinct B-cell populations. The development of stem-cell populations is shown vertically, while the maturation of B cells is shown from left to right. Stem cells in fetal mice give rise to progenitors that have little or no terminal deoxynucleotidyl transferase (TdT), which in turn give rise to CD5 B cells. These cells lack N-nucleotides in their V(D)J junctions and are self-renewing. At birth, stem cells in the bone marrow give rise to CD5⁻ B cells that are nevertheless like the CD5 B cells in being self-renewing but express some TdT and have diverse receptors. Finally, adult bone marrow stem cells give rise only to conventional B cells that have high junctional diversity and a short life span, being replaced continuously from the bone marrow because they are not self-renewing.

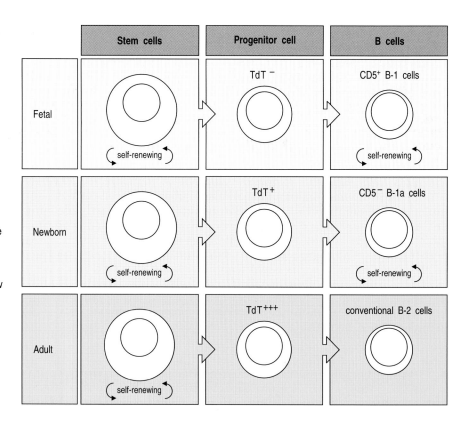

receptors of CD5 B cells are dominated by the V_H gene segments that lie closest to the D gene segments, presumably because V_H gene segments closest to the enhancer are the first to become accessible to recombinases during development. Because TdT is not active early in B-cell development, these heavy-chain gene rearrangements are accompanied by few, if any, N-nucleotide insertions. The V(D)J junctions of CD5 B cells are thus far less diverse than those of conventional B cells. The specificity of the receptors on CD5 B cells also differs from those of conventional B cells. CD5 B-cell receptors and the antibodies these cells produce tend to bind numerous different ligands, a property known as **polyspecificity**, with a preference for binding common bacterial polysaccharides. Indeed, the V gene segments that encode CD5 B-cell receptors may have been selected in evolution to recognize common bacterial antigens, allowing them to contribute to early phases of immunity, which we shall describe in detail in Chapter 9.

After birth, a transitional period occurs during which self-renewing B cells are still produced from the bone marrow. This population uses a more diverse repertoire of V genes and their rearranged immunoglobulin genes have abundant N-nucleotides. This transitional population is thus intermediate between the CD5 B cells made before birth and the mature, conventional B cells, and is termed **B-1a cells.**

As mice develop, the bone marrow stem cells seem to undergo a developmental change such that only conventional B cells or **B-2 cells** are produced (see Fig. 5.18). In adult animals, CD5 B cells maintain themselves by continuing division in peripheral tissues where they are the source of a very common tumor of self-renewing B cells called chronic lymphocytic leukemia. The γ:δ T cells that arise early in ontogeny are strikingly similar to CD5 B cells in many aspects of their biology, as we shall see when we consider T-cell development in Chapter 6.

5-15 | **B cells at different developmental stages are found in different anatomical sites.**

As B cells mature, they leave the bone marrow and migrate to the lymphoid follicles of lymph nodes and spleen, and other peripheral lymphoid tissues. Mature B cells are not sessile but form part of the recirculating lymphocyte pool, passing from blood into primary lymphoid follicles and then back into peripheral blood. Many B cells are found in the gut-associated lymphoid tissues, where very large lymphoid follicles known as Peyer's patches appear to provide specialized sites where B cells mature to secrete IgA.

If B cells encounter antigen and appropriate helper T cells on entering the lymphoid tissue and become activated, they proliferate first in the T-cell areas and then some proliferating cells migrate to the center of the lymphoid follicles to establish **germinal centers**. Germinal centers are sites of intense B-cell proliferation, where somatic hypermutation of rearranged antibody variable-region genes occurs (see Chapter 8). The proliferating B cells eventually give rise to antibody-secreting plasma cells. Plasma cells are found predominantly in the medullary cords of lymph nodes, in red pulp in the spleen, and in the bone marrow. The bone marrow can be an important site of antibody production. In hyperimmune individuals (those exposed to repeated stimulation by antigen) up to 90% of the antibody production can derive from the plasma cells in the bone marrow, because of the migration of mature antibody-secreting cells to this site and their persistence there. The localization of these different B-cell populations is shown schematically in Fig. 5.19.

5-16 | **B-cell tumors and their normal counterparts often occupy the same site.**

Tumors retain many of the characteristics of the cell type from which they arose, especially when the tumor is relatively differentiated and slow-growing. This is clearly illustrated in the case of B-cell tumors. B-cell tumors corresponding to essentially all stages of B-cell development have been found in humans, from the earliest stages to the myelomas that represent malignant outgrowths of plasma cells (Fig. 5.20). Furthermore, each type of tumor retains its characteristic homing properties. Thus, a tumor that resembles mature, naive B cells homes to follicles in lymph nodes and spleen, giving rise to a follicular center cell

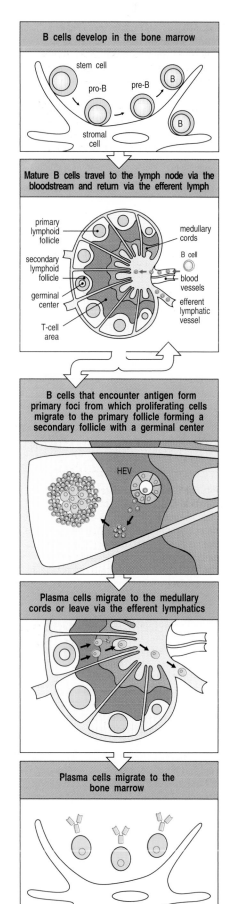

Fig. 5.19 The distribution of B cells. B cells are found in bone marrow, blood, lymphoid organs, and lymph. B cells develop in the bone marrow in adult mammals, migrate via the blood to the lymphoid organs, where they leave the circulation through the high endothelial venules (HEV) and enter the cortex of the lymphoid organ. In the absence of antigen, they migrate through primary follicles and return to the circulation via the lymphatic system, which joins the blood through the thoracic duct. In the presence of antigen, B cells are activated by helper T cells to form primary foci of proliferating cells from which the B cells then migrate to form the germinal center of a secondary follicle. These are sites of rapid B-cell proliferation and differentiation into plasma cells, which in turn migrate to the medullary cords of the lymph node, or to bone marrow, where 90% of antibody is produced in hyperimmune individuals. We have illustrated a lymph node here: the other major peripheral lymphoid tissues are the spleen and Peyer's patches of the gut.

Fig. 5.20 B-cell tumors represent clonal outgrowths of B cells at various stages of development. Each type of tumor cell has a normal cell equivalent, homes to similar sites, and has behavior similar to that cell. Thus, myeloma cells, whose growth is very aggressive, look much like the plasma cells from which they derive, secrete immunoglobulin, and are found predominantly in the bone marrow.

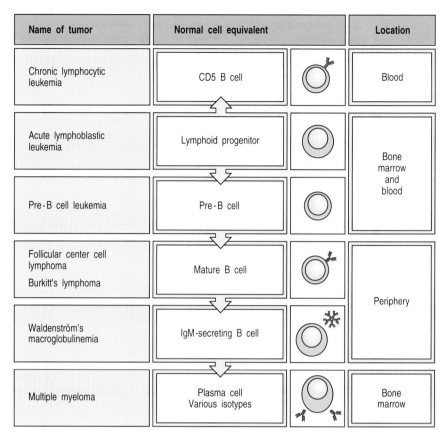

Name of tumor	Normal cell equivalent		Location
Chronic lymphocytic leukemia	CD5 B cell		Blood
Acute lymphoblastic leukemia	Lymphoid progenitor		Bone marrow and blood
Pre-B cell leukemia	Pre-B cell		
Follicular center cell lymphoma Burkitt's lymphoma	Mature B cell		Periphery
Waldenström's macroglobulinemia	IgM-secreting B cell		
Multiple myeloma	Plasma cell Various isotypes		Bone marrow

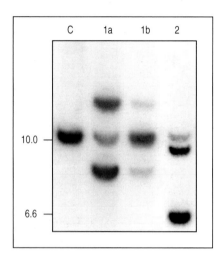

Fig. 5.21 Clonal analysis of B-cell tumors. DNA analysis of white blood cells by Southern blotting can be used to detect lymphoid malignancy. In a sample from a healthy person (lane C), immuno-globulin genes are in the germline configuration in non-B cells, so a digest of their DNA with HindIII restriction endonuclease yields a single 'germline' DNA fragment when probed with a sequence corresponding to an Ig heavy-chain J region (J_H). Normal B cells (also present in sample C) make many different rearrangements to J_H, so that no pattern other than germline is seen. By contrast, in samples from B-cell malignancies (1a and 2), where a single cell has given rise to all the cells, one or two extra predominant bands are seen. These result from the rearrangement of one or both alleles of the J_H gene in that cell. Each tumor gives a unique pattern of bands, and the intensity of the bands, compared with the germline signal, gives an indication of the abundance of the tumor cells in the sample. In lanes 1a and 1b, the same patient is analyzed before and after treatment. Note the reduction in the intensity of the tumor-specific bands after treatment. Photograph courtesy of T J Vulliamy and L Luzzatto.

lymphoma, while plasma cell tumors are usually found in many different sites in bone marrow, giving rise to their clinical name of multiple myeloma (tumor of bone marrow). These similarities reflect the expression by both the normal B cell and its malignant counterpart of cell-surface molecules that determine B-cell localization. The analysis of these molecules on B-cell tumors will be crucial for the understanding of these complex homing processes.

5-17   Tumors of B lymphocytes represent clonal outgrowths of B cells.

Tumors represent the clonal outgrowth of a single, malignantly transformed cell; this general conclusion is very clearly illustrated by tumors of B cells. All the cells in a B-cell tumor have the same immunoglobulin gene rearrangements, decisively documenting their origin from a single progenitor cell. This has clinical diagnostic utility, as the presence or absence of tumor cells can be detected by sensitive assays for these homogeneous rearrangements (Fig. 5.21).

Because tumors of B cells are a source of large numbers of cells with identical immunoglobulin gene rearrangements, they have proved invaluable for studying B-cell development, homing, and antibody production. Tumors of mature, antibody-secreting plasma cells provided the means for understanding the genetic basis of antibody diversity and isotype switching; tumors of less-mature B cells have illustrated the steps through which B-cell development proceeds. Some tumors representing B cells at early stages of development retain the ability to rearrange their immunoglobulin genes, and much of what we know about gene rearrangement has come from studying these B-cell tumor lines.

5-18 | Malignant B cells frequently carry chromosomal translocations that join immunoglobulin loci to genes that regulate cell growth.

The unregulated growth that is the most striking characteristic of tumor cells is caused by mutations that release the cell from the normal restraints on its growth. In addition to their unique, clonal immunoglobulin gene rearrangements, many B-cell tumors have rearrangements of immunoglobulin loci to genes on other chromosomes that control cell growth, thus disrupting normal growth controls. Many of the genes that control cell growth, division, and differentiation were first discovered because they were carried by RNA tumor viruses that could transform cells directly; these viral genes were therefore named **oncogenes**. It was later found that the viral oncogenes were derived from normal cellular genes that perform key roles in normal cells but cause cancer when their function or expression is disrupted by mutation. These normal cellular genes are termed **proto-oncogenes**.

The interchromosomal gene rearrangements (translocations) between immunoglobulin loci and proto-oncogenes give rise to visible chromosomal abnormalities that are characteristic of tumors of different types. That the immunoglobulin loci, sites in which double-stranded DNA breaks occur normally in B cells, are sites of chromosomal translocation is not surprising.

The analysis of chromosomal abnormalities has revealed much about the regulation of B-cell growth and the disruption of growth control in tumor cells. In Burkitt's lymphoma cells, recombination of the c-*myc* proto-oncogene on chromosome 8 with an immunoglobulin locus on chromosome 14 (heavy chain), 2 (κ light chain), or 22 (λ light chain) occurs. These rearrangements deregulate expression of the Myc protein (Fig. 5.22), which is involved in the regulation of the cell cycle in normal cells. Deregulation of Myc protein expression as a result of the chromosomal translocation leads to increased proliferation of B cells, although other mutations elsewhere in the genome are also needed before a B-cell tumor results.

Other B-cell lymphomas bear a chromosomal translocation resulting from recombination of immunoglobulin genes with the proto-oncogene *bcl-2*, increasing production of Bcl-2 protein. The Bcl-2 protein prevents the programmed cell death that is the usual fate of developing B cells. Like the change in c-*myc* expression, this abnormal *bcl-2* expression allows some B cells to survive and accumulate beyond their normal life span. During this time, further genetic changes occur that lead to malignant transformation, and mice carrying an expressed *bcl-2* transgene tend to develop B-cell lymphomas late in life. Much remains to be learned both about cancer and about normal B-cell development from the careful analysis of B-cell lymphomas and leukemias.

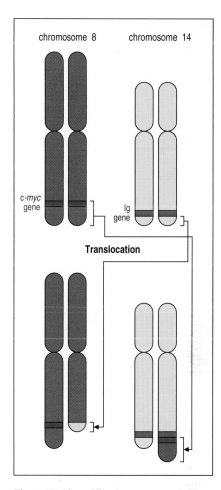

Fig. 5.22 Specific chromosomal rearrangements are common in mouse plasma-cell tumors and in Burkitt's lymphoma. Chromosomal rearrangements in B-cell tumors frequently involve joining of one of the immunoglobulin genes to a cellular proto-oncogene, usually resulting in the aberrant expression of the proto-oncogene under the control of the immunoglobulin regulatory sequences. In the example shown, from Burkitt's lymphoma, the translocation of the proto-oncogene c-*myc* from chromosome 8 to the immunoglobulin heavy-chain locus on chromosome 14 results in the deregulated expression of c-*myc* and the unregulated growth of the B cell. The immunoglobulin gene located on the normal chromosome 14 is usually productively rearranged and the tumors that result from such translocations generally have a mature phenotype and express immunoglobulin.

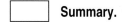 **Summary.**

B cells are not a single, homogeneous population. Rather, there are two major subpopulations that appear to arise from distinct stem cells and have distinctive properties. CD5 B cells first arise early in ontogeny and, in adults, form a self-renewing population of B cells whose functions and specificity are still being determined. Conventional B cells appear later in ontogeny and are replaced by new cells from bone marrow throughout life. Conventional B cells can also be divided into several subpopulations. These populations tend to represent stages in the maturation of these cells, the final stage being the antibody-secreting plasma cell. Each cell type also has a distinctive location in lymphoid tissue, suggesting important microenvironmental factors that act on cells at different stages of development. Much has been learned already about B-cell development and maturation, and more remains to be learned, by studying the behavior of B-cell tumors. These tumors are readily identified by their unique immunoglobulin gene rearrangements. The behavior of different tumor types often reflects the normal behavior of the cells from which they arose. These clonal outgrowths of normal B-cell types provide a unique window on minor lymphocyte populations by providing large numbers of cells of the same distinctive phenotype and identical rearranged immunoglobulin genes. Analysis of the growth and differentiation requirements of B cells may also lead to novel biological therapies for these tumors.

Summary to Chapter 5.

In adult mammals, B cells develop in the bone marrow and are produced throughout life. The development of human B cells is summarized in Fig. 5.23. The stages of B-cell development are marked by a series of irreversible changes in the immunoglobulin genes, which contribute to the diversity of antibodies, and by changes in immunoglobulin gene expression that depend upon the regulation of transcription and RNA splicing: these are summarized in Fig. 5.24. The major irreversible changes that generate complete immunoglobulin genes from the separate V, D, and J gene segments occur in regulated steps, which result in the monospecificity of most B cells. The heavy-chain genes become rearranged first, and as soon as a functional heavy-chain gene is generated, it is expressed on the cell surface with a surrogate light chain and further heavy-chain gene rearrangement ceases. Light-chain gene rearrangement is similarly halted by the expression of a complete light-chain protein. The completion of immunoglobulin gene rearrangement results in an immature B cell expressing IgM. The generation of the receptor repertoire in this way is essentially random and independent of encounter with antigen. Once surface immunoglobulin is expressed, however, it can function as an antigen receptor, and immature B cells that bind antigen in the bone marrow or periphery will die, change their receptor, or become anergic there; this is important for self tolerance. Self tolerance in mature B cells is further assured by the dependence of most B-cell responses on signals from helper T cells. Mature naive B cells, which co-express IgM and IgD, leave the bone marrow to circulate through the lymphoid organs, including Peyer's patches in the gut, until they encounter antigen. Upon interaction with antigen and specific helper T cells in a primary focus, the progeny B cells accumulate in the lymphoid follicles and form germinal centers in which they undergo vigorous proliferation and further changes to the immunoglobulin variable-region genes by somatic hypermutation. The B cells then differentiate into plasma cells, which secrete large amounts of antibody, or long-lived memory cells, which contribute to lasting protective immunity. Many plasma cells migrate to the bone marrow, while some remain in the medullary cords of the lymphoid organs. B-cell tumors can arise from cells at many of these stages of development and are found at sites characteristic of the normal cell. Thus, B-cell development provides the necessary raw material for clonal selection in the adaptive humoral immune response. Before we can understand that response in its entirety, however, the development and activation of T cells must be described. This will occupy the next two chapters of this book.

Fig. 5.23 A summary of the development of human B cells. The stages in B-cell development, their location, the state of the immunoglobulin genes, the expression of cell-surface molecules, and the expression of essential intracellular proteins are all shown.

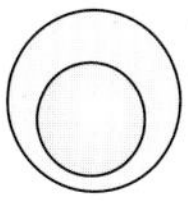

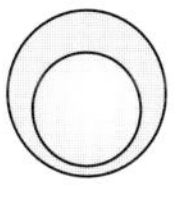

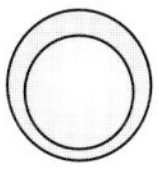

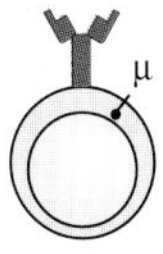

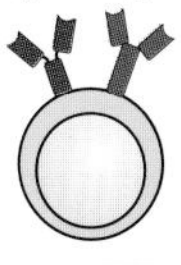

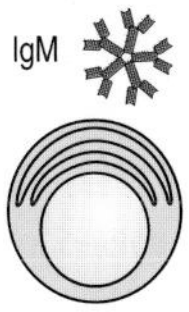

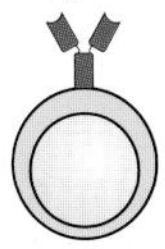

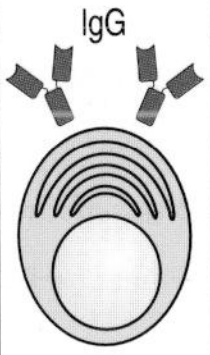

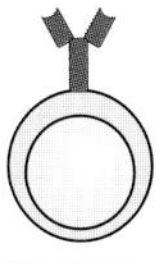

Fig. 5.24 Changes in immunoglobulin genes that accompany B-cell development and differentiation. Those that establish immunological diversity are all irreversible, as they involve changes in B-cell DNA. However, changes in expression of enhancer and promoter binding proteins can regulate immunoglobulin expression. Those that regulate immunoglobulin gene expression are reversible, as they involve changes in transcription or RNA processing.

Event	Process	Nature of change
V-region assembly	Somatic recombination of DNA	Irreversible
Junctional diversity	Imprecise joining, N-sequence insertion in DNA	Irreversible
Transcriptional activation	Activation of promoter by proximity to the enhancer	Irreversible but regulated
Switch recombination	Somatic recombination of DNA	Irreversible
Somatic hypermutation	DNA point mutation	Irreversible
IgM, IgD expression on surface	Differential splicing of RNA	Reversible, regulated
Membrane vs secreted form	Differential splicing of RNA	Reversible, regulated

General references.

Kantor, A.B., and Herzenberg, L.A.: **Origin of murine B-cell lineages.** *Ann. Rev. Immunol.* 1993, **11**:501-538.

Shatz, D.G., Oettinger, M.A., and Schlissel, M.S.: **V(D)J recombination: molecular biology and regulation.** *Ann Rev. Immunol.* 1993, **10**:359-830.

Osmond, D.G.: **The turnover of B-cell populations.** *Immunol. Today* 1993, **14**:34-37.

Moller, G. (ed.): **The B-cell antigen receptor complex.** *Immunol. Rev.* 1993, **132**:5-206.

Nossal, G.J.V.: **B-cell selection and tolerance.** *Curr. Opin. Immunol.* 1991, **3**:193-198.

Spangrude, G.J., Heinfeld, S., and Weissman, I.L.: **Purification and characterization of mouse hematopoietic stem cells.** *Science* 1988, **241**:58-62.

Alt, F.W., Oltz, E.M., Young, F., Gorman, J., Taccioli, G., and Chen, J.: **VDJ recombination.** *Immunol. Today* 1992, **13**:306-314.

Weill, J.-C., and Reynaud, C.-A.: **Early B-cell development in chickens, sheep, and rabbits.** *Curr. Opin. Immunol.* 1992, **4**:177-180.

Chen, J., and Alt, F.W.: **Gene rearrangement and B-cell development.** *Curr. Opin. Immunol.* 1993, **5**:194-200.

Cosy, S.: **Regulation of lymphocyte survival by the bck-Z gene.** *Annu. Rev. Immunol.* 1995, **13**:513-543.

Melchers, F., Haasner, D., Grawunder, U., Kalberer, C., Karasuyama, H., Winkler, T., and Rolink, A.G.:**The role of IgN and L chains and of surrogate H and L chains in the development of cells of the B lymphocyte lineage.** *Ann. Rev. Immunol.* 1994, **12**:209-225.

Section references.

5-1 | **The bone marrow provides an essential microenvironment for B-cell development.**

Hardy, R.R., Carmack, C.E., Shinton, S.A., Kemp, J.D., and Hayakawa, K.: **Resolution and characterization of pro-B and pre-pro-B cell stages in normal mouse bone marrow.** *J. Exper. Med.* 1991, **173**:1213-1225.

Tsubata, T., and Nishikawa, S.-I.: **Molecular and cellular aspects of early B-cell development.** *Curr. Opin. Immunol.* 1991, **3**:186-192.

Hayashi, S.I., Kunishada, T., Ogawa, M., Sudo, T., Kodama, H., Suda, T., Nishikawa, S., and Nishikawa, S.I.: **Stepwise progression of B-lineage differentiation supported by interleukin-7 and other stromal cell molecules.** *J. Exper. Med.* 1990, **171**:1683-1695.

Kincade, P.W., Lee, G., Pietrangeli, C.E., Hayashi, S.I., and Gimble, J.M.: **Cells and molecules that regulate B lymphopoiesis in bone marrow.** *Ann. Rev. Immunol.* 1993, **7**:111-143.

5-2 | **B-cell development depends on the productive, sequential rearrangement of a heavy- and a light-chain gene.**

Alt, F.W., Rosenberg, N., Lewis, S., Thomas, E., and Baltimore, D.: **Organization and reorganization of immunoglobulin genes in A-MuLV-transformed cells: rearrangement of heavy- but not light-chain genes.** *Cell* 1981, **27**:381-390.

Hieter, P.A., Korsmeyer, S.J., Waldmann, T.A., and Leder, P.: **Human immunoglobulin κ light-chain genes are deleted or rearranged in λ-producing B cells.** *Nature* 1981, 290:**368-372.**

Chen, J., Trounstine, M., Kurahara, C., Young, F., Kuo, C.C., Xu, Y., Loring, J.F., Alt, F.W., and Huszar, D.: **B-cell development in mice that lack one or both immunoglobulin κ genes.** *EMBO J* 1993, **12**:821-830.

5-3 | **The expression of the enzymes involved in immunoglobulin gene rearrangements is developmentally programmed.**

Oettinger, M.A., Schatz, D.G., Gorka, C., and Baltimore, D.: **RAG-1 and RAG-2, adjacent genes that synergistically activate V(D)J recombination.** *Science* 1990, **248**:1517-1523.

Ma, A., Fisher, P., Dildrop, R., Oltz, E., Rathbun, G., Achacoso, P., Stall, A., and Alt, F.W.: **Surface IgM-mediated regulation of RAG gene expression in E-N-myc B-cell lines.** *EMBO J* 1992, **11**:2727-2734.

5-4 | **Gene rearrangement in B cells is controlled by proteins that regulate the state of chromatin.**

Schlissel, M.S., and Baltimore, D.: **Activation of immunoglobulin κ-gene rearrangement correlates with induction of germline κ-gene transcription.** *Cell* 1989, **58**:1001-1007.

Takeda, S., Zou, Y.-R., Bluethmann, H., Kitamura, D., Muller, W., and Rajewsky, K.: **Deletion of the immunoglobulin κ-chain intron enhancer abolishes κ-chain gene rearrangement in *cis* but not λ chain gene rearrangements in *trans*.** *EMBO J* 1993, **12**:2329-2336.

5-6   Partial immunoglobulin molecules combine with invariant chains in the developing B cell to direct gene rearrangement.

Gu, H., Kitamura, D., and Rajewsky, K.: **B-cell development regulated by gene rearrangement — arrest of maturation by membrane-bound Dμ protein and selection of D$_H$ element reading frames.** *Cell* 1991, **65**:47-54.

Kitamura, D., Roes, J., Kuhn, R., and Rajewsky, K.: **A B cell-deficient mouse by targeted disruption of the membrane exon of the immunoglobulin μ chain.** *Nature* 1991, **350**:423-426.

Kitamura, D., Kudo, A., Schaal, S., Muller, W., Melchers, F., and Rajewsky, K.: **A critical role of λ5 protein in B-cell development.** *Cell* 1992, **69**:823-831.

Nishimoto, N., Kubagawa, H., Ohno, T., Gartland, G.L., Stankovic, A.K., and Cooper, M.D.: **Normal pre-B cells express a receptor complex of μ heavy chains and surrogate light-chain proteins.** *Proc. Natl. Acad. Sci. USA* 1991, **88**:6284-6288.

5-7   The immunoglobulin gene rearrangement program leads to monospecificity of B-cell receptors.

Nussenzweig, M.C., Shaw, A.C., Sinn, E., Danner, D.B., Holmes, K.I., Morse, H.C., and Leder, P.: **Allelic exclusion in transgenic mice that express the membrane form of immunoglobulin.** *Science* 1987, **236**:816-819.

5-9   Immature B cells can be eliminated or inactivated by contact with self antigens.

Nemazee, D., and Burki, K.: **Clonal deletion of B lymphocytes in a transgenic mouse bearing anti-MHC class I antibody genes.** *Nature* 1989, **337**:562-566.

5-10   Some potentially self-reactive B cells may be rescued by further immunoglobulin gene rearrangement.

Radic, M.Z., Erikson, J., Litwin, S., and Weigert, M.: **B lymphocytes may escape tolerance by revising their antigen receptors.** *J. Exper. Med.* 1993, **177**:1165-1173.

Gay, D., Saunders, T., Camper, S., and Wegert, M.: **Receptor editing: an approach by autoreactive B cells to escape tolerance.** *J. Exper. Med.* 1993, **177**:999-1008.

Tiegs, S.L., Russell, D.M., and Nemazee, D.: **Receptor editing in self-reactive bone marrow B cells.** *J. Exper. Med.* 1993, **177**:1009-1020.

5-11   In some species, most immunoglobulin gene diversification occurs after gene rearrangement.

Becker, R.S., and Knight, K.L.: **Somatic diversification of immunoglobulin heavy-chain VDJ genes: evidence for somatic gene conversion in rabbits.** *Cell* 1990, **63**:987-997.

McCormack, W.T., Tjoelker, L.W., and Thompson, C.B.: **Avian B-cell development: generation of an immunoglobulin repertoire by gene conversion.** *Ann. Rev. Immunol.* 1993, **9**:219-241.

5-12   Mature self-reactive B cells can be silenced in the periphery.

Cyster, J.G., Hartley, S.B., and Goodnow, C.C.: **Competition for follicular niches excludes self-reactive cells from the recirculating B-cell repertoire.** *Nature* 1994, **371**:389-395.

Cooke, M.P., Heath, A.W., Shokat, K.M., Zeng, Y.J., Finkelman, F.D., Linsley, P.S., Howard, M., and Goodnow, C.C.: **Immunoglobulin signal transduction guides the specificity of B-cell - T-cell interactions and is blocked in tolerant self-reactive B cells.** *J. Exper. Med.* 1994, **179**,425-438.

Goodnow, C.C., Crosbie, J., Jorgensen, H., Brink, R.A., and Basten, A.: **Induction of self-tolerance in mature peripheral B lymphocytes.** *Nature* 1989, **342**:385-391.

Russel, D.M., Dembic, Z., Morahan, G., Miller, J.F.A.P., Burki, K., and Nemazee, D.: **Peripheral depletion of self-reactive B cells.** *Nature* 1991, **354**:308-311.

5-13   B cells are produced continuously but only some contribute to a relatively stable peripheral pool.

Forster, I., and Rajewsky, K.: **The bulk of the peripheral B-cell pool in mice is stable and not rapidly renewed from the bone marrow.** *Proc. Natl. Acad. Sci. USA* 1990, **87**:4781-4784.

5-14   CD5 B cells have a distinctive repertoire.

Herzenberg, L.A., and Kantor, A.B.: **B-cell lineages exist in the mouse.** *Immunol. Today* 1993, **14**:79-83.

5-15   B cells at different developmental stages are found in different anatomical sites.

Rouse, R.V., Reichert, R.A., Gallatin, W.M., Weissman, I.L., and Butcher, E.C.: **Localization of lymphocyte subpopulations in peripheral lymphoid organs: directed lymphocyte migration and segregation into specific micro-environments.** *Am. J. Anat.* 1984, **170**:391.

Liu, Y.J., Johnson, G.D., Gordon, J., and MacLennan, I.C.: **Germinal centers in T cell-dependent antibody responses.** *Immunol. Today* 1992, **13**:17-21.

5-16   B-cell tumors and their normal counterparts often occupy the same site.

Greaves, M.F.: **Differentiation-linked leukemogenesis in lymphocytes.** *Science* 1986, **234**:697-704.

Waldmann, T.A.: **The arrangement of immunoglobulin and T-cell receptor genes in human lymphoproliferative disorders.** *Adv. Immunol.* 1987, **40**:247-321.

5-17   Tumors of B lymphocytes represent clonal outgrowths of B cells.

Korsmeyer, S.J.: **B-lymphoid neoplasms: immunoglobulin genes as molecular determinants of clonality, lineage, differentiation, and translocation.** *Adv. Intern. Med.* 1988, **33**:1-15.

Waldmann, T.: **Immune receptors: targets for therapy of leukemia/lymphoma, autoimmune diseases, and for prevention of allograft rejection.** *Ann. Rev. Immunol.* 1993, **10**:675-704.

5-18   Malignant B cells frequently carry chromosomal translocations that join immunoglobulin loci to genes that regulate cell growth.

Korsmeyer, S.J.: **Chromosomal translocations in lymphoid malignancies reveal proto-oncogenes.** *Ann. Rev. Immunol.* 1993, **10**:785-807.

Rabbitts, T.H.: **Chromosomal translocations in human cancer.** *Nature* 1994, **372**:143-149.

The Thymus and the Development of T Lymphocytes

6

T-cell development has much in common with B-cell development. Like B cells, T cells derive from bone marrow stem cells and undergo gene rearrangements in a specialized microenvironment to produce a unique antigen receptor on each cell. However, unlike B cells, T cells do not differentiate in the bone marrow but rather migrate at a very early stage to the **thymus**, a central lymphoid organ that provides the specialized microenvironment where receptor gene rearrangement and maturation of T cells occur. There is a further crucial difference in T- and B-cell development that reflects the distinct ways in which T cells and B cells recognize antigen. Because T cells are MHC restricted and recognize foreign antigen only in the form of peptide fragments bound to molecules encoded by the MHC, only those T cells able to recognize the body's own MHC molecules will be capable of contributing to adaptive immune responses. It is thus essential that each individual's T cells are able to recognize foreign antigenic peptides when they are bound to his or her own MHC molecules; that is, that they should be self MHC restricted. It is equally important, however, that T cells should be unable to recognize self peptides bound to self MHC molecules; that is, they must also be self tolerant.

T cells are selected to fulfill these dual requirements for self MHC restriction and self tolerance during their maturation in the thymus (Fig. 6.1). Here, once the immature T cells have rearranged their antigen-receptor genes and the receptor is expressed on the cell surface, they undergo the two selective processes known as **positive selection**, in which they are screened for self MHC restriction, and **negative selection**, which eliminates those cells that are specific for self peptides bound to self MHC.

How T cells are selected for self restriction but not self recognition during T-cell maturation is one of the most intriguing problems in immunobiology and, in consequence, one of the most active areas of research. In this chapter we shall describe what is known about the development of T cells and what mechanisms might explain positive and negative selection. Because developmental studies depend largely on experimental manipulation of the developing system, virtually all the information that we have about T-cell development in the thymus has been gained from experiments with mice. We shall comment on the development of human T cells where information exists.

Fig. 6.1 T-cell precursors migrate to the thymus to mature. T cells derive from bone marrow stem cells, whose progeny migrate from the bone marrow to the thymus (left panel), where the development of the T cell takes place. Mature T cells leave the thymus and recirculate from the bloodstream through secondary lymphoid tissues (right panel) such as lymph nodes, spleen or Peyer's patches, where they may encounter antigen. It is the developmental process within the thymus that is the subject of this chapter.

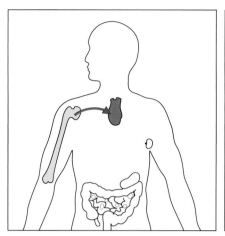 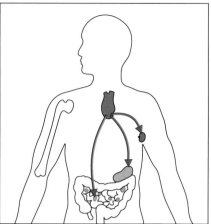

The development of T cells in the thymus.

T cells develop from bone marrow stem cells, and their progenitors migrate to the thymus where they mature: for that reason they are called **thymus-dependent (T) lymphocytes** or **T cells**. In the thymus, the immature T cells, or **thymocytes**, proliferate and differentiate, passing through a series of discrete phenotypic stages that can be identified by distinctive patterns of expression of various cell-surface proteins. It is during their development as thymocytes that the cells undergo the gene rearrangements that produce the T-cell receptor, and the positive and negative selection that shapes the mature receptor repertoire. These processes depend upon interactions of the developing cells with the cells of the thymic microenvironment. We shall therefore begin with a general overview of the stages of thymocyte development and its relationship to thymic architecture, before going on in the later sections of this chapter to consider the rearrangement of the T-cell receptor genes and the selection of the receptor repertoire.

6-1 | T cells develop in the thymus.

T lymphocytes develop in the thymus, a lymphoid organ in the upper anterior thorax, just above the heart. In young individuals, the thymus contains many developing T-cell precursors embedded in an epithelial network known as the **thymic stroma**, which provides a unique microenvironment for T-cell development. The thymus consists of numerous lobules, each clearly differentiated into an outer cortical region, the **thymic cortex**, and an inner **medulla**. The thymic stroma arises early in embryonic development from the endodermal and ectodermal layers of the embryonic structures known as the third pharyngeal pouch and third branchial cleft. From studies in embryonic mice it appears that the ectodermal layers give rise to epithelial cells in the thymic cortex, while the endodermal layers give rise to the epithelial component of the medulla. Together these epithelial tissues form a rudimentary thymus, or **thymic anlage** (Fig. 6.2). The thymic anlage then attracts cells of hematopoietic origin, which colonize it; these include dendritic cells and macrophages in addition to the thymocyte precursors.

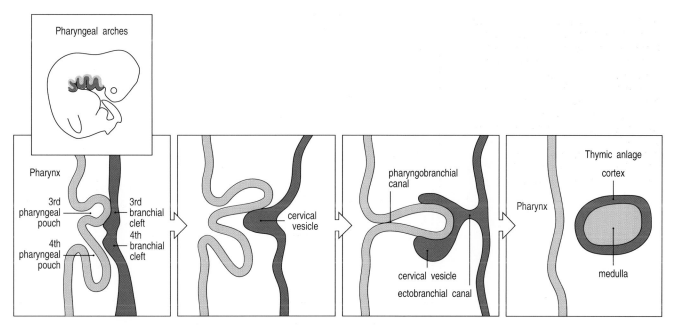

Fig. 6.2 The thymus forms from a fold of tissue in the pharyngeal region of the embryo, here illustrated for the mouse. Two discrete layers of embryonic tissues are involved, the ectoderm (blue) of the third branchial cleft and the endoderm (orange) of the third pharyngeal pouch (first panel). Starting at about 9 days (second panel), the endoderm of the third pharyngeal pouch and the ectoderm of the branchial cleft grow inwards, forming a structure known as the cervical vesicle. With the continued invagination of these structures the two layers come together and the ectodermal layer begins to surround the endodermal layer (third panel). At this stage, by about 11 days, the invaginations close, eventually isolating the thymic rudiment (last panel). Comparisons of thymus development in normal and mutant (nude) mice that lack a normal thymus, suggest that the ectodermal layer forms the cortical epithelial tissues of the thymus, while the endodermal layer forms the medullary tissues.

The human thymus is fully developed before birth and consists of cortical and medullary epithelia, which together with connective tissue form the thymic stroma, and very large numbers of bone marrow derived cells. The bone marrow derived cells are differentially distributed between the thymic cortex and medulla; the cortex contains only immature thymocytes and scattered macrophages, whereas more mature thymocytes, along with the dendritic cells and most of the macrophages, are found in the medulla (Fig. 6.3). We shall see that this reflects the different developmental events that occur in these two compartments.

The rate of T-cell production by the thymus is greatest before puberty. After puberty, the thymus begins to shrink and the production of new T cells in adults is lower. However, data from the measurement of CD4 T-cell expansion in patients with AIDS suggest that the ability of CD4 T cells to expand, at least in the periphery, may be retained. (see Chapter 10 for details).Moreover, in both mice and humans, removal of the thymus is not accompanied by any notable loss of T-cell function, and it seems that once the T-cell repertoire is established, immunity can be sustained without the production of large numbers of new T cells, provided these are not removed by infection with the human immunodeficiency virus.

6-2   **The thymus is required for T-cell maturation.**

The importance of the thymus in T-cell development was first discovered through observations on immunodeficient children, and much evidence has accumulated since to confirm and extend these observations. Thus, for example, in the **DiGeorge syndrome** in humans, and in mice with the ***nude*** mutation (which also causes hairlessness), the

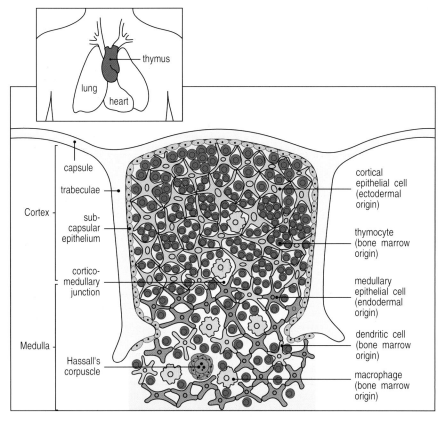

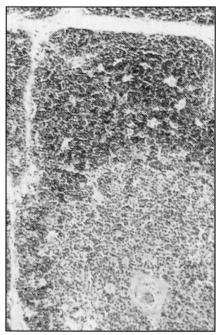

Fig. 6.3   The cellular organization of the thymus. The thymus, which lies in the midline of the body, above the heart, is made up from several lobules, each of which contains discrete cortical (outer) and medullary (central) regions. The cortex consists of immature thymocytes (dark blue), branched cortical epithelial cells (pale blue), with which the immature cortical thymocytes are closely associated, and scattered macrophages (yellow) involved in clearing apoptotic thymocytes. The medulla consists of mature thymocytes (dark blue), and medullary epithelial cells (orange), along with macrophages (yellow) and dendritic cells (yellow) of bone marrow origin. Hassall's corpuscles found in the human thymus are probably also sites of cell destruction. The thymocytes in the outer cortical cell layer are proliferating immature cells, while the deeper cortical thymocytes are mainly cells undergoing thymic selection. The photograph shows the equivalent section of a human thymus, stained with hematoxylin and eosin. Photograph courtesy of C J Howe.

thymus fails to form and the affected individual produces B lymphocytes but no T lymphocytes. Surgical removal of the thymus (thymectomy) of mice at birth, when no mature T cells have left the thymus, likewise results in a mouse with B cells but no T cells.

The crucial role of the thymic stroma in inducing the differentiation of bone marrow derived precursor cells can be demonstrated using two mutant mice, each lacking mature T cells for a different reason. In *nude* mice, the thymic epithelium fails to differentiate; while in *scid* mice, which we encountered in Section 3-16, the thymic stroma is normal but both B and T lymphocytes fail to develop because of a defect in receptor gene recombination. Reciprocal grafts of thymus and bone marrow between these immunodeficient strains show that *nude* bone marrow precursors develop normally in a *scid* thymus (Fig. 6.4). We shall see later that thymic grafts between different strains of mice have been instrumental in defining the role of the thymus in selecting the mature T-cell repertoire.

6-3   **Developing T cells proliferate in the thymus but most die there.**

T-cell precursors arriving in the thymus from the bone marrow enter a phase of intense proliferation. In a young adult mouse, where the thymus contains about $1–2 \times 10^8$ thymocytes, about 5×10^7 cells are newly

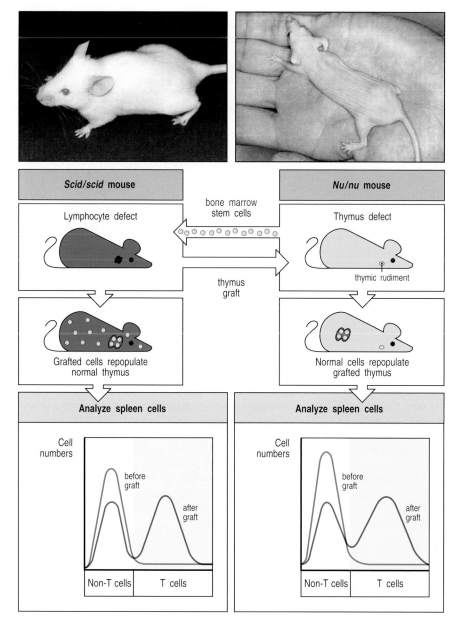

Fig. 6.4 The thymus is critical for the maturation of bone marrow derived cells into T cells. Mice with the *scid* mutation (upper left) have a defect that prevents lymphocyte maturation, while mice with the *nude* mutation (upper right) have a defect that affects the development of the cortical epithelium of the thymus. T cells do not develop in either strain of mouse: this can be demonstrated by staining spleen cells with antibodies specific for mature T cells and analyzing them in a flow cytometer (see Chapter 2), as represented by the graphs in the bottom panels. Bone marrow cells from *nude* mice can restore T cells to *scid* mice, showing that the *nude* bone marrow cells are intrinsically normal and capable, in the right environment, of producing T cells. Thymic epithelial cells from *scid* mice can induce the maturation of T cells in *nude* mice, demonstrating that the thymus is the essential environment for T-cell development.

generated each day. However, only about 10^6 (roughly 2%) of these will leave the thymus as mature T cells. Despite the disparity between the numbers of T cells generated continuously in the thymus and the number leaving, the thymus does not continue to grow in size or in cell number. This is because approximately 98% of the thymocytes generated each day die within the thymus. No widespread damage is seen, indicating that death is occurring by apoptosis rather than necrosis.

Apoptosis is a common feature of many developmental pathways, and one of its features is that changes in the membrane of cells undergoing apoptosis lead to their rapid phagocytosis. Indeed, apoptotic bodies, which are residual condensed chromatin, are seen inside macrophages throughout the thymic cortex (Fig. 6.5); as a result of the ready staining of the apoptotic bodies these macrophages are sometimes referred to as 'tingible body macrophages'. The apparently profligate wastefulness of this massive cell death is a crucial part of T-cell development, as it reflects the intensive screening that each new T cell undergoes for self MHC restriction and self tolerance.

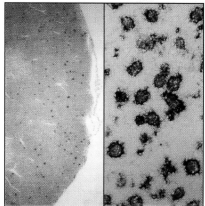

Fig. 6.5 Developing T cells that undergo apoptosis are ingested by macrophages in the thymic cortex. Apoptotic cells are stained red in the photographs above, and can be seen predominantly within the thymic cortex (left panel). At higher power (right panel), the apoptotic cells can be seen to be contained within macrophages, revealed when the thymus sections are stained also for a macrophage marker (in blue). Apoptosis changes the surface properties of cells so that they are readily injested by macrophages. Photographs courtesy of J Sprent and C Surh.

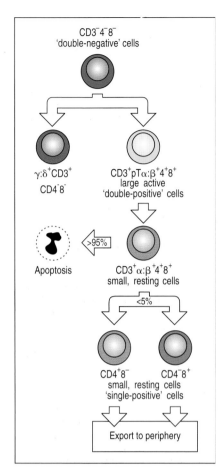

CD3⁻4⁻8⁻
'double-negative' cells

γ:δ⁺CD3⁺
CD4⁻8⁻

CD3⁺pTα:β⁺4⁺8⁺
large active
'double-positive' cells

Apoptosis   >95%

CD3⁺α:β⁺4⁺8⁺
small, resting cells

<5%

CD4⁺8⁻   CD4⁻8⁺
small, resting cells
'single-positive' cells

Export to periphery

Fig. 6.6 Changes in cell-surface molecules allow thymocyte populations at different stages of maturation to be distinguished. The most important cell-surface molecules in identifying thymocyte subpopulations have been the CD4, CD8, and T-cell receptor molecules. The earliest cell population in the thymus does not express any of these. Since these cells do not express CD4 or CD8, they are called 'double-negative'. (In the thymus, γ:δ T cells do not express CD4 or CD8 but these are a minor population.) Maturation of α:β T cells occurs through a stage where both CD4 and CD8, as well as low levels of the T-cell receptor are expressed by the same cell. These cells are known as 'double-positive' thymocytes. Most of these cells become small double-positive cells and die in the thymus. Those whose receptors bind self MHC molecules lose expression of either CD4 or CD8 and increase the level of expression of the T-cell receptor. The outcome of this process is the mature, 'single-positive' T cell that is exported from the thymus.

6-4 | **Successive stages in the development of thymocytes are marked by changes in cell-surface molecules.**

As thymocytes proliferate and mature into T cells, they pass through a series of distinct phases marked by changes in the status of T-cell receptor genes and in the expression of the T-cell receptor, the co-receptors CD4 and CD8, and other cell-surface molecules that reflect the state of functional maturation of the cell. Specific combinations of these cell-surface molecules can thus be used as markers of T cells at different stages of differentiation: the principal stages are summarized in Fig. 6.6.

When progenitor cells first enter the thymus from the bone marrow, they lack most of the surface molecules characteristic of mature T cells and their receptor genes are unrearranged. Once the progenitor cell arrives in the thymus, interactions with the thymic stroma trigger rapid proliferation and the expression of the first T-cell specific surface molecules CD2 and (in mice) Thy-1. At the end of this phase, the immature thymocytes bear distinctive markers of the T-cell developmental lineage but they do not express any of the three cell-surface markers that define mature T cells, namely the CD3:T-cell receptor complex, and CD4 or CD8. Because of the absence of CD4 and CD8, such cells are called '**double-negative**' thymocytes. In the fully developed thymus, double-negative cells form a small, highly heterogeneous pool of cells (about 5% of thymocytes), which includes several early stages in T-cell development.

Some of the double-negative cells (representing about 20% of all the double-negative cells in the thymus) have rearranged and are expressing the genes encoding the rare γ:δ receptor; these cells represent a separate developmental lineage of CD4⁻ CD8⁻ thymocytes (see Section 6-7). A second double-negative population expresses the α:β T-cell receptor; the role of these cells is unknown. We shall use the term 'double-negative thymocyte' to describe the remaining 75% of early thymocytes that are committed to the major α:β T-cell lineage but have not yet rearranged their α or β T-cell receptor genes.

These cells can be further subdivided on the basis of expression of the adhesion molecule CD44 and the α chain of the IL-2 receptor, CD25 (see Fig. 6.7, top right panel). The earliest thymocytes are CD44⁺ CD25⁻, and the β chain of the T-cell receptor is in the germline configuration. As the cells mature further, they begin to rearrange the T-cell receptor and express CD25 on their surface. Although CD25 is the α chain of the IL-2 receptor, mice in which the IL-2 gene has been deleted by gene knockout (see Section 2-38) have normal T-cell development. Thus, the exact significance of CD25 expression at this phase is unknown. The transition to CD44⁻ CD25⁺ cells is accompanied by productive rearrangement of the β chain; cells with incomplete or out-of-frame rearrangements of the β-chain gene remain in the CD44⁺ CD25⁺ stage, while in cells that have lost CD44, most β-chain gene rearrangements are complete and in frame. The remaining out-of-frame β-chain joins in CD44⁻ cells are those on the other chromosome.

The functional β chain is found paired with a surrogate α chain called pTα (pre-T cell α), together with CD3 molecules. Expression of this complex induces rapid loss of CD25, cell proliferation, and the expression of both CD8 and CD4; these cells are therefore called '**double-positive**' thymocytes. It is not known whether simply expressing this complex in the cell membrane is sufficient to induce the subsequent cell proliferation and the rearrangement of the α chain, or whether the β:pTα complex must bind a ligand, the nature of which is unknown. The expression of CD8 precedes that of CD4 in some strains of mice, while in

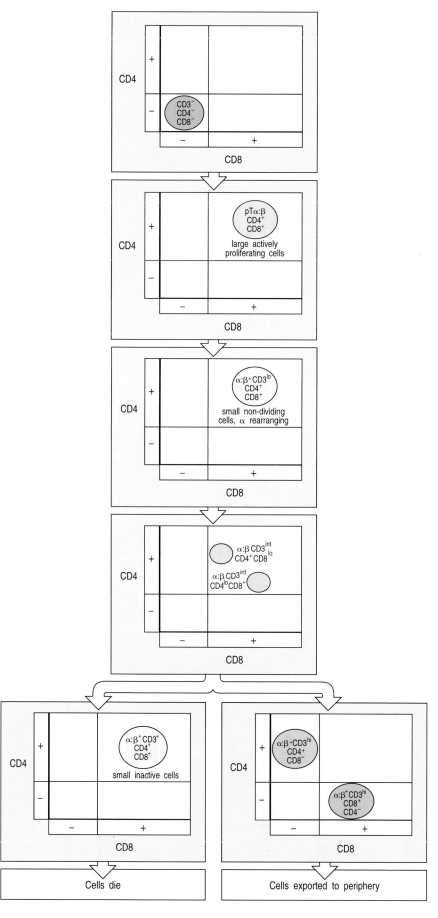

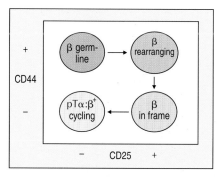

Fig. 6.7 The pathways of T-cell development. The fate of a single cohort of thymocytes stained for CD4 and CD8, from a FACS analysis. The progenitor thymocytes do not express CD3, CD4, or CD8 (top left panel). From these cells develop both the γ:δ T cells (which remain CD4⁻ CD8⁻ in the thymus) and the α:β T cells. The first steps in development of α:β T cells are best studied in terms of expression of CD44 and CD25 (top right panel). A productively rearranged β chain is finally expressed with a surrogate α chain, pTα (second panel on left). These cells proliferate rapidly, express CD4 and CD8, and then rearrange the α chain. These double-positive cells express low levels of α:β:CD3 (third panel). They become small inactive cells, most of which die (bottom left panel) as the consequence of failing positive selection. Successfully selected cells randomly down-regulate expression of CD4 or CD8 (fourth panel), and mature into single-positive thymocytes, increase T-cell receptor expression and lose either CD4 (if the receptor is restricted by MHC class I) or CD8 (if restricted by MHC class II). They then leave the thymus (middle bottom panel). Bottom right panel: percentage of the different populations of thymocytes in the thymus of young adult mice. (Of the three classes of CD4 CD8 double-negative cells, 1% bear γ:δ T-cell receptors, 1% bear α:β receptors, and 3% are immature progenitor cells.)

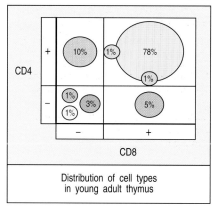

others CD4 is expressed first; it is not known if this is of any significance. Because these rapidly proliferating cells phosphorylate RAG-2 protein and degrade it, there is no gene rearrangement; once the cells cease to proliferate and become small double-positive cells, RAG-2 protein levels increase and the α-chain genes can rearrange and may produce a complete α:β T-cell receptor.

Small double-positive thymocytes express only low levels of the T-cell receptor, and most (more than 95%) are destined to die. These are the cells that express receptors that cannot recognize self MHC and thus fail positive selection. Those double-positive cells that recognize self MHC, however, mature to express high levels of T-cell receptor and subsequently cease to express one or other of the two co-receptor molecules, becoming either CD4 or CD8 **'single-positive' thymocytes**. Thymocytes also undergo negative selection during the double-positive stage in development. Those that survive this dual screening mature to single-positive T cells that are rapidly exported from the thymus to join the peripheral T-cell repertoire. Fig. 6.7 shows these steps in T-cell development represented as a FACS analysis (see Chapter 2) of thymocytes at each stage in their maturation.

6-5	**Thymocytes at different developmental stages are found in distinct parts of the thymus.**

We have seen that the thymus is divided into two main regions, a peripheral cortex and a central medulla (see Fig. 6.3). Most T-cell development takes place in the cortex; only mature single-positive thymocytes are seen in the medulla. At the outer edge of the cortex, in the subcapsular region of the thymus, large immature double-negative thymocytes proliferate vigorously (Fig. 6.8); these cells are thought to represent the thymic progenitors that give rise to all subsequent thymocyte populations. Deeper in the cortex, most of the thymocytes are small double-positive cells. The stroma of the cortex is composed of epithelial cells with long branching processes that express MHC class II as well as MHC class I molecules on their surface. The thymic cortex is densely

Fig. 6.8 Thymocytes of different developmental stages are found in distinct parts of the thymus. The earliest cells to enter the thymus are found in the subcapsular region of the cortex. As these cells proliferate and mature into double-positive thymocytes, they migrate deeper into the thymic cortex. Finally, the medulla contains only mature single-positive T cells, which eventually leave the thymus and enter the bloodstream.

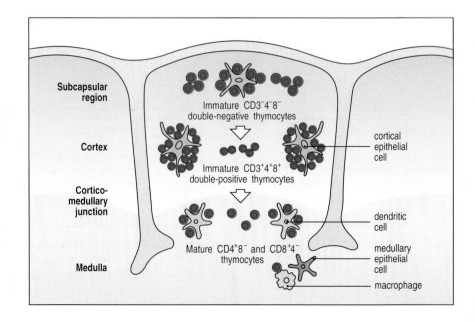

packed with thymocytes, and the branching processes of the thymic cortical epithelial cells make contact with most cortical thymocytes. Contact between the MHC molecules on cortical epithelial cells and the receptors of developing T cells plays a crucial part in positive selection, as shown later.

The medulla of the thymus is less well characterized. It contains relatively few thymocytes, and those that are present are single-positive cells resembling mature T cells. These cells may be newly mature cells that are leaving the thymus through the medulla, or they may represent some other population of mature T cells that remain within the medulla or return to it from the periphery to perform some specialized function, such as elimination of infectious agents within the thymus. At some point during their development in the thymic cortex and before their appearance in the medulla, therefore, the developing thymocytes must undergo negative selection. We shall see that this selective process is mainly carried out by the dendritic cells, which are particularly numerous at the cortico-medullary junction, and by the macrophages which are scattered in the cortex but are also abundant in the thymic medulla.

Before discussing in more detail the succession of interactions whereby double-negative thymocytes mature into a population of self MHC-restricted and self-tolerant T cells, we must turn to the gene rearrangements that generate the random receptor repertoire on which positive and negative selection act.

Summary

The thymus provides a sequestered and architecturally organized microenvironment for the development of mature T cells. Precursors of T cells migrate from the bone marrow and mature in the thymus, passing through a series of stages that can be distinguished by the differential expression of CD44 and CD25, the CD3:T-cell receptor complex proteins, and the co-receptor proteins, CD4 and CD8. T-cell development is accompanied by extensive cell death, reflecting the intense selection of T cells and the elimination of those with inappropriate receptor specificities. Most steps in T-cell differentiation occur in the cortex of the thymus. The thymic medulla contains only mature cells.

T-cell receptor gene rearrangements and receptor expression.

In the early stages of thymocyte maturation, the receptor genes of T cells go through a programmed series of rearrangements that produce large numbers of immature T cells each expressing receptors of a single specificity. This process is similar in many ways to that which occurs in B cells, with two important differences. First, rearrangement of two different sets of receptor genes distinguishes two T-cell lineages, one expressing $\alpha{:}\beta$ and the other $\gamma{:}\delta$ receptors. Second, there is much greater scope for repeated rearrangements of T-cell receptor genes at a single locus, allowing rescue of many cells in which the initial rearrangements have been unproductive. The end result of this process in the $\alpha{:}\beta$ T-cell lineage is a double-positive thymocyte expressing T-cell receptors on which positive and negative selection can then act.

| 6-6 | **T cells with α:β or γ:δ receptors arise from a common progenitor.** |

The γ:δ T cells arise from hematopoietic precursor cells, as do the α:β T cells, but differ in their specificity, the pattern of expression of the CD4 and CD8 co-receptors, and in their anatomical distribution. The two types of T cells also differ in function, although very little is known about the function of γ:δ T cells.

At present, the mechanism by which T-cell precursors become committed to one or the other of these cell types is not known. It appears that the two lineages of T cells share a common precursor, since productively rearranged β-chain genes can be found in mice in which the α-chain genes have been inactivated by homologous recombination and α:β T cells often contain rearranged δ-chain genes, presumably as extrachromosomal DNA circles following α-chain rearrangement (see Fig. 6.11).

One model that is consistent with these observations is that there is simultaneous rearrangement of the β, γ and δ genes and that cells in which there are successful rearrangements of the γ and δ genes produce a functional γ:δ receptor, which signals the cell to differentiate into the γ:δ lineage. Precursors in which there was a successful rearrangement of a β-chain gene would make a functional β-chain protein that could pair with pTα and signal the cell to enter the α:β lineage and to start rearranging the α-chain genes, thus deleting the δ-chain genes again as extrachromosomal circles.

The signals that initiate the decision to become an α:β T cell or a γ:δ T cell are unknown, nor is it known whether this signal has to be delivered within the thymus. Certainly, γ:δ cells seem able to develop in the absence of a functioning thymus and are present in, for example, *nude* mice.

| 6-7 | **Cells expressing particular γ:δ genes arise first in embryonic development.** |

The first T cells to appear during embryonic development carry γ:δ T-cell receptors (Fig. 6.9). In the mouse, where the development of the immune system can be studied in detail, γ:δ T cells first appear in discrete waves or bursts, with the T cells in each wave homing to distinct sites in the adult animal.

The first wave of γ:δ T cells homes specifically to the epidermis, where they are called **dendritic epidermal cells (dEC)**, whereas the second wave homes to the epithelial layers of the reproductive tract. The receptors expressed by these early waves of γ:δ T cells are essentially homogeneous: all the cells in each wave express the same Vγ and Vδ sequences and the same J regions. There are no N-nucleotides to contribute additional diversity at the junctions between V, D, and J gene segments, reflecting the absence of the enzyme terminal deoxynucleotidyl transferase (TdT) in these early T cells.

Later in development, T cells are produced continuously rather than in waves, and α:β T cells predominate, making up more than 95% of thymocytes. The γ:δ T cells produced at this stage are different from those of the early waves, with considerably more diverse receptors containing several different V gene segments and abundant N-region additions. Most of these γ:δ T cells, like α:β T cells, are found in

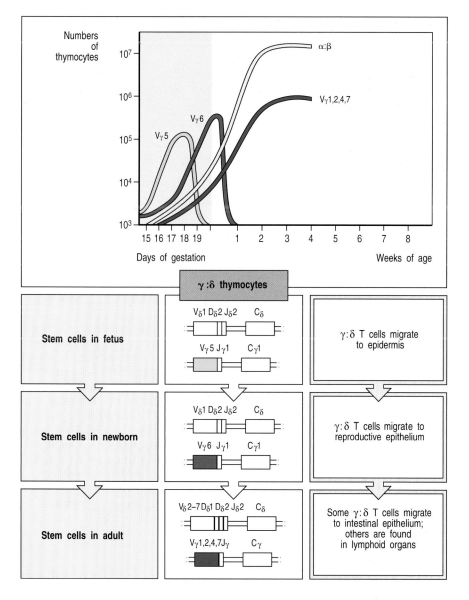

Fig. 6.9 The rearrangement of T-cell receptor γ and δ genes in the mouse proceeds in waves of cells expressing different V gene segments (upper panel). At about two weeks of gestation, the $C_\gamma 1$ locus is expressed with its closest V gene ($V_\gamma 5$). After a few days $V_\gamma 5$-bearing cells decline and are replaced by cells expressing the next most proximal gene, $V_\gamma 6$. Both these rearranged γ chains are expressed with the same rearranged δ-chain gene, as shown in the lower panels, and there is no junctional diversity. As a consequence, all of the γ:δ T cells produced in each of these early waves have the same specificity, although the nature of the antigen recognized by the early γ:δ T cells is not known. The $V_\gamma 5$- bearing cells migrate selectively to the epidermis while the $V_\gamma 6$-bearing cells migrate to the epithelium of the reproductive tract. After birth, the α:β T-cell lineage becomes dominant and, while γ:δ T cells are still produced, they are a much more heterogeneous population with high junctional diversity.

peripheral lymphoid tissues rather than in the specific epithelial sites to which the early γ:δ T cells preferentially home.

The developmental changes in V gene segment usage and N-nucleotide additions in γ:δ T cells parallel changes in B-cell populations during fetal development (see Section 5-13) and are believed to reflect a developmental program operating in hematopoietic stem cells. Similar changes occur in erythrocyte development, where different globin genes are expressed by red blood cells during different stages of development (Fig. 6.10).

It should be emphasized that most of what we know about γ:δ T-cell development comes from studies in mice, and we do not know whether similar changes in the pattern of receptors expressed by γ:δ T cells occur in humans. Certainly, the γ:δ T cells that home to the skin of mice, the dendritic epidermal cells, do not seem to have exact human counterparts. The functional significance of this fact, like the functional significance of the γ:δ T cells themselves, is unclear.

Fig. 6.10 Properties of mouse hematopoietic stem cells. The earliest hematopoietic stem cells arise in the yolk sac, where they give rise to erythrocytes containing embryonic hemoglobins. It is not known whether these embryonic stem cells give rise to lymphocytes. Later in development the site of hematopoiesis moves to the fetal liver, and stem cells give rise to erythrocytes making fetal hemoglobins, T lymphocytes making simple rearrangements of γ and δ T-cell receptor genes, and CD5⁺ B lymphocytes. In both early γ:δ T cells and early CD5⁺ B cells, the receptor rearrangements lack N-nucleotides, suggesting that the enzyme terminal deoxynucleotidyl transferase (TdT) is inactive. Around the time of birth, the site of hematopoiesis moves to the bone marrow, and adult stem cells produce erythrocytes with adult hemoglobins, and lymphocytes with highly diverse receptors containing abundant N-nucleotides in the junctions. It is not known whether the changes in the cell types produced by the stem cells result from maturation of the stem cell itself, or from the different environments in which hematopoiesis occurs.

Site of stem cell	Erythrocytes	Lymphocytes
Embryonic stem cells (yolk sac)	Embryonic hemoglobins	?
Fetal stem cells (fetal liver)	Fetal hemoglobins	CD5⁺ B1 B cells $V_\gamma 5$ and $V_\gamma 6$ γ:δ T cells No N-nucleotides
Adult stem cells (bone marrow)	Adult hemoglobins	CD5⁻ B2 B cells V_γ 1,2,4,7,γ:δ T cells α:β T cells N-nucleotide additions

6-8   Productive β-chain gene rearrangement triggers α-chain gene rearrangement.

T cells expressing α:β receptors first appear a few days after the earliest γ:δ T cells and rapidly become the most abundant type of thymocyte (see Fig. 6.9). The rearrangement of β- and α-chain genes during T-cell development (Fig. 6.11) closely parallels the rearrangement of immunoglobulin heavy- and light-chain genes during B-cell development (see Section 5-2). The β-chain genes rearrange first (Fig. 6.11). Dβ gene segments rearrange to Jβ gene segments, and this is followed by Vβ to DJβ gene rearrangement. If no functional β chain can be synthesized from these rearrangements, the cell will not be able to produce a receptor and will die. Unlike B cells with non-productive immunoglobulin heavy-chain gene rearrangements, however, thymocytes with non-productive β-chain VDJ rearrangements can be rescued by subsequent rearrangements, because of the organization of the Dβ and Jβ gene segments into two clusters. This increases the likelihood of a productive β-chain VDJ join from 55% for immunoglobulin heavy chains to more than 80% for T-cell receptor β chains (Fig. 6.12).

Once a productive β-chain gene rearrangement has occurred, the β-chain protein is expressed on the cell surface together with an invariant partner chain called pTα. Like the pre-B cell receptor complex in B-cell development, this β:pTα heterodimer is a functional receptor that triggers rapid proliferation of the cells; it also halts β-chain gene rearrangement and induces the expression of the co-receptor proteins CD4 and CD8. The induction of proliferation and of CD4 and CD8 expression, and the arrest of β-chain gene rearrangement, all require the protein tyrosine kinase Lck, which later associates with the co-receptor proteins; in Lck-deficient mice, T-cell development is arrested before the double-positive stage. The role of the β chain in suppressing further β-chain gene rearrangement can be demonstrated in transgenic mice containing a rearranged β-chain transgene: these mice express the transgenic β chain on most or all their T cells and rearrangement of the endogenous β-chain genes is strongly suppressed.

During the proliferative phase triggered by the expression of the β:pTα heterodimer, the *RAG-1* and *RAG-2* genes that mediate receptor gene recombination remain transcriptionally active, but RAG-2 protein is not active because it is phosphorylated and degraded in the rapidly cycling cells. Hence, no rearrangement of α-chain genes occurs until the proliferative phase ends, allowing RAG-2 protein to accumulate again. This ensures that each successful rearrangement of a β-chain gene gives rise

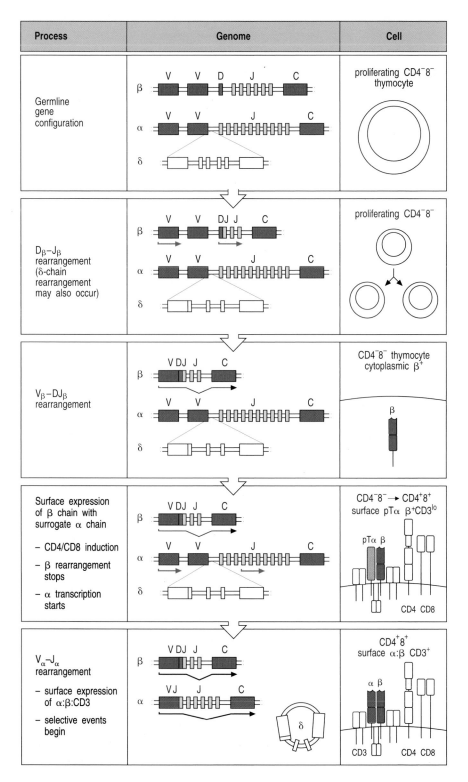

Fig. 6.11 The stages of gene rearrangement in α:β T cells. The sequence of gene rearrangements is shown, together with an indication of the stage at which the events take place and the nature of the cell-surface receptor molecules expressed at each stage. The T-cell receptor (TCR) β-chain genes rearrange first, in CD4⁻CD8⁻ double-negative thymocytes. As with immuno-globulin heavy-chain genes, D to J rearrangements precede V to DJ rearrangements (second and third panels). Since there are four D gene segments and two sets of J gene segments, it is possible to make up to four attempts to generate a productive rearrangement of the β-chain genes. The productively rearranged gene is expressed initially within the cell and then at low levels on the cell surface in a complex with the CD3 chains as a β:pTα heterodimer (fourth panel), where pTα is a 33 kDa surrogate α chain equivalent to λ5 in B-cell development. The expression of the TCR β chain:CD3 complex signals via the tyrosine kinase Lck to the developing thymocyte both to express CD4 and CD8 and to rearrange the α-chain genes, as well as to halt β-chain gene rearrangement. The first α-chain gene rearrangement deletes all δ chain D, J, and C gene segments on that chromosome, although these are retained as a circular DNA, proving that these are non-dividing cells (bottom panel). This inactivates the δ-chain genes. The α-chain gene rearrangement can proceed through many cycles, because of the large number of V and J gene segments, until a functional α chain is produced that pairs efficiently with the β chain. Finally, with the expression of a functional α:β receptor capable of recognizing peptides in association with self MHC molecules, the CD3^low CD4⁺ CD8⁺ thymocyte is ready to undergo selection.

to many CD4 CD8 double-positive thymocytes, each of which inde-pendently rearranges its α-chain genes once the cells stop dividing, so that a single β chain is associated with many different α chains in the resulting progeny. During the period of α-chain gene rearrangement, α:β heterodimeric T-cell receptors are first expressed, and selection by peptide:MHC complexes in the thymus can begin. The events leading to this point are summarized in Fig. 6.11.

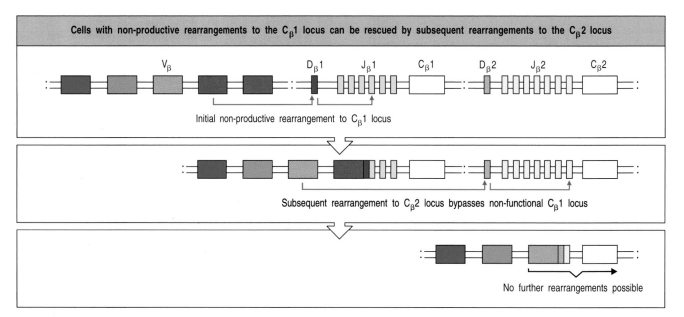

Fig. 6.12   Rescue of non-productive β-chain gene rearrangements. Successive rearrangements can rescue an initial non-productive β-chain gene rearrangement only if that rearrangement involved the $C_{\beta}1$ locus. A second rearrangement is then possible in which a second V_{β} gene segment rearranges to a DJ segment in the $C_{\beta}2$ locus, deleting the $C_{\beta}1$ locus and the non-productively rearranged gene.

6-9   **T-cell receptor α-chain genes can undergo several successive rearrangements.**

The T-cell receptor α-chain genes are comparable with the immunoglobulin κ light-chain genes, in that they do not have D gene segments and are the second of the two receptor-chain genes to undergo rearrangement during normal T-cell development. However, the presence of at least 50 J_{α} gene segments spread over some 80 kilobases of DNA allows many successive VJ_{α} gene rearrangements, conferring a far greater capacity to rescue cells with non-productive rearrangements than is the case for κ-chain genes (Fig. 6.13).

The potential for successive α-chain gene rearrangements on both chromosomes virtually guarantees that α-chain proteins will be produced in every developing T cell. Indeed, many T cells have in-frame rearrangements on both chromosomes and produce two α-chain proteins. Thus, in the strict sense, T-cell receptor α chains are not subject to allelic exclusion (see Section 5-7). However, as we shall see in the next part of this chapter, even T cells with two cell-surface α:β T-cell receptors have only a single receptor that can recognize peptide:self MHC complexes, and the cell therefore effectively expresses only a single receptor specificity. We shall see that even after production of a cell-surface receptor, however, the rearrangement of α-chain genes can continue and it only ceases when positive selection has occurred or the cell dies. This process lasts three to four days in the mouse.

Summary

In differentiating T cells, receptor genes rearrange according to a defined program, which is similar to that in B cells with the added complication that individual precursor cells can follow one of two distinct lines of development — either leading to cells bearing γ:δ receptors or to cells bearing α:β receptors. Early in ontogeny, γ:δ T cells predominate,

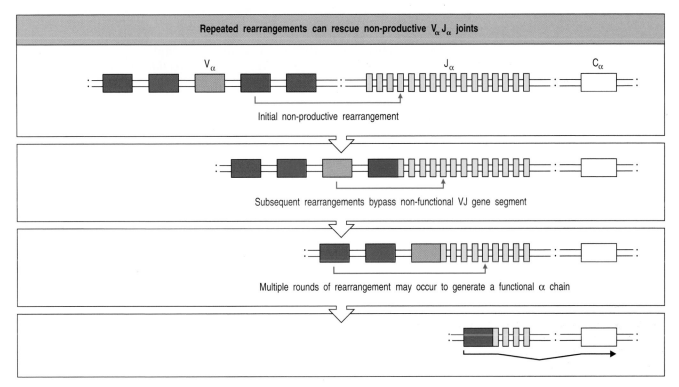

Fig. 6.13 Several successive gene rearrangement events can allow the replacement of one T-cell receptor α chain by another. For the T-cell receptor α chains, the multiplicity of V and J gene segments allows successive rearrangement events to 'leapfrog' over non-productively rearranged VJ segments, deleting any intervening gene segments. This process can continue until either a productive rearrangement occurs or there are no more V or J gene segments available for rearrangement. The α-chain rescue pathway resembles that of immunoglobulin κ light-chain genes (see Section 5-2).

but from birth onwards more than 90% of thymocytes express α:β receptors. The two T-cell lineages home to different tissues and perform different functions, although the function of γ:δ T cells is not yet fully established. In precursors destined to become γ:δ T cells, the γ and δ genes seem to rearrange virtually simultaneously. In cells of the α:β lineage, the β-chain genes rearrange first and the expression of a functional β chain at the cell surface signals for CD4 and CD8 expression and for the subsequent rearrangement of the α chain in CD4 CD8 double-positive thymocytes. In α:β T cells, α-chain gene rearrangement occurs continuously during selection, but mature T cells with two expressed α chains appear to have only one receptor restricted to self MHC expressed at one time.

Positive and negative selection of T cells.

We saw in the first section of this chapter that T cells first enter the thymus as double-negative cells, expressing neither the T-cell receptor nor either of the two co-receptor molecules, CD4 and CD8. During a phase of vigorous proliferation in the subcapsular zone, these immature thymocytes differentiate into double-positive cells, expressing low levels of the T-cell receptor and both co-receptor molecules, and enter the thymic cortex. Here they undergo positive selection for self MHC restriction and start to lose one of their two co-receptor molecules. The double-positive cells must also undergo negative selection in which potentially self-reactive cells are eliminated. By the time single-positive thymocytes are ready to emigrate, autoreactive T cells have been deleted. This sequence of events is summarized in Fig. 6.14.

Most of the evidence on the role of the thymus in the selection of the T-cell receptor repertoire has come from studies on chimeric or transgenic mice (see Sections 2-32 and 2-38). In this section, we shall see how these studies have defined the crucial interactions between developing thymocytes and the different thymic components that contribute to the selection of the mature T-cell repertoire, and will discuss the mechanisms by which these distinctive selective processes generate a self MHC-restricted and self-tolerant repertoire of T cells.

Fig. 6.14   The development of T cells can be considered as a series of discrete phases. Thymocyte progenitors enter the thymus in the subcapsular region. At this stage, they express neither the antigen receptor nor either of the two co-receptors CD4 and CD8, and are known as double-negative cells. As double-negative cells, the thymocytes proliferate and begin the process of gene rearrangement that culminates in the expression of the pre-T cell-surface receptor along with the co-receptors CD4 and CD8, to produce double-positive cells. As the cells mature, they move deeper into the thymus. These cells then rearrange α-chain genes and become sensitive to peptide:MHC complexes. These double-positive cells are found in the thymic cortex where they undergo positive selection and negative selection. Negative selection is thought to be most stringent at the corticomedullary junction, where nearly mature thymocytes encounter plentiful bone marrow derived dendritic cells. Finally, surviving thymocytes mature and exit to the peripheral circulation from the medulla.

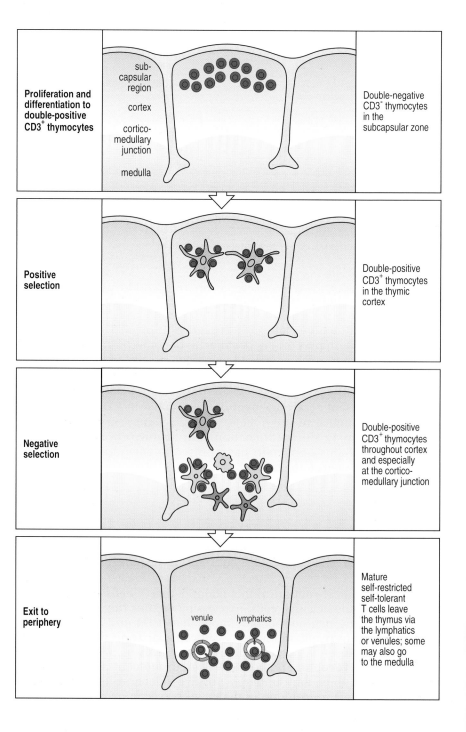

6-10	**Only T cells specific for peptides bound to self MHC molecules mature in the thymus.**

Positive selection was first shown clearly by transferring bone marrow cells from a mouse of one MHC genotype into an irradiated mouse of a different MHC genotype. Irradiation destroys all the lymphocytes and bone marrow progenitor cells in the host animal, so that all the cells derived from bone marrow are of the donor genotype. This includes all lymphocytes and antigen-presenting cells. Mice whose bone marrow derived cells have been replaced by those of a donor mouse are known as **bone marrow chimeras** (see Section 2-32). The donor mice used in the experiments on positive selection were F1 hybrids derived from MHC^a and MHC^b parents, and thus were of the MHC^{axb} genotype, while the irradiated recipients were one of the parental strains, either MHC^a or MHC^b (Fig. 6.15).

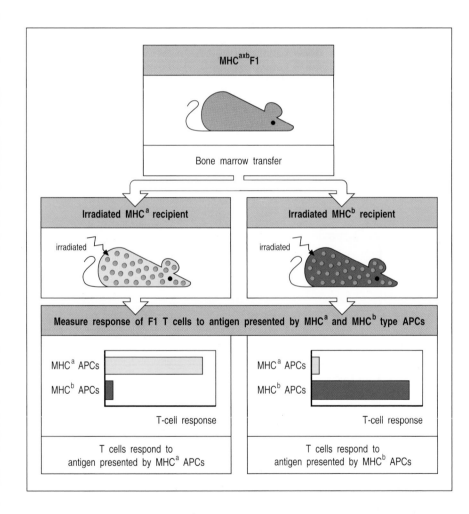

Fig. 6.15 Positive selection is revealed by bone marrow chimeric mice. T cells in MHC^{axb} F1 mice can be primed to respond to antigen presented by antigen-presenting cells (APCs) of both type *a* and type *b* MHC. If bone marrow from such an F1 hybrid mouse is transferred to a lethally irradiated recipient mouse of either parental MHC type (MHC^a or MHC^b), the T cells that mature are positively selected in that recipient's thymus, as shown by their response to antigen. When tested *in vitro* with APCs of type *a* or type *b*, T cells from such chimeric animals only respond to antigen presented by the MHC molecules of the recipient MHC type, as shown in the bottom panel.

Individual T cells in MHC^{axb} F1 hybrid mice will recognize antigen presented by either MHC^a or MHC^b, but not both, because their receptors are MHC restricted in antigen recognition. When T cells of MHC^{axb} genotype develop in a parental MHC^a thymus and are then immunized, they will be presented with antigen bound to both MHC^a and MHC^b, as the antigen-presenting cells in the chimera are of bone marrow origin and thus MHC^{axb}. However, these T cells recognize antigen only when it is presented by MHC^a molecules (Fig. 6.15). This experiment thus shows clearly that the environment in which the T cells mature determines the MHC molecules to which they become restricted.

A further experiment demonstrates that the host component responsible for the positive selection of developing T cells is the thymic stroma. For this experiment, the recipient animals were athymic nude or thymecto-mized mice of the MHC^{axb} genotype with thymic stromal grafts of the MHC^a genotype, so that all of their cells carried both MHC^a and MHC^b except those of the thymic stroma. The MHC^{axb} bone marrow cells of these mice also mature into T cells that recognize antigens presented by MHC^a, but not antigens presented by MHC^b. Thus, what mature T cells consider to be self MHC is determined by the MHC molecules expressed by the thymic stromal cells they encounter during intrathymic development. We shall see later that the thymic cortical epithelial cell is the critical cell that governs the specificity of positive selection.

The chimeric mice used to demonstrate positive selection produce normal T-cell responses to foreign antigens. By contrast, chimeras made by injecting MHC^a bone marrow cells into MHC^b animals cannot make normal T-cell responses. This is because the T cells in these animals have been selected to recognize peptides only when they are presented by MHC^b, while the antigen-presenting cells that they encounter as mature T cells in the periphery are bone marrow derived MHC^a cells. The T cells will therefore fail to recognize antigen presented by antigen-presenting cells of their own MHC type, and T cells can be activated in these animals only if antigen-presenting cells of the MHC^b type are injected together with the antigen. Thus, for a bone marrow graft to reconstitute immunity, there must be at least one MHC molecule in common between donor and recipient (Fig. 6.16). This can be an important consideration when bone marrow grafts are used in the treatment of human diseases such as leukemias.

Fig. 6.16 Summary of T-cell responses in bone marrow chimeric mice. T cells can make immune responses only if the antigen-presenting cells (APCs) present in the host share at least one MHC molecule with the thymus in which the T cells developed.

Bone marrow donor	Recipient	Mice contain APC of type:	T-cell responses to antigen presented *in vitro* by APC of type:	
			MHC^a APC	MHC^b APC
MHC^{axb}	MHC^a	MHC^{axb}	Yes	No
MHC^{axb}	MHC^b	MHC^{axb}	No	Yes
MHC^a	MHC^b	MHC^a	No	No
MHC^a	MHC^b + MHC^b APC	MHC^a + MHC^b	No	Yes

6-11   Cells that fail positive selection die in the thymus.

Bone marrow chimeras and thymic grafting provided the first crucial evidence for the central importance of the thymus in positive selection, but more detailed investigation of the process has generally required the use of T-cell receptor transgenic mice. When rearranged T-cell receptor genes of known specificity are introduced into the genomes of mice, rearrangement of the endogenous genes is inhibited, so that most developing T cells express the receptor encoded by the α- and β-chain transgenes. By introducing the transgenes into mice of known MHC genotype, it is possible to establish the effect of MHC molecules on the maturation of thymocytes with known recognition properties. Such a T-cell receptor transgenic mouse was used to establish the fate of T cells that fail positive selection. In this case, rearranged receptor genes from a mature T cell restricted to a particular MHC molecule were introduced into a recipient mouse lacking that molecule, and the fate of the thymocytes was investigated directly by staining with clonotypic antibodies specific for the transgenic receptor. Antibodies to other molecules such as CD4 and CD8 were used at the same time to mark the stages of T-cell development. In this way it was shown that cells that do not encounter their restricting MHC molecule on the thymic epithelium never progress further than the double-positive stage and die in the thymus within three or four days of their last division.

The total potential receptor repertoire must be capable of recognizing all of the hundreds of different allelic variants of MHC molecules present in the population since, prior to receptor gene rearrangement and surface expression of an α:β T-cell receptor, the MHC molecules expressed in the thymus cannot be detected by the thymocyte. As a given thymus will express only a few of these many distinct MHC molecules, only a relatively small proportion of the thymocytes in each animal will be capable of recognizing an MHC molecule, so that most of the 50×10^6 thymocytes that die each day in the thymus presumably do so because they fail positive selection. It has been estimated that 95% of thymocytes die because they are not rescued by a signal received from their T-cell receptor.

6-12 **Positive selection also regulates α-chain gene rearrangement.**

We have seen that in B cells, the expression of a receptor on the cell surface shuts off further rearrangement of the receptor genes; this is accompanied by the disappearance of the expression of RAG-1 and RAG-2. In the case of T cells, however, receptor expression is not sufficient to shut off gene rearrangement. Instead, the rearrangement machinery, including RAG-1, RAG-2, and TdT, is active, and rearrangement of the α-chain genes continues until the cells are positively selected or die. In this way, several different α chains can be tested for self MHC recognition with the β chain of each developing T cell. If positive selection does not occur within three to four days of the initial expression of an α:β receptor, the cell dies.

Because α-chain gene rearrangement occurs continuously, and because positive selection is such a rare event, it seemed likely that a significant percentage of mature T cells would express two T-cell receptors, sharing a β chain but differing in α-chain expression. Indeed, one can predict that if positive selection is sufficiently rare, one should have roughly one cell in three with two α chains at the cell surface. This was confirmed recently for human and mouse T cells. However, only one of these receptor chains was functional, as only one of the two T-cell receptors could recognize peptide presented by self MHC. It remains to be shown whether the situation in which two T-cell receptors are both restricted by the same self specificity can arise.

Thus, positive selection not only selects cells for further maturation, but it also regulates the rearrangement of T-cell receptor α-chain genes. The ability of a single developing thymocyte to express several different rearranged α-chain genes during the time it is susceptible to positive selection must increase the yield of useful T cells significantly. Without this mechanism even more thymocytes would die because they fail positive selection. The rate of rescue of T cells by subsequent α-chain gene rearrangements has been estimated in TCR transgenic mice to be very small but significant.

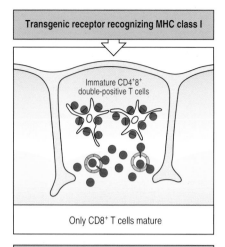

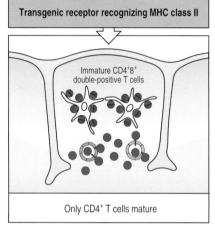

Fig. 6.17 Positive selection determines co-receptor specificity. In mice transgenic for T-cell receptors restricted by an MHC class I molecule (top panel), the only mature T cells to develop have the CD8 (red) phenotype. In mice transgenic for receptors restricted by an MHC class II molecule (bottom panel), all the mature T cells have the CD4 (blue) phenotype. In both cases, normal numbers of immature, double-positive thymocytes are found. The specificity of the T-cell receptor determines the outcome of the developmental pathway, ensuring that the only T cells that mature are those equipped with a co-receptor that is able to bind the same self MHC molecule as the T-cell receptor.

6-13 ## The expression of CD4 and CD8 on mature cells is determined by positive selection.

At the time of positive selection, a thymocyte expresses both the CD4 and the CD8 co-receptor molecules. At the end of the selection process, mature thymocytes ready for export to the periphery express only one of these two co-receptors; moreover, all mature T cells that express CD4 have receptors that recognize peptides bound to self MHC class II molecules, whereas all those that express CD8 have receptors that recognize peptides bound to self MHC class I molecules. Thus, positive selection also determines the cell-surface phenotype of the mature T cell, equipping it with the co-receptor that it requires for efficient antigen recognition. Again, experiments with mice made transgenic for rearranged T-cell receptor genes show clearly that it is the specificity of the T-cell receptor for self MHC molecules that determines which co-receptor a mature T cell will express. If the T-cell receptor transgenes encode a receptor specific for antigen presented by self MHC class I molecules, all mature T cells that express the transgenic receptor are also CD8 T cells. Similarly, in mice made transgenic for a receptor that recognizes antigen with self MHC class II molecules, all mature T cells that express the transgenic receptor also express CD4 (Fig. 6.17).

The importance of MHC molecules in such selective events can also be seen in the class of human immunodeficiency diseases known as **bare lymphocyte syndromes**, which are caused by mutations that lead to absence of MHC molecules on lymphocytes and thymic epithelial cells. People who selectively lack MHC class II molecules have CD8 T cells but only a few highly abnormal CD4 T cells, and a similar result has been obtained in mice in which MHC class II expression has been eliminated by targeted gene disruption (see Sections 2-37 and 2-38). Likewise, mice and humans that lack MHC class I molecules lack CD8 T cells. Thus, MHC class II molecules are required for CD4 T-cell development, while MHC class I molecules are required for CD8 T-cell development.

6-14 ## Thymic cortical epithelial cells mediate positive selection.

The ability of thymic stromal cells to determine co-receptor specificity has been used as the basis for experiments aimed at identifying the stromal cell type that is critical in positive selection of thymocytes. An obvious candidate, on the basis of circumstantial evidence, is the thymic cortical epithelial cell. Thymic cortical epithelial cells form a web of processes that make close contacts with the double-positive T cells undergoing positive selection and, at these sites of contact, T-cell receptors can be seen clustering with MHC molecules. Direct evidence that thymic cortical epithelial cells mediate positive selection comes from an ingenious manipulation of mice whose MHC class II genes have been eliminated by targeted gene disruption.

As we have already seen, mutant mice that lack MHC class II molecules do not produce CD4 T cells. To test the role of the thymic epithelium in positive selection, therefore, an MHC class II transgene was introduced into such mutant mice. The MHC class II coding region of the transgene was placed under the control of a promoter that restricted its expression to thymic cortical epithelial cells. In these mice, CD4 T cells develop normally (Fig. 6.18). When MHC class II genes are expressed in other tissues but are not expressed in thymic cortical epithelial cells, however, few CD4 T cells develop. Thus, positive selection normally requires MHC molecule expression on the thymic cortical epithelial

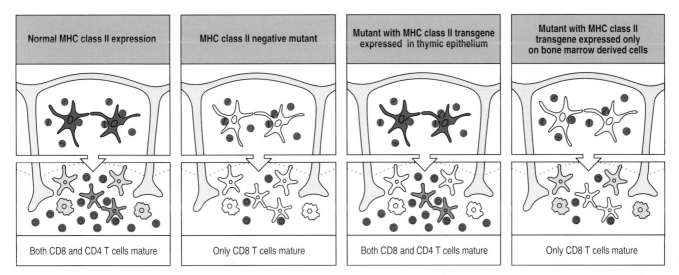

Normal MHC class II expression	MHC class II negative mutant	Mutant with MHC class II transgene expressed in thymic epithelium	Mutant with MHC class II transgene expressed only on bone marrow derived cells
Both CD8 and CD4 T cells mature	Only CD8 T cells mature	Both CD8 and CD4 T cells mature	Only CD8 T cells mature

Fig. 6.18   Mice lacking MHC class II molecules fail to develop CD4 T cells. The expression of MHC class II molecules in the thymus of normal and mutant strains of mice is shown, where the stromal cells are colored only if they are expressing MHC class II molecules. In the thymus of normal mice (first column), which express MHC class II molecules on epithelial cells in the thymic cortex (blue) as well as on medullary epithelial cells (orange) and bone marrow derived cells (yellow), both CD4 (blue) and CD8 (red) T cells mature. Double-positive thymocytes are shown as half red/half blue. The second column represents mutant mice in which MHC class II expression has been eliminated by targeted gene disruption; in these mice, no CD4 T cells develop, although CD8 T cells develop normally. In MHC class II-negative mice containing an MHC class II transgene engineered so that it is expressed only on the epithelial cells of the thymic cortex (third column), normal numbers of CD4 T cells mature. In MHC class II-negative mice containing an MHC class II transgene expressed only on bone marrow derived cells (fourth column), which in thymus are found predominantly in the medulla, no CD4 T cells develop. Thus, the cortical epithelial cells are the critical cell type mediating positive selection.

determined by the genotype of the MHC molecules expressed on these epithelial cells. While other cells injected into the thymus may influence the specificity of positive selection (see Section 6-19), they apparently do so only in the presence of thymic cortical epithelial cells. Thus it appears that some survival signal, possibly contact dependent, delivered by thymic cortical epithelial cells is essential for positive selection to occur, while recognition of MHC molecules, which are optimally expressed on cortical epithelial cells but can, nevertheless, be expressed on other cells, is required to ensure the specificity of positive selection.

6-15   Co-receptor selection occurs in two stages.

We have seen that the specificity of a developing thymocyte for MHC class I or MHC class II molecules determines which co-receptor will be retained by the mature single-positive T cell. Although the mechanism whereby the receptor MHC specificity dictates the choice of co-receptor is not understood in detail, recent evidence suggests that selection for co-receptor specificity occurs in two stages: in the first, the expression of either CD4 or CD8 is decreased at random, while the second is a selective step requiring the interaction of both the antigen receptor and the co-receptor with the appropriate class of MHC molecule (Fig. 6.19). The first step occurs when the antigen receptor on a developing double-positive thymocyte first binds to its specific MHC molecule on a cortical epithelial cell. This gives rise to cells that are either $CD8^{high}CD4^{low}$, or $CD4^{high}CD8^{low}$, but are still double-positive. It is likely that these cells have ceased to transcribe one of their co-receptor genes but still retain some of the corresponding protein. This step may be accompanied by programming for the different T-cell effector functions of CD4

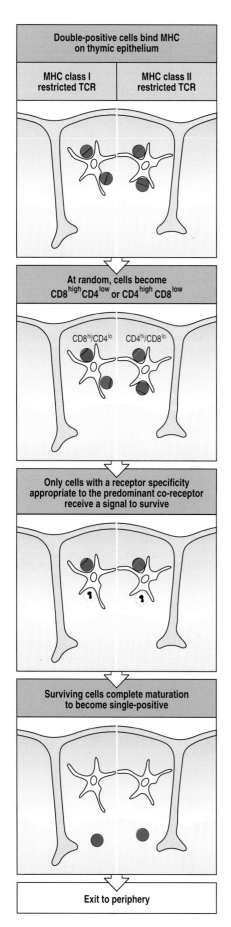

Double-positive cells bind MHC on thymic epithelium

| MHC class I restricted TCR | MHC class II restricted TCR |

At random, cells become CD8^high CD4^low or CD4^high CD8^low

CD8^hi/CD4^lo   CD4^hi/CD8^lo

Only cells with a receptor specificity appropriate to the predominant co-receptor receive a signal to survive

Surviving cells complete maturation to become single-positive

Exit to periphery

Fig. 6.19 Selection for co-receptor expression occurs in two stages. The first stage is triggered by specific recognition of self MHC molecules by the T-cell receptor (top panel). The cells become either CD4^{high} CD8^{low} and probably programmed for CD4 effector functions, or CD8^{high} CD4^{low} and programmed for CD8 effector functions (second panel). The choice of pathway appears to be independent of antigen-receptor specificity for MHC class I or MHC class II. In the second step, the CD4^{high} CD8^{low} T cells mature into CD4 single-positive cells only if the T-cell receptors on the cells bind to self MHC class II molecules, while CD8^{high} CD4^{low} cells only mature into CD8 single-positive cells if their T-cell receptors are specific for self MHC class I molecules (third and fourth). Cells with the inappropriate co-receptor undergo programmed cell death.

and CD8 cells. The cells must also have an antigen receptor that can bind self MHC, but it is immaterial whether the receptor binds MHC class I or MHC class II molecules: thus both types of intermediate double-positive cells are seen in mice that lack one or other class of MHC molecule.

These cells, however, will now die unless their antigen receptors and the remaining co-receptor are able to bind the same self MHC molecule. Binding by the antigen receptor and the co-receptor rescues the developing T cell by activating unknown genes that are able to inhibit programmed cell death. Bcl-2, which is known to rescue both B and T cells from apoptosis at other times, does not appear to play a part in this process. In mice that lack the *bcl-2* gene as a result of targeted gene disruption, positive selection operates fairly normally in young mice, although all the mature lymphocytes disappear at about 3 weeks, at which time puberty occurs and a wave of steroid hormones is produced.Because many genes encoding proteins that interact with Bcl-2 are being identified, it will be necessary to knock out several of these genes before we have decisive evidence of the gene activation events that accompany positive selection.

The only CD4^{high} CD8^{low} cells to mature are those whose antigen receptors recognize self MHC class II molecules and, conversely, CD8^{high} CD4^{low} cells mature only if their antigen receptors recognize self MHC class I molecules. As expression of CD4 or CD8 occurs at random, about half of the developing T cells that enter these intermediate populations will survive. The cells thus selected differentiate into single- positive thymocytes.

Although the evidence for the stochastic/selective process of T-cell development is strong, there may, in addition, be a role for differential signals delivered by CD4 or CD8. In this case one could argue for an inductive model of T-cell development, and evidence for this model has been obtained in mice transgenic for both a class I-restricted T-cell receptor and a CD8 molecule expressed constitutively in T cells. The stochastic model would predict the development of T cells expressing both endogenous CD4 and the transgenic CD8, but these are not seen. These observations led to the suggestion that, in this case, signals transduced by co-ligation of CD8 and the class I-restricted receptor were inducing the double-positive thymocyte to switch off CD4 expression and to acquire the phenotype of a CD8 T cell. Other recent data have also challenged the stochastic/selection model, at least for CD8 T cells, which appear to derive not only from CD4^{low} CD8$^+$ thymocytes but also from CD4$^+$ CD8^{low} cells. Obviously, further studies of this problem are needed. It is possible that for some T-cell receptors, direct interactions with either CD4 or CD8 at the surface of the T cell could allow such effects to occur, while for other receptors, stochastic selection would predominate.

6-16   T cells specific for self antigens are deleted in the thymus.

When a mature T cell in the periphery encounters the antigen for which its receptor is specific, it is usually stimulated to proliferate and produce effector cells. In contrast, when a developing T cell in the thymus encounters the antigen it recognizes, it dies. This response of thymocytes to antigen is the basis of negative selection and has been demonstrated clearly in experiments with transgenic mice bearing receptors of known specificity on all their T cells. For example, in mice transgenic for a T-cell receptor that recognizes a specific foreign peptide in association with self MHC molecules, injection of the peptide into the mouse results in apoptotic death of the thymocytes, while peripheral T cells are activated (Fig. 6.20).

In unmanipulated mice, developing T cells in the thymus will encounter a large selection of self peptides bound to self MHC molecules on thymic cells, and the developing cells with receptors specific for these self peptides will be deleted from the repertoire. The self peptides encountered by developing thymocytes are thought to be derived from proteins expressed in the thymus as well as from ubiquitous proteins that are brought to the thymus by the bloodstream. The deletion of T cells recognizing self peptides in the thymus can be demonstrated experimentally in mice made transgenic for rearranged genes encoding receptors that are specific for a cell-surface antigen expressed only in male mice. Thymocytes bearing these receptors disappear from the developing T-cell population in male mice at the CD4 CD8 double-positive stage of development, and no single-positive cells bearing anti-male antigen receptors mature in these mice. In female mice, by contrast, the cells mature normally. Similar experiments have been carried out with other kinds of antigens, with similar results.

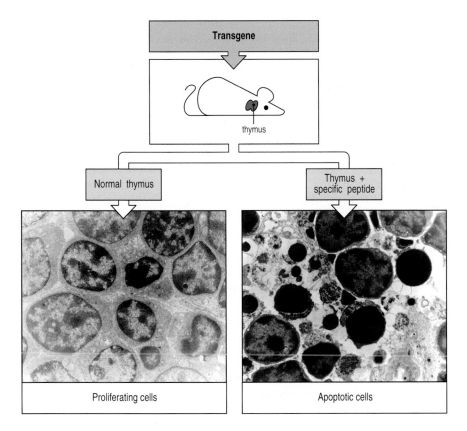

Fig. 6.20 T cells specific for self antigens are deleted in the thymus. In mice transgenic for a T-cell receptor that recognizes a known peptide antigen with self MHC, all of the T cells have the same specificity; in the absence of the peptide, their thymocytes mature (bottom left panel) and migrate to the periphery. When the mice are injected with the specific peptide antigen, immature T cells in the same animal (bottom right panel) undergo apoptosis and die. Photographs courtesy of K Murphy.

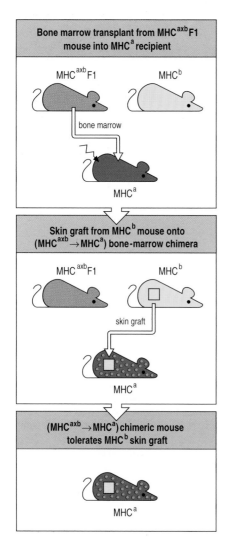

Bone marrow transplant from MHC^{axb}F1 mouse into MHC^a recipient

MHC^{axb}F1   MHC^b

bone marrow

MHC^a

Skin graft from MHC^b mouse onto (MHC^{axb}→MHC^a) bone-marrow chimera

MHC^{axb}F1   MHC^b

skin graft

MHC^a

(MHC^{axb}→MHC^a) chimeric mouse tolerates MHC^b skin graft

MHC^a

Fig. 6.21 Bone marrow derived cells mediate negative selection in the thymus. When MHC^{axb}F1 bone marrow is injected into an irradiated strain A mouse, the T cells mature on thymic epithelium expressing only type a MHC molecules (MHC^a). Nonetheless, the chimeric mice are tolerant to skin grafts expressing MHC^b molecules. This implies that the T cells whose receptors recognize antigens presented by MHC^b have been eliminated in the thymus. Since the transplanted MHC^{axb}F1 bone marrow cells are the only source of MHC^b molecules in the thymus, bone marrow derived cells must be able to induce negative selection.

Clonal deletion in the thymus cannot, however, eliminate T cells whose receptors recognize proteins found exclusively at other sites in the body and which are not presented in the thymus. Thus, proteins that are expressed only in other tissues or only at certain times in development, such as after puberty, cannot cause the deletion of potentially autoreactive thymocytes; immunological tolerance to such antigens is maintained by inactivation or deletion of T cells in the periphery rather than by their deletion before they mature. This mechanism will be discussed in the next chapter (see Section 7-10).

6-17 Negative selection is driven most efficiently by antigen-presenting cells.

Whereas thymic cortical epithelial cells mediate positive selection, negative selection in the thymus can be mediated by several different cell types. The most important of these are the bone marrow derived macrophages and dendritic cells. These are the professional antigen-presenting cells that also activate mature T cells in peripheral lymphoid tissues. The self antigens presented by these cells are, therefore, the most important source of potential autoimmune responses, and T cells responding to such self peptides must be eliminated in the thymus.

Bone marrow chimera experiments have clearly shown the role of thymic macrophages and dendritic cells in negative selection. Thus, if MHC^{axb}F1 bone marrow is grafted into the parental strains (MHC^a or MHC^b), T cells developing in the grafted animals will tolerate skin grafts from animals of both MHC^a and MHC^b strains (Fig. 6.21). This means they must have become tolerant not only to host MHC^a antigens but also to the donor-specific MHC^b antigens carried on cells derived from the grafted marrow. As the only cells that could present donor antigens are the bone marrow derived cells, these cell types are assumed to have a crucial role in negative selection.

It is interesting to note that in some mouse strain combinations, such skin grafts are rejected. This occurs because some proteins expressed in skin are not expressed by bone marrow derived cells, and hence the mouse is not tolerant to peptides derived from them. We shall see in Chapter 11 that responses to such **minor histocompatibility antigens** are important in human tissue transplantation. Although bone marrow derived cells are the principal mediators of negative selection, both thymocytes themselves and thymic epithelial cells also have the ability to cause the deletion of self-reactive cells. Such reactions may normally be of little significance. In patients undergoing bone marrow transplantation from an unrelated donor, however, where all the thymic macrophages and dendritic cells are of donor type, negative selection mediated by thymic epithelial cells may assume a special importance in maintaining tolerance to the recipient's own self tissue antigens.

6-18 Superantigens mediate negative selection of T-cell receptors derived from particular V$_\beta$ gene segments.

It is virtually impossible to demonstrate directly the negative selection of T cells specific for any particular self antigen in the normal thymus because such T cells will be too few to detect. There is, however, one case in which negative selection can be seen on a large scale in normal mice, and the point at which it occurs in T-cell development can be identified. In the most striking examples, T cells expressing receptors encoded by particular V$_\beta$ gene segments are virtually eliminated in the affected mouse strains. This occurs as the consequence of the interaction of immature thymocytes with endogenous superantigens present in those strains. We learned in Chapter 4 that superantigens are viral or bacterial proteins that bind tightly to both MHC class II molecules and particular V_β domains, irrespective of the antigen specificity of the receptor and the peptide bound by the MHC molecule (see Fig. 4-33).

The endogenous superantigens of mice are encoded by mouse mammary tumor virus genomes that have become inserted into the mouse chromosomes, where they are inherited by successive generations of mice along with mouse genes. Like the bacterial superantigens, these viral antigens induce strong T-cell responses; indeed, they were originally designated **minor lymphocyte stimulating (Mls)** antigens because, although they are not MHC proteins (hence minor), they stimulate exceptionally strong primary T-cell responses when T cells from a strain lacking the superantigen gene are stimulated by B cells from MHC-identical mice that do express it.

T-cell receptors containing V_β regions to which the Mls proteins bind are signaled during intrathymic maturation in Mls$^+$ strains, causing apoptosis and thus elimination of such T cells. For example, one variant of the Mls antigen (Mls-1^a) deletes all thymocytes expressing the $V_\beta6$ variable region (and also those expressing $V_\beta8.1$ and $V_\beta9$), whereas such cells are not deleted in mice that lack Mls-1^a. Thus, the expression of endogenous superantigens in mice has a profound impact on the repertoire of T-cell receptors. This sort of deletion has not yet been seen in any other species, including humans, despite the presence of retroviral sequences in the genomes of many mammals.

Cells expressing superantigen-responsive receptors are found among double-positive thymocytes, and are abundant in thymic cortex but absent from the thymic medulla and the periphery in mice that express the superantigen and are tolerant to it. This suggests that superantigens may delete relatively mature cells as they migrate out of the cortex into the medulla, where a particularly dense network of dendritic cells marks the corticomedullary junction (Fig. 6.22).

Although clonal deletion by superantigens is a powerful tool for examining negative selection in normal mice, it must be remembered that superantigen-driven clonal deletion may not be representative of clonal deletion by self peptide:self MHC complexes. What is clear is that clonal deletion by either superantigens or self peptide:self MHC complexes generates a repertoire of T cells that does not respond to the self-antigens expressed by its own professional antigen-presenting cells.

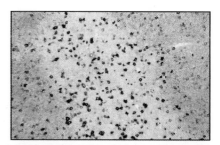

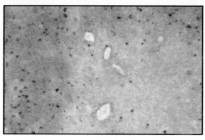

Fig. 6.22   Clonal deletion by Mls-1^a occurs late in the development of thymocytes. T cells with Mls-1^a responsive receptors encoded by $V_\beta6$ are seen in both the cortex and medulla of Mls-1^b mice (left panel, cells stained with anti-$V_\beta6$ antibody). Note that the mature cells in the medulla express higher levels of the receptor and thus stain more darkly than the immature cells in the cortex. In Mls-1^a mice, the mature cells are not found; instead only the immature, cortical cells express the $V_\beta6$ receptor (right panel). Photographs courtesy of H Hengartner.

6-19   The signals for negative and positive selection must differ.

In the preceding sections we have described some of the experiments that have contributed to the large body of evidence that T cells are selected both for self MHC restriction and for self tolerance by MHC molecules expressed on cells in the thymus. We now turn to the central question posed by positive and negative selection: how can the same receptor, interacting with the same thymic MHC:peptide complexes, lead both to further maturation during positive selection, and to cell death during negative selection?

There are two issues to be resolved. First, the interaction of the T-cell receptor with self MHC:peptide complexes that leads to positive selection must differ from that for negative selection. Were this not so, all the cells that are positively selected in the thymic cortex would subsequently be eliminated by negative selection, and no T cells would ever leave the thymus (Fig. 6.23). Second, the consequences of the interaction must differ, so that the cells that recognize self MHC on cortical

Fig. 6.23 The specificity or affinity of positive selection must differ from that of negative selection. Immature T cells are positively selected to remove those thymocytes whose receptors are not capable of recognizing self MHC molecules, giving rise to a self-restricted population of thymocytes. Negative selection removes those T cells whose receptors recognize the complex of self MHC molecules with self peptides to give a self-tolerant population of thymocytes. If the specificity of positive and negative selection is the same (left column), then all the T cells that survive positive selection will be deleted during negative selection. Only if the specificity or affinity of negative selection is different from that of positive selection (right column) can thymocytes mature into T cells.

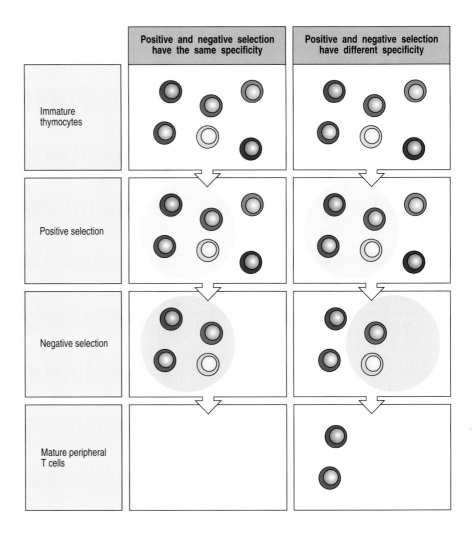

epithelial cells mature, whereas those whose receptors might confer autoreactivity are negatively selected and die.

Two main hypotheses have been proposed to account for these differences between positive and negative selection. The first is the **avidity hypothesis**, which states that the outcome of MHC:peptide binding by T-cell receptors of thymocytes depends upon the strength of the signal delivered by the receptor on binding, and that this will in turn depend upon both the affinity of the T-cell receptor for the MHC:peptide complex and the density of the complex on the antigen-presenting cell (usually a thymic cortical epithelial cell). Thymocytes that are signaled weakly are rescued from programmed cell death and therefore positively selected, whereas thymocytes that are signaled strongly are driven to programmed cell death and therefore negatively selected.

Alternatively, self peptides that deliver incomplete activating signals could account for positive selection: we shall call this the **differential signaling hypothesis.** Under this hypothesis, it is the nature of the signal delivered by the receptor, rather than the number of receptors engaged, that distinguishes positive from negative selection. Thus, the avidity hypothesis would predict that the same signaling complex could drive positive or negative selection depending on its density on the cell surface, whereas the differential signaling hypothesis would predict that different complexes drive positive and negative selection.

A new approach to testing these hypotheses has opened up with the recent description of antagonist peptides. Antagonist peptides, which we discussed in Chapter 4 (see section 4-29), are variants of the peptide component of an MHC:peptide complex that, when substituted for the original peptide, bind the T-cell receptor and block the response of the T cell to the original MHC:peptide complex. Some peptide variants which act as antagonists may deliver a partial signal to the T cell that produces a subset of the full response (for example, proliferation or cytokine secretion but not both). Since positive selection is thought to entail the delivery of a weak signal to developing thymocytes, it seemed possible that antagonist peptides that deliver partial signals might reflect the same mechanism that operates in positive selection. Using thymic lobe cultures from mice transgenic for a known T-cell receptor, it has been possible to test the effect of antagonist peptides on thymic selection of developing T cells bearing receptors recognizing a specific MHC:peptide complex.

The cultured thymic lobes used for the experiments were taken from so-called knock-out mice (see section 2-38), genetically engineered to lack either β_2-microglobulin or the TAP transporter, and therefore unable to express MHC class I molecules on the cell surface. Expression of class I MHC can be restored to such thymic tissue by the addition either of an appropriate peptide, or of peptide with β_2-microglobulin in the case of mice deficient in β_2-microglobulin. In this way it is possible to generate a thymic environment in which only one MHC class I:peptide complex is displayed.

Using this system, developing thymocytes of known specificity have been tested for their response to four types of MHC:peptide complex. In each case the MHC molecule was the self MHC molecule that presents peptide to the T-cell receptor being tested. If the added peptides were unrelated to the peptide recognized by the cells, the thymocytes died because they failed positive selection. If the added peptides were identical to the peptide recognized by the cells, the thymocytes died because they were negatively selected. If, however, they were antagonist or partial agonist variants of the peptide for which the cells were specific, the thymocytes were positively selected and survived (Fig. 6.24).

In some experiments, attempts have been made directly to test the avidity hypothesis by varying the dose of agonist or partial agonist peptides and

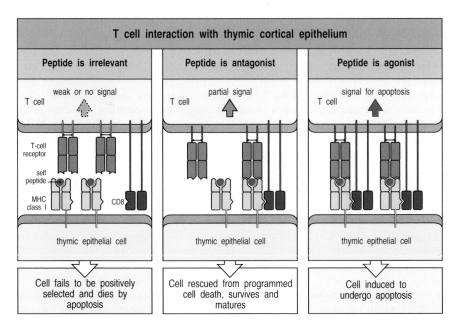

Fig. 6.24 **Effects of peptides acting as agonists, antagonists or neither on thymic selection.** Thymocytes encounter self MHC:self peptide complexes that have different effects depending upon the specificity of the T-cell receptor. For some receptors, no self peptide bound to self MHC molecules will signal at all (left panel), and cells with these receptors undergo programmed cell (death by neglect). For other receptors, a self peptide bound by self MHC acts as an agonist, triggering programmed cell death (right panel) (death as a result of activation). Some cells, however, bear receptors that are partially signaled by self peptides bound to self MHC molecules. These peptides are equivalent to antagonist peptides and rescue the cells from programmed cell death, leading to positive selection.

showing that at high doses of peptide the cells died, whereas at lower doses they could survive. However it is not clear that the surviving cells in these experiments are functional: in some experiments aimed at addressing this question it has been shown that although the cells may appear to mature, they express a low level of CD8 and cannot respond to complexes containing the peptide for which the receptor is normally specific.

Antagonist or partial agonist peptides, as we saw in Chapter 4, seem to be unable to deliver a full activating signal to T cells. These experiments therefore imply that in a normal animal, thymocytes may be positively selected by an MHC:peptide complex that delivers only a partial activating signal, but negatively selected by one that delivers a full activating signal. Whether the strength of the signal is determined by the avidity of binding, as predicted by the avidity hypothesis, or by some special characteristic of the peptide, as predicted by the differential signaling hypothesis, remains to be determined.

Finally, it is known that the level of signal required for negative selection in the thymus is lower than that required for activation in the periphery. This is likely to be important in preventing the autoreactivity that would otherwise be a risk if a peptide or MHC molecule is overexpressed in peripheral tissues.

6-20 The requirements of T-cell activation and of thymic selection may explain why the MHC is highly polymorphic and not highly polygenic.

As we saw in Chapter 4, the MHC locus is highly polymorphic, with hundreds of different allelic variants within the human population. There are several different genes for each class of MHC molecule (each of which is highly polymorphic), and so the MHC is also somewhat polygenic. All these allelic and non-allelic MHC variants preferentially bind different antigenic peptides. The polymorphism and polygenism of the MHC is believed to reflect both the selective advantage to the species of individuals able to bind different sets of peptides, and the selective advantage to each individual of expressing several variants able to bind peptides from a broad range of pathogens.

From the individual's point of view, it would seem that the greater the number of different MHC genes — the greater the polygeny at the locus — the better the protection from infectious organisms. However, an obvious disadvantage of polygeny arises from the need for some minimum number of identical MHC:peptide complexes on the surface of any given cell if it is to be able to successfully stimulate a T cell. This minimum has been estimated at approximately 100 copies. But the greater the number of different MHC molecules expressed by a cell, the fewer the copies of each different MHC molecule that can be expressed, and hence, the fewer the copies of each unique peptide:MHC complex. In the extreme case, a cell expressing a large number of different MHC molecules would not display sufficient numbers of one specific peptide:MHC complex to be able to stimulate any T cells.

A consideration of the constraints of thymic selection also suggests why polymorphism in a limited number of genes may be preferable to the expression in one individual of a large number of different genes. It seems likely that around 5% of T cells can recognize self peptides presented by a given MHC molecule and must be deleted in the thymus to avoid reactivity to self. (This estimate is based on the frequency of T cells that respond to a given non-self MHC molecule: see Section 4-18.) Thus, each new MHC molecule expressed will cost the animal 5% of its T-cell receptor repertoire. A normal human expresses up to 15 different MHC molecules, and thus may delete a substantial portion (up to 75%) of the positively selected T cells that develop. This effect will be partly counterbalanced by the advantage of gaining new MHC molecules that can drive positive selection, but it seems unlikely that the individual will improve his or her ability to respond by adding MHC genes.

Thus, both because of the requirements of T-cell activation and for reasons of selection, it seems that polymorphism rather than polygenism provides the greater adaptive advantage.

6-21 A range of tumors of immune system cells throws light on different stages of T-cell development.

We saw in Chapter 5 that tumors of lymphoid cells corresponding in phenotype to intermediate stages in the development of the B cell can provide an invaluable tool in the analysis of B-cell differentiation. Tumors of T cells and other cells involved in T-cell development have been identified but, unlike the malignancies of B cells, few that correspond to intermediate stages in T-cell development have been identified in humans. Instead, the tumors resemble either mature T cells or, in the case of common acute lymphoblastic leukemia, the earliest type of lymphoid progenitor (Fig. 6.25). One possible reason for the rarity of tumors corresponding to intermediate stages is that immature T cells are programmed to die unless rescued within a very narrow time window by positive selection (see Section 6-11). It may therefore be that thymocytes simply do not linger long enough at the intermediate stages of their development to provide an opportunity for malignant transformation. Thus, only cells that are already transformed at earlier stages, or that do not become transformed until the T cell has matured, are ever seen as tumors.

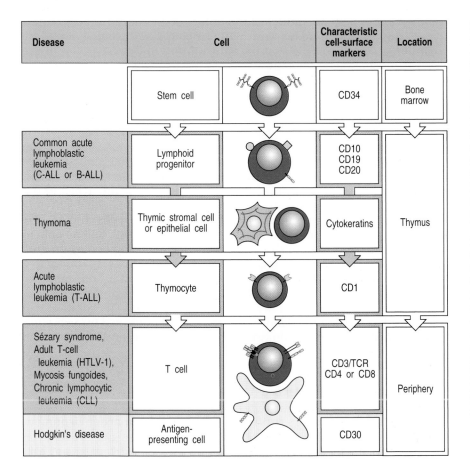

Disease	Cell			Characteristic cell-surface markers	Location
	Stem cell			CD34	Bone marrow
Common acute lymphoblastic leukemia (C-ALL or B-ALL)	Lymphoid progenitor			CD10 CD19 CD20	
Thymoma	Thymic stromal cell or epithelial cell			Cytokeratins	Thymus
Acute lymphoblastic leukemia (T-ALL)	Thymocyte			CD1	
Sézary syndrome, Adult T-cell leukemia (HTLV-1), Mycosis fungoides, Chronic lymphocytic leukemia (CLL)	T cell			CD3/TCR CD4 or CD8	Periphery
Hodgkin's disease	Antigen-presenting cell			CD30	

Fig. 6.25 T-cell tumors represent monoclonal outgrowths of normal cell populations. Each distinct T-cell tumor has a normal equivalent, as also seen with B cells, and retains many of the properties of the cell from which it develops. Some of these tumors represent massive outgrowth of a rare cell type with, for example, common acute lymphoblastic leukemia being derived from the lymphoid progenitor cell. Thus, T-cell tumors provide valuable information about the phenotype, homing properties and receptor gene rearrangements of normal cell types. Two T-cell related tumors are also included. Thymomas derive from thymic stromal or epithelial cells, while the malignantly transformed cell in Hodgkin's disease is thought to be an antigen-presenting cell. Some characteristic cell-surface markers for each stage are also shown. For example, CD10 (common acute lymphoblastic leukemia antigen or CALLA) is a widely-used marker for acute lymphoblastic leukemia. Note that T-cell chronic lymphocytic leukemia (CLL) cells express CD8, while the other T-cell tumors mentioned express CD4.

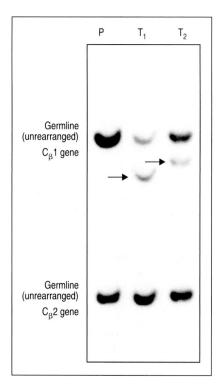

Fig. 6.26   The unique rearrangement in each T cell can identify tumors of T cells. Tumors are the outgrowth of a single transformed cell. Thus, each cell in a tumor will have an identical pattern of rearranged T-cell receptor genes. The gels show DNA fragments probed with the T-cell receptor β chain constant regions. P, DNA from the placenta, a tissue in which the T-cell receptor genes are not rearranged. T_1 and T_2, DNA from peripheral blood lymphocytes from two patients suffering from T-cell tumors. Bands corresponding to the unrearranged $C_\beta 1$ and $C_\beta 2$ genes can be seen in all lanes. Additional bands corresponding to specific rearrangements can be seen in each of the tumor samples. Photograph courtesy of T Diss.

An understanding of the normal development of the immature T cell may help in understanding the pathology of the tumors that arise from such cells. For example, cutaneous T cell lymphomas, which home to the skin and proliferate slowly, are clonal outgrowths of a CD4 T cell that, when activated, homes to the skin. The most complex lymphoid tumor is known as Hodgkin's disease, and appears in several forms. The malignantly transformed cell seems to be an antigen-presenting cell, so that in some patients the disease is dominated by T cells that are stimulated by the tumor cells. This form of the disease is called Hodgkin's lymphoma. Other patients have no lymphocytic abnormalities and show a proliferation of a reticular cell, a condition known as nodular sclerosis. The differences between these two manifestations of Hodgkin's disease may reflect a real heterogeneity in the transformed cell or, more probably, differences in the T-cell responses of individual patients to the transformed cells. The prognosis of Hodgkin's lymphoma is far better than that of nodular sclerosis, suggesting that the responding cells may be controlling tumor growth. Control of tumors by T cells will be considered in Chapter 12.

As with B-cell tumors, T-cell lymphomas can be shown to be monoclonal outgrowths of a single transformed cell by examination of the rearrangements of their receptor genes (Fig. 6.26). When tissues or cells from patients are examined, the proportion of cells showing the same rearrangements is a measure of the proportion of transformed cells in the sample. The sensitivity of this approach can be increased by using the polymerase chain reaction (see Section 2-27) to identify the tumor-specific rearrangement, allowing the identification of very small numbers of tumor cells remaining in a tissue. This can be of particular importance in cases where a patient's own bone marrow has been taken for re-injection after radiotherapy. If the marrow contains any transformed cells, then returning the marrow would re-transplant the tumor into the patient and defeat the object of the therapy. Techniques exist to deplete the bone marrow of tumor cells and the efficiency of the treatments can be monitored by determining the persistence of the tumor-specific rearrangement.

Summary

T-cell development involves two types of selection: positive selection for recognition of self MHC:self peptide complexes that provide a still ill-defined positive survival signal, and negative selection for recognition of self peptide:self MHC complexes that would trigger the T cell in the periphery. The first process is normally mediated exclusively by thymic epithelial cells and the second largely by dendritic cells and macrophages. Positive selection ensures that all mature T cells will be able to respond to foreign peptides presented by self MHC molecules on antigen-presenting cells, and negative selection eliminates self-reactive cells. The paradox that recognition of the same ligand by the same receptor leads to two conflicting effects, namely positive and negative selection, is one of the central mysteries of immunology. Its solution will rest in understanding the ligands, the receptors, the signal transduction mechanisms and the physiology of each step of the process.

Summary to Chapter 6.

T-cell development occurs in the special inductive microenvironment of the thymic cortex. In this location, T-cell receptor gene rearrangement is induced separately for the two lineages of T cells, γ:δ and α:β.

This specialized environment also selects for those α:β T cells having useful receptors, by contact of the receptor and its co-receptor with self MHC molecules on thymic cortical epithelial cells. Also within the thymus, professional antigen-presenting cells from the bone marrow delete all T cells whose receptors recognize antigens normally expressed by these cells, thus assuring self tolerance. In this way, a useful and non-damaging repertoire of T-cell receptors is generated.

General references.

Adkins, B., Mueller, C., Okada, C.Y., Reichert, R.A., Weissman, I.L., and Spangrude, G.J.: **Early events in T-cell maturation.** *Ann. Rev. Immunol.* 1987, **5**:325.

Fowlkes, B.J., and Pardoll, D.M.: **Molecular and cellular events of T cell development.** *Adv. Immunol.* 1989, **44**:207-264.

Kruisbeek, A.M.: **Development of αβ T cells.** *Curr. Opin. Immunol.* 1993, **5**:227-234.

Möller, G (ed).: **Positive T-cell selection in the thymus.** *Immunol. Rev.* 1993, **135**:5-242.

von Boehmer, H.: **Developmental biology of T cells in T-cell receptor transgenic mice.** *Ann. Rev. Immunol.* 1990, **8**:531-556.

von Boehmer, H.: **The developmental biology of T lymphocytes.** *Ann. Rev. Immunol.* 1993, **6**:309-326.

von Boehmer, H., and Kisielow, P.: **Lymphocyte lineage commitment: instruction versus selection.** *Cell* 1993, **73**:207-208.

von Boehmer, H.: **Thymic selection: a matter of life and death.** *Immunol. Today* 1992, **13**:742-744.

Zinkernagel, R.M. and Doherty, P.: **MHC-restricted cytotoxic T cells: Studies on the biological role of polymorphic major transplantation antigens determining T-cell restriction-specificity, function, and responsiveness.** Adv. *Immunol* 1979, **27**:51.

Section references.

| 6-1 | T cells develop in the thymus. |

Cordier, A.C., and Haumont, S.M.: **Development of thymus, parathyroids, and ultimobranchial bodies in NMRI and nude mice.** *Am. J. Anat.* 1980, **157**:227.

Owen, J.T., and Jenkinson, E.J.: **Embryology of the immune system.** *Prog. Allergy* 1981, **29**:1-34.

van Ewijk, W.: **T-cell differentiation is influenced by thymic microenvironments.** *Annu. Rev. Immunol.* 1991, **9**:591-615.

von Gaudecker, B.: **Functional histology of the human thymus.** *Anat. Embryol.* 1991, **183**:1-15.

| 6-2 | The thymus is required for T-cell maturation. |

Fulop, G.M., and Phillips, R.A.: **Use of SCID mice to identify and quantitate lymphoid-restricted stem cells in long-term bone marrow cultures.** *Blood* 1989, **74**:1537-1544.

Hong, R.: **The DiGeorge anomaly.** *Immunodef. Rev.* 1991, **3**:1-14.

Pritchard, H., and Micklem, H.S.: **Haemopoeitic stem cells and progenitors of functional T lymphocytes in the bone marrow of nude mice.** *Clin. Exper. Immunol.* 1973, **14**:597.

| 6-3 | Developing T cells proliferate in the thymus but most die there. |

Shortman, K., Egerton, M., Spangrude, G.J., and Scollay, R.: **The generation and fate of thymocytes.** *Semin. Immunol.* 1990, **2**:3-12.

| 6-4 | Successive stages in the development of thymocytes are marked by changes in cell-surface molecules. |

Crispe, I.N., Shimonkevitz, R.P., Husmann, L.A., Kimura, J., and Allison, J.P.: **Expression of T-cell antigen receptor β chains on subsets of mouse thymocytes. Analysis by three-color flow cytometry.** *J. Immunol.* 1987, **139**:3585-3589.

Crispe, I.N., Moore, M.W., Husmann, L.A., Smith, L., Bevan, M.J., and Shimonkevitz, R.P.: **Differentiation potential of subsets of CD4-8-thymocytes.** *Nature* 1987, **329**:6137.

Petrie, H.T., Hugo, P., Scollay, R., and Shortman, K.: **Lineage relationships and developmental kinetics of immature thymocytes: CD3, CD4, and CD8 acquisition** *in vivo* **and** *in vitro*. *J. Exper. Med.* 1990, **172**:1583-1588.

Scollay, R.: **T-cell subsets in thymocyte development.** *Curr. Opin. Immunol.* 1991, **3**:204-209.

| 6-5 | Thymocytes at different developmental stages are found in distinct parts of the thymus. |

Picker, L.J., and Siegelman, M.H.: **Lymphoid Tissues and Organs.** *In: Fundamental Immunology,* 1993, 3rd edn. Raven Press Ltd., New York, (Paul, W.E., Ed.), pp 152-161.

| 6-6 | T cells with α:β or γ:δ receptors arise from a common progenitor. |

Lauzurica, P., and Krangel, M.S.: **Temporal and lineage-specific control of T-cell receptor α/δ gene rearrangement by T-cell receptor α and δ enhancers.** *J. Exp. Med.* 1994, **179**:193-1921.

Livak, F., Petrie, H.T., Crispe, I.N., and Schatz, D.G.: **In-frame TCR δ gene rearrangements play a critical role in the αβ/γδ T cell lineage decision.** *Immunity* 1995, **2**: In press

Raulet, D.H., Spencer, D.M., Hsiang, Y.-H., *et al.*: **Control of γδ T-cell development.** *Immunol. Rev.* 1991, **120**:185-204.

| 6-7 | Cells expressing particular γ:δ genes arise first in embryonic development. |

Haas, W., and Tonegawa, S.: **Development and selection of γδ T cells.** *Curr. Opin. Immunol.* 1992, **4**:147-155.

Itohara, S., Nakanishi, N., Kanagawa, O., Kubo, R., and Tonegawa, S.: **Monoclonal antibodies specific to native murine T cell receptor γδ analysis of** γδ T cells in thymic ontogeny and peripheral lymphoid organs. *Proc. Natl. Acad. Sci. USA* 1989, **86**:5094-5098.

| 6-8 | Productive β-chain gene rearrangement triggers α-chain gene rearrangement. |

Dudley, E.C., Petrie, H.T., Shah, L.M., Owen, M.J., and Hayday, A.C.: **T-cell receptor β chain gene rearrangement and selection during thymocyte development in adult mice.** *Immunity,* 1994, **1**:83-93.

Mombaerts, P., Clarke, R., Rudnicki, M.A., Iacomini, J., Itohara, S., Lafaille, J.J., Ichikawa, Y., Jaenisch, R., Hooper, M.I., and Tonegawa, S.: **Mutations in T cell antigen receptor genes α and β block thymocyte development at different stages.** *Nature* 1992, **360**:255-258.

Molina, T.J., Kishihara, K., Siderovski, D.P., Van Ewijk, W., Narendran, A., Timms, A., Wakeham, A., Paige, C.J., Hartmann, K.-U., Veillette, A., Davidson, D., and Mak, T.W.: **Profound block in thymocyte development in mice lacking p56^{lck}.** *Nature* 1992, **357**:161-164.

Philpott, K.I., Viney, J.L., Kay, G., Rastan, S., Gardiner, E.M., Chae, S., Hayday, A.C., and Owen, M.J.: **Lymphoid development in mice congenitally lacking T cell receptor α β-expressing cells.** *Science* 1992, **256**:1448-1453.

Saint-Ruf, C., Ungewiss, K., Groetrrup, M., Bruno, L., Fehling, H.J., and von Boehmer, H.: **Analysis and expression of a cloned pre-T-cell receptor gene.** *Science* 1994, **266**:1208.

| 6-9 | T-cell receptor α- chain genes can undergo several successive rearrangements. |

Padovan, E., Casorati, G., Dellabona, P., Meyer, S., Brockhaus, M., and Lanzavecchia, A.: **Expression of two T-cell receptor α chains: Dual receptor T cells.** *Science* 1993 **262**:422-424.

Hardardottir, F., Baron, J.L., and Janeway, C.A. Jr.: **T cells with two functional antigen-specific receptors.** *Proc. Natl. Acad Sci.* 1995, **92**:354-358.

Petrie, H.T., Livak, F., Schatz, D.G., Strasser, A., Crispe, I.N., and Shortman, K.: **Multiple rearrangements in T-cell receptor α-chain genes maximize the production of useful thymocytes.** *J. Exp. Med.* 1993, **178**:615-622.

| 6-10 | Only T cells specific for peptides bound to self MHC molecules mature in the thymus. |

Fink, P.J., and Bevan, M.J.: **H-2 antigens of the thymus determine lymphocyte specificity.** *J. Exper. Med.* 1978, **148**:766-775.

Sprent, J., Lo. D., Gao, E.-K., and Ron, Y.: **T-cell selection in the thymus.** *Immunol. Rev.* 1989, **10**:57-61.

Zinkernagel, R.M., Callahan, G.N., Klein, J., and Dennert, G.: **Cytotoxic T cells learn specificity for self H-2 during differentiation in the thymus.** *Nature* 1978, **271**:251-253.

| 6-11 | Cells that fail positive selection die in the thymus. |

Huessman, M., Scott, B., Kisielow, P., and von Boehmer, H.: **Kinetics and efficacy of positive selection in the thymus of normal and T-cell receptor transgenic mice.** *Cell* 1991, **66**:533-562.

Shortman, K., Vremec, D., and Egerton, M.: **The kinetics of T-cell antigen receptor expression by subgroups of CD4$^+$8$^+$3^{2+} thymocytes as post-selection intermediates leading to mature T cells.** *J. Exper. Med.* 1991, **173**:323-332.

Teh, H.S., Kisielow, P., Scott, B., Kishi, H., Uematsu, Y., Bluthmann, H., and von Boehmer, H.: **Thymic major histocompatibility complex antigens and the αβ T-cell receptor determine the CD4/CD8 phenotype of cells.** *Nature* 1988, **335**:6187.

| 6-12 | Positive selection also regulates α-chain gene rearrangement. |

Borgulya, P., Kishi, H., Uematsu, Y., and von Boehmer, H.: **Exclusion and inclusion of α and β T-cell receptor alleles.** *Cell* 1992, **65**:529-537.

Malissen, M., Trucy, J., Jouvin-Marche, E., Cazenave, P.A., Scollay, R., and Malissen, B.: **Regulation of TCR α and β chain gene allelic exclusion during T-cell development.** *Immunol. Today* 1992, **13**:315-322.

| 6-13 | The expression of CD4 and CD8 on mature cells is determined by positive selection. |

Kaye, J., Hsu, M.L., Sauvon, M.E., Jameson, S.C., Gascoigne, N.R.J., and Hedrick, S.M.: **Selective development of CD4$^+$ T cells in transgenic mice expressing a class II MHC-restricted antigen receptor.** *Nature* 1989, **341**:746-748.

von Boehmer, H., Kisielow, P., Lishi, H., Scott, B., Borgulya, P., and Teh, H.S.: **The expression of CD4 and CD8 accessory molecules on mature T cells is not random but correlates with the specificity of the αβ receptor for antigen.** *Immunol. Rev.* 1989, **109**:143-151.

| 6-14 | Thymic cortical epithelial cells mediate positive selection. |

Cosgrove, D., Chan, S.H., Waltzinger, C., Benoist, C., and Mathis, D.: **The thymic compartment responsible for positive selection of CD4$^+$ T cells.** *Intl. Immunol.* 1992, **4**:707-710.

| 6-15 | Co-receptor selection occurs in two stages. |

Chan, S.H., Benoist, C., and Mathis, D.: **A challenge to the instructive model of positive selection.** *Immunol. Rev.* 1993, **135**:119-131.

Chan, S.H., Cosgrove, D., Waltzinger, C., Benoist, C., and Mathis, D.: **Another view of the selective model of thymocyte selection.** *Cell* 1993, **73**:225-236.

Davis, C.B., Killeen, N., Casey Crooks, M.E., Raulet, D., and Littman, D.R.: **Evidence for a stochastic mechanism in the differentiation of mature subsets of T lymphocytes.** *Cell* 1993, **73**:237-247.

Suzuki, H., Punt, J.A., Granger, L.G., and Singer, A.: **Asymmetric signaling requirements for thymocyte commitment to the CD4$^+$ versus CD8$^+$ T cell lineages: A new perspective on thymic commitment and selection.** *Immunity* 1995, **2**:413-524.

Lundberg, K., Heath, W., Kontgen, F., Carbone, F.R., and Shortman, K.: **Intermediate steps in positive selection: Differentiation of CD4$^+$8^{int}TCR^{int} thymocytes into CD4$^-$8$^+$TCR^{hi} thymocytes.** *J. Exp. Med.* 1995, **181**:1643-1651.

| 6-16 | T cells specific for self antigens are deleted in the thymus. |

Surh, C.D. and Sprent, J.: **T-cell apoptosis detected *in situ* during positive and negative selection in the thymus.** *Nature* 1994, **372**:100-103.

Zal, T., Volkmann, A., and Stockinger, B.: **Mechanisms of tolerance induction in major histocompatibility complex class II-restricted T cell specific for a blood-borne self antigen.** *J. Exp. Med.* 1994, **180**:2089-2099.

| 6-17 | Negative selection is driven most efficiently by antigen-presenting cells. |

Sprent, J., and Webb, S.R.: **Intrathymic and extrathymic clonal deletion of T cells.** *Curr. Op. Immunol.* 1995, **7**:196-205.

Matzinger, P., and Guerder, S.:**Does T cell tolerance require a dedicated antigen-presenting cell?** *Nature.* 1989. **338**:74-76.

6-18 Superantigens mediate negative selection of T-cell receptors derived from particular Vβ gene segments.

Kappler, J.W., Roehm, N., and Marrack, P.: **T-cell tolerance by clonal elimination in the thymus.** *Cell* 1987, **49**:273-280.

MacDonald, H.R., Schneider, R., Lees, R.K., Howe, R.C., Acha-Orbea, H., Festenstein, H., Zinkernagel, R.M., and Hengartner, H.: **T-cell receptor Vβ use predicts reactivity and tolerance to Mls[a]-encoded antigens.** *Nature* 1988, **332**:40-45.

6-19 The signals for negative and positive selection must differ.

Ashton-Rickardt, P.G., Van Kaer, L., Schumacher, T.N.M., Ploegh, H.L., and Tonegawa, S.: **Peptide contributes to the specificity of positive selection of CD8+ T cells in the thymus.** *Cell* 1993, **73**:1041-1049.

Ashton-Rickardt, P.G., Bandeira, A., Delaney, J.R., Van Kaer, L., Pircher, H.P., Zinkernagel, R.M., and Tonegawa, S.: **Evidence for a differential avidity model of T-cell selection in the thymus.** *Cell* 1994.

Elliott, J.I.: **Thymic selection reinterpreted.** *Immunol. Rev.* 1993, **135**:227-242.

Hogquist, K.A., Gavin, M.A., Bevan, M.J.: **Positive selection of CD8[+] T cells induced by major histocompatibility complex binding peptides in fetal thymus organ culture.** *J. Exper. Med.* 1993, **177**:1464-1473.

Hogquist, K.A., Jameson, S.C., Heath, W.R., Howard, J.L., Bevan, M.J., and Carbane, F.R.: **T-cell receptor antagonist peptides induce positive selection.** *Cell* 1994, **76**:17-27.

Janeway, C.A.Jr.: **Ligands for the T-cell receptor: hard times for avidity models.** *Immunol. Today.* 1995, **16**:223-225.

Jameson, S.C., Hogquist, K.A., and Bevan, M.J:**Specificity and flexibility in thymic selection.** *Nature.* 1994, **369**:750-753.

Fowlkes, B.J. and Schweighoffer, E.: **Positive selection of T cells.** *Curr. Op. Immunol.* 1995, **7**:188-195.

6-20 The requirements of T cell activation and of thymic selection may explain why the MHC is highly polymorphic and not highly polygenic.

Calitutti, S., Muller, S., Cella, M., Padovan, E., and Lanzavecchia, A.: **Serial triggering of many T-cell receptors by a few peptide-MHC complexes.** *Nature.* 1995, **375**:148-151.

Harding, C.V., and Unanue, E.R.: **Quantitation of antigen-presenting cell MHC class II/peptide complexes necessary for T cell stimulation.** *Nature* 1990, **346**:574-576.

Demotz, S., Grey, H.M., and Sette, A.: **The minimal number of class II MHC-antigen complexes needed for T cell activation.** *Science* 1990, **249**:1028-1030.

6-21 A range of tumors of immune system cells throws light on different stages of T-cell development.

Rabbitts, T.H.: **Chromosomal translocations in human cancer.** *Nature* 1994, **372**:143-149.

PART IV

THE ADAPTIVE IMMUNE RESPONSE

T-Cell Mediated Immunity

Once they have completed their development in the thymus, T cells enter the bloodstream, from which they migrate through the peripheral lymphoid organs, returning to the bloodstream to recirculate until they encounter antigen. To participate in an adaptive immune response, these **naive T cells** must be induced to proliferate and differentiate into cells capable of contributing to the removal of pathogens; we shall term these **armed effector T cells** because they can act immediately or very rapidly after encountering MHC:peptide complexes on other cells. Effector T cells, as we learned in Chapter 4, fall into three functional classes that detect antigens derived from different types of pathogens presented by the two different classes of MHC molecule. Antigens derived from pathogens that multiply within the cell are carried to the cell surface by MHC class I molecules and presented to CD8 **cytotoxic T cells** that kill the infected cell; antigens derived from pathogens multiplying in intracellular vesicles, and those derived from ingested extracellular bacteria and toxins, are carried to the cell surface by MHC class II molecules and presented to CD4 T cells that can differentiate into two types of effector T cell: **inflammatory T cells (T$_H$1)** that activate infected macrophages to destroy intracellular pathogens; and **helper T cells (T$_H$2)** that activate specific B cells to produce antibody (Fig. 7.1). The cells on which armed effector T cells act will be referred to as **target cells**.

In this chapter, we shall see how naive T cells are activated to proliferate and differentiate into armed effector cells the first time they encounter their specific antigen on the surface of a **professional antigen-presenting cell (APC)**. These specialized antigen-presenting cells are distinguished by surface molecules that synergize with specific antigen in the activation of naive T cells. Professional antigen-presenting cells are concentrated in the peripheral lymphoid organs, where they trap antigen and present its peptide fragments to recirculating T cells. The most important professional antigen-presenting cells are the highly specialized **dendritic cells**, whose only known function is to present antigen, and **macrophages**, which are also important as phagocytic cells in providing a first line of defense against infection and as targets for

Fig. 7.1   The role of effector T cells in cell-mediated and humoral immunity to representative pathogens. Cell-mediated immunity involves the destruction of infected cells by cytotoxic T cells, or the destruction of intracellular pathogens by macrophages activated by inflammatory (T$_H$1) CD4 T cells, and is directed principally at intracellular parasites. Humoral immunity depends upon the production of antibody by B cells activated by helper (T$_H$2) CD4 T cells, and is directed principally at extracellular pathogens. Note, however, that both cell-mediated and humoral immunity play a role in many infections, such as the response to *Pneumocystis carinii*, which requires antibody for ingestion by phagocytes and macrophage activation for effective destruction of the ingested pathogen.

	Cell-mediated immunity		Humoral immunity
Typical pathogens	Vaccinia virus Influenza virus Rabies virus *Listeria* *Toxoplasma gondii*	*Mycobacterium tuberculosis* *Mycobacterium leprae* *Leishmania donovani* *Pneumocystis carinii*	*Clostridium tetani* *Staphylococcus aureus* *Streptococcus pneumoniae* *Polio virus* *Pneumocystis carinii*
Location	Cytosol	Macrophage vesicles	Extracellular fluid
Effector T cell	Cytotoxic CD8 T cell	T$_H$1 inflammatory CD4 T cell	T$_H$2 helper CD4 T cell
Antigen recognition	Peptide:MHC class I on infected cell	Peptide:MHC class II on infected macrophage	Peptide:MHC class II on specific B cell
Effector action	Killing of infected cell	Activation of infected macrophages	Activation of specific B cell to make antibody

activation by armed effector T cells. B cells can also serve as professional antigen-presenting cells in some circumstances. The first encounter of naive T cells with antigen on a professional antigen-presenting cell results in a **primary immune response**, and at the same time generates immunological memory, which provides protection from subsequent challenge by the same pathogen. The generation of memory T cells — long-lived cells that respond to antigen with an accelerated reponse — is much less well understood than the initial activation of T cells, and will be dealt with in Chapter 9.

Armed effector T cells differ in many ways from their naive precursors, and these changes equip them to respond quickly and efficiently when they encounter antigen on their target cells. In the final sections of the chapter, we shall describe the specialized mechanisms of T-cell mediated cytotoxicity and of macrophage activation by armed effector T cells, the major components of **cell-mediated immunity**. We shall leave the activation of B cells by helper T cells until Chapter 8, where the humoral or antibody-mediated immune response is discussed.

The production of armed effector T cells.

Activation of naive T cells requires recognition of a foreign peptide fragment bound to a self MHC molecule but this is not on its own sufficient for activation; it also requires the simultaneous delivery of a **co-stimulatory signal** by a specialized antigen-presenting cell. Only professional antigen-presenting cells (APCs) are able to express both classes of MHC molecules as well as the co-stimulatory surface molecules that drive the clonal expansion of naive T cells and their differentiation into armed effector T cells. The activation of naive T cells on initial encounter with antigen on the surface of a professional antigen-presenting cell is often called **priming**, to distinguish it from the responses of armed effector T cells to antigen on their target cells, and the responses of primed memory T cells.

7-1   The initial interaction of naive T cells with antigen occurs in peripheral lymphoid organs.

Adaptive immune responses are not initiated at the site where a pathogen first establishes a focus of infection. They occur in the organized peripheral lymphoid tissues, such as the lymph nodes, to which the pathogen or its products are transported in the lymph that is produced continuously by filtration of extracellular fluid from the blood. Pathogens infecting peripheral sites will be trapped in the lymph nodes directly downstream of the site of infection; those that enter the blood will be trapped in the spleen; and pathogens infecting mucosal surfaces will accumulate in Peyer's patches or tonsils (as we saw in Chapter 1). All these lymphoid organs contain antigen-presenting cells specialized for capturing antigen and activating T cells. Naive T lymphocytes circulate continuously from the bloodstream to the lymphoid organs, and back to the blood, making contact with many antigen-presenting cells every day. This ensures that each naive T cell has a high probability of encountering antigens derived from pathogens at any site of infection.

Naive T cells leave the blood by crossing the walls of specialized venules known as **high endothelial venules**, which deliver them to the cortical region of a lymph node. The continual passage of naive T cells past antigen-presenting cells in the lymph node is crucial for adaptive immunity. As only one naive T cell in 10^5 is likely to be specific for a particular antigen, most of these passing T cells will not recognize the antigen, and these T cells eventually reach the medulla of the lymph node and are carried by the efferent lymphatics back to the blood so that they can continue recirculating through other lymphoid organs. Naive T cells that recognize their specific antigen on the surface of a professional antigen-presenting cell cease to migrate, and embark on the steps that will lead to the generation of armed effector cells (Fig. 7.2).

The three main types of specialized antigen-presenting cells present in the peripheral lymphoid organs are macrophages, dendritic cells, and B cells. Each of these cell types is specialized to process and present antigens from different sources to naive T cells. Two of them, the macrophages and the B cells, are also the targets of subsequent actions of armed effector T cells. Only these three cell types express the specialized co-stimulatory molecules that enable them to activate naive T cells, although macrophages and B cells express these molecules only when suitably activated by infection. The three types of antigen-presenting cell are distributed differently in the lymphoid organs (Fig. 7.3). Macrophages are found in all areas of the lymph node and actively ingest microbes and particulate antigens. As most pathogens are particulate, macrophages stimulate immune responses to many sources of infection. Dendritic cells, also known in lymphoid tissues as **interdigitating reticular cells**, are present only in the T-cell areas of the lymph node. These cells, which we mentioned in Chapter 6 because of their

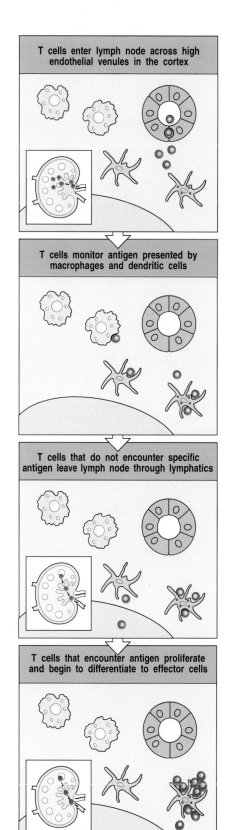

T cells enter lymph node across high endothelial venules in the cortex

T cells monitor antigen presented by macrophages and dendritic cells

T cells that do not encounter specific antigen leave lymph node through lymphatics

T cells that encounter antigen proliferate and begin to differentiate to effector cells

Fig. 7.2 Naive T cells encounter antigen during their recirculation through lymphoid organs. Naive T cells recirculate through peripheral lymphoid organs, such as the lymph node shown here, entering through specialized regions of vascular endothelium called high endothelial venules. On leaving the blood vessel, the T cells enter the cortex of the lymph node, where they encounter many antigen-presenting cells (mainly dendritic cells and macrophages). T cells (colored green) that do not encounter their specific antigen leave the lymph node through the lymphatics and return to the circulation. T cells that encounter antigen (colored blue) on the antigen-presenting cells are activated to proliferate and to differentiate into effector cells. Once this process is completed, these armed effector T cells leave the lymph node via the efferent lymphatics and enter the circulation.

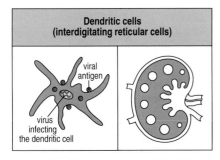

Dendritic cells (interdigitating reticular cells)

viral antigen

virus infecting the dendritic cell

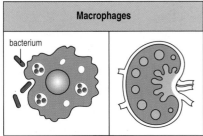

Macrophages

bacterium

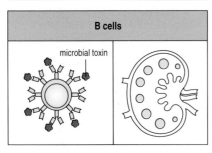

B cells

microbial toxin

Fig. 7.3 Professional antigen-presenting cells are distributed differentially in the lymph node. Dendritic cells, also called interdigitating reticular cells, are found throughout the cortex of the lymph node in the T-cell areas. Macrophages are distributed throughout the lymph node. B cells are found mainly in the follicles. The three types of professional antigen-presenting cells are thought to be adapted to present different types of pathogens or products of pathogens.

role in negative selection of thymocytes, are the most potent antigen-presenting cells for naive T cells and are thought to be especially important in presenting viral antigens. Finally, the B cells in the lymphoid follicles are particularly efficient at taking up soluble antigens, such as bacterial toxins, through binding specifically to their cell-surface immunoglobulin molecules. Degraded fragments of these antigens can reach the B-cell surface on MHC class II molecules and allow B cells to play a part in the activation of naive CD4 T cells.

The generation of effector cells from a naive T cell takes several days. At the end of this period, the armed effector T cells leave the lymphoid organ, and re-enter the bloodstream so that they can migrate to sites of infection.

7-2   Lymphocyte migration, activation, and effector function depend on cell-adhesion molecules.

All the steps that lead from a recirculating naive T cell to a clone of antigen-specific armed effector T cells, including the migration of the cells through the lymph nodes and their initial interactions with antigen-presenting cells, involve antigen non-specific interactions of the lymphocyte with other cells. Similar interactions eventually guide the effector T cells into the peripheral tissues and play an important part in their interactions with target cells. These binding reactions are controlled by a varying array of adhesion molecules on the surface of the T lymphocyte that recognize a complementary array of adhesion molecules on the surface of the cells with which the T cell interacts. The main classes of adhesion molecules that play a part in lymphocyte interactions are the selectins, the integrins, members of the immunoglobulin superfamily, and some **mucin**-like molecules. Some of these molecules are concerned mainly with lymphocyte homing and migration, which we shall describe in more detail in Chapter 9, where we present an integrated view of the immune response; others have broader roles in the generation of immune responses and the interactions of armed effector T cells with their target cells, which will be discussed here.

The nomenclature of the adhesion molecules is confusing, because most were first defined either as cell-surface molecules recognized by monoclonal antibodies or in functional assays of cell–cell interactions, and were biochemically characterized only later. For this reason, the names of many of the adhesion molecules bear no relationship to the structural families to which they belong. A brief explanation of the terminology can be found in the legend to Fig. 7.4, where the main classes of leukocyte adhesion molecules are summarized. We begin our discussion, however, with a small family of molecules, the **selectins**, whose nomenclature reflects their structural characteristics.

The selectins are particularly important for leukocyte homing to specific tissues, and can be expressed either on leukocytes (**L-selectin**) or on vascular endothelium (**P-selectin** and **E-selectin**, which are discussed in Chapter 9). Selectins are cell-surface molecules with a similar core structure, distinguished by the presence of a lectin-like domain in their extracellular portion (Fig. 7.5). Lectins are molecules that bind to specific sugar groups, and each selectin binds to a cell-surface carbohydrate molecule. L-selectin, which is expressed on naive T cells and binds to the carbohydrate moiety, sulfated sialyl Lewis x, of mucin-like molecules called **vascular addressins**, which are expressed on vascular endothelium. Two of these, **CD34** and **GlyCAM-1**, are expressed on high endothelial venules in lymph nodes. A third, **MAdCAM-1**, is

		Name	Tissue distribution	Ligand
Selectins Bind carbohydrates Initiate leukocyte: endothelial interaction	L-selectin	L-selectin (MEL-14, CD62L)	Naive and some memory lymphocytes, neutrophils, monocytes, eosinophils	Sulfated Sialyl Lewis x GlyCAM-1 CD34 MAdCAM-1
		P-selectin (PADGEM, CD62P)	Activated endothelium	Sialyl Lewis x PSGL-1
		E-selectin (ELAM-1, CD62E)	Activated endothelium	Sialyl Lewis x
Mucin-like vascular addressins Bind to L-selectin Initiate leukocyte: endothelial interaction	CD34	CD34	Endothelium	L-selectin
		GlyCAM-1	High endothelial venules	L-selectin
		MAdCAM-1	Mucosal lymphoid tissue venules	L-selectin, VLA-4
Integrins Bind to cell-adhesion molecules and extracellular matrix Strong adhesion	LFA-1	$\alpha_L\beta_2$ (LFA-1, CD11a/CD18)	Monocytes	ICAMs
		$\alpha_M\beta_2$ (Mac-1, CR3, CD11b/CD18)	Neutrophils, monocytes	ICAMs, iC3b
		$\alpha_X\beta_2$ (CR4, p150.95, CD11c/CD18)	Dendritic cells, macrophages	iC3b
		$\alpha_4\beta_1$ (VLA-4, LPAM-1, CD49d/CD29)	Lymphocytes, monocytes	VCAM-1
		$\alpha_5\beta_1$ (VLA-5, CD49d/CD29)	T cells?	Fibronectin
		$\alpha_4\beta_7$ (LPAM-2)	B cells	MAdCAM-1
Immunoglobulin superfamily Various roles in cell adhesion Target for integrins	CD2	CD2 (LFA-2)	T cells	LFA-3
		ICAM-1 (CD54)	Activated vessels, lymphocytes	LFA-1
		ICAM-2 (CD102)	Resting vessels	LFA-1
		ICAM-3 (CD50)	Antigen-presenting cells	LFA-1
		LFA-3 (CD58)	Lymphocytes, antigen-presenting cells	CD2
		VCAM-1 (CD106)	Activated endothelium	VLA-4

Fig. 7.4 Adhesion molecules in leukocyte interactions. Several structural families of adhesion molecules play a part in leukocyte migration, homing and cell–cell interactions: the selectins and mucin-like vascular addressins; the integrins; proteins of the immunoglobulin superfamily. The figure shows schematic representations of an example from each family, a list of other family members that participate in leukocyte interactions, their cellular distribution, and their partners in adhesive interactions. The family members shown here are limited to those we consider in this text but include some that will not be encountered until Chapter 9. The nomenclature of the different molecules in these families is confusing because it often reflects the way in which the molecules were first identified rather than their related structural characteristics. Thus while all the ICAMs are immunoglobulin-related, and all the VLA molecules are b1 integrins, the CD nomenclature reflects the characterization of leukocyte cell-surface molecules by monoclonal antibodies raised against them (Appendix I contains details of all the CD molecules mentioned in this book). Thus CD molecules comprise a large and diverse collection of cell-surface molecules including adhesion molecules in all the structural families. The LFA molecules were defined through experiments in which cytotoxic T-cell killing could be blocked by monoclonal antibodies against cell-surface molecules on the interacting cells and there are LFA molecules in both the integrin and the immunoglobulin families. Alternative names for each of the molecules shown are given in parentheses. Sialyl Lewis x, which is recognized by P- and E-selectin, is an oligosaccharide present on cell-surface glycoproteins of circulating leukocytes.

expressed on endothelium in mucosa, and guides lymphocyte entry into mucosal lymphoid tissue such as that of the gut (see Fig. 7.5).

The interaction between L-selectin and the vascular addressins is responsible for the specific homing of naive T cells to lymphoid organs but does not, on its own, enable the cell to cross the endothelial barrier into the lymphoid tissue; for this, molecules of two other families, the integrins and the immunoglobulin superfamily, are required. These two families of molecules also play a critical part in the subsequent interactions of lymphocytes with antigen-presenting cells and later with their target cells.

The **integrins** comprise a large family of molecules that mediate adhesion between cells, and of cells to the extracellular matrix, in immune and inflammatory responses; they are also important in many aspects of tissue organization and cell migration during development. Integrins consist of a large α chain that has several cation-binding sites usually occupied by calcium ions, paired non-covalently with a smaller β chain. There are several subfamilies of integrins, broadly defined by their common β chains. We shall be concerned chiefly with the **leukocyte intergrins**, which

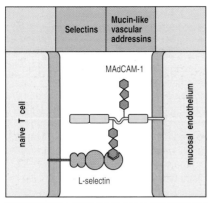

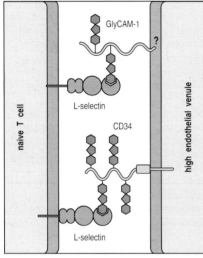

Fig. 7.5   L-selectin and the mucin-like vascular addressins direct naive lymphocyte homing to lymphoid tissues. L-selectin is expressed on naive T cells, which bind to the vascular addressins CD34 and GlyCAM-1 on high endothelial venules to enter lymph nodes. The relative importance of CD34 and GlyCAM-1 in this interaction is not clear. GlyCAM-1 is expressed exclusively on high endothelial venules but has no transmembrane region and it is unclear how it is attached to the membrane; CD34 has a transmembrane anchor and is expressed on endothelial cells but not exclusively on high endothelial venules. However, CD34 is appropriately glycosylated in HEV only. The addressin MAdCAM-1 is expressed on mucosal endothelium and guides entry into mucosal lymphoid tissue. L-selectin recognizes carbohydrate moieties on the vascular addressins.

have a common β_2 chain with distinct α chains (Fig. 7.6). All T cells express a leukocyte integrin known as lymphocyte function-associated antigen-1 (LFA-1). This is thought to be the most important adhesion molecule for lymphocyte activation as antibodies to LFA-1 effectively inhibit the activation of both naive and armed effector T cells. Leukocyte integrins are also expressed on neutrophils and macrophages; immunity to infection with extracellular bacteria is severely impaired because of defective neutrophil and macrophage function in **leukocyte adhesion deficiency**, an inherited immunodeficiency disease resulting from a defect in the synthesis of the common β_2 chain. Surprisingly, T-cell responses can be normal in such patients. This is probably because T cells also express other adhesion molecules, including CD2 and members of the β_1 integrin family, which may be able to compensate for the absence of LFA-1. Expression of the β_1 integrins increases significantly late in T-cell activation, and they are thus often called **VLA** for **very late antigen**; we shall see in Chapter 9 that they play an important part in directing armed effector T cells to their target tissues.

Many cell-surface adhesion molecules are members of the immunoglobulin superfamily, which also includes the antigen receptors of T and B cells, the co-receptors CD4, CD8, and CD19, and the invariant domains of MHC molecules. At least five adhesion molecules of the immunoglobulin superfamily are especially important in T-cell activation (Fig. 7.7). Three very similar **intercellular adhesion molecules (ICAMs)**, **ICAM-1**, **ICAM-2**, and **ICAM-3**, all bind to the T-cell integrin LFA-1. ICAM-1 and ICAM-2 are expressed on endothelium as well as on antigen-presenting cells; binding to these molecules enables lymphocytes to migrate through blood vessel walls. ICAM-3 is expressed only on leukocytes and is thought to play an important part in adhesion between T cells and antigen-presenting cells. The interaction of LFA-1 with ICAM-1, -2, and -3 synergizes with a second adhesive interaction. This

Fig. 7.6   Integrins are important in leukocyte adhesion. Integrins are heterodimeric proteins containing a β chain, which defines the class of integrin, and an α chain, which defines the different integrins within a class. The α chain is larger than the β chain and contains binding sites for divalent cations that may be important in signaling. Most integrins expressed on leukocytes have a common β chain, β_2, but different α chains. LFA-1 and VLA-4, which is a β_1 integrin, are expressed on T cells and are important in the migration and activation of these cells. Mac-1 is also a complement receptor (CR3) whose function will be discussed in Chapter 8; the function of p150.95, which also binds complement, is unknown.

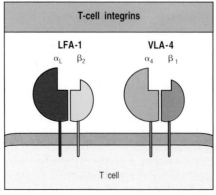

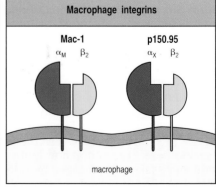

involves the immunoglobulin superfamily members **CD2** and **LFA-3**; CD2 is expressed on the T-cell surface, and LFA-3 is expressed on the antigen-presenting cell (Fig. 7.7).

| 7-3 | The initial interaction of T cells with antigen-presenting cells is also mediated by cell-adhesion molecules. |

As they migrate through the cortical region of the lymph node, naive T cells bind transiently to each antigen-presenting cell they encounter. Professional antigen-presenting cells, and dendritic cells in particular, bind naive T cells very efficiently through interactions between LFA-1 and CD2 on the T cell, and ICAM-1, -2, and -3 and LFA-3 on the antigen-presenting cell. These molecules synergize in the binding of lymphocytes to antigen-presenting cells and the exact role of each has been difficult to distinguish. People lacking LFA-1 can have normal T-cell responses, and this also seems to be the case for genetically engineered mice lacking CD2. It would not be surprising if there was sufficient redundancy in the molecules mediating T-cell adhesive interactions to enable immune responses to occur in the absence of any one of them; such molecular redundancy has been observed in other complex biological processes.

The transient binding of naive T cells to professional antigen-presenting cells is crucial in providing time for T cells to sample large numbers of MHC molecules on the surface of each antigen-presenting cell for the presence of specific peptide. In those rare cases in which a naive T cell recognizes its specific peptide:MHC ligand, signaling through the T-cell receptor induces a conformational change in LFA-1, which greatly increases its affinity for ICAM-1, -2, and -3. The mechanism of this conformational change in LFA-1 is not known; the binding of Mg^{2+} rather than Ca^{2+} to its divalent cation-binding sites is thought to play a part. These changes stabilize the association between the antigen-specific T cell and the cell-presenting antigen (Fig. 7.8). The association can persist for several days during which the naive T cell proliferates and its progeny differentiate into armed effector T cells.

Most T-cell encounters with antigen-presenting cells, however, do not result in recognition of specific antigen. In these encounters, the T cells must be able to separate efficiently from the antigen-presenting cells so that they can continue to migrate through the lymph node, eventually leaving via the efferent lymphatic vessels to re-enter the blood and continue to recirculate. Dissociation, like stable binding, may also involve signaling between the T cell and the antigen-presenting cells but little is known of its mechanism.

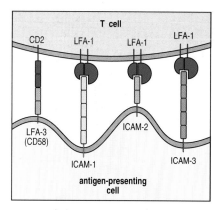

Fig. 7.7 Cell-surface molecules of the immunoglobulin superfamily are important in the interactions of lymphocytes with antigen-presenting cells. In the initial encounter of T cells with antigen- presenting cells, CD2 binding to LFA-3 on the antigen-presenting cell synergizes with LFA-1 binding to ICAMs 1, 2, and 3 on the antigen-presenting cell. Similar adhesive interactions occur between effector T cells and their targets (not shown).

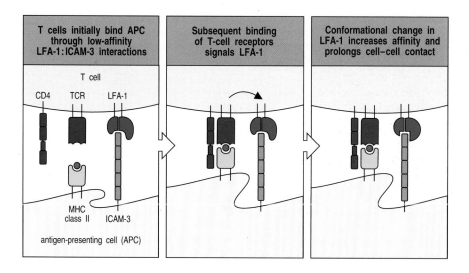

Fig. 7.8 Transient adhesive interactions between T cells and antigen-presenting cells are stabilized by specific antigen recognition. When a T cell binds to its specific ligand on an antigen-presenting cell (APC), intracellular signaling through the T-cell receptor (TCR) induces a conformational change in LFA-1 that causes it to bind with higher affinity to ICAM-3 on the antigen-presenting cell. The cell shown here is a CD4 T cell.

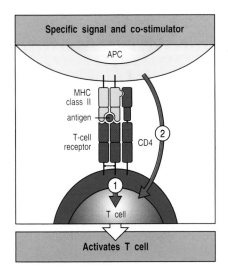

Specific signal and co-stimulator

APC

MHC class II

antigen

T-cell receptor

CD4

1

2

T cell

Activates T cell

Fig. 7.9   Activation of naive T cells requires two independent signals. The binding of the peptide:MHC complex by the T-cell receptor and, in this example, the CD4 co-receptor transmits a signal (signal 1 indicated by arrow 1) to the T cell that antigen has been recognized. Activation of naive T cells requires a second signal (signal 2 indicated by arrow 2), the co-stimulatory signal, which is delivered by the same antigen-presenting cell (APC).

7-4   Both specific ligand and co-stimulatory signals provided by a professional antigen-presenting cell are required for the clonal expansion of naive T cells.

We saw in Chapter 4 that effector T cells are triggered when their antigen-specific receptors and either the CD4 or the CD8 co-receptors bind to peptide:MHC complexes. But ligation of the T-cell receptor and co-receptor does not, on its own, stimulate naive T cells to proliferate and differentiate into armed effector T cells. The antigen-specific clonal expansion of naive T cells requires a second, co-stimulatory, signal (Fig. 7.9) which, in the case of CD4 T cells, is delivered by the same antigen-presenting cell on which the T cell recognizes its specific antigen. Activation of CD8 T cells also requires both signals on a single cell, although on occasion it may be less direct, as we shall see later.

The best characterized co-stimulatory molecules on antigen-presenting cells are the structurally related glycoproteins **B7.1** and **B7.2**. These are homodimeric members of the immunoglobulin superfamily found exclusively on the surface of cells capable of stimulating T-cell growth. Their role in co-stimulation has been demonstrated by transfecting fibroblasts with the B7.1 and B7.2 genes and showing that the fibroblasts could then co-stimulate growth of naive T cells. The receptor for B7 molecules on the T cell is **CD28**, yet another member of the immunoglobulin superfamily (Fig. 7.10). Ligation of CD28 by B7.1 or B7.2 or by anti-CD28 antibodies will co-stimulate the growth of naive T cells, while antibodies to the B7 molecules, which inhibit their binding to CD28, inhibit T-cell responses.

On naive T cells, CD28 is the only receptor for B7.1 and B7.2. Once T cells are activated, however, they express an additional receptor called **CTLA-4**, which binds B7 molecules with a higher affinity than does CD28. CTLA-4 closely resembles CD28 in sequence, and the two molecules are encoded by closely linked genes. CTLA-4 binds more avidly than CD28 but appears to play a negative role in the activation of the T cell expressing it (Fig. 7.11); the activated progeny of a naive T cell become less sensitive to stimulation by antigen than the naive T cells. This may help to limit the early proliferative response of the T cells to antigen and B7 molecules on the surface of antigen-presenting cells. Although other molecules have been reported to co-stimulate naive T cells, to date only B7.1 and B7.2 binding to CD28 has been shown definitively to provide co-stimulatory signals in normal immune responses.

The requirement for simultaneous delivery of antigen-specific and co-stimulatory signals in the activation of naive T cells means that only professional antigen-presenting cells can initiate T-cell responses. This is important because not all potentially self-reactive T cells are deleted in the thymus; peptides derived from proteins made only in specialized cells in the peripheral tissues may not be encountered during the negative selection of thymocytes. Self tolerance could be broken if naive, autoreactive T cells could recognize self antigens on tissue cells and then be co-stimulated by a professional antigen-presenting cell, either locally or at a distant site. Thus, the requirement that the same cell

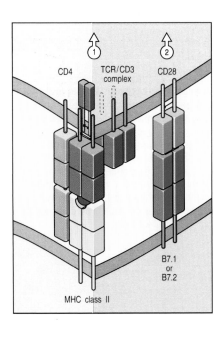

Fig. 7.10   The principal co-stimulatory signal expressed on professional antigen-presenting cells is B7, which binds the T-cell protein CD28. Binding of the T-cell receptor (TCR) and its co-receptor CD4 to the peptide:MHC class II complex delivers a signal (signal 1) that can only induce clonal expansion of T cells when the co-stimulatory signal (signal 2) is given by binding of CD28 to B7. Both CD28 and B7 are members of the immunoglobulin superfamily. B7 is a homodimer each of whose chains has one V-like domain and one C-like domain. CD28 is a disulfide-linked homodimer in which each chain has one domain, resembling an immunoglobulin V-domain.

CD4   TCR/CD3 complex   CD28

1   2

B7.1 or B7.2

MHC class II

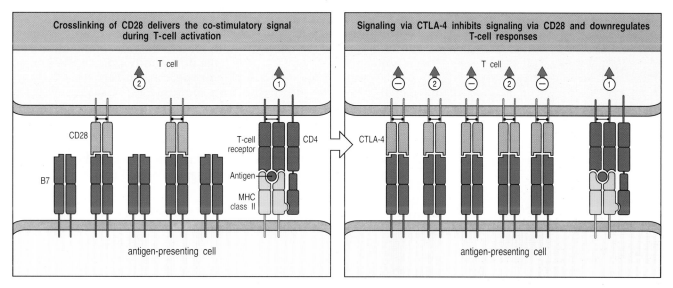

Fig. 7.11 T-cell activation through the T-cell receptor and CD28 leads to increased expression of CTLA-4, an alternative receptor for B7 molecules. CTLA-4 has a higher affinity for B7 molecules than does CD28 and makes the cell more sensitive to stimulation by B7. CTLA-4 binding to B7 molecules appears to play a negative role in T-cell activation.

presents both the specific antigen and the co-stimulatory signal plays an important part in preventing destructive immune responses to self tissues. Indeed, antigen binding to the T-cell receptor in the absence of co-stimulation not only fails to activate the cell but also leads to a state called **anergy**, in which the T cell becomes refractory to activation (Fig. 7.12).

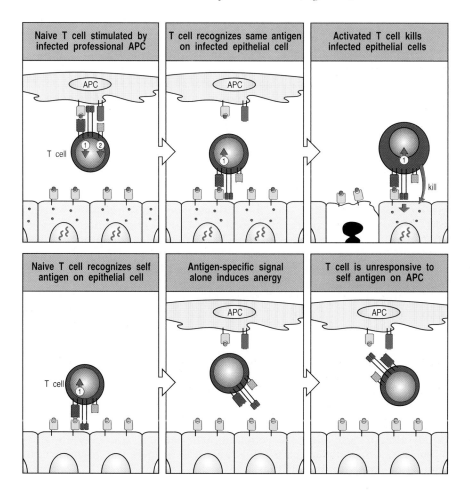

Fig. 7.12 The requirement for one cell to deliver both the antigen-specific signal and the co-stimulatory signal plays a crucial role in preventing immune responses to self antigens. In this example of the initiation of an immune response to a virus, a T cell recognizes a viral peptide on a professional antigen-presenting cell (APC) and is activated to proliferate and differentiate into an effector cell capable of eliminating any virus-infected cell (upper panels). Naive T cells that recognize antigen on cells that cannot provide co-stimulation become anergic, as when a T-cell recognizes a self antigen expressed by an uninfected epithelial cell (lower panels). This T cell does not differentiate into an armed effector cell, and cannot be stimulated further by professional antigen-presenting cells (see Fig. 7.20).

As well as B7.1 and B7.2, professional antigen-presenting cells must express adhesion molecules like ICAM-3 and they must be able to process antigen for presentation on both classes of MHC molecules. The three types of antigen-presenting cells differ both in their co-stimulatory and in their antigen-processing properties, and are thus likely to have distinctive functions in initiating immune responses.

7-5   Macrophages are scavenger cells that can be induced by pathogens to present foreign antigens to naive T cells.

Many of the microorganisms that enter the body are readily engulfed and destroyed by phagocytes that provide an innate, antigen non-specific first line of defense against infection. Microorganisms that are destroyed by phagocytes do not cause disease and do not require an adaptive immune response. Pathogens, by definition, have developed mechanisms to avoid elimination by innate immune mechanisms, and the recognition and removal of such pathogens is the function of the adaptive immune response. Mononuclear phagocytes, or macrophages, contribute to the adaptive immune response as professional antigen-presenting cells.

Professional antigen-presenting cells must be capable of presenting peptide fragments of the antigen on both classes of MHC molecules, and of delivering a co-stimulatory signal, probably through B7 molecules. Resting macrophages, however, have few or no MHC class II molecules on their surface, and do not express B7. Expression of both MHC class II and B7 molecules is induced in these cells by the ingestion of microorganisms.

Macrophages have a variety of receptors, including the macrophage mannose receptor, that recognize bacterial carbohydrates and other microbial constituents and enable the macrophage to bind and engulf microorganisms displaying these compounds. The ingested microorganisms are degraded in the endosomes and lysosomes, generating peptides that can be presented by MHC class II molecules on the cell surface. At the same time, MHC class II and B7 molecules are induced on the surface of the macrophage.

Little is known about most of the receptors that allow macrophages to recognize microbial constituents; the same receptors probably mediate both pathogen ingestion and the induction of co-stimulatory activity since exposure to a single microbial constituent can induce B7 molecules on most macrophages. It seems likely that these receptors evolved originally to allow the phagocytic cells in primitive eukaryotic organisms to recognize microorganisms by binding to structures such as bacterial carbohydrates or lipopolysaccharide that are not found in eukaryotes. Macrophage receptors still serve this function in innate immunity as well as playing an important part in the initiation of adaptive immune responses.

The induction of co-stimulator activity by common microbial constituents is believed to allow the immune system to distinguish antigens borne by infectious agents from antigens associated with innocuous proteins, including self proteins. Indeed, many foreign proteins do not induce an immune response when injected on their own, presumably because they fail to induce co-stimulatory activity in antigen-presenting cells. When such protein antigens are mixed with bacteria, however, they become immunogenic, because the bacteria induce the essential co-stimulatory activity in cells that ingests the protein (Fig. 7.13). Bacteria

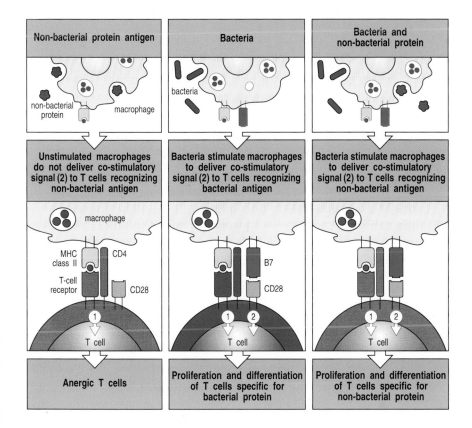

Fig. 7.13 Many microbial substances can induce co-stimulatory activity in macrophages. If protein antigens are taken up and presented by macrophages in the absence of bacterial components that induce co-stimulatory activity in the macrophage, T cells specific for the antigen will become anergic (refractory to activation). Many bacteria induce expression of co-stimulators by antigen-presenting cells, and macrophages can present peptide antigens derived by degradation of such bacteria. When bacteria are mixed with protein antigens, the protein antigens are rendered immunogenic because the bacteria induce co-stimulatory activity (e.g. the expression of B7 molecules) in the antigen-presenting cells. Such added bacteria act as adjuvants.

used in this way are known as adjuvants (see Section 2-3). We shall see in Chapter 11 how self-tissue proteins mixed with bacterial adjuvants can induce autoimmune diseases, illustrating the crucial importance of the regulation of co-stimulatory activity in self:non-self discrimination.

It is particularly important that macrophages should not normally be capable of activating T cells in the absence of microbial infection because macrophages continuously scavenge dead or senescent cells. The Kupffer cells of the liver sinusoids and the macrophages of the splenic red pulp, in particular, remove large numbers of dying cells from the blood daily. Kupffer cells express little MHC class II and expression is not increased by ingestion of dead cells in the absence of infection or inflammation. Moreover, they are not located at sites through which large numbers of naive T cells pass. Thus, although they generate large amounts of self peptides in their endosomes and lysosomes, these macrophages are not likely to elicit an autoimmune response.

7-6   Dendritic cells are highly efficient inducers of T-cell activation.

It is of crucial importance that all infections be detected by T cells but many dangerous pathogens, including many viruses, do not induce MHC class II and co-stimulatory molecules on macrophages. Viruses use the biosynthetic machinery of the host to synthesize their proteins, nucleic acids, carbohydrates, and membranes, and are therefore more difficult to distinguish from self than are bacteria. It seems likely that dendritic cells, which are found in the T-cell areas of lymphoid tissues, evolved to cope with this potential chink in the armor of the body.

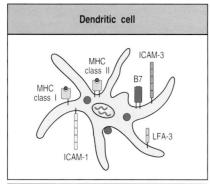

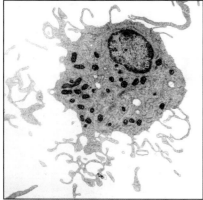

Fig. 7.14 Dendritic cells in lymphoid tissue have co-stimulatory activity. To activate naive T cells, antigen-presenting cells must be capable of processing antigen from extracellular and intracellular pathogens and presenting it on MHC class I and MHC class II molecules, and they must also express co-stimulatory molecules, probably in the form of B7. Dendritic cells in lymphoid tissue express all these surface molecules as well as high levels of the adhesion molecules ICAM-3 and LFA-3. However, their ability to take up antigen is limited. Photograph courtesy of J Barker.

These cells can arise from either bone marrow progenitors cultured with the cytokine GM-CSF (see Section 7-17) or from a lymphoid-specific progenitor. This suggests that some dendritic cells may have appeared after T and B lymphocytes in evolution and is consistent with their apparently exclusive function of presenting antigen to T cells. Several specializations equip them for this function.

The dendritic cells that are concentrated in the lymphoid tissues express high levels of MHC class I and MHC class II molecules as well as the co-stimulatory molecules B7.1 and B7.2, and the adhesion molecules ICAM-1, ICAM-3, and LFA-3 (Fig. 7.14). Not surprisingly, they are very potent activators of naive T cells. The lymphoid dendritic cells, however, are non-phagocytic and do not readily take up antigen from the extracellular milieu. This suggests that they may be specialized to present peptides of viruses and possibly cellular toxins, which have their own means of entering cells.

Most cells are susceptible to only a limited range of viruses but dendritic cells can be infected by many different viruses and efficiently present peptides derived from the viral proteins on their abundant surface MHC molecules. These peptides may be presented either on MHC class I molecules, where they are recognized by naive CD8 T cells (which will differentiate into cytotoxic effector cells) or on MHC class II molecules, where they are recognized by CD4 T cells (which give rise to inflammatory and helper T cells). Helper T cells initiate the production of antibodies which, as we shall see in Chapter 8, are important in blocking viral entry into cells.

Most viral proteins are produced in the cytosol; peptides derived from them are transported to the surface by MHC class I molecules for recognition by CD8 T cells. However, viral envelope proteins are translocated into the endoplasmic reticulum, from where they are delivered to the cell surface and can then enter endosomes. Peptides of these proteins are delivered to the cell surface by MHC class II molecules and stimulate CD4 T cells. Thus, dendritic cells are able to prime both CD8 and CD4 T cells in many viral infections.

Cells that resemble dendritic cells are found in many sites in the body and it is thought that the interdigitating reticular dendritic cells of the lymphoid tissues are derived from these tissue dendritic cells. The best studied tissue dendritic cells are those of the skin. These are called Langerhans' cells, and differ from those found in lymphoid tissues in two crucial respects.

First, they can ingest antigen, and second, they lack co-stimulatory activity. These cells can be triggered by infection to migrate through the lymph to the lymphoid organs, where they differentiate into dendritic cells that cannot ingest antigen but have potent co-stimulatory activity (Fig. 7.15). It is likely that their role in physiological immune responses is to transport antigens from sites of infection to the lymphoid tissues, where they efficiently activate recirculating T lymphocytes. Whether all lymphoid dendritic cells are derived from phagocytic precursors in the peripheral tissues is not known.

Once in the lymphoid tissue, it is important that dendritic cells do not readily take up extracellular antigens or scavenge self cells or protein, since their constitutively expressed co-stimulatory activity enables them to present to T cells any antigen they can internalize or synthesize. Dendritic cells do, of course, efficiently present peptides derived from their own proteins. However, these do not elicit autoimmune responses because, as we saw in Section 6-17, dendritic cells in the thymus efficiently delete developing T cells specific for these peptides.

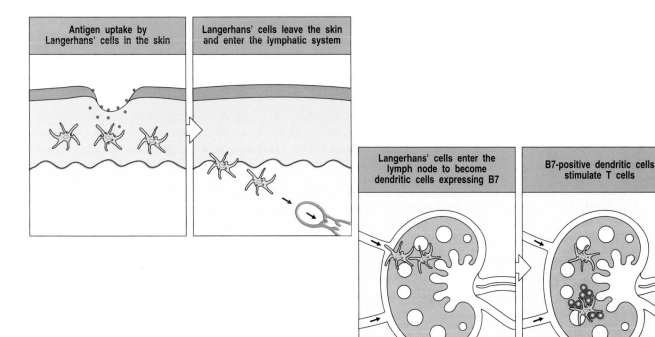

Fig. 7.15 Langerhans' cells take up antigen in the skin and migrate to lymphoid organs where they present it to T cells. Langerhans' cells can ingest antigen but have no co-stimulatory activity. In the presence of infection, they take up antigen locally in the skin and then migrate to the lymph nodes where they differentiate into dendritic cells that can no longer ingest antigen but now have co-stimulatory activity.

Much of the evidence for the importance of tissue dendritic cells comes from their role in inducing the rejection of tissue grafts, as we shall see in Chapter 11. In experimental animals, grafts depleted of dendritic cells are well tolerated by recipients, at least until repopulated with host antigen-presenting cells.

7-7   B cells are highly efficient at presenting antigens that bind to their surface immunoglobulin.

Neither macrophages nor dendritic cells can efficiently take up soluble antigens. B cells, by contrast, are uniquely adapted to bind soluble molecules through their cell-surface immunoglobulin and this is critical to their ability to serve as targets for antigen-specific armed helper T cells (see Chapter 8). However, B cells can also function as professional antigen-presenting cells by internalizing soluble antigens bound by their surface immunoglobulins and then presenting peptide fragments of these antigens as MHC:peptide complexes. It is not clear how important T-cell priming by B cells is in natural immune responses.

Soluble protein antigens are not abundant during natural infections; most natural antigens, such as bacteria and viruses, are particulate, while soluble bacterial toxins act by binding to cell surfaces and are thus present only at low concentrations in solution. However, there are some natural immunogens that enter the body as soluble molecules; examples are insect toxins, anticoagulants injected by blood-sucking insects, snake venoms, and many allergens. Moreover, much of what we know about the immune system in general, and about T-cell responses in particular, has been learned from the study of immune responses to soluble protein immunogens such as ovalbumin, hen egg-white lysozyme, and cytochrome *c*. CD4 T-cell responses to these soluble protein antigens seem to require B cells as antigen-presenting cells. They also depend on adjuvants to elicit co-stimulator activity.

When an antigen is bound by an immunoglobulin molecule on the surface of a B cell, the complex of immunoglobulin and antigen is internalized and degraded. Because this mechanism of antigen uptake is highly efficient and B cells constitutively express high levels of MHC class II molecules, high levels of specific peptide:MHC class II complexes are generated at the B-cell surface (Fig. 7.16).

Fig. 7.16   B cells can use their immunoglobulin receptor to present specific antigen very efficiently to T cells. Surface immunoglobulin allows B cells to bind and internalize specific antigen very efficiently. The internalized antigen is processed in cellular vesicles where it binds to MHC class II molecules, which transport the antigenic fragments to the cell surface where they can be recognized by T cells. When the protein antigen is not recognized specifically by the B cell, its internalization is inefficient and only a low density of antigenic fragments of any given protein is subsequently presented at the B-cell surface.

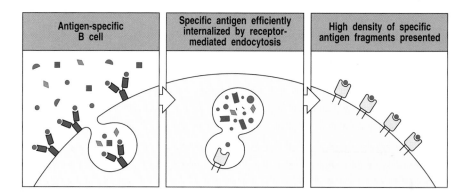

| Antigen-specific B cell | Specific antigen efficiently internalized by receptor-mediated endocytosis | High density of specific antigen fragments presented |

B cells do not constitutively express co-stimulatory activity but they can be induced by various microbial constituents to express B7.1 and especially B7.2. Indeed, B7.1 was first identified as a molecule expressed on B cells activated by microbial lipopolysaccharide. This requirement that B cells be activated in order to activate naive T cells underlies the experimental observation that to produce immune responses to soluble protein antigens, which can only be ingested effectively by antigen-specific B cells, it is essential to inject the protein with a bacterial adjuvant.

It also helps to explain why, although B cells efficiently present soluble proteins, they are unlikely to induce responses to soluble self proteins in the absence of infection; in the absence of co-stimulatory activity, antigen not only fails to activate naive T cells but causes them to become anergic, or non-responsive (see Fig. 7.12). This provides an additional safeguard to the mechanisms discussed in Chapter 5 whereby potentially self-reactive B cells are eliminated or inactivated in the bone marrow. However, it is also true that binding of certain antigens to B cells can, via the B-cell receptor, signal for induction of B7.2. How this relates to self tolerance is not known and is well worth studying.

Thus T-cell responses are primed by three distinct classes of professional antigen-presenting cells. Each is optimally equipped to present a particular class of antigen to naive T cells: those that can present ingested antigens express co-stimulatory activity only when this is induced by microbial particles; only dendritic cells, which are probably specialized to present viral antigens, constitutively express co-stimulatory activity. These properties allow professional antigen-presenting cells to present peptides of pathogens while avoiding immunization against self (Fig. 7.17).

	B cells	Macrophages	Dendritic cells
Antigen uptake	Antigen-specific receptor (Ig) ++++	Phagocytosis +++	+++ Phagocytosis by tissue dendritic cells ++++ Viral infection
MHC expression	Constitutive Increases on activation +++ to ++++	Inducible by bacteria and cytokines – to +++	Constitutive ++++
Co-stimulator delivery	Inducible – to +++	Inducible – to +++	Constitutive ++++
Antigen presented	Toxins Viruses Bacteria	Extracellular and vesicular bacteria	Viruses (allergens?)
Location	Lymphoid tissue Peripheral blood	Lymphoid tissue Connective tissue Body cavities	Lymphoid tissue Connective tissue Epithelia

Fig. 7.17 The properties of professional antigen-presenting cells. B cells, macrophages and dendritic cells are the main cell types involved in the initial presentation of exogenous antigens to naive T cells. These cells vary in their means of antigen uptake, MHC class II expression, co-stimulator expression, the antigens they appear to be crucial for presenting, and their locations in the body.

7-8	**Activated T cells synthesize the T-cell growth factor interleukin-2 and its receptor.**

Naive T cells can live for many years without dividing. These small resting cells have condensed chromatin and a scanty cytoplasm and are synthesizing little RNA or protein. On activation, they must re-enter the cell cycle and divide rapidly to produce large numbers of progeny that will differentiate into armed effector T cells. Their proliferation and differentiation is driven by a protein growth factor or cytokine called **interleukin-2 (IL-2)**, which is produced by the activated T cell itself.

The initial encounter with specific antigen in the presence of the required co-stimulatory signal triggers the entry of the T cell into the G1 phase of the cell cycle and, at the same time, induces the synthesis of IL-2 along with the α chain of the IL-2 receptor. Resting T cells express a low-affinity receptor for IL-2, composed of β and γ chains. Association of these with the α chain creates a receptor with a much higher affinity for IL-2 (Fig. 7.18). Binding of IL-2 to the high-affinity receptor then triggers progression through the rest of the cell cycle. T cells activated in this way can divide two to three times a day for several days, allowing one cell to give rise to thousands of progeny, all bearing an identical receptor for antigen. IL-2 also promotes the differentiation of these cells into armed effector T cells (Fig. 7.19).

Activation of T cells also causes the expression on the T-cell surface of the molecule called CD40 ligand, because it binds to the B-cell surface molecule CD40. The binding of CD40 ligand to CD40 activates CD40+ cells and induces surface expression of B7.1 and B7.2, further driving the T-cell response.

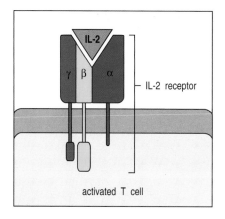

Fig. 7.18 IL-2 receptors are three-chain structures composed of an α, a β and a γ chain expressed fully only on activated T cells. On resting T cells, only the β and γ chains are expressed. They bind IL-2 with moderate affinity, allowing resting T cells to respond to very high concentrations of IL-2. Activation of T cells induces the synthesis of the α chain and the formation of the heterotrimeric receptor, which has a high affinity for IL-2 and allows the T cell to respond to very low concentrations of IL-2. The β and γ chains show amino acid similarities to cell-surface receptors for growth hormone and prolactin, all of which regulate cell growth and differentiation.

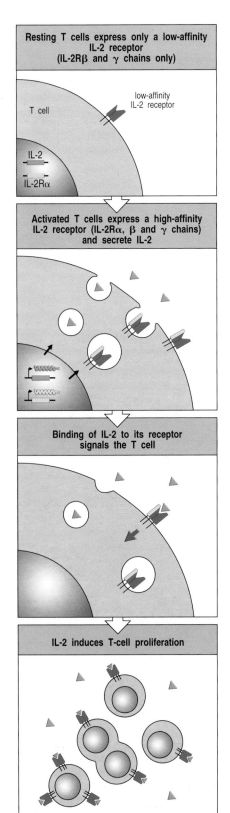

Resting T cells express only a low-affinity IL-2 receptor (IL-2Rβ and γ chains only)

T cell

low-affinity IL-2 receptor

IL-2

IL-2Rα

Activated T cells express a high-affinity IL-2 receptor (IL-2Rα, β and γ chains) and secrete IL-2

Binding of IL-2 to its receptor signals the T cell

IL-2 induces T-cell proliferation

Fig. 7.19 Activated T cells secrete and respond to interleukin-2 (IL-2). Activation of naive T cells by the recognition of a peptide:MHC complex accompanied by co-stimulation induces expression and secretion of IL-2 and the expression of high-affinity IL-2 receptors. IL-2 binds to the IL-2 receptors to promote T-cell growth in an autocrine fashion.

7-9   The co-stimulatory signal is necessary for the synthesis and secretion of IL-2.

The production of IL-2 determines whether a T cell will proliferate and become an armed effector cell, and the most important function of the co-stimulatory signal is to promote the synthesis of IL-2. Antigen recognition by the T-cell receptor ultimately induces several transcription factors (see Chapter 4). One of these factors, NF-AT (nuclear factor of activation in T cells), binds to the promoter region of the IL-2 gene and is necessary to activate its transcription. IL-2 gene transcription on its own, however, does not lead to the production of IL-2. This requires in addition CD28 ligation by B7 molecules. The main effect of signaling through CD28 is thought to be the stabilization of IL-2 mRNA. Cytokine mRNAs are very unstable, because of an 'instability sequence' in their 3' untranslated region, as we shall see later in this chapter. This instability prevents sustained cytokine release and enables cytokine activity to be tightly regulated. The stabilization of IL-2 mRNA increases IL-2 synthesis by 20- to 30-fold, and at the same time CD28 ligation increases transcription of IL-2 mRNA by about three-fold. These two effects together increase IL-2 production by 100-fold. When a T cell recognizes specific antigen in the absence of co-stimulation through its CD28 molecule, little IL-2 is produced and the T cell does not induce its own proliferation.

The requirements for expression of the IL-2 receptor are less stringent than those for IL-2 synthesis. For example, T-cell receptor ligation alone is frequently sufficient to induce expression of high-affinity IL-2 receptors on T cells. This can allow IL-2 made by one cell to act on IL-2 receptors expressed on neighboring antigen-specific cells. Later in this chapter we shall see how this may be important in the priming of CD8 T cells.

The central importance of IL-2 in initiating adaptive immune responses is well illustrated by the drugs that are most commonly used to suppress undesirable immune responses such as the rejection of tissue grafts. The drugs cyclosporin A and FK506 inhibit IL-2 production by disrupting signaling through the T-cell receptor. The drug rapamycin inhibits signaling through the IL-2 receptor. Cyclosporin A and rapamycin act synergistically to inhibit immune responses by preventing the IL-2 driven clonal expansion of T cells. The mode of action of these drugs will be considered in detail in Chapter 12.

7-10   Antigen recognition in the absence of co-stimulation leads to T-cell tolerance.

Antigen recognition in the absence of co-stimulation inactivates naive T cells, inducing a state known as anergy (Fig. 7.20). The most important change in anergic T cells is their inability to produce IL-2: this prevents them from proliferating and differentiating into effector cells when they encounter antigen, even if the antigen is subsequently presented by professional antigen-presenting cells. This helps ensure tolerance of T cells to self-tissue antigens.

As we saw in Section 6-16, any protein synthesized by all cells will be presented by professional antigen-presenting cells in the thymus and

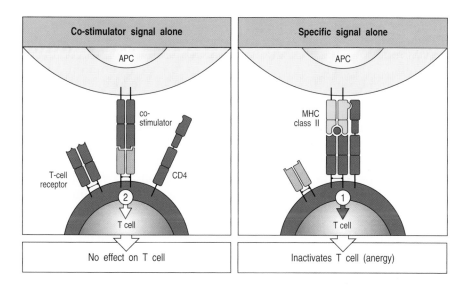

Fig. 7.20 T-cell tolerance to antigens expressed on tissue cells results from antigen recognition in the absence of co-stimulation. Antigen-presenting cells (APC) neither activate nor inactivate T cells if specific antigen is not present on that surface, even if they express a co-stimulatory molecule and can deliver signal 2. However, when T cells recognize antigen in the absence of co-stimulatory molecules, they receive signal 1 alone and are inactivated. This allows self antigens expressed on tissue cells to induce tolerance in T cells.

will cause clonal deletion of T cells reactive to these ubiquitous self proteins. However, many proteins have specialized functions and are made only by the cells of certain tissues. Because MHC class I molecules present only those peptides derived from proteins synthesized within the cell, such tissue-specific peptides will not be displayed on the MHC molecules of thymic cells and cells recognizing them are unlikely to be deleted in the thymus. An important factor in avoiding autoimmune responses to such tissue-specific proteins is the absence of co-stimulator activity on tissue cells. Naive T cells recognizing self peptides on tissue cells are not activated; instead they may be induced to enter a state of anergy.

The induction of anergy to antigens expressed on peripheral tissues has been demonstrated in a series of experiments on transgenic animals that also confirm the importance of B7.1 and B7.2. In addition, these experiments show that the induction of IL-2 is a critical function of B7.1 and B7.2 binding by CD28. In these experimental animals, a transgene encoding a non-self MHC allele is placed under the control of a tissue-specific promoter so that it is expressed only in the cells of a peripheral tissue (in this case, the pancreas). The transgenic mice are tolerant to this 'pseudo-self' antigen, and the mechanism of this tolerance can be explored by breeding them to mice transgenic for genes encoding a T-cell receptor that recognizes the 'pseudo-self' MHC protein (Fig. 7.21). Although all the T cells in the double transgenic offspring can recognize the 'pseudo-self' antigen, no autoimmune response develops. In these mice, mature T cells capable of responding to the pseudo-self protein

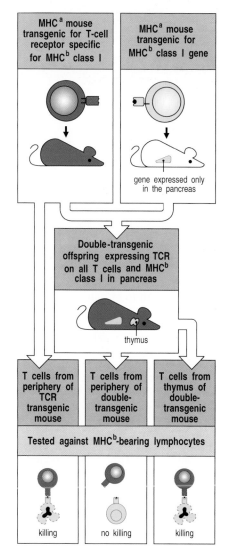

Fig. 7.21 T-cell tolerance can be induced by antigen-dependent inactivation of mature T cells in the periphery. MHC^a mice are made transgenic for an MHC^b class I gene under the control of the rat insulin 1 promoter and thus expressed only in insulin-producing pancreatic β cells. Other MHC^a mice are made transgenic for rearranged T-cell receptor genes that recognize the MHC^b class I product. Double-transgenic offspring express the transgenic T-cell receptor (TCR) on all

their T cells and MHC^b class I molecules in the pancreas. The T cells do not respond to the MHC^b molecules expressed in the pancreas and there is little or no infiltration of the islets by T cells. Circulating T cells from these mice do not respond to MHC^b cells in mixed lymphocyte culture (lower middle panel). T cells taken from the thymus, by contrast, respond to cells bearing MHC^b (lower right panel). Tolerance must therefore be acquired in the periphery.

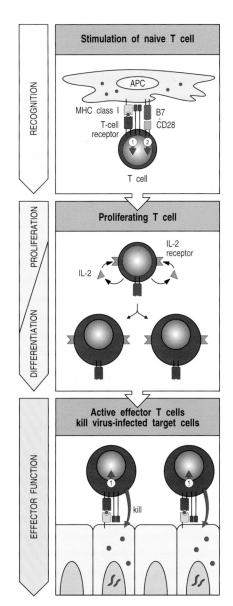

RECOGNITION

PROLIFERATION

DIFFERENTIATION

EFFECTOR FUNCTION

Stimulation of naive T cell

APC

MHC class I   B7
T-cell   CD28
receptor

T cell

Proliferating T cell

IL-2
receptor

IL-2

**Active effector T cells
kill virus-infected target cells**

kill

**Fig. 7.22 Clonal expansion precedes
differentiation to effector function.**
A naive T cell that recognizes antigen on
the surface of a professional antigen-
presenting cell (APC) and receives the
required two signals (arrows 1 and 2, top
panel) becomes activated and both
secretes and responds to IL-2. It
proliferates, and clonal expansion
(middle panel) is followed by the
differentiation of the T cells to armed
effector cell status. Once the cells have
differentiated into effector T cells, any
encounter with specific antigen triggers
their effector actions without the need
for co-stimulation. Thus, as illustrated
here, a cytotoxic T cell can kill targets
that express only the peptide:MHC
ligand and not co-stimulatory signals
(bottom panel).

are found in the thymus, indicating that they are not deleted during thymic ontogeny; but responsive T cells are not seen in the peripheral blood, showing that they are subsequently inactivated. If the mice also carry either the IL-2 gene or the gene encoding B7.1 attached to the same tissue-specific promoter as the 'pseudo-self' antigen, however, the T cells become activated and destroy the tissue. This shows that IL-2 is necessary and sufficient for the differentiation of naive T cells into armed effector cells in the presence of specific antigen, and suggests that the principal function of B7.1 binding by CD28 is to induce the production of IL-2.

While deletion of potentially autoreactive T cells is readily understood as a simple way to maintain self tolerance, the retention of anergic T cells specific for tissue antigens is less easy to understand. It would seem more economical and efficient to eliminate such cells; indeed, binding of the T-cell receptor on peripheral T cells in the absence of co-stimulators can lead to programmed cell death as well as to anergy. Nevertheless, some T cells persist in an anergic state *in vivo*. One possible explanation for this is that such anergic T cells have a role in preventing responses by naive, non-anergic T cells to foreign antigens that mimic self peptide:self MHC complexes. The persisting anergic T cells could recognize and bind to such peptide:MHC complexes on professional antigen-presenting cells without responding, and thus could compete with naive, potentially autoreactive cells of the same specificity. In this way, anergic T cells could serve to prevent the accidental activation of autoreactive T cells by infectious agents, thus actively contributing to tolerance.

**7-11   Proliferating T cells differentiate into armed effector T cells with
altered surface properties that do not require co-stimulation to act.**

The combination of antigen and co-stimulator induces naive T cells to express IL-2 and its receptor; IL-2 then induces clonal expansion of the naive T cell and the differentiation of its progeny into armed effector T cells. Late in the proliferative phase of the response, after 4–5 days of rapid growth, these T cells differentiate into armed effector T cells that are able to synthesize all the proteins required for their specialized functions as helper, inflammatory, and cytotoxic T cells. As well as acquiring the capacity to synthesize the appropriate arsenal of specialized effector molecules when they encounter antigen on target cells, all classes of armed effector T cells undergo several changes that distinguish them from naive T cells. One of the most critical is in the activation requirements of the cells: once a T cell has differentiated into an armed effector cell, further encounter with its specific antigen results in immune attack without the need for co-stimulation (Fig. 7.22).

This change in the requirement for triggering applies to all classes of armed effector T cells. Its importance is particularly easy to understand in the case of cytotoxic CD8 T cells, which must be able to act on any cell infected with a virus, whether or not the infected cell can express co-stimulatory molecules. However, even B cells and macrophages that have taken up antigen often have too little co-stimulatory activity to activate a naive CD4 T cell. Effector CD4 T cells must be able to activate these B cells and macrophages efficiently, and the change from co-stimulator dependence to independence ensures that any cell displaying antigen can trigger an appropriate T-cell response.

In addition to the reduced stringency of their activation requirements, all armed effector T cells have an increased sensitivity to activation. This is, in part, because of an increase in the numbers of LFA-1 and CD2

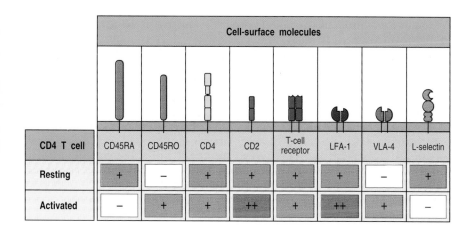

Fig. 7.23　Activation of T cells changes the expression of several cell-surface molecules. Resting naive T cells express L-selectin, through which they home to lymph nodes, with relatively low levels of adhesion molecules, such as CD2 and LFA-1. Upon activation of the T cell, the expression of these molecules changes. Activated T cells express higher densities of the adhesion molecules CD2 and LFA-1, increasing the avidity of the interaction of the activated T cell with potential target cells. Expression of the L-selectin homing receptor is lost and instead increased amounts of the integrin VLA-4 are expressed. VLA-4 acts as a homing receptor for vascular endothelium in sites of inflammation and ensures that activated T cells recirculate through peripheral tissues where they may encounter sites of infection. Finally, the isoform of the CD45 molecule expressed by activated cells changes, by alternative splicing of the RNA transcript of the CD45 gene, so that activated T cells now express the CD45RO isoform that associates with CD4 or CD8 co-receptors and the T-cell receptors. The consequences of this change in CD45 make the T cell more sensitive to stimulation by low concentrations of peptide:MHC complexes.

molecules on their surface, allowing more effective adhesion to target cells. This change is important because most cells in the body do not express the high levels of ICAMs or LFA-3 found on professional antigen-presenting cells.

Finally, in humans, about half of the armed effector T cells lose their cell-surface L-selectin and thus cease to recirculate through lymph nodes. Instead, they express the integrin VLA-4, which allows them to bind to vascular endothelium at sites of inflammation. The T cells are now able to migrate to sites of infection in the peripheral tissues where their armory of effector proteins can be put to use. These changes in the T-cell surface are summarized in Fig. 7.23.

7-12　**The differentiation of CD4 T cells into helper (T$_H$2) or inflammatory (T$_H$1) effector cells is the crucial event in determining whether humoral or cell-mediated immunity will predominate.**

Naive CD8 T cells emerging from the thymus are already predestined to become cytotoxic cells, even though they are not yet expressing any of the differentiated functions of armed effector cells. The case of CD4 T cells, however, is more complex. They can become either inflammatory (T$_H$1) cells, or helper (T$_H$2) cells, and the final decision on which fate the cell will follow is made during its first encounter with antigen. As CD4 T cells differentiate, they are thought to go through an intermediate stage, known as T$_H$0. T$_H$0 cells express some differentiated effector functions of both the inflammatory and helper T cells (Fig. 7.24).

The factors that determine whether a proliferating CD4 T cell will differentiate into an inflammatory T cell or a helper T cell are not fully understood. The cytokines elicited by infectious agents, principally the interleukins **IL-12** and **IL-4**, the co-stimulators used to drive the response, and the nature of the peptide:MHC ligand all have an effect. In particular, since the decision to differentiate into T$_H$1 versus T$_H$2 cells occurs early in the immune response, the ability of pathogens to stimulate cytokine production by cells of the innate, non-adaptive immune system plays an important part in shaping the subsequent adaptive response; we shall learn more about this in Chapter 9. However, the consequences of this decision are profound; selective activation of inflammatory T cells leads to cell-mediated immunity, while selective production of helper T cells provides humoral immunity.

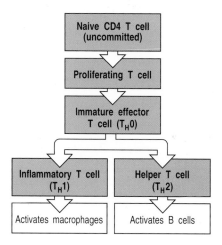

Fig. 7.24　The stages of activation of CD4 T cells. Naive CD4 T cells first respond to peptide:MHC class II complexes by making IL-2 and proliferating. These cells then differentiate into a cell type known as T$_H$0. The T$_H$0 cell has the potential to become either an inflammatory CD4 T cell (T$_H$1) or a helper CD4 T cell (T$_H$2). T$_H$0 cells may have some effector actions in their own right.

A striking example of the difference this can make to the outcome of infection is seen in leprosy, a disease caused by infection with *Mycobacterium leprae*. *M. leprae*, like *M. tuberculosis*, grows in macrophage vesicles, and effective host defense requires macrophage activation by inflammatory T cells. In patients with tuberculoid leprosy, in which inflammatory T cells are preferentially induced, few live bacteria are found, little antibody is produced, and although skin and peripheral nerves are damaged by the inflammatory responses associated with macrophage activation, the disease progresses slowly and the patient usually survives. However, when helper T cells are preferentially induced, the main response is humoral, the antibodies cannot reach the intracellular bacteria, and the patients develop lepromatous leprosy, in which the *M. leprae* grows abundantly in macrophages, causing gross tissue destruction, which is eventually fatal.

7-13 | Naive CD8 T cells can be activated in different ways to become armed cytotoxic effector cells.

Naive CD8 T cells can differentiate only into cytotoxic cells, and perhaps because the effector actions of these cells are so destructive, they require more co-stimulatory activity to activate them than naive CD4 T cells. This requirement can be met in two ways. The simplest is activation by antigen-presenting cells, such as dendritic cells, that have high intrinsic co-stimulatory activity. These cells can directly stimulate CD8 T cells to synthesize the IL-2 that drives their own proliferation and differentiation (Fig. 7.25).

Cytotoxic T-cell responses to some viruses and tissue grafts, however, seem to require the presence of CD4 T cells during the priming of the naive CD8 T cell. In these responses, both the naive CD8 T cell and the CD4 T cell must recognize antigen on the surface of the same antigen-presenting cell. It is thought that, in this case, the actions of the CD4 T cell may be necessary to compensate for co-stimulation by the antigen-presenting cell that is inadequate for direct activation of the CD8 T cell. This compensatory effect could occur in either of two ways. If the CD4 T cell is an armed effector cell, it may activate the antigen-presenting cell to express higher levels of co-stimulatory activity (we shall see that this is one of the actions of the specialized molecules produced by effector CD4 T cells). This would enable the antigen-presenting cell to co-stimulate the CD8 T cell (Fig. 7.26, left panels).

Alternatively, the CD4 T cell may be a naive or memory T cell secreting IL-2 in response to antigen and low levels of co-stimulatory molecules. As IL-2 receptors can be induced by receptor ligation alone, the CD8 T cell may express IL-2 receptors even though it cannot produce the IL-2 it needs to drive its own proliferation. The IL-2 in this case comes instead from the adjacent responding CD4 T cell (Fig. 7.26, right panels). It is known that adding IL-2 can eliminate the need for a co-stimulatory signal for CD8 T-cell activation in experimental situations, in keeping with the general finding that the crucial role of co-stimulation of T cells is the production of sufficient IL-2 to drive their clonal expansion, allowing them to differentiate into armed effector T cells.

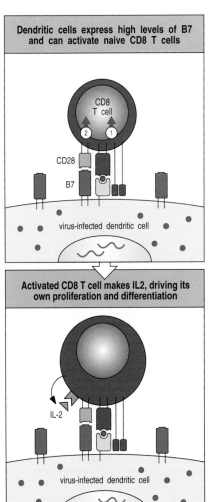

Dendritic cells express high levels of B7 and can activate naive CD8 T cells

CD8 T cell

CD28

B7

virus-infected dendritic cell

Activated CD8 T cell makes IL2, driving its own proliferation and differentiation

IL-2

virus-infected dendritic cell

Fig. 7.25 Naive CD8 T cells can be activated directly by potent antigen-presenting cells. Naive CD8 T cells that encounter peptide:MHC class I complexes on the surface of dendritic cells, which express high levels of co-stimulatory molecules (top panel), are activated to produce IL-2 (bottom panel) and proliferate in response to it, eventually differentiating into armed cytotoxic CD8 T cells (not shown).

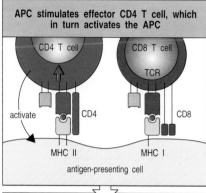

APC stimulates effector CD4 T cell, which in turn activates the APC

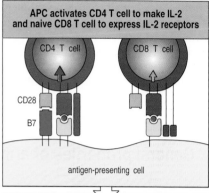

APC activates CD4 T cell to make IL-2 and naive CD8 T cell to express IL-2 receptors

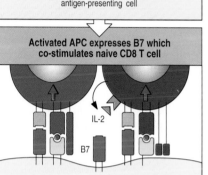

Activated APC expresses B7 which co-stimulates naive CD8 T cell

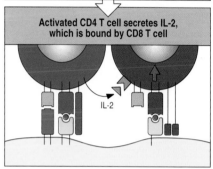

Activated CD4 T cell secretes IL-2, which is bound by CD8 T cell

Fig. 7.26   Some CD8 T-cell responses require CD4 T cells. CD8 T cells recognizing antigen on weakly co-stimulating cells may become activated only in the presence of CD4 T cells bound to the same antigen-presenting cell (APC). There are two ways in which CD4 T cells may contribute to the activation of CD8 T cells. Left panels: an effector CD4 T cell may recognize antigen on the antigen-presenting cell and be triggered to induce increased levels of co-stimulatory activity on the antigen-presenting cell, which in turn activates the CD8 T cell to make its own IL-2. Right panels: alternatively, a naive CD4 T cell activated by the antigen-presenting cell may provide the IL-2 required for the proliferation and differentiation of the CD8 T cell. Which of these two mechanisms operates *in vivo* is not known.

Summary.

The crucial first step in adaptive immunity is the activation of naive antigen-specific T cells by professional antigen-presenting cells. The most distinctive feature of professional antigen-presenting cells is the expression of co-stimulatory activities, of which the B7.1 and B7.2 molecules are the best characterized. Naive T cells will respond to antigen only when one cell presents both specific antigen to the T-cell receptor, and a B7 molecule to CD28, the receptor for B7 on the T cell. The three cell types that can serve as professional antigen-presenting cells are macrophages, dendritic cells, and B cells. Each of these cells has a distinct function in eliciting immune responses. Macrophages efficiently ingest particulate antigens and are induced by infectious agents to express MHC class II molecules and co-stimulatory activity. Dendritic cells express both MHC class II molecules and co-stimulatory activity constitutively, and may be specialized to present pathogens, such as some viruses, that do not induce co-stimulatory activity in macrophages. The unique ability of B cells to bind and internalize soluble protein antigens via their receptors may be important in activating T cells to this class of antigen, provided that co-stimulatory molecules are also induced on the B cell. The activation of T cells by a professional antigen-presenting cell leads to their proliferation and the differentiation of their progeny into armed effector T cells. The proliferation and differentiation of T cells depends on the production of cytokines such as the T-cell growth factor IL-2 and its binding to a high-affinity receptor on the activated T cell. T cells whose antigen receptors are ligated in the absence of co-stimulatory signals fail to make IL-2 and instead become anergic. This dual requirement for both receptor ligation and co-stimulation helps to prevent naive T cells from responding to antigens on self tissue cells, which lack co-stimulator activity. Proliferating T cells develop into armed effector T cells, the critical event in most adaptive immune responses. Once an expanded clone of T cells achieves effector function, its progeny can act on any target cell that displays antigen on its surface. This allows armed effector T cells to recognize any cell that is displaying antigen, whether it is a professional antigen-presenting cell or not. Effector T cells can mediate a variety of functions, the most important of which are the killing of infected cells by CD8 cytotoxic T cells and the activation of macrophages by inflammatory CD4 T cells (T_H1), which together make up cell-mediated immunity. Helper CD4 T cells (T_H2) are needed to activate B cells to produce antibody, thus driving the humoral immune response.

General properties of armed effector T cells.

All T-cell effector functions involve the interaction of an armed effector T cell with a target cell displaying specific antigen (Fig. 7.27). The effector proteins released by these T cells are focused on the appropriate target cell by mechanisms that are activated by the specific recognition of antigen on the target cell surface. The focusing mechanism is common to all types of effector T cells, while their effector actions depend upon the array of membrane and secreted proteins they express upon receptor ligation and are specific to the different effector cell types.

Fig. 7.27 There are three classes of effector T cells, specialized to deal with three classes of pathogens. CD8 cytotoxic cells or cytotoxic T lymphocytes (CTL) (left panels) kill target cells that display antigenic fragments of cytosolic pathogens, most notably viruses, bound to MHC class I molecules at the cell surface. Inflammatory CD4 T cells (T_H1) (middle panels) and helper CD4 T cells (T_H2) (right panels) both express the CD4 co-receptor and recognize fragments of antigens degraded within intracellular vesicles, displayed at the cell surface by MHC class II molecules. The inflammatory CD4 T cells, upon activation, activate macrophages, allowing them to destroy intracellular microorganisms more efficiently. Helper CD4 T cells, on the other hand, activate B cells to differentiate and secrete immunoglobulins, the effector molecules of the humoral immune response.

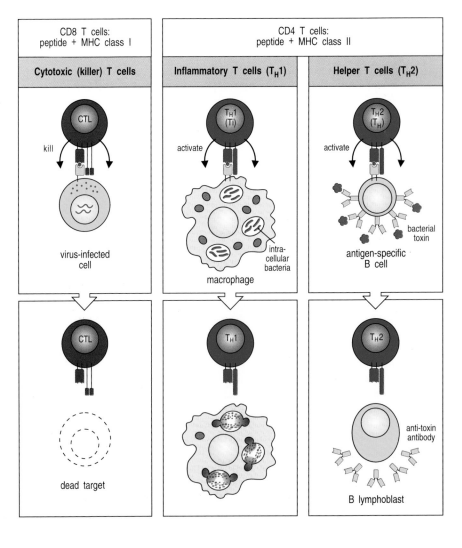

7-14 Effector T-cell interactions with target cells are initiated by antigen non-specific cell-adhesion molecules.

Once an effector T cell has completed its differentiation in the lymphoid tissues it must find the target cells that are displaying the specific peptide:MHC complex that it recognizes. This occurs in two steps. First, the armed effector T cells emigrate from their site of activation in the lymphoid tissues and enter the blood. Second, because of the cell-surface changes that have occurred during differentiation, they migrate into the peripheral tissues, particularly at sites of infection to which they are guided by changes in adhesion molecules expressed on the endothelium of the local blood vessels (see Chapter 9).

The initial binding of an effector T cell to its target, like that of naive T cells to antigen-presenting cells, is an antigen non-specific interaction mediated by the LFA-1 and CD2 adhesion molecules. However, the level of LFA-1 and CD2 is two- to four-fold higher on armed effector T cells than on naive T cells and, therefore, armed effector T cells can bind efficiently to target cells that have lower levels of ICAMs amd LFA-3 on their surface than do antigen-presenting cells. This interaction, again like that of naive T cells with antigen-presenting cells, is normally transient unless specific recognition of antigen on the target cell triggers a change in the affinity of LFA-1 for its ligands on the target cell surface. This change causes the T cell to bind more tightly to its target, and to remain bound for long enough to release its specific effector molecules. Armed CD4 effector T cells, which activate macrophages or induce B cells to secrete antibody, must maintain contact with their targets for relatively long periods, as we shall see when we consider the distinctive features of each type of effector cell action. Cytotoxic T cells, by contrast, can be observed under the microscope attaching to and dissociating from successive specific targets relatively rapidly as they kill them (Fig. 7.28). This may reflect a unique function of CD8, which binds more tightly to MHC class I molecules after T-cell receptor ligation and provides for additional adhesion to the target cell. Killing the target, or some local change in the T cell, then allows the effector T cell to detach and address new targets. How armed CD4 effector T cells disengage from their targets is not known, although some evidence suggests that CD4 binding directly to MHC class II molecules on target cells that are not displaying antigen provides a signal for detachment.

7-15 The T-cell receptor complex directs the release of effector molecules and focuses them on the target cell.

The binding of the T-cell receptor to antigen on a target cell not only increases the strength with which the T cell binds its target, it also signals a reorganization of the cytoskeleton in the T cell. This polarizes the effector cell so as to focus the release of effector molecules at the site

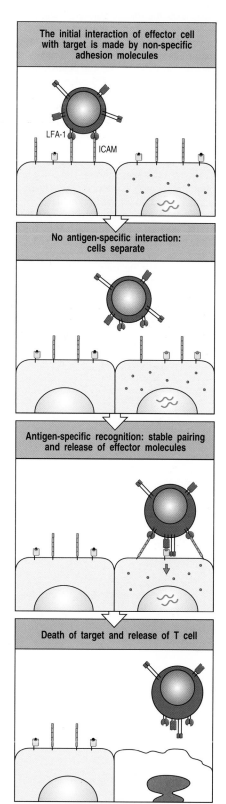

The initial interaction of effector cell with target is made by non-specific adhesion molecules

LFA-1   ICAM

No antigen-specific interaction: cells separate

Antigen-specific recognition: stable pairing and release of effector molecules

Death of target and release of T cell

Fig. 7.28 Interactions of T cells with their targets are mediated initially by non-specific adhesion molecules. The major initial interaction is between LFA-1 expressed by the T cell, illustrated here as a CD8 cytotoxic T cell, and ICAM-1, ICAM-2, or ICAM-3 expressed by the target cell (top panel). This binding allows the T cell to remain in contact with the target cell and to scan its surface for the presence of specific peptide:MHC complexes. If the target cell does not express the specific antigen, the T cell disengages (second panel) and can scan other potential targets. If the target cell expresses the specific antigen (third panel), signaling through the T-cell receptor increases the strength of the adhesive interactions, prolonging the contact between the two cells, and stimulating the T cell to deliver its effector molecules. The T cell then disengages (bottom panel).

Fig. 7.29 The polarization of T cells during specific antigen recognition allows cytokine release and effector molecule expression to be focused on the antigen-bearing target cell. T cells, like all nucleated cells, contain several subcellular organelles such as the Golgi apparatus, the microtubule-organizing center (MTOC) and various populations of vesicles, as shown in the upper right panel. Binding of a T cell to its target causes the T cell to become polarized (illustrated here for a CD8 cytotoxic cell): the cytoskeleton is reoriented to align the Golgi apparatus and the microtubule-organizing center towards the target cell. Protein secretion is thus specifically directed onto the target cell; this is shown here for granules released by a cytotoxic T cell (left panels). The photomicrograph in panel a shows lytic granules stained for the fragmentin granzyme A (green) clustered around the MTOC stained with anti-tubulin antibody (red). Panel b shows a cytotoxic T cell killing a target cell, where the granules are localized at the interface with the target cell; panel c shows the release of granules from the cytotoxic T cell. Panels a and b courtesy of G Griffiths. Panel c courtesy of E Podack.

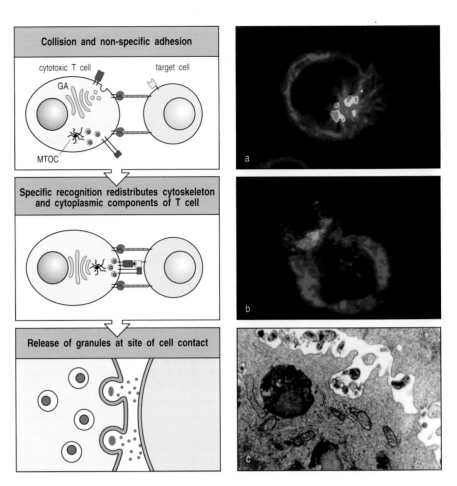

of contact with the target cell (Fig. 7.29). Thus, the antigen-specific T-cell receptor controls the effector action of the T cell in three ways: it induces stable binding of effector cells to their targets, forming a narrow space within which effector molecules can be concentrated; it triggers the release of the effector molecules; and it focuses the delivery of these effector molecules onto the antigen-bearing target. All these mechanisms result in selective action of the effector molecules on cells bearing specific antigen. In this way, effector T-cell action is highly selective for those target cells that display antigen, although the effector molecules themselves are not antigen-specific.

7-16   The effector functions of T cells are mediated by induced expression of both membrane-bound and secreted molecules.

Most of the best understood functions of armed effector T cells are mediated by secreted molecules whose release is stimulated by specific recognition of antigen. These molecules fall into two broad classes: cytotoxins, which are released by CD8 cytotoxic T cells and by some inflammatory CD4 T cells; and cytokines, which are released by all effector T cells and are the principal mediators of CD4 T-cell effector actions. The cytotoxins are not specific and can act on any cell; the cytokines act through specific receptors on the target cell and the main effector actions of CD4 cells are therefore directed at specialized cells expressing those receptors.

As well as these secreted mediators, which we discuss in more detail later, all three classes of effector T cells express membrane-associated effector molecules, which, like cytokines, are induced by recognition of antigen on the target cell. For this reason, supernatants of activated T cells rarely reproduce the full effect of the cells from which they are derived, even when used at very high concentrations. Some of these cell-surface effector molecules are membrane-bound forms of molecules belonging to the tumor necrosis factor (TNF) family of proteins, and their receptors on the target cells are members of the TNF-receptor family. This is known to be the case, however, only for helper T cells and cytotoxic T cells. For example, for particular helper T cells the TNF-related partner is a T-cell membrane molecule called the **CD40 ligand**, which binds to a receptor called **CD40** on the B cell. For CD8 cytotoxic T cells, the TNF-related partner is a molecule called the **Fas ligand**, which binds to a receptor called **Fas** on the target cell. Some CD4 T cells are cytotoxic, and these also express the Fas ligand; they do not however, express the non-specific cytotoxic molecules secreted by CD8 cytotoxic T cells. We shall discuss the CD40 ligand further in Chapter 8 where we deal with the effector action of helper T cells. The effector actions and main effector molecules of all three functional classes of effector T cells are summarized in Fig. 7.30. The cytokines themselves are a diverse group of molecules and will be reviewed briefly next, before we discuss the T-cell cytokines and their contributions to the effector actions of cytotoxic and inflammatory T cells.

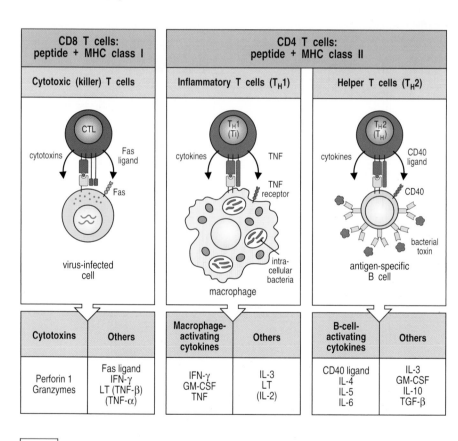

Fig. 7.30 **The three main types of armed effector T cell produce distinct sets of effector molecules.** CD8 T cells are predominantly killer T cells that recognize pathogen-derived peptides bound to MHC class I molecules. They release perforin 1 (which creates holes in the target-cell membranes), granzymes (which are proteases), and often the cytokine IFN-γ. A membrane-bound effector molecule on CD8 T cells is believed to be a ligand for Fas, a receptor whose activation induces apoptosis. CD4 T cells recognize peptides bound to MHC class II molecules and are of two functional types: inflammatory CD4 T cells (T$_H$1); and helper CD4 T cells (T$_H$2). Inflammatory CD4 T cells are specialized for activation of macrophages that contain or have ingested pathogens; they secrete IFN-γ as well as other effector molecules, and are thought to express membrane-bound TNF. Helper CD4 T cells are specialized for B-cell activation; they secrete the growth factors IL-4, IL-5 and IL-6, all of which play a part in the activation and differentiation of B cells. T$_H$2 cells express the membrane-bound effector molecule CD40 ligand, which binds to CD40 on the B cell and induces proliferation.

7-17   Cytokines can act locally or at a distance.

Cytokines are small soluble proteins produced by one cell that alter the behavior or properties of another cell. They are released by many cells in addition to those of the immune system. The cytokines released by phagocytic cells are discussed in Chapter 9 where we deal with the inflammatory reactions that play an important part in innate immunity; here we shall be concerned mainly with the cytokines that mediate the effector functions of CD4 T cells. Cytokines produced by lymphocytes are often called **lymphokines** but this nomenclature can be confusing because some lymphokines are also secreted by non-lymphoid cells;

we shall therefore use the generic term 'cytokine' for all of them. Many cytokines produced by T cells are given the name **interleukin (IL)** followed by a number; we have already encountered **interleukin-2 (IL-2)**. Cytokines of immunological interest are listed in Appendix II.

Most cytokines have a multitude of different biological effects when tested at high concentration in biological assays *in vitro*, making simple statements about their function difficult, although targeted disruption of cytokine genes in gene knock-out mice (see Section 2-38) has helped to clarify their physiological roles. The major actions of the cytokines produced by effector T cells are given in Fig. 7.31. As the effect of a cytokine varies depending on the target cell, the actions are listed according to the major target cell types — B cells, T cells, macrophages, tissue cells, and hematopoietic cells.

Cytokine	Produced by	Effects on				
		B cells	T cells	Macrophages	Hematopoietic cells	Other somatic cells
Interleukin-4 (IL-4)	T_H2	Activation, growth IgG1, IgE response ↑MHC class II induction	Growth Survival	Inhibits macrophage activation	↑Growth of mast cells	–
Interleukin-5 (IL-5)	T_H2	Differentiation IgA synthesis	–	–	↑Eosinophil growth and differentiation	–
Interleukin-6 (IL-6)	T_H2	Growth and differentiation	Co-stimulator (Fig. 9.14)	–	Induces colony-stimulating factor	Acute-phase protein release (Fig. 9.15)
Interleukin-10 (IL-10)	T_H2	↑MHC class II	Inhibits T_H1	Inhibits cytokine release	Co-stimulates mast cell growth	–
Interleukin-2 (IL-2)	T_H1, some CTL	Stimulates growth and J-chain synthesis	Growth	–	Stimulates NK cell growth	–
Interferon-γ (IFN-γ)	T_H1, CTL	Differentiation IgG2a synthesis	Kills	Activation ↑MHC class I and class II	Activates NK cells	Antiviral ↑MHC class I and class II
Lymphotoxin (LT, TNF-β)	T_H1, some CTL	Inhibits	Kills	Activates, induces NO production	Activates neutrophils	Kills fibroblasts and tumor cells
Interleukin-3 (IL-3)	T_H1, T_H2, some CTL	–	–	–	Growth factor for progenitor hematopoietic cells (multi-CSF)	–
Tumor necrosis factor-α (TNF-α)	T_H1, some T_H2, some CTL	–	–	Activates, induces NO production		
Granulocyte-macrophage colony-stimulating factor (GM-CSF)	T_H1, some T_H2, some CTL	Differentiation	Inhibits growth	Activation	Stimulates production of granulocytes and macrophages (myelopoiesis)	–
Transforming growth factor-β (TGF-β)	T cells Macrophages	Inhibits growth IgA switch factor	–	Inhibits activation	Activates neutrophils	Inhibits/ stimulates cell growth

Fig. 7.31 The nomenclature and functions of well-defined T-cell cytokines. The major actions are noted in boxes. Each cytokine has multiple activities on different cell types. The mixture of cytokines secreted by a given cell type produces many effects through what is called a 'cytokine network'. Major activities of effector cytokines are highlighted in red. (↑ = increase; CTL = cytotoxic T lymphocyte.)

Fig. 7.32 Inflammatory CD4 T cells (TH1), helper CD4 T cells (TH2), and their TH0 precursor secrete distinct but overlapping sets of cytokines. GM-CSF and IL-3, which are secreted by both inflammatory and helper CD4 T cells, have distant effects on hematopoietic cells in the bone marrow. The cytokines released only by inflammatory CD4 T cells activate macrophages; those released only by helper CD4 T cells activate B cells. See Fig. 7.31 for cytokine abbreviations.

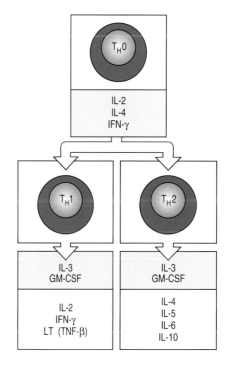

A major cytokine produced by CD8 effector T cells is **interferon-γ (IFN-γ)**, which can block viral replication. The principal cytokines produced by the different classes of CD4 effector T cells are indicated in Fig. 7.32. Helper and inflammatory T cells release different but overlapping sets of cytokines, which define their distinct actions in immunity; the **TH0 cells** from which both these functional classes are thought to derive also secrete cytokines (other than IL-2) and may have some effector function. Most cytokines have local actions that synergize with those of membrane-bound effector molecules. Helper (TH2) T cells secrete **IL-4**, **IL-5**, **IL-6**, and **IL-10**, all of which activate B cells; inflammatory (TH1) T cells secrete IFN-γ and **tumor necrosis factor-α (TNF-α)**, which are the main macrophage-activating cytokines, and **lymphotoxin (LT or TNF-γβ)**, which is directly cytotoxic for some cells. Growth of TH2 clones is driven by IL-4, while growth of cloned TH1 and TH0 cells is mainly or exclusively driven by IL-2.

Some cytokines, however, have more distant effects. **IL-3** and **granulocyte-macrophage colony-stimulating factor (GM-CSF)**, for example, which are released by both types of CD4 effector T cell, help to recruit effector cells in infection by acting on bone marrow cells to stimulate **myelopoiesis**, the production of macrophages and granulocytes. These are important effector cells in both humoral and cell-mediated immunity. How the local and more distant effects of the cytokines may reflect the amounts of cytokine released and the stability of the cytokine *in vivo* is not yet known.

Cytokines act on receptors that can be grouped into four families of structures with genetic, structural, and functional similarity (Fig. 7.33). Similarly, cytokines themselves can be grouped into families based on their structure, the linkage of their genes, and the cells that make them. For instance, IL-3, IL-5, and GM-CSF are related structurally, their genes are closely linked in the genome, and they are major cytokines produced by helper T cells. In addition, they bind to closely related receptors; IL-3, IL-5, and GM-CSF receptors share a common β chain. This is also true of other groups of cytokines, suggesting that cytokines and their receptors may have diversified together in the evolution of increasingly specialized effector functions.

Fig. 7.33 Cytokine receptors belong to four families of receptor proteins, each with a distinctive structure. Some cytokine receptors are members of the immunoglobulin superfamily, some are members of the hematopoietin receptor family, some are members of the tumor necrosis factor (TNF) receptor family and some are members of the chemokine receptor family. Each family member is a variant with a distinct specificity, performing a particular function on the cell that expresses it. In the case of the hematopoietin receptor family, the α chain often defines the ligand specificity of the receptor, while the β chain confers the intracellular signaling function. For the TNF receptor family, the ligands may be associated with the cell membrane rather than being secreted. Of the receptors listed here, some have been mentioned already in this book, some will occur in later chapters, and some are important examples from other biological systems. The diagrams indicate the representations of these receptors you will encounter throughout this book. MIP-1, Macrophage inflammatory protein-1; PF4, Platelet factor 4.

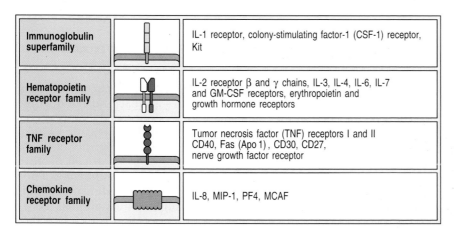

Immunoglobulin superfamily		IL-1 receptor, colony-stimulating factor-1 (CSF-1) receptor, Kit
Hematopoietin receptor family		IL-2 receptor β and γ chains, IL-3, IL-4, IL-6, IL-7 and GM-CSF receptors, erythropoietin and growth hormone receptors
TNF receptor family		Tumor necrosis factor (TNF) receptors I and II CD40, Fas (Apo 1), CD30, CD27, nerve growth factor receptor
Chemokine receptor family		IL-8, MIP-1, PF4, MCAF

	Summary.

Interactions between armed effector T cells and their targets are initiated by transient non-specific adhesion between the cells. T-cell effector functions are only elicited when peptide:MHC complexes on the surface of the target cell are recognized by the receptor on an armed effector T cell. This recognition event triggers the armed effector T cell to adhere more strongly to the antigen-bearing target cell and to release its effector molecules directly at the target cell, leading to the activation or death of the target. The consequences of antigen recognition by an armed effector T cell are determined largely by the set of effector molecules it produces when stimulated. Effector T cells mediate many of their effects by secreting cytokines; helper CD4 T cells (T_H2) secrete B-cell-activating cytokines, while inflammatory CD4 T cells (T_H1) secrete cytokines that activate macrophages, and CD8 killer T cells release IFN-γ. CD8 T cells also release cytotoxins, which are the principal effector molecules of CD8 cells. The cytokines act on cytokine receptors expressed locally on the target cell or at a distance on hematopoietic cells. The action of cytokines on cells via cytokine receptors, together with that of the cytotoxins that are released by CD8 cells, account for effector functions of T cells.

T-cell mediated cytotoxicity.

All viruses, and some bacteria, multiply in the cytoplasm of infected cells; indeed, the virus is a highly sophisticated parasite that has no bio-synthetic or metabolic apparatus of its own and, in consequence, can only replicate inside cells. Once inside cells, these pathogens are not accessible to antibodies and can be eliminated only by the destruction of the infected cells on which they depend. This role in host defense is fulfilled by cytotoxic CD8 T cells. The critical role of cytotoxic T cells in limiting such infections is seen in the increased susceptibility of animals artificially depleted of these T cells, or of mice or humans that lack the MHC class I molecules that present antigen to CD8 cells. As well as controlling infection by viruses and cytoplasmic bacteria, CD8 T cells are important in controlling some protozoal infections and are crucial, for example, in host defense against the protozoon *Toxoplasma gondii*, a cytoplasmic parasite. The elimination of infected cells without destruction of healthy tissue requires the cytotoxic mechanisms of CD8 T cells to be both powerful and accurately targeted.

7-18	Cytotoxic T cells can induce target cells to undergo programmed cell death.

Cells can die in either of two different ways. Physical or chemical injury, such as the deprivation of oxygen that occurs in heart muscle during a heart attack, or membrane damage with antibody and complement, leads to cell disintegration or **necrosis**. The dead or necrotic tissue is taken up and degraded by phagocytic cells, which eventually clear the damaged tissue and heal the wound. The other form of cell death is known as **programmed cell death** or **apoptosis**. Apoptosis is a normal cellular response that is crucial in the tissue remodeling that occurs during development and metamorphosis in multicellular animals. As we saw in Chapter 6, most thymocytes die an apoptotic death when they fail positive selection or are negatively selected as a result of recognizing self antigens. The first changes seen in apoptotic cell death are fragmentation of the DNA, disruption of the nucleus, and alterations in cell morphology. The cell then destroys itself from within, shrinking and degrading itself until little is left. A hallmark of this type of cell death is the fragmentation of nuclear DNA into 200 base pair (bp) fragments through the activation of endogenous nucleases that cleave between nucleosomes, each of which contains about 200 bp of DNA.

There is good evidence that cytotoxic effector T cells kill their targets largely by programming them to undergo apoptosis. When cytotoxic T cells are mixed with target cells and rapidly brought into contact by centrifugation, they can program specific target cells to die within 5 minutes, although death may take hours to become fully evident. An early feature of T-cell killing is degradation of target cell DNA, while later effects include the loss of membrane integrity, which may also be induced by other cytotoxic mechanisms. The short period required by cytotoxic T cells to program their targets to die is believed to reflect the release of preformed effector molecules by the T cell which activates an endogenous apoptotic pathway within the target cell (Fig. 7.34).

The apoptotic mechanism, as well as killing the host cell, may also act directly on cytosolic pathogens. For example, the nucleases that are activated in apoptosis to destroy cellular DNA can also degrade viral DNA, preventing the assembly of virions and thus the release of virus and the infection of nearby cells. Other enzymes activated as part of

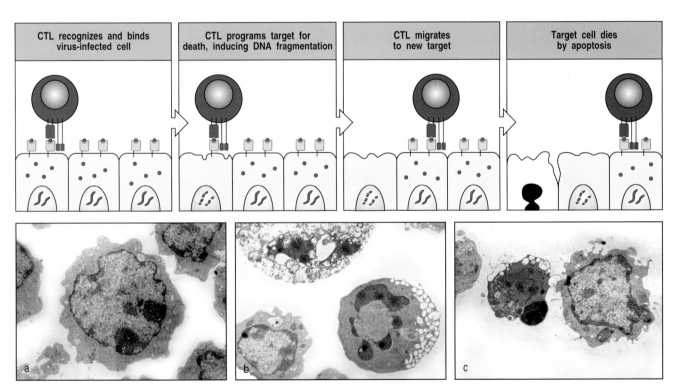

Fig. 7.34　Cytotoxic CD8 T cells can induce programmed cell death (apoptosis) in target cells. Specific recognition of peptide:MHC complexes on a target cell (top panels) by a cytotoxic CD8 T cell (CTL) leads to the death of the target cell by apoptosis. Cytotoxic T cells can recycle to kill multiple targets. Each killing event requires the same series of steps, including receptor binding and directed release of cytotoxic mediators. The process of apoptosis is shown in the micrographs (bottom panels), where panel a shows a healthy cell with a regular nucleus. Early in apoptosis (panel b) the chromatin becomes condensed and, although the cell sheds membrane vesicles, the integrity of the cell membrane is retained, in contrast to the necrotic cell in the upper part of the same field. In late stages of apoptosis (panel c), the cell nucleus is very condensed, no mitochondria are visible and the cell has lost much of its cytoplasm and membrane through the shedding of vesicles. Photographs (x 3 500) courtesy of R Windsor and E Hirst.

Protein released by cytotoxic T cells	Actions on target cells
Perforin 1 (P1)	Polymerizes to form a pore in target membrane
Granzymes (fragmentins)	Serine proteases, required for some killing
Lymphotoxin (TNF-β)	? Induces apoptosis

Fig. 7.35   Several cytotoxic proteins released by cytotoxic T cells have a role in killing target cells.

apoptosis may destroy other cytosolic pathogens before the plasma membrane disintegrates and they are released from the cell. Apoptosis is therefore preferable to necrosis as a means of killing cells as, in necrosis, intact pathogens are released by the dead cell to continue infection or are ingested by healthy phagocytes, which may then become parasitized.

<table>
<tr><td>7-19</td><td>Cytotoxic T cells store cytotoxic proteins in preformed granules that they release by directed exocytosis upon recognizing antigen on a target cell.</td></tr>
</table>

The principal mechanism through which cytotoxic T cells act is by the release of secretory granules upon recognition of antigen on the surface of a target cell. These secretory granules contain at least two distinct classes of **cytotoxins** that are expressed selectively in cytotoxic T cells (Fig. 7.35). One of these, **perforin**, can polymerize to generate transmembrane pores in cell membranes. The other class comprises at least three proteases called **granzymes** or **fragmentins**, which belong to the same family of enzymes (the serine proteases) as the digestive enzymes trypsin and chymotrypsin. Granules that store perforin can be seen in armed CD8 cytotoxic effector cells in tissue lesions (Fig. 7.36), and the *in vitro* combination of perforin and fragmentins can mimic the action of cytotoxic effector T cells.

Secretory granules are found in many cell types, such as neurons, pancreatic acinar cells and mast cells, which are specialized for the rapid release of secreted proteins on stimulation by a specific signal. After stimulation, the contents of the granule are released promptly by fusion of the granule and plasma membranes. In similar fashion, the release of granules from cytotoxic T cells occurs almost immediately after receptor ligation and requires no new protein or RNA synthesis. This allows cytotoxic T cells to act very rapidly on their targets, programming them for eventual lysis in a matter of minutes.

When purified granules from cytotoxic T cells are added to target cells *in vitro*, they lyse the cells by creating pores in the lipid bilayer. The pores consist of polymers of perforin 1, which is a major constituent of these granules. On release from the granule, perforin 1 polymerizes into a cylindrical structure that is lipophilic on the outside and hydrophilic down a hollow center of inner diameter of 16 nm. This structure can insert into lipid bilayers, forming a pore that allows water and salts to pass rapidly into the cell (Fig. 7.37). With the integrity of the cell membrane destroyed, the cells die rapidly. Purified granules can kill target cells *in vitro* without inducing fragmentation of cellular DNA but this

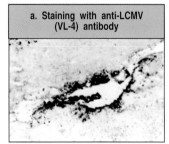
a. Staining with anti-LCMV (VL-4) antibody

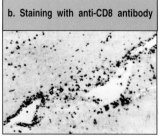
b. Staining with anti-CD8 antibody

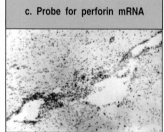
c. Probe for perforin mRNA

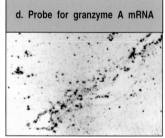
d. Probe for granzyme A mRNA

Fig. 7.36   CD8 T cells expressing perforin and granzymes can be seen in viral infections. In brains of mice infected with the lymphocytic choriomeningitis virus (LCMV) the presence of virus-infected cells can be demonstrated using antibodies specific for viral proteins (panel a). CD8 T cells are detected by staining with a CD8-specific antibody (panel b). These CD8 T cells are making both perforin (panel c) and granzymes (panel d) as can be revealed using radiolabeled probes for perforin and granzyme mRNAs and a photographic emulsion to show the location of the radiolabeled probes. Photographs courtesy of E Podack.

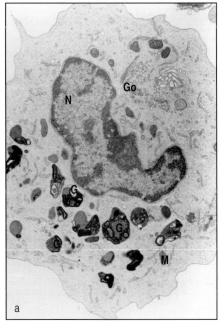
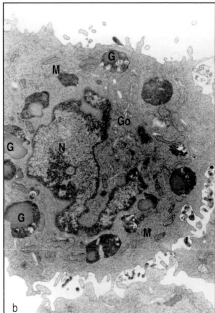
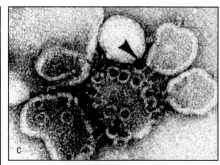
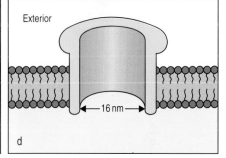

Fig. 7.37 Cytotoxic T cells can kill by inserting perforin into the target-cell membrane. Perforin molecules, as well as several other effector molecules, are contained in the granules of cytotoxic T cells (panel a: G, granules; N, nucleus; M, mitochondria; Go, Golgi apparatus). When a CD8 cytotoxic T cell recognizes its target, the granules are released onto the target cell (panel b, bottom right quadrant). The perforin molecules released from the granules polymerize and insert into the membrane of the target cell to form pores. The structure of these pores is best visualized when purified perforin is added to synthetic lipid vesicles (panel c: pores are seen both end on, as circles, and sideways on, arrow). The pores span the target cell membrane (panel d). Photographs courtesy of E Podack.

lytic mechanism of cell killing probably occurs only at artificially high levels of perforin that do not reflect the physiological activity of cytotoxic T cells. Instead, it is thought that *in vivo* a limited number of perforin pores serves to allow the entry of fragmentins into the target cell and that these are responsible for inducing apoptosis.

Evidence for this comes from *in vitro* studies in which the contents of secretory granules were added separately to target cells. When one of the fragmentins is added directly to target cells, it has no effect, but when the same fragmentin is added to target cells together with a limited amount of perforin, fragmentation of cellular DNA into oligomers of 200 bp occurs rapidly, as in apoptosis. It should be noted that fragmentins are proteases and, therefore, cannot be directly responsible for the fragmentation of DNA. They are thought to act by inducing the cell's endogenous apoptotic program, perhaps by mimicking the action of proteases that form part of the apoptotic pathway. A protease closely related to interleukin-1β converting enzyme, or ICE, is known to be involved in programmed cell death and has a similar specificity to the fragmentin, granzyme B. It is possible that granzyme B cleaves the same substrates as ICE and thus is able to activate apoptosis.

7-20   Membrane proteins of CD8 T cells can also activate apoptosis.

The release of granule contents accounts for most of the cytotoxic activity of CD8 effector T cells, as shown by the loss of most killing activity in perforin gene knock-out mice. Furthermore, granule-mediated killing is strictly calcium-dependent, yet some cytotoxic action of CD8 T cells survives calcium depletion. Finally, some CD4 cells are also capable of killing other cells, yet do not contain granules and make neither perforin nor fragmentins. These observations imply that there is a second independent mechanism of cytotoxicity. This mechanism is believed to involve the activation of Fas, a receptor of the TNF receptor family, in the target cell membrane. Fas, also known as Apo-1 (see Fig. 7.33), is known to induce apoptosis when activated by antibodies against it. The Fas ligand, which is induced in the cytotoxic T cell membrane has been identified as a membrane-bound member of the TNF family.

7-21   Cytotoxic T cells selectively kill targets expressing specific antigen.

When cytotoxic T cells are offered an equal mixture of two target cells, one bearing specific antigen and the other not, they kill only the target cell bearing the specific antigen. The 'innocent bystander' cell and the cytotoxic T cell itself are not killed, despite the fact that cloned cytotoxic T cells can be recognized and killed by other cytotoxic T cells like any tissue cell. At first sight, this may seem surprising, since the effector molecules released by cytotoxic T cells lack any specificity for antigen. The explanation probably lies in the highly polar release of the effector molecules. We have seen (Fig. 7.29) that cytotoxic T cells orient their secretory apparatus to focus it on the point of contact with a target cell (Fig. 7.38); indeed, cytotoxic T cells attached to several different target cells reorient their secretory apparatus towards each cell in turn and kill them one by one, strongly suggesting that the mechanism whereby cytotoxic mediators are released allows attack at only one focal point of contact at any one time. This may reflect, in part, the focal expression of cell-surface effector molecules in the vicinity of crosslinked receptors: such localized expression of membrane molecules can be seen clearly in the case of B-cell activation by helper T cells. The narrowly focused action of cytotoxic CD8 T cells allows them to kill single infected cells in a tissue without creating widespread tissue damage (Fig. 7.39) and is of critical importance in tissues where cell regeneration does not occur, as in neurons of the central nervous system, or is very limited, as in the pancreatic islets.

7-22   Cytotoxic T cells also act by releasing cytokines.

Although the secretion of perforin and fragmentins is known to be a major mechanism by which CD8 cytotoxic T cells eliminate infection, with expression of Fas L playing a lesser role, most cytotoxic CD8 T cells also release IFN-γ and TNF-α, which contribute to host defense in several other ways. IFN-γ directly inhibits viral replication, and also induces increased expression of MHC class I and peptide transporter molecules

Time 0

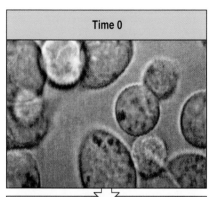

After 1 minute

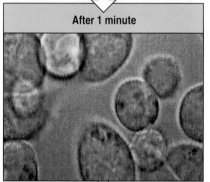

After 4 minutes

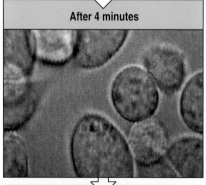

After 40 minutes

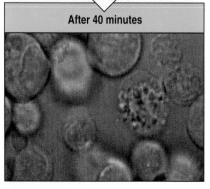

Fig. 7.38 Effector molecules are released from T-cell granules in a highly polar fashion. The granules of cytotoxic T cells can be labeled with fluorescent dyes, allowing them to be seen under the microscope, and their movements followed by time-lapse photography. Here, we show a series of pictures taken during the interaction of a cytotoxic T cell with a target cell, which is eventually killed. In the top panel, at time 0, the T cell (upper left) has just made contact with the target cell (lower right). At this time, the granules of the T cell, labeled with a red fluorescent dye, are distant from the point of contact. In the second panel, after 1 minute has elapsed, the granules have now begun to move towards the target cell, a move that has essentially been completed in the third panel, after 4 minutes. After 40 minutes, in the last panel, the granule contents have been released into the space between the T cell and the target, which has begun to undergo apoptosis (note the fragmented nucleus). The T cell will now disengage from the target cell and can recognize and kill other targets. Photographs courtesy of G Griffiths.

in infected cells, thus increasing the chance that infected cells will be recognized as target cells for cytotoxic attack. IFN-γ also activates macrophages, recruiting them to sites of infection, both as effector cells and as antigen-presenting cells. The activation of macrophages by IFN-γ is a critical component of the host immune response to intracellular protozoan pathogens such as *Toxoplasma gondii*. IFN-γ has a secondary role in reducing the tryptophan concentration within treated cells and thus can kill intracellular parasites, effectively by starvation. TNF-α and TNF-β (lymphotoxin) are also produced by cytotoxic CD8 T cells; TNF-α or TNF-β can synergize with IFN-γ in killing some target cells by a cytokine-mediated pathway as well as in macrophage activation. Thus, armed cytotoxic CD8 effector T cells act in a variety of ways to limit the spread of cytosolic pathogens. The relative importance of these mechanisms remains to be determined.

Summary.

Armed CD8 cytotoxic effector T cells are essential in host defense against pathogens that live in the cytosol, the commonest of which are viruses. Cytotoxic T cells can kill any cell harboring such pathogens by recognizing foreign peptides that are transported to the cell surface bound to MHC class I molecules. CD8 cytotoxic T cells carry out their killing function by releasing of two types of preformed cytotoxins — the fragmentins, which seem able to induce apoptosis in any type of target cell, and the pore-forming protein perforin, which punches holes in the target-cell membrane through which the fragmentins can enter. A membrane-bound molecule, the Fas ligand, on CD8 T cells is also capable of inducing apoptosis by binding to Fas on target cells. These properties allow the cytotoxic T cell to attack and destroy virtually any cell that is infected with a cytosolic pathogen. Cytotoxic CD8 T cells also produce interferon-γ, which is an inhibitor of viral replication and an important inducer of MHC class I expression and macrophage activation. Cytotoxic T cells kill infected targets with great precision, sparing adjacent normal cells. This precision is critical in minimizing tissue damage, while allowing the eradication of infected cells. Some CD4 T cells are also cytotoxic but do not secrete either perforin or fragmentins.

Macrophage activation by armed inflammatory CD4 T cells.

Some microorganisms, such as mycobacteria, the causative agents of tuberculosis and leprosy, are intracellular pathogens that grow primarily in the vesicles, called phagolysosomes, of macrophages where they are shielded from the effects of both antibodies and cytotoxic T cells. These microbes maintain themselves in the usually hostile environment of the phagocyte by inhibiting lysosomal fusion to the phagolysosomes in which they grow or by preventing the acidification of these vesicles that is required to activate lysosomal proteases. Such microorganisms are eliminated when the macrophage is activated by an inflammatory CD4 T cell. Armed inflammatory T cells act by synthesizing and secreting a range of cytokines whose local and distant actions coordinate the immune response to these intracellular pathogens. Macrophages that have recently ingested pathogens can also be assisted in killing them by T-cell mediated activation.

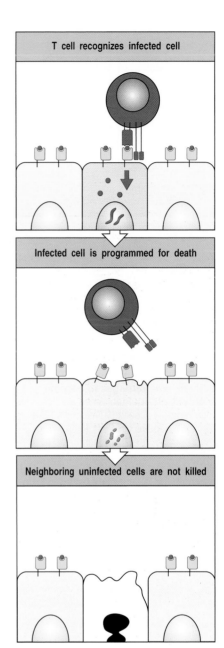

Fig. 7.39 Cytotoxic T cells kill target cells bearing specific antigen while sparing neighboring uninfected cells. All of the cells in a tissue are susceptible to lysis by T cells but only the infected cells are killed. Specific recognition by the T-cell receptor identifies which target cell to kill, and the polarized release of granules (not shown) ensures that neighboring cells are spared.

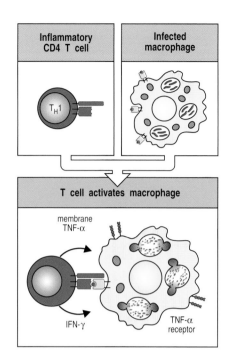

Fig. 7.40 Inflammatory CD4 T cells activate macrophages to become highly bacteriocidal. When an inflammatory T cell (T$_H$1) specific for a bacterial peptide contacts an infected macrophage, the T cell is induced to secrete macrophage-activating factors, the most important of which is IFN-γ. The macrophage is sensitized by this cytokine to respond to cell-surface molecules, probably TNF-α, on the T cell.

7-23 **Armed inflammatory CD4 T cells have a central role in macrophage activation.**

Macrophages can recognize and ingest many extracellular bacteria, thereby destroying the bacteria and at the same time presenting peptides derived from them to CD4 T cells. This can lead to the generation of armed effector CD4 T cells specific for the ingested microorganism. An important function of these armed effector T cells is to act back on the macrophages themselves, enhancing their ability to kill ingested bacteria, many of which have evolved strategies for surviving and proliferating inside phagocytic cells. The induction of antibacterial mechanisms in macrophages is known as **macrophage activation**, and is the principal effector action of inflammatory CD4 T cells. Among the extracellular pathogens that are killed when macrophages are activated is *Pneumocystis carinii*, which, because of the deficiency of CD4 T cells, is a common cause of death in people with AIDS. Macrophage activation can be measured by the ability of activated macrophages to damage helminthic parasites and certain tumor cells. This ability to act on extracellular targets extends to healthy self cells, which means that macrophages must normally be maintained in a non-activated state.

Macrophages require two signals for activation, only one of which need be delivered by the armed inflammatory T cell. The first signal, which sensitizes the macrophage to respond to the second signal, is delivered by the macrophage-activating cytokine IFN-γ (Fig. 7.40). IFN-γ is the most characteristic cytokine produced by armed inflammatory T cells. CD8 T cells are also an important source of IFN-γ, and mice lacking class I molecules (and which therefore have no CD8 T cells) show increased susceptibility to some parasite infections. The second signal can be delivered either by membrane-bound molecules induced on armed effector CD4 T cells when they encounter specific antigen on the macrophage surface, or by very small amounts of bacterial lipopolysaccharide. This latter pathway may be particularly important when CD8 T cells are the primary source of the IFN-γ. The likely identity of the membrane-bound signal delivered by the triggered CD4 T cell is a form of TNF-α. Soluble TNF-α at high concentration can substitute for the membrane-bound signal in macrophage activation, and, conversely, antibody to TNF-α can inhibit macrophage activation. This role for TNF-α would be consistent with the evidence for membrane-bound members of the TNF family as effector molecules on the other classes of effector T cells. Helper (T$_H$2) CD4 T cells, which do not produce IFN-γ, are inefficient macrophage activators, although they can deliver a contact-dependent signal required to activate macrophages primed by IFN-γ.

7-24 **The expression of cytokines and membrane-associated molecules by armed inflammatory CD4 T cells requires new RNA and protein synthesis.**

Within minutes of the recognition of specific antigen by armed cytotoxic effector CD8 T cells, directed exocytosis of preformed perforins and fragmentins programs the target cell to die by an apoptotic pathway. In contrast, when armed inflammatory CD4 T cells encounter their specific ligand, they must synthesize *de novo* the cytokines and cell-surface molecules that mediate their effects. This process requires several hours, so inflammatory T cells must adhere to their target cells for far longer than cytotoxic T cells.

Recognition of its target by an inflammatory T cell rapidly induces transcription of cytokine genes and new protein synthesis begins within an hour of receptor triggering. The newly synthesized cytokines are then delivered directly through the microvesicles of the constitutive secretory pathway to the site of contact between the T-cell membrane and the macrophage. It is thought that the newly synthesized cell-surface molecules are also expressed in a polarized fashion. This means that, although all macrophages have receptors for IFN-γ, the macrophage actually displaying antigen to the T cell is far more likely to become activated by it than neighboring, uninfected macrophages.

Activated macrophages can be very destructive to host tissues. It is therefore important not only that delivery of IFN-γ be focused on the infected cells but that its production is shut off immediately the T cell loses contact with the infected macrophage. This seems to be achieved in two ways. First, the mRNA encoding IFN-γ contains a sequence in its 3′ untranslated region that greatly reduces its half-life and serves to limit the period of cytokine production. This is characteristic of the mRNAs of all cytokines. Second, activation of the T cell appears to induce production of a new protein that promotes cytokine mRNA degradation: treatment of activated effector T cells with the protein synthesis inhibitor cyclo-heximide greatly increases the level of cytokine mRNA. The rapid destruction of cytokine mRNA, together with the focal delivery of IFN-γ at the point of contact between the activated inflammatory T cell and its target, thus limits the action of the effector T cell to the infected macro-phage. We shall see in Chapter 8, when we consider the activation of B cells by helper T cells, that the same mechanisms direct and limit T-cell help to the specific antigen-binding B cell.

7-25   Activation of macrophages by inflammatory T cells promotes bacterial killing and must be tightly regulated to avoid damage to host tissues.

Macrophage activation through cell contact and the secretion of IFN-γ by an armed inflammatory T cell generates a series of biochemical responses that converts the macrophage into a potent antibacterial effector cell (Fig. 7.41). Activated macrophages fuse their lysosomes more efficiently to phagosomes, exposing intracellular or recently ingested bacteria to a variety of bacteriocidal lysosomal enzymes. Activated macrophages make oxygen radicals and nitric oxide (NO), both of which have potent antibacterial activity, as well as antibacterial peptides.

Additional changes in the activated macrophage help to amplify the immune response. The number of MHC class II molecules and of receptors for TNF-α on the macrophage surface increases, making the cell both more effective at presenting antigen to fresh T cells, which may thereby be recruited as effector cells, and more responsive to TNF-α. TNF-α syner-gizes with IFN-γ in macrophage activation, particularly in the induction of the reactive nitrogen metabolite NO, which has broad antimicrobial activity. Activated macrophages secrete IL-12, which directs the differen-tiation of activated naive CD4 T cells into effector inflammatory T cells. Finally, macrophages, as well as helper T cells, secrete IL-10, which inhibits the production of IFN-γ and serves to dampen the potentially damaging effects of uncontrolled macrophage activation in host tissues.

These and many other surface and secreted molecules of activated macrophages are instrumental in the effector actions of macrophages in cell-mediated as well as humoral immune responses, which we shall dis-cuss in Chapter 8, and in recruiting other immune cells to sites of infection, a function to which we return in Chapter 9.

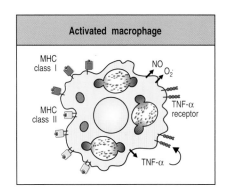

Fig. 7.41 Activated macrophages undergo changes that greatly increase their antibacterial effectiveness and amplify the immune response. The expression of surface MHC class II molecules is increased in activated macrophages, which also express TNF-α receptors and secrete TNF-α. This autocrine stimulus synergizes with IFN-γ secreted by inflammatory CD4 T cells to increase the antibacterial action of the macrophage, in particular by inducing the production of nitric oxide (NO) and oxygen radicals (O$_2$).

Since activated macrophages are extremely effective in destroying pathogens, one may ask why macrophages are not simply maintained in a state of constant activation. Besides the fact that macrophages consume large quantities of energy to maintain the activated state, macrophage activation *in vivo* is usually associated with localized tissue destruction that apparently results from the release of antibacterial mediators such as oxygen radicals, NO and proteases, which are also toxic to host cells.

The ability of activated macrophages to release toxic mediators is important in host defense because it enables them to attack large extracellular pathogens that they cannot ingest, such as parasitic worms. This can only be achieved, however, at the expense of tissue damage. Tight regulation of the activity of macrophages by inflammatory T cells thus allows the specific and effective deployment of this potent means of host defense, while minimizing local tissue damage and energy consumption.

In addition to the mechanisms controlling IFN-γ synthesis already discussed, macrophage activation itself is markedly inhibited by cytokines such as transforming growth factor-β (TGF-β), IL-4, IL-10, and IL-13. Since several of these inhibitory cytokines are produced by helper T cells, the induction of CD4 cells belonging to this subset represents an important pathway for controlling (by cross-regulation) the effector functions of activated macrophages.

7-26   Inflammatory CD4 T cells coordinate the host response to intracellular bacteria and parasites.

The activation of macrophages by IFN-γ secreted by armed inflammatory T cells is central to the host response to pathogens that proliferate in macrophage vesicles. In mice in which the IFN-γ gene has been destroyed by targeted gene disruption, production of antimicrobial agents by macrophages is impaired, and the animals succumb to sublethal doses of *Mycobacteria* spp, *Leishmania* spp, and vaccinia virus. Mice lacking a TNF-α receptor also show increased susceptibility to these pathogens. But while IFN-γ and TNF-α are probably the most important cytokines secreted by inflammatory T cells, the immune response to pathogens that proliferate in macrophage vesicles is complex, and other cytokines secreted by inflammatory T cells have a crucial role in coordinating these responses (Fig. 7.42).

Macrophages that are chronically infected with intracellular bacteria may lose the ability to become activated. Such cells would provide a reservoir of infection that is shielded from immune attack. Activated inflammatory T cells can kill a limited range of target cells upon activation, and they may destroy these infected cells. This cytotoxic activity is thought to be caused by the synergistic action of TNF-β (lymphotoxin) and IFN-γ, both products of inflammatory T cells. This combination of cytokines also synergizes effectively in killing fibroblasts, a major constituent of connective tissue, and may be important in allowing access of cells to sites of infection.

Another very important function of inflammatory T cells is recruitment of phagocytic cells to sites of infection. While some intravesicular bacteria pose a hazard by incapacitating chronically infected macrophages, others, including some mycobacteria and *Listeria*, can escape cell vesicles and enter the cytoplasm where they are not susceptible to macrophage activation. Their presence can, however, be detected by CD8 cytotoxic T cells, which can release them by killing the cell. The pathogens released when macrophages are killed either by inflammatory CD4

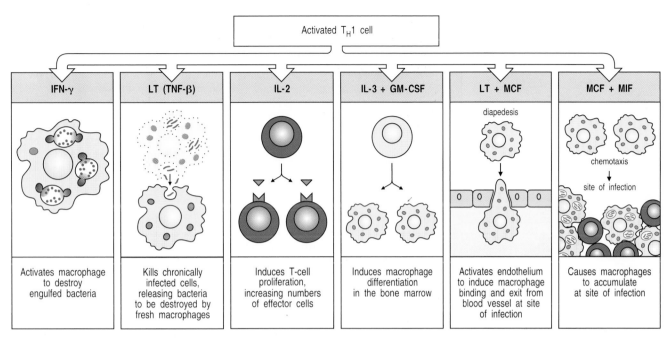

Fig. 7.42   The immune response to intracellular bacteria is coordinated by activated inflammatory CD4 T cells. The activation of inflammatory CD4 T cells (T$_H$1) by infected macrophages results in the release of cytokines that both activate the macrophage and coordinate the immune response to intracellular bacteria. IFN-γ activates the macrophage and allows it to kill engulfed bacteria. Chronically infected macrophages lose the ability to kill intracellular bacteria, and TNF-β (LT, lymphotoxin) produced by the inflammatory T cell can kill these macrophages, releasing the bacteria, which are taken up and killed by fresh macrophages. Thus, IFN-γ and TNF-β synergize in the removal of intracellular bacteria. IL-2 produced by the inflammatory T cells induces T-cell proliferation and potentiates the release of other cytokines. IL-3 and GM-CSF stimulate the production of new macrophages by acting on hematopoietic stem cells in the bone marrow. New macrophages are recruited to the site of infection by the action of lymphokines such as TNF-β on vascular endothelium that signal macrophages to leave the bloodstream and enter the tissues. A chemokine with macrophage chemotactic activity (MCF) signals macrophages to migrate into sites of infection and together with a second chemokine, migration inhibition factor (MIF), causes the accumulation of macrophages at sites of infection. Thus, the inflammatory T cell coordinates a macrophage response that is highly effective in engulfing and destroying local infectious agents.

T cells or by CD8 cytotoxic T cells can be taken up by freshly recruited macrophages still capable of activation to antibacterial activity.

Inflammatory T cells recruit macrophages by two mechanisms. First, they make the hematopoietic growth factors IL-3 and GM-CSF, which stimulate the production of new phagocytic cells in the bone marrow. Second, TNF-α and TNF-β (lymphotoxin), which are secreted by inflammatory T cells at sites of infection, change the surface properties of endothelial cells so that phagocytes adhere to them, while other cytokines produced in the inflammatory response serve to direct the migration of these phagocytic cells.

When microbes effectively resist the bacteriocidal effects of activated macrophages, chronic infection with inflammation can develop. Often, this has a characteristic pattern, consisting of a central area of macrophages surrounded by activated lymphocytes. This pathological pattern is called a **granuloma** (Fig. 7.43). Giant cells consisting of fused macrophages usually form the center of these granulomas. This serves to 'wall-off' pathogens that resist destruction. Helper CD4 T cells appear to participate in granulomas along with inflammatory CD4 T cells, perhaps by regulating their activity and preventing widespread tissue damage. In tuberculosis, the center of the large granulomas can become isolated and the cells there die, probably from a combination of lack of oxygen and the cytotoxic effects of activated macrophages. As the dead tissue in the center resembles cheese, this process is called **caseation necrosis**.

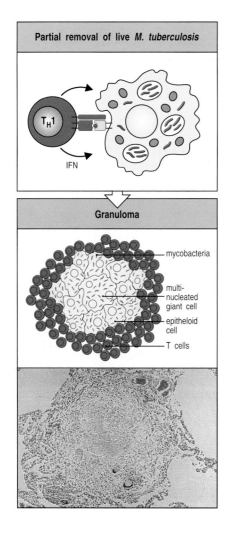

Partial removal of live *M. tuberculosis*

T$_H$1

IFN

Granuloma

mycobacteria

multi-
nucleated
giant cell

epitheloid
cell

T cells

Fig. 7.43 Granulomas form when an intracellular pathogen or its constituents cannot be totally eliminated. When mycobacteria (red) resist the effects of macrophage activation, a characteristic localized inflammatory response called a granuloma develops. This consists of a central core of infected macrophages. The core may include multinucleated giant cells, which are fused macrophages, surrounded by large macrophages often called epithelioid cells.

Mycobacteria can persist in the cells of the granuloma. The central core is surrounded by T cells, many of which are CD4-positive. The exact mechanisms by which this balance is achieved, and how it breaks down, are unknown. Granulomas, as seen in the bottom panel, also form in the lungs and elsewhere in a disease known as sarcoidosis, which may be caused by occult mycobacterial infection. Photograph courtesy of J Orrell.

Thus, activation of inflammatory T cells can cause significant pathology. Its absence, however, leads to the more serious consequence of death from disseminated infection. This is now seen frequently in patients with AIDS and mycobacterial infection.

Summary.

CD4 T cells that can activate macrophages play a critical role in host defense against those intracellular pathogens that resist killing in non-activated macrophages. Macrophage activation is mediated by membrane-bound signals delivered by the inflammatory CD4 T cells, as well as by the potent macrophage-activating cytokine IFN-γ, which is secreted by these cells. Once activated, the macrophage can kill intracellular bacteria. Activated macrophages can also cause local tissue damage, which explains why this activity must be strictly regulated by T cells. Inflammatory T cells produce a range of cytokines that not only activate infected macrophages but can also kill senescent macrophages to release engulfed bacteria, stimulate bone marrow production of new macrophages, and recruit fresh macrophages to sites of infection. Thus, inflammatory T cells have a central role in controlling and coordinating host defense against certain intracellular pathogens. It is likely that the absence of this function explains the preponderance of intracellular infections in adult AIDS patients.

Summary to Chapter 7.

Armed effector T cells play a critical role in almost all adaptive immune responses. Immune responses are initiated when naive T cells encounter specific antigen on the surface of a professional antigen-presenting cell that also expresses effective co-stimulatory molecules, usually B7.1 and B7.2. The activated T cells produce IL-2, which drives them to proliferate and differentiate into armed effector T cells. All T-cell effector functions involve cell interactions. When armed effector T cells recognize specific antigen on target cells, they release mediators that act directly on the target cell, altering its behavior. The triggering of armed effector T cells by peptide:MHC complexes is independent of co-stimulation, so that any infected target cell can be activated or destroyed by an armed effector T cell. CD8 cytotoxic T cells kill target cells infected with cytosolic pathogens, removing sites of pathogen replication. Inflammatory CD4 T cells (T$_H$1) activate macrophages to kill intracellular parasites. Helper CD4 T cells (T$_H$2) are essential in the activation of B cells to secrete the antibodies that mediate humoral immune responses directed against extracellular pathogens, as will be seen in Chapter 8. Thus, effector T cells control virtually all known effector mechanisms of the adaptive immune response through their interactions with target cells.

General references.

Dustin, M.L. and Springer, T.A.: **The role of lymphocyte adhesion receptors in transient interactions and cell locomotion.** *Annu. Rev. Immunol.* 1993, 9:27-66.

Schwartz, R.H.: **Co-stimulation of T lymphocytes: the role of CD28, CTLA-4, and B7/BB1 in interleukin-2 production and immunotherapy.** *Cell* 1992, 71:1065-1068.

Linsley, P.S. and Ledbetter, J.A.: **The role of the CD28 receptor during T-cell responses to antigen.** *Annu. Rev. Immunol.* 1993, 11:191-221.

Knight, S.C. and Stagg, A.J.: **Antigen-presenting cell types.** *Curr. Opin. Immunol.* 1993, 5:374-382.

Bottomly, K: **A functional dichotomy in CD4+ T lymphocytes.** *Immunol. Today* 1988, 9:268-273.

Mosmann, T.R. and Coffman, R.L.: **T$_H$1 and T$_H$2 cells: Different patterns of lymphokine secretion lead to different functional properties.** *Annu. Rev. Immunol.* 1993, 7:145-173.

Thomson, A. (ed.): *The Cytokine Handbook*, 2nd edn. Academic Press, San Diego 1994.

Kupfer, A. and Singer, S.J.: **Cell biology of cytotoxic and helper T-cell functions.** *Annu. Rev. Immunol.* 1993, 7:309-337.

Cohen, J.J., Duke, R.C., Fadok, V.A., and Sellins, K.S.: **Apoptosis and programmed cell death in immunity.** *Annu. Rev. Immunol.* 1993, 10:267-293.

Stout, R.D.: **Macrophage activation by T cells: cognate and non-cognate signals.** *Curr. Opin. Immunol.* 1993, 5:398-403.

Pigott, R., and Power C.: *The Adhesion Molecule Facts Book.* Academic Press, London, 1993.

Section references.

7-1 The initial interaction of naive T cells with antigen occurs in peripheral lymphoid organs.

Picker, L.J. and Butcher, E.C.: **Physiological and molecular mechanisms of lymphocyte homing.** *Annu. Rev. Immunol.* 1993, 10:561-591.

Barker, C.F. and Billingham, R.E.: **The role of regional lymphatics in the skin homograft response.** *Transplantation* 1967, 5:692.

Tilney, N.L. and Gowans, J.L.: **The sensitization of rats by allografts transplanted to allymphatic pedicles of skin.** *J. Exper. Med.* 1971, 113:951.

7-2 Lymphocyte migration, activation, and effector function depend on cell-adhesion molecules.

Hogg, N. and Landis, R.C.: **Adhesion molecules in cell interactions.** *Curr. Opin. Immunol.* 1993, 5:383-390.

Hynes, R.S. and Lander, A.D.: **Contact and adhesive specificities in the associations, migrations, and targeting of cells and axons.** *Cell* 1992, 68:303-322.

7-3 The initial interaction of T cells with antigen-presenting cells is also mediated by cell-adhesion molecules.

Shimizu, Y., van Seventer, G., Horgan, K.J., and Shaw, S.: **Roles of adhesion molecules in T-cell recognition: fundamental similarities between four integrins on resting human T cells (LFA-1, VLA-4, VLA-5, VLA-6) in expression, binding, and co-stimulation.** *Immunol. Rev.* 1990, 114:109-143.

Dustin, M.L. and Springer, T.A.: **T-cell receptor crosslinking transiently stimulates adhesiveness through LFA-1.** *Nature* 1989, 341:619-624.

Hahn, W.C., Rosenstein, Y., Clavo, V., Burakoff, S.J., and Bierer, B.: **A distinct cytoplasmic domain of CD2 regulates ligand avidity and T-cell responsiveness to antigen.** *Proc. Natl. Acad. Sci. USA* 1992, 89:7179-7183.

7-4 Both specific ligand and co-stimulatory signals provided by a professional antigen-presenting cell are required for the clonal expansion of naive T cells.

Freeman, G.J., Gribben, J.G., Boussitis, V.A., Ng, J.W., Restive, V.A. Jr., Lombard, L.A., Gray, G.S., and Nadler, L.M.: **Cloning of B7-2: CTLA-4 counter receptor that co-stimulates human T-cell proliferation.** *Science* 1993, 262:907-909.

Liu, Y. and Janeway, C.A. Jr.: **Cells that present both specific ligand and co-stimulatory activity are the most efficient inducers of clonal expansion of normal CD4 T cells.** *Proc. Natl. Acad. Sci. USA* 1992, 89:3845-3949.

Linsley, P.S., Brady, W., Grosmaire, L., Aruffo, A., Damle, N.K., and Ledbetter, J.A.: **Binding of the B-cell activation antigen B7 to CD28 co-stimulates T-cell proliferation and interleukin 2 mRNA accumulation.** *J. Exper. Med.* 1991, 173:721-730.

7-5 Macrophages are scavenger cells that can be induced by pathogens to present foreign antigens to naive T cells.

Razi-Wolf, Z., Freeman, G.J., Galvin, F., Benacerraf, B., Nadler, L., and Reiser, H.: **Expression and function of the murine B7 antigen, the major co-stimulatory molecule expressed by peritoneal exudate cells.** *Proc. Natl. Acad. Sci. USA* 1992, 89:4210-4214.

Liu, Y., and Janeway, C.A. Jr.: **Microbial induction of co-stimulatory activity for CD4 T-cell growth.** *Intl. Immunol.* 1991, 3:323-332.

7-6 Dendritic cells are highly efficient inducers of T-cell activation.

Schon-Hegard, M.A., Oliver, J., McMenamin, P.G., and Holt, P.G.: **Studies on the density, distribution, and surface phenotype of intraepithelial class II major histocompatibility complex (Ia) antigen-bearing dendritic cells in the conducting airways.** *J. Exper. Med.* 1991, 173:1345-1356.

Austyn, J.M., Kupiec, Weglinski, J.W., Hankins, D.F., and Morris, P.J.: **Migration patterns of dendritic cells in the mouse: homing to T-cell-dependent areas of spleen, and binding within marginal zone.** *J. Exper. Med.* 1988, 167:646-651.

Steinman, R.M.: **The dendritic cell system and its role in immunogenicity.** *Annu. Rev. Immunol.* 1993, 9:271-296.

7-7 B cells are highly efficient at presenting antigens that bind to their surface immunoglobulin.

Lanzavecchia, A.: **Receptor-mediated antigen uptake and its effect on antigen presentation to class II-restricted T lymphocytes.** *Annu. Rev. Immunol.* 1993, 8:773-793.

7-8 Activated T cells synthesize the T-cell growth factor interleukin-2 and its receptor.

Minami, Y., Kono, T., Miyazaki, T., and Taniguchi, T.: **The IL-2 receptor complex: its structure, function, and target genes.** *Annu. Rev. Immunol.* 1993, 11:245-267.

Smith, K.A.: **Interleukin 2.** *Annu. Rev. Immunol.* 1984, 2:319-333.

7-9 The co-stimulatory signal is necessary for the synthesis and secretion of IL-2.

Fraser, J.D., Irving, B.A., Grabtree, G.R., and Weiss, A.: **Regulation of interleukin-2 gene enhancer activity by the T-cell accessory molecule CD28.** *Science* 1991, **251**:313-316.

Lindsten, T., June, C.H., Ledbetter, J.A., Stella, G., and Thompson, C.B.: **Regulation of lymphokine messenger RNA stability by a surface-mediated T-cell activation pathway.** *Science* 1989, **244**:339-342.

7-10 Antigen recognition in the absence of co-stimulation leads to T-cell tolerance.

Eynon, E.E. and Parker, D.C.: **Small B cells as antigen-presenting cells in the induction of tolerance to soluble protein antigens.** *J. Exper. Med.* 1993, **175**:131-138.

Lenschow, D.J., Zeng, Y., Thistlethwaite, J.R., Montag, A., Brady, W., Gibson, M.G., Linsley, P.S., and Bluestone, J.A.: **Long-term survival of xenogenic pancreatic islet cell grafts induced by CTLA-4lg.** *Science* 1992, **257**:789-792.

Guerder, S. Meyerhoff, J, and Flavell, R.A.: **The role of the T cell costimulator B7.1 in autoimmunity and the induction and maintenance of tolerance to peripheral antigen.** *Immunity* 1994: **1**:155-166.

7-11 Proliferating T cells differentiate into armed effector T cells with altered surface properties that do not require co-stimulation to act.

Wong, S.F., Visintin, I., Wen, L, Flavell, R.A., and Janeway, C.A. Jr. **CD8 T cell clones from young NOD islets can transfer rapid onset of diabetes in NOD mice in the absence of CD4 cells.** *J. exp. Med.* 1995. In press.

7-12 The differentiation of CD4 T cells into helper (T_H2) or inflammatory (T_H1) effector cells is the crucial event in determining whether humoral or cell-mediated immunity will predominate.

Salgame, P.R., Abrams, J.S., Clayberger, C., Goldstein, H., Convit, J., Modlin, R.L., and Bloom, B.R.: **Differing lymphokine profiles of functional subsets of human CD4 and CD8 T-cell clones.** *Science* 1991, **254**:279-289.

Kamogawa, Y., Minasi, L.A., Carding, S.R., Bottomly, K., and Flavell, R.A. **The relationship of IL-4 and IFN-γ producing T cells studied by lineage ablation of IL-4-producing cells.** *Cell* 1993 **75**:985-995.

7-13 Naive CD8 T cells can be activated in different ways to become armed cytotoxic effector cells.

Macatonia, S.E., Taylor, P.M., Knight, S.C., and Askonas, B.A.: **Primary stimulation by dendritic cells induces antiviral proliferation and cytotoxic T-cell responses** *in vitro*. *J. Exper. Med.* 1988, **169**:1255-1264.

Guerder, S. and Matzinger, P.: **Activation versus tolerance: a decision made by T helper cells.** *Cold Spring Harbor Symp. on Quant. Biol.* 1989, **54**:799-805.

Azuma, M., Cayabyab, M., Buck, D., Phillips, J.H., Lanier, L.L.: **CD28 interaction with B7 co-stimulates primary allogeneic proliferative responses and cytotoxicity mediated by small, resting T lymphocytes.** *J. Exper. Med.* 1992, **175**:353-360.

7-14 Effector T-cell interactions with target cells are initiated by antigen non-specific cell-adhesion molecules.

van Seventer, G.A., Simuzi, Y., and Shaw, S.: **Roles of multiple accesory molecules in T-cell activation.** *Curr. Opin. Immunol.* 1991, **3**:294-303.

Rodrigues, M., Nussezwieg, R.S., Romero, P., and Zavala, F.: **The** *in vivo* **cytotoxic activity of CD8⁺ T-cell clones correlates with their levels of expression of adhesion molecules.** *J. Exper. Med.* 1992, **175**:895-905.

O'Rourke, A.M. and Mescher, M.F.: **Cytotoxic T lymphocyte activation involves a cascade of signaling and adhesion events.** *Nature* 1992, **358**:253-255.

7-15 The T-cell receptor complex directs the release of effector molecules and focuses them on the target cell.

Geiger, B., Rosen, D., and Berke, G.: **Spatial relationships of microtubule-organizing centers and the contact area of cytotoxic T lymphocytes and target cells.** *J. Cell Biol.* 1982, **95**:137-143.

Poo, W.J., Conrad, L., and Janeway, C.A. Jr.: **Receptor-directed focusing of lymphokine release by helper T cells.** *Nature* 1988, **332**:378.

7-16 The effector functions of T cells are mediated by induced expression of both membrane-bound and secreted molecules.

Brian, A.A.: **Stimulation of B-cell proliferation by membrane-associated molecules from activated T cells.** *Proc. Natl. Acad. Sci. USA* 1988, **85**:564.

Armitage, R.J., Fanslow, W.C., Strockbine, L., Sato, T.A., Cliffors, K.N., MacDuff, B.M., Anderson, D.M., Gimpel, S.D., Davis Smith, T., Maliszewski, C.R.: **Molecular and biological characterization of a murine ligand for CD40.** *Nature* 1992, **357**:80-82.

7-17 Cytokines can act locally or at a distance.

Arai, K., Lee, F., Miyajima, A., Miyatake, S., Arai, N., Yokota, T.: **Cytokines: co-ordinators of immune and inflammatory responses.** *Annu. Rev. Biochem.* 1990, **59**:783.

7-18 Cytotoxic T cells can induce target cells to undergo programmed cell death.

Apasov, S., Redegeld, F., and Sitkovsky, M.: **Cell-mediated cytotoxicity: contact and secreted factors.** *Curr. Opin. Immunol.* 1993, **5**:404-410.

Berke, G.: **Lymphocyte-triggered internal target disintegration.** *Immunol. Today* 1991, **12**:396-399.

7-19 Cytotoxic T cells store cytotoxic proteins in preformed granules that they release by directed exocytosis upon recognizing antigen on a target cell.

Shiver, J.W., Su, L., and Henkart, P.A.: **Cytotoxicity with target DNA breakdown by rat basophilic leukemia cells expressing both cytolysin and granzyme A.** *Cell* 1992, **71**:315-322.

Kagi, D., Ledermann, B., Burki, K., Seiler, P., Odermatt, B., Olsen, K.J., Podack, E.R., Zinkernagel, R.M., and Hengartner, H. **Cytotoxicity mediated by T cells and natural killer cells is greatly impaired in perforin-deficient mice.** *Nature* 1994 **369**: 31-37.

7-20 Membrane proteins of CD8 T cells can also activate apoptosis.

Rouvier, E., Luciani, M.-F., and Golstein, P.: **Fas involvement in Ca²⁺ independent T-cell-mediated cytotoxicity.** *J. Exper. Med.* 1993, **177**:195-200.

Suda, T., Takahashi, T., Goldstein P., and Nagata, S.: **Molecular cloning and expression of the Fas ligand, a novel member of the tumor necrosis factor family.** *Cell* 1993 **75**:1169-1178.

Watanbe Fukunaga, R., Branna, C.I., Copeland, N.G., Jenkins, N.A., and Nagata, S.: **Lymphoproliferation disorder in mice explained by defects in Fas antigen that mediates apoptosis.** *Nature* 1992, **356**:314-317.

Fisher, G.H., Rosenberg, E.J., Straus, S.E., Dale, J.K., Middleton, L.A., Lin, A.Y., Strober, W., Leonardo, M.J., amd Puck, J.M. **Dominant interfering Fas gene mutations impair apoptosis in a human autoimmune lymphoproliferative syndrome.** *Cell* 1995 **81**:935-946.

7-21 Cytotoxic T cells selectively kill targets expressing specific antigen.

Kuppers, R.C. and Henney, C.S.: **Studies on the mechanism of lymphocyte-mediated cytolysis. IX. Relationships between antigen recognition and lytic expression in killer T cells.** *J. Immunol.* 1977, **118**:71-76.

7-22 Cytotoxic T cells also act by releasing cytokines.

Ramshaw, I., Ruby, J., Ramsay, A., Ada, G., and Karupiah, G.: **Expression of cytokines by recombinant vaccinia viruses: a model for studying cytokines in virus infections** *in vivo. Immunol. Rev.* 1992 ,**127**:157-182.

7-23 Armed inflammatory CD4 T cells have a central role in macrophage activation.

Stout, R. and Bottomly, K.: **Antigen-specific activation of effector macrophages by interferon-gamma producing (T$_H$1) T-cell clones: failure of IL-4 producing (T$_H$2) T-cell clones to activate effector functions in macrophages.** *J. Immunol.* 1989, **142**:760.

Munoz Fernandez, M.A., Fernandez, M.A., and Fresno, M.: **Synergism between tumor necrosis factor-alpha and interferon-gamma on macrophage activation for the killing of intracellular** *Trypanosoma crusi* **through a nitric oxide-dependent mechanism.** *Eur. J. Immunol.* 1992, **22**:301-307.

7-24 The expression of cytokines and membrane-associated molecules by armed inflammatory CD4 T cells requires new RNA and protein synthesis.

Shaw, G., and Karmen, R.: **A conserved UAU sequence from the 3′ untranslated region of GM-CSF mRNA mediates selective mRNA degradation.** *Cell* 1986, **46**:659.

7-25 Activation of macrophages by inflammatory T cells promotes bacterial killing and must be tightly regulated to avoid damage to host tissues.

Paulnock, D.M.: **Macrophage activation by T cells.** *Curr. Opin. Immunol.* 1992, **4**:344-349.

7-26 Inflammatory CD4 T cells coordinate the host response to intracellular bacteria and parasites.

Oppenheim, J.J., Zachariae, C.O.C., Mukaida, W., and Matsushima, K.: **Properties of the novel proinflammatory supergene intercrine cytokine family.** *Annu. Rev. Immunol.* 1991, **9**:617.

Kindler, V., Sappino, A.-P., Grau, G.E., Piquet, P.-F., Vassali, P.: **The inducing role of tumor necrosis factor in the development of bactericidal granulomas during BCG development.** *Cell* 1989, **56**:731-740.

McInnes, A. and Rennick, D.M.: **Interleukin 4 induces cultured monocytes/ macrophages to form giant multinucleated cells.** *J. Exper. Med.* 1988, **167**:598-611.

Yamamura, M., Uyemura, K., Deans, R,J., Weinberg, K., Rea, T.H., Bloom, B.R., and Modlin, R.L.: **Defining protective responses to pathogens: cytokine profiles in leprosy lesions.** *Science* 1991, **254**:277-279.

The Humoral Immune Response

8

Many of the bacteria that are most important in human infectious disease multiply in the extracellular spaces of the body, and most intracellular pathogens must spread by moving from cell to cell through the extracellular fluids. The humoral immune response leads to the destruction of extracellular microorganisms and prevents the spread of intracellular infections. This is achieved by antibodies secreted by B lymphocytes.

There are three main ways in which antibodies contribute to immunity (Fig. 8.1). Viruses and intracellular bacteria, which need to enter cells in order to grow, spread from cell to cell by binding to specific molecules on their target cell surface. Antibodies that bind to the pathogen can prevent this and are said to **neutralize** the pathogen. Neutralization by antibodies is also important in protection from toxins. Other types of bacteria multiply outside cells, and antibodies protect against these pathogens mainly by facilitating their uptake into phagocytic cells that are specialized to destroy ingested bacteria. There are two ways in which this can occur. In the first case, bound antibodies coating the pathogen are recognized by specific **Fc receptors** on the surface of phagocytic cells. Coating the surface of a pathogen to enhance phagocytosis in this way is called **opsonization**. Alternatively, antibodies binding to the surface of a pathogen may activate the proteins of the **complement** system. Complement proteins bound to the pathogen also opsonize it by binding **complement receptors** on phagocytes. Other complement components recruit phagocytic cells to the site of infection, and the terminal components of complement can lyse certain microorganisms directly by forming pores in their membranes. The effector mechanism that is recruited in a particular response is determined by the **isotype** of the antibodies produced.

The activation of B cells and their differentiation into antibody-secreting cells is triggered by antigen and often requires **helper T cells (T_H2)**. Helper T cells also control **isotype switching** and play a role in initiating **somatic hypermutation** of antibody variable-region genes, which is required for the affinity maturation of antibodies that occurs during the course of a humoral immune response. In the first part of this chapter, we shall describe the interactions of B cells with helper T cells and the mechanism of affinity maturation in the specialized microenvironment of peripheral lymphoid tissues. In the rest of the chapter we shall discuss in detail the mechanisms whereby antibodies contain and eliminate infections.

Fig. 8.1 The humoral immune response is mediated by antibody molecules that are secreted by plasma cells. Antigen binding to surface antibody signals B cells and is, at the same time, internalized and processed into peptides that activate helper T cells (T$_H$2). Signals from the bound antigen and from the helper T cell induce the B cell to proliferate and differentiate into a plasma cell secreting specific antibody (top two panels). There are three main ways in which these antibodies protect the host from infection (bottom panels). They may inhibit the toxic effects or infectivity of pathogens by binding to them: this is termed neutralization (left panel). By coating the pathogens, they may enable accessory cells that recognize the Fc piece of arrays of antibodies to ingest and kill the pathogen, a process called opsonization (middle panel). Antibodies can also trigger the complement cascade of proteins, which strongly enhance opsonization and can directly kill some bacterial cells (right panel).

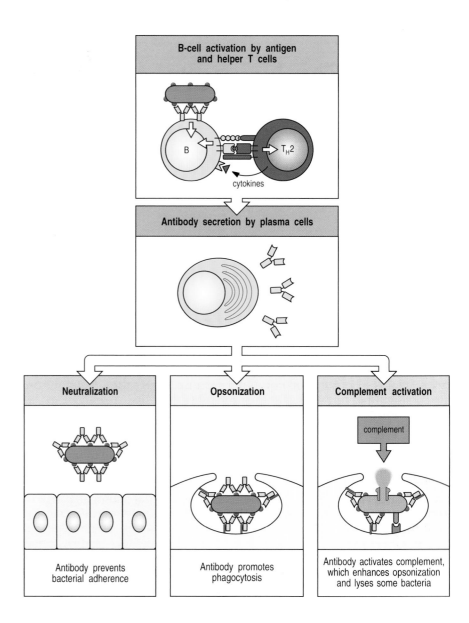

Antibody production by B lymphocytes.

The surface immunoglobulin that serves as the antigen receptor on B lymphocytes plays two roles in their activation. First, like the antigen receptor on T cells, when it binds antigen it directly transmits a signal to the cell's interior. Second, it delivers the antigen to intracellular sites where it is degraded and from which it is returned to the B-cell surface as peptides bound to MHC class II molecules. The peptide:MHC class II complex can then be recognized by antigen-specific armed helper T cells, triggering them to make molecules that, in turn, cause the B cell to proliferate and its progeny to differentiate into antibody-secreting cells. Some microbial antigens can directly activate B cells in the absence of T-cell help, and provide a means whereby antibodies can be produced rapidly against many important bacterial pathogens. However, the changes in the functional properties of antibody molecules that result from isotype switching, and the changes in the variable region that underlie affinity maturation, depend upon the interaction of antigen-stimulated B cells with helper T cells and other cells in the peripheral lymphoid organs. Antibodies induced by microbial antigens alone are therefore less variable and less functionally versatile than those induced with T-cell help.

8-1   The antibody response is initiated when B cells bind antigen and are signaled by helper T cells or by certain microbial antigens.

It is a general rule in adaptive immunity that naive antigen-specific lymphocytes cannot be activated by antigen alone. Naive T cells require a co-stimulatory signal from professional antigen-presenting cells; naive B cells require accessory signals that may come either from an armed helper T cell or, in some cases, directly from microbial constituents (Fig. 8.2).

Antibody responses to protein antigens require T-cell help. B cells become effective targets for armed helper T cells when antigen bound by surface immunoglobulin is internalized and returned to the cell surface as peptides bound to MHC class II molecules. Helper T cells that recognize the peptide:MHC complex then deliver activating signals to the B cell. Thus, protein antigens binding to B cells provide both a specific signal to the B cell and a focus for T-cell help (Fig. 8.2 top two panels). Antigens that require T-cell help to activate B cells are called **thymus-dependent** or **TD antigens** because animals or humans in which the thymus fails to develop cannot make functional T cells and thus do not make antibody responses to these antigens.

Although armed helper T cells are required for B-cell responses to protein antigens, many constituents of microbes, such as bacterial polysaccharides, can directly induce B cells to produce antibody in the absence of helper T cells (Fig. 8.2 bottom panel). These microbial antigens are known as **thymus-independent** or **TI antigens**. Thymus-independent antibody responses can be seen in individuals who lack functional T lymphocytes and help account for the fact that, while such individuals are susceptible to viral infections and to intracellular pathogens, they are relatively resistant to infections with most extracellular bacteria. We shall return at the end of this section to the special characteristics of TI antigens that enable them to activate naive B cells without engaging armed helper T cells.

8-2   Armed helper T cells activate B cells that recognize the same antigen.

Thymus-dependent antibody responses depend upon the activation of B cells by helper T cells that respond to the same antigen; this is called **linked recognition**. This means that before B cells can be induced to make antibody to a given pathogen in an infection, a CD4 T cell that is specific for peptides of the pathogen must first be activated to produce appropriate armed helper T cells. Although the epitope recognized by the armed helper T cell must therefore be linked to that recognized by the B cell, the two cells need not recognize identical epitopes. Indeed, we saw in Chapter 4 that T cells can recognize internal peptides in proteins that are quite distinct from the surface epitopes recognized by B cells on the same molecule (see Fig. 4.5). In the case of more complex natural antigens, such as viruses, the T cell and the B cell may not even recognize the same protein. It is, however, crucial that the peptide recognized by the T cell be a part of the antigen or antigenic complex recognized by the B cell, which can thereby produce the appropriate peptide on internalization of antigen bound to its surface immunoglobulin.

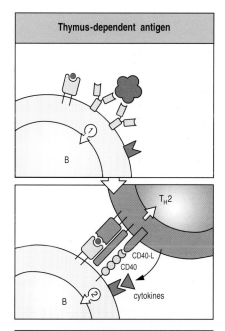

Thymus-dependent antigen

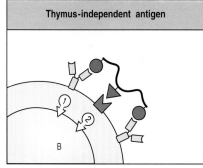

Thymus-independent antigen

Fig. 8.2 A second signal is required for B-cell activation either by thymus-dependent or by thymus-independent antigens. The first signal required for B-cell activation is delivered through the antigen receptor. In the case of thymus-dependent antigens, the second signal is delivered by a helper T cell that recognizes degraded fragments of antigen bound as peptides to MHC class II molecules on the B-cell surface. In the case of thymus-independent antigens, the second signal is delivered by the antigen itself.

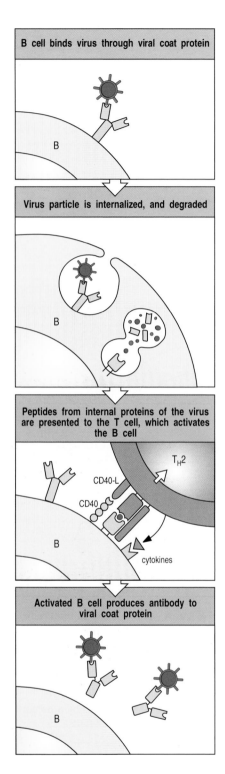

B cell binds virus through viral coat protein

Virus particle is internalized, and degraded

Peptides from internal proteins of the virus are presented to the T cell, which activates the B cell

T$_H$2

CD40-L

CD40

B

cytokines

Activated B cell produces antibody to viral coat protein

Fig. 8.3 B cells and helper T cells must recognize epitopes of the same molecular complex in order to interact. An epitope on a viral coat (spike) protein is recognized by the surface immunoglobulin on a B cell and the virus is internalized and degraded. Peptides derived from viral proteins including an internal protein of the virus are returned to the B-cell surface bound to MHC class II molecules where they are recognized by helper T cells, which activate the B cells to produce antibody against the coat protein.

The specific activation of the B cell by T cells sensitized to the same antigen then depends upon the ability of the antigen-specific B cell to concentrate the appropriate peptides on its surface MHC class II molecules. B cells binding a specific antigen are 10 000-fold more efficient at displaying peptide fragments of the antigen on their surface MHC class II molecules than B cells that do not bind the antigen specifically. Armed helper T cells will thus help only B cells whose receptors bind to the antigen containing the peptide that they recognize.

For example, B cells can internalize particles as large as viruses whose coat proteins are recognized by their surface immunoglobulin. After internalization, the virus is degraded and peptides from internal proteins as well as coat proteins may be displayed by the surface MHC class II molecules of the B cell. Helper T cells that have been primed earlier in an infection by macrophages or dendritic cells presenting these same internal peptides can then activate the B cell to make antibodies that recognize the coat protein (Fig. 8.3).

The requirement for linked recognition has important consequences for the regulation and manipulation of the humoral immune response. One of these is to help ensure self tolerance. A B cell that binds a self antigen will present peptides derived from it on self MHC class II molecules. As long as T cells that recognize peptides derived from self proteins are either eliminated in the thymus or inactivated in the periphery, however, no T-cell help will be available to activate such a B cell. Thus, T-cell tolerance provides a mechanism for preventing the production of self-reactive antibodies by B cells that have themselves escaped deletion or inactivation. Such potentially self-reactive B cells are known to exist, because self-reactive antibodies are sometimes produced in the course of an immune response to infection. In this case, the self-reactive B cell is thought to bind to an epitope on the infectious microorganism that resembles an epitope on the self protein. This enables the B cell to internalize the antigen and generate microbial peptides, which can then be displayed on MHC class II molecules on its surface. Armed helper T cells already primed against the microbial peptides can activate these B cells to produce antibody that recognizes both the microorganism and the self antigen. Antibodies induced against self antigens in this way usually disappear again when the infection subsides, since, in the absence of infection, only the self antigen will be presented and helper T cells remain tolerant to self peptides.

An important application of linked recognition is in the design of vaccines, such as that used to immunize infants against *Haemophilus influenzae* B. This is a bacterial pathogen that can infect the lining of the brain, or meninges, causing meningitis and, in severe cases, neurological damage or death. Protective immunity against this pathogen is mediated by antibodies to its capsular polysaccharide. Adults make very effective T-cell independent responses to these polysaccharide antigens, but T-cell independent responses are weak in the immature immune system of the infant. To make an effective vaccine for use in infants, therefore, the polysaccharide is chemically linked to tetanus toxoid, a foreign protein to which infants are routinely and

Fig. 8.4 Protein antigens attached to polysaccharide antigens allow T cells to help polysaccharide-specific B cells. *Haemophilus influenzae* B vaccine is a conjugate of bacterial polysaccharide and the tetanus toxoid protein. The B cell recognizes and binds the polysaccharide, internalizes and degrades the toxoid protein to which it is attached, and displays peptides derived from it on surface MHC class II molecules. Helper T cells generated in response to earlier vaccination against the toxoid recognize the complex on the B-cell surface and activate the B cell to produce antibody against the polysaccharide. This antibody can then protect against *H. influenzae* B infection.

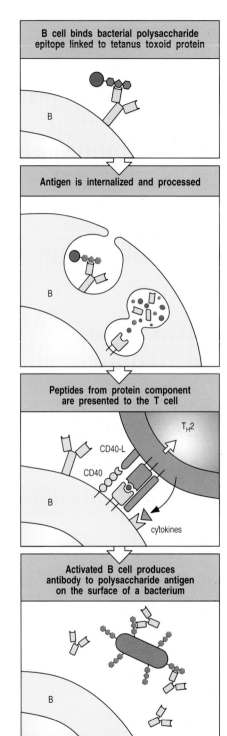

successfully vaccinated (see Fig.1.31). B cells that bind the polysaccharide component of the vaccine can be activated by helper T cells specific for peptides of the linked toxoid (Fig. 8.4).

Linked recognition was originally discovered through studies on the production of antibodies to haptens, as described in Chapter 2. Haptens are small chemical groups that cannot elicit antibody responses because they cannot recruit T-cell help. When coupled to a carrier protein, however, they become immunogenic, because T cells can be primed to peptides derived from the protein. This effect is responsible for allergic responses of many people to the powerful antibiotic penicillin, which reacts with host proteins to form a hapten that can stimulate an antibody response, as we shall learn in Chapter 11.

8-3 | **Peptide:MHC class II complexes on a B cell trigger armed helper T cells to make membrane and secreted molecules that activate the B cell.**

Armed helper T cells activate B cells when they recognize the appropriate peptide:MHC class II complex on the B-cell surface. As with inflammatory CD4 T cells (T_H1) acting on macrophages, peptide:MHC class II on B cells triggers armed helper CD4 T cells to synthesize both cell-bound and secreted effector molecules that synergize in B-cell activation. The most important effector molecule in the early phases of the B-cell response is a T-cell surface molecule of the TNF family that is known as the **CD40 ligand** because it binds to the B-cell surface molecule CD40. **CD40** is a member of the TNF-receptor family of cytokine receptors and is analogous to the TNF receptor on macrophages and Fas on cytotoxic T-cell targets. Binding of CD40 by CD40 ligand helps to drive the resting B cell into the cell cycle and is essential for B-cell responses to thymus-dependent antigens; patients with mutations that affect CD40 ligand make very weak and ineffective antibody responses and suffer from severe humoral immunodeficiency, as we shall see in Chapter 10.

B cells are stimulated to proliferate *in vitro* when they are exposed to a mixture of artificially synthesized CD40 ligand and the cytokine IL-4. IL-4 is also made by armed helper T cells when they recognize their specific ligand on the B-cell surface, and IL-4 and CD40 ligand are thought to synergize in driving the clonal expansion that precedes antibody production *in vivo*. IL-4 is secreted in a polar fashion by the helper T cell and is directed at the site of contact with the B cell (Fig. 8.5) so that it acts selectively on the antigen-specific target B cell.

The initial steps in the activation of B cells by helper T cells are strikingly analogous to those of the activation of macrophages by inflammatory T cells. However, while the activation of infected macrophages leads directly to the destruction of the pathogen, naive B cells, like naive T cells,

Fig. 8.5 When an armed helper T cell encounters an antigen-binding B cell, it is triggered to express CD40 ligand (CD40-L) and secrete IL-4 and other cytokines. These are released at the point of contact with the antigen-binding B cell, as shown by staining for IL-4 (bottom right panel). The bottom right panel shows the IL-4 confined to the space between the B cell and the helper T cell. In the middle right panel, the helper T cell is stained for the cytoskeletal protein talin, showing that the cytoskeleton in the helper T cell is polarized, directing the secretion of the IL-4 to the point of contact between the cells. Photographs courtesy of A Kupfer.

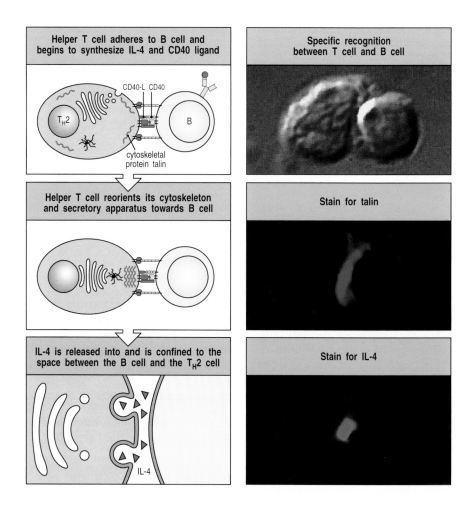

must undergo clonal expansion before they can differentiate into effector cells. The immediate effect of activation by helper T cells is therefore to trigger B-cell proliferation. This is then followed by differentiation of the B cells into antibody-secreting plasma cells (Fig. 8.6). Two additional cytokines, IL-5 and IL-6, both secreted by helper T cells, contribute to these later stages in B-cell activation.

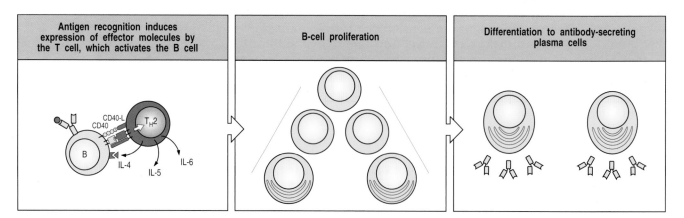

Fig. 8.6 Armed helper T cells stimulate first the proliferation and then the differentiation of antigen-binding B cells. The specific interaction of an antigen-binding B cell with an armed helper T cell leads to the expression of the B-cell stimulatory molecule CD40 ligand (CD40-L) on the helper T-cell surface and to the secretion of the B-cell stimulatory cytokines, IL-4, IL-5, and IL-6, which drive the proliferation and differentiation of the B cell into antibody-secreting plasma cells.

8-4	Isotype switching requires expression of CD40 ligand by the helper T cell and is directed by cytokines.

Antibodies are remarkable, as we saw in Chapter 3, not only for the diversity of their antigen-binding sites but also for their versatility as effector molecules. The specificity of an antibody response is determined by the antigen-binding site, comprising the two variable domains; however, the effector action of the antibody is determined by the isotype of its heavy-chain constant domains; and a given heavy-chain variable domain can become associated with the constant region of any isotype through **isotype switching**. We shall see later in this chapter how antibodies of each isotype contribute distinctively to the elimination of pathogens. The DNA rearrangements that underlie isotype switching and confer this functional diversity on the humoral immune response are directed by cytokines, especially those released by armed CD4 effector T cells.

All mature naive B cells express cell-surface IgM and IgD, yet IgM comprises less than 10% of the immunoglobulin found in plasma, where the most abundant isotype is IgG. Much of the antibody in plasma, therefore, has been produced by B cells that have undergone isotype switching. Little IgD antibody is produced at any time, so the early stages of the antibody response are dominated by IgM antibodies. Later, IgG and IgA are the predominant isotypes, with IgE contributing a small but biologically important part of the response. The overall predominance of IgG is due, in part, to its longer lifetime in the plasma (see Fig. 3.23). These changes do not occur in individuals who make a defective CD40 ligand, which is necessary for interactions between B cells and helper T cells; such individuals make only IgM antibodies and have abnormally high levels of IgM in their plasma, perhaps induced by thymus-independent antigens (see Sections 8-9 and 8-10).

Most of what is known about the regulation of isotype switching by helper T cells has come from experiments in which mouse B cells are stimulated with purified cytokines *in vitro*. These experiments show that different cytokines preferentially induce switching to different isotypes. Some of these cytokines are the same as those that drive B-cell proliferation in the initiation of a B-cell response. In the mouse, IL-4 preferentially induces switching to IgG1 and IgE, while TGF-β induces switching to IgG2b and IgA. T_H2 cells make both of these cytokines as well as IL-5, which induces IgA secretion by cells that have already undergone switching. Although T_H1 cells are poor initiators of antibody responses, they do participate in isotype switching by releasing IFN-γ, which preferentially induces switching to IgG2a and IgG3. The cytokines that direct B cells to make the different isotypes of antibody are summarized in Fig. 8.7.

Cytokines induce isotype switching by making the switch recombination sites that lie 5′ to each C_H gene (see Fig. 3.29) accessible to switch recombinases. When activated B cells are exposed to IL-4, for example, transcription from DNA upstream of the switch regions of $C_\gamma1$ and $C\varepsilon$ can be detected a day or two before switching occurs (Fig. 8.8), indicating that the chromatin at these sites is accessible to DNA-binding proteins. The transcriptional activation of the switch regions that precedes isotype switching is analogous to the transcription that precedes the somatic recombination of immunoglobulin gene segments during the generation of intact variable-region exons in developing B cells (see Chapter 5). Each of the cytokines that induce switching appears to induce a change in chromatin conformation in the switch regions of two different C_H genes, promoting specific recombination to one or other of these genes only. Such a directed mechanism is supported by the observation

Fig. 8.7 Different cytokines induce switching to different isotypes. The individual cytokines induce (violet) or inhibit (red) production of certain isotypes. Much of the inhibitory effect is probably the result of directing switching to a different isotype. These data are drawn from experiments with mouse cells.

Role of cytokines in regulating Ig isotype expression							
Cytokines	IgM	IgG3	IgG1	IgG2b	IgG2a	IgA	IgE
IL-4	Inhibits	Inhibits	Induces		Inhibits		Induces
IL-5						Augments production	
IFN-γ	Inhibits	Induces	Inhibits		Induces		Inhibits
TGF-β	Inhibits	Inhibits		Induces		Induces	

that individual B cells frequently undergo switching to the same C$_H$ gene on both chromosomes, even though only one of the chromosomes is producing the expressed antibody. Thus, helper T cells regulate both the production of antibody by B cells and the isotype that determines the effector function of the antibody that is ultimately produced. How the balance between different isotypes is regulated in the humoral immune response to a given pathogen is not understood.

Fig. 8.8 Isotype switching is preceded by chromatin changes seen as transcriptional activation of C$_H$ genes. Resting naive B cells transcribe the μ and δ loci at a low rate, giving rise to surface IgM and IgD. Bacterial lipopolysaccharide (LPS), which can activate B cells independently of antigen (see Section 8.9), induces IgM secretion. In the presence of IL-4, however, C$_{\gamma 1}$ and C$_\varepsilon$ are transcribed at a low rate, presaging switches to IgG1 and IgE production. The transcripts originate in the region to which switching occurs, and do not code for protein. Similarly, TGF-β gives rise to C$_{\gamma 2b}$ and C$_\alpha$ transcripts and drives switching to IgG2b and IgA. It is not known what determines which of the two transcriptionally activated C$_H$ gene segments undergoes switching. Arrows indicate transcription.

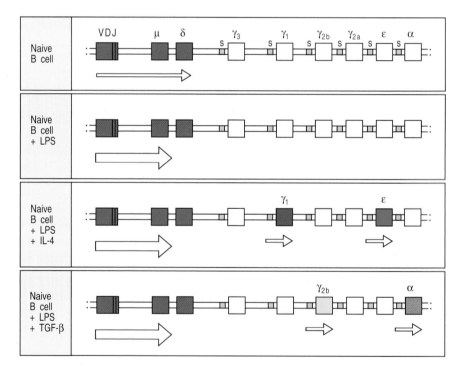

8-5 Activated B cells proliferate extensively in the specialized microenvironment of the germinal center.

In cultures of suspensions of lymphocytes, the interaction of naive, antigen-binding B cells and specific, armed helper T cells can lead to the production of antibody of all isotypes. However, although B-cell proliferation and differentiation (including isotype switching) can all be induced in this way *in vitro*, interactions with T cells in suspension culture cannot reproduce, either in magnitude or in complexity, the responses obtained using the same cells cultured with fragments of spleen, or the antibody response achieved *in vivo*. In particular, the gradual increase in the affinity of antibodies for the inducing antigen that is seen in the course of an immune response requires specialized features of lymphoid tissue. This phenomenon, which is known as **affinity maturation**, is the consequence of somatic hypermutation of the immunoglobulin genes followed by selection of B cells with high-affinity surface immunoglobulin, and depends upon the interaction of activated B cells with cells in the specialized microenvironment of the **germinal center**, which forms after antigen stimulation and which we have already mentioned in Chapter 5 as a site of intense B-cell proliferation in the lymph nodes and spleen (Fig. 8.9).

Germinal centers are formed a week or so after antigen stimulation. B cells that have been activated by T$_H$2 in the T-cell areas of lymphoid tissues can follow either of two fates. Some differentiate into plasma cells secreting IgM or IgG, thus providing an early source of circulating antibodies; however, others migrate into the **primary follicles** and form germinal centers (Fig. 8.9). Primary follicles contain resting B cells clustered around a dense network of processes extending from a specialized cell type, the **follicular dendritic cell**, which is thought to make a central contribution to the selective events that underlie the antibody response.

The cellular origins of follicular dendritic cells are obscure; they are unrelated to the dendritic cells that activate T cells, sharing with them only their branched morphology (dendritic means 'branched'). Their role in driving the maturation of the humoral immune response depends chiefly on their ability to hold intact antigens on their surfaces for long

Schematic representation of a germinal center	Light micrograph of germinal center (high power)	Germinal center (low power) stained to show follicular dendritic cells
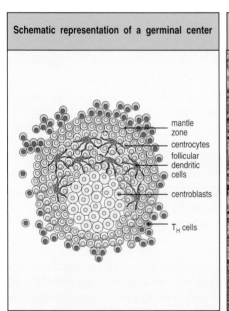	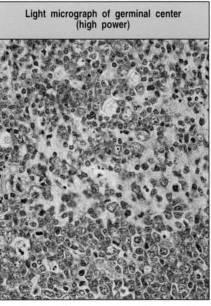	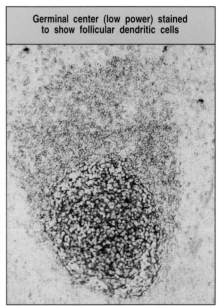

Fig. 8.9 Germinal centers are formed when activated B cells enter lymphoid follicles. The germinal center is a specialized microenvironment in which B-cell proliferation, somatic hypermutation, and selection for antigen binding all occur. Rapidly proliferating B cells in germinal centers are called centroblasts. Closely packed centroblasts form the so-called 'dark zone' of the germinal center, as can be seen in the lower part of the center panel, which shows a section through a germinal center. As these cells mature, they stop dividing and become small centrocytes, moving out into an area of the germinal center called the 'light zone' (the upper part of the center panel), where the centrocytes make contact with a dense network of follicular dendritic cell processes. The follicular dendritic cells are not stained in the center panel but can be seen clearly in the right panel where both follicular dendritic cells (stained blue with an antibody to Bu10, a marker specific for follicular dendritic cells) in the germinal center as well as the mature B cells in the mantle zone (stained brown with an antibody to IgD) can be seen. The plane of this section reveals mostly the dense network of follicular dendritic cells in the light zone, although the less-dense network in the dark zone can just be seen at the bottom of the figure. Photographs courtesy of I MacLennan.

periods. Because follicular dendritic cells are difficult to isolate, the nature of the receptors that hold antigen on their surface is not yet characterized, although it seems likely to be similar to the Fc receptor that holds antibody-bound antigen on the surface of B cells (see Section 8-16). Other specialized properties of follicular dendritic cells, for example, the ability to attract B cells to the follicles, are poorly characterized because this cell type is difficult to study outside an intact lymphoid organ.

When activated B cells enter the primary lymphoid follicle, they start dividing to form germinal centers. The proliferating B cells in germinal centers divide about once every six hours and can be distinguished by their morphological characteristics, which are typical of blast cells (see Fig. 1.16): thus they are large cells with an expanded cytoplasm, which stains intensely for RNA, and diffuse chromatin in the nucleus. These B-cell blasts are called **centroblasts**. The visible focus of centroblasts that forms in a few days within a primary lymphoid follicle is called the germinal center, the remaining B cells that are not specific for antigen being pushed to the outside to form the **mantle zone**.

The rapid proliferation of cells in the germinal center greatly increases the number of B cells specific for the pathogen that initiated the antibody response. By dissecting out individual germinal centers and even individual B cells, and using the polymerase chain reaction to analyze the DNA encoding expressed immunoglobulin chains, it has been possible to demonstrate that all of the B cells in each germinal center are derived from only one or a few founder cells. This technique has also revealed that the germinal centers are the site of somatic hypermutation of immunoglobulin variable-domain genes.

8-6 | **Somatic hypermutation occurs in the rapidly dividing centroblasts in the germinal center.**

Affinity maturation in the course of an immune response can be viewed as a Darwinian process, requiring first the generation of variability in B-cell receptors and then selection for those with the highest affinity for antigen. The variability is generated by somatic hypermutation of the immunoglobulin variable-domain genes, and selection by antigen occurs on the surface of the follicular dendritic cell.

Somatic hypermutation takes place in dividing centroblasts, whose rearranged immunoglobulin variable-region genes accumulate mutations at a rate of about one base pair per 10^3 per cell division. (The mutation rate of all other known somatic cell DNA is one base pair per 10^{12} per division.) As there are about 360 base pairs encoding each of the expressed heavy- and light-chain variable-region genes in a B cell, and as about three out of every four base changes results in an altered amino acid, every second cell will acquire a mutation in its receptor at each division.

Somatic hypermutation affects all the rearranged variable-region genes in a B cell, whether they are expressed in immunoglobulin chains or not. These mutations also affect some DNA flanking the rearranged V gene but they do not extend into the constant-region exons. Thus, the rearranged variable-region genes in a B cell are somehow targeted for the introduction of random somatic point mutations. The resulting mutant receptors are expressed on the progeny of the rapidly dividing centroblasts, which are small cells called **centrocytes**, all derived from the few antigen-specific progenitors that founded the germinal center. As the number of centrocytes increases in the germinal center, two distinct regions begin to be distinguished; the dark zone, where proliferating centroblasts are packed closely together and where there are few follicular dendritic cells, and the light zone, where less-densely packed centrocytes make contact with numerous follicular dendritic cells (see Fig. 8.9).

The centrocytes eventually give rise to memory B cells and antibody-secreting plasma cells. By comparing the expressed and the non-expressed variable-region genes in these cells, the effects of selection can be separated from those resulting from mutation alone, as we shall see later.

| 8-7 | **Non-dividing centrocytes with the best antigen-binding receptors are selected for survival by binding antigen on a follicular dendritic cell.** |

Centrocytes are programmed to die within a fixed period unless their surface immunoglobulin is bound to antigen. It is not known whether follicular dendritic cells play any part in inducing somatic hypermutation in centroblasts; however, they are thought to have a crucial role in the selection of centrocytes for high-affinity binding to antigen.

The evidence implicating the follicular dendritic cells in the selection of centrocytes in the germinal center is circumstantial but strong. We have already mentioned that one of their specialized features is the ability to hold intact antigen on their surface for long periods, possibly in the form of antigen:antibody complexes, bound to Fc receptors. Alternatively, if complement components have been deposited on the surface of the antigen (see Sections 8-24 to 8-27), these may bind to a complement receptor, CR2 (see Section 8-27), which is expressed by follicular dendritic cells. CR2, as well as being a complement receptor, is part of the co-receptor complex of B cells, along with CD19 and TAPA-1, and simultaneous binding of CR2 and surface immunoglobulin to complement-coated antigens increases the sensitivity of B cells to antigen by 100-fold. Follicular dendritic cells may also stimulate B cells through CR2 in the absence of complement components. This they do by means of CD23, which is also able to bind to CR2 and deliver a co-stimulatory signal. Thus the conjoint display of antigen, either with complement components or with CD23 on the surface of follicular dendritic cells, may increase greatly the sensitivity of selection of antigen-binding centrocytes.

After somatic hypermutation, the surface immunoglobulin on the centrocytes derived from a single progenitor B cell may bind antigen either better or less well than the immunoglobulin expressed on the progenitor. Some will inevitably lose the ability to bind antigen at all, and centrocytes bearing these mutations die: a characteristic feature of germinal centers is the presence of **tingible body macrophages**, phagocytes engulfing apoptotic cells. If, on the other hand, the mutant surface immunoglobulin of the centrocyte binds antigen well, the cell is induced to express the *bcl-2* gene, whose product inhibits apoptotic cell death, and the cell is rescued (Fig. 8.10).

Those B cells whose receptors now have a lower affinity for antigen will have to compete not only with these cells but also, and more importantly, with secreted antibody for binding to antigen displayed on follicular dendritic cells. In a primary response, the level of secreted antibody is initially low and the selective pressure on cells with surface immunoglobulin of moderate affinity correspondingly weak. Hence, affinity maturation occurs late in the primary response and is much more prominent in secondary and subsequent responses, as we shall see in Chapter 9.

Fig. 8.10 After somatic hyper-mutation, B cells with high-affinity receptors for antigen are selected by antigen on the surface of follicular dendritic cells. Somatic hypermutation occurs during the proliferation of centroblasts in germinal centers. The centroblasts give rise to small, non-dividing centrocytes. These interact with follicular dendritic cells (FDC) that display antigen in a complex with antibody and complement on their surface. Centrocytes whose receptors no longer bind antigen die by apoptosis, while centrocytes with receptors that bind well are induced to express Bcl-2 and survive. The higher the affinity of the receptor for antigen, the better the centrocyte will compete with other centrocytes and with existing antibodies for binding to antigen and the more likely it is to survive. Binding of the B cell co-receptor complex (CR2:CD19) to complement displayed together with antigen on the follicular dendritic cell surface is thought to amplify the signal from the antigen receptor. This process allows selection of B cells of progressively higher affinity to contribute to the response.

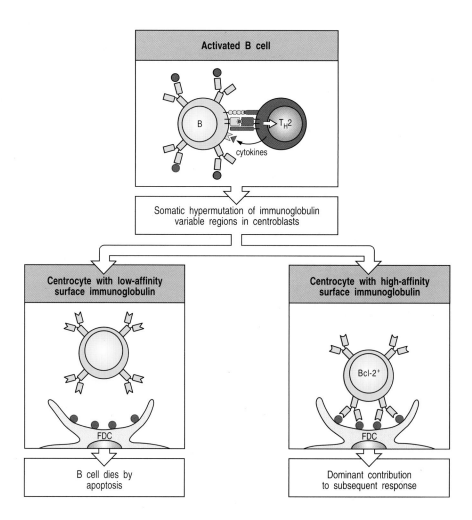

Because the centrocytes are selected in this way for antigen binding, the mutations in the expressed immunoglobulin genes of the surviving cells change amino acids mainly in the complementarity determining regions, while mutations in sequences encoding framework residues, which might affect the stability of the variable domain, tend to be silent, as we saw in Chapter 3. By contrast, in the rearranged V genes that are not expressed, replacement and silent mutations are distributed randomly throughout the exon encoding the V-domain.

The selection of centrocytes in germinal centers resembles, in some respects, the positive selection of thymocytes. However, B cells are selected during the response to foreign antigen instead of during ontogeny, and the selecting antigen is the foreign antigen itself, providing a direct check on the ability of each cell to produce antibodies that can bind the invading pathogen at the time when they are needed. This selective step can be abolished by abnormal expression of the *bcl-2* gene, which, as we learned in Chapter 5, can give rise to B-cell tumors that resemble cells in germinal centers.

As might be expected, mice that express protein Bcl-2 constitutively from a transgene make much larger amounts of antibody for much longer periods after antigenic stimulation, since antigen-binding B cells that would normally be programmed to die instead survive. Because the antibody-producing cells are no longer subjected to selection, however, the antibody produced in these prolonged responses is likely to be of lower average affinity for antigen than that produced in normal mice.

8-8 | B cells leaving the germinal center differentiate into antibody-secreting plasma cells or memory B cells.

B cells that have successfully bound antigen and survived selection leave the germinal center to become either memory B cells or antibody-secreting plasma cells. Which of these two fates a given B cell follows is believed to be determined by signals from follicular dendritic cells and T cells as the B cells leave the germinal center (Fig. 8.11).

Although the signal for plasma-cell differentiation not known for certain, it is thought that CD23 on the surface of follicular dendritic cells plays a part; CD23 is also released from follicular dendritic cells in a soluble form that may contribute to the signal. The differentiation of a B cell into a plasma cell is accompanied by many morphological changes that reflect its commitment to the production of large amounts of secreted antibody (Fig. 8.12). Plasma cells have abundant cytoplasm that is dominated by multiple layers of rough endoplasmic reticulum (see Fig. 1.16). The nucleus shows a characteristic pattern of peripheral chromatin condensation, a prominent perinuclear Golgi apparatus is visible, and the cysternae of the endoplasmic reticulum are rich in immunoglobulin, which makes up 10–20% of all the protein synthesized. Surface immunoglobulin and MHC class II molecules are low or absent, so plasma cells can no longer interact with antigen or helper T cells and antibody secretion is independent of both antigen and T-cell regulation. Plasma cells have a life span of about four weeks in bone marrow or the lamina propria of epithelial surfaces after their final differentiation, and this helps to limit the duration of antibody responses.

The alternative fate of B cells leaving the germinal center is to become memory B cells that do not secrete antibody in the primary response but can be rapidly activated upon subsequent challenge with the same antigen. It is not known exactly what decides whether a given B cell will become a memory or a plasma cell; one possibility is that B cells that have survived selection at the follicular dendritic cell surface become plasma cells unless they encounter CD40 ligand, in which case they are diverted into the memory B-cell pool (see Fig. 8.11).

Germinal centers contain scattered CD4 T cells that express CD40 ligand, and it may be these cells, or CD4 T cells in surrounding T-cell areas, that induce the differentiation of B cells into memory cells as they pass out of the germinal center. CD40 ligand is also capable of inducing *bcl-2* expression in B cells, and this may contribute to the survival of memory B cells. We shall consider the role of these cells in memory responses in Chapter 9.

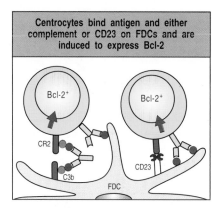

Centrocytes bind antigen and either complement or CD23 on FDCs and are induced to express Bcl-2

Fig. 8.11 Surviving centrocytes migrate out of the germinal center to become either antibody-secreting plasma cells or memory B cells. Some centrocytes differentiate into plasma cells that secrete antibodies in large quantities under the influence of cytokines and possibly soluble or bound CD23 . Others, possibly as a result of stimulation by CD40 ligand (CD40-L), persist as small lymphocytes with high-affinity receptors that can contribute to memory responses to the same antigen.

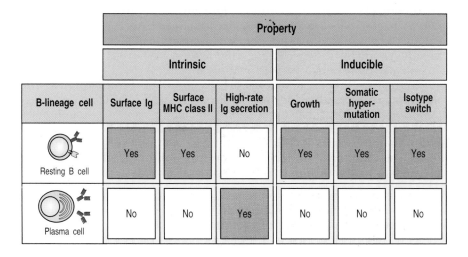

Property					
Intrinsic			Inducible		
B-lineage cell	Surface Ig	Surface MHC class II	High-rate Ig secretion	Growth	Somatic hyper-mutation	Isotype switch
Resting B cell	Yes	Yes	No	Yes	Yes	Yes
Plasma cell	No	No	Yes	No	No	No

Fig. 8.12 Plasma cells secrete antibody at a high rate but can no longer respond to antigen or helper T cells. B cells can take up antigen and present it to helper T cells, which induce them to grow, switch isotype or undergo somatic hypermutation; however, they do not secrete significant amounts of antibody. Plasma cells are terminally differentiated B cells with a finite life span that secrete antibodies. They can no longer interact with helper T cells because they lack surface Ig receptors and MHC class II molecules. They have also lost the ability to change isotype or undergo somatic hypermutation.

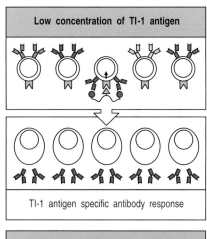

Low concentration of TI-1 antigen

TI-1 antigen specific antibody response

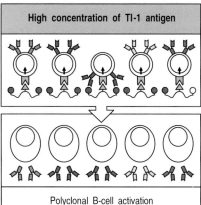

High concentration of TI-1 antigen

Polyclonal B-cell activation

Fig. 8.13 T-cell independent type I antigens are polyclonal B-cell activators at high concentrations. At low concentrations, only specific antigen-binding B cells bind enough of the TI-1 antigen to focus its B-cell activating properties on the B cell; this gives a specific antibody response to epitopes on the TI-1 antigen (top two panels). At high concentrations, the signal delivered by the B-cell activating moiety on TI-1 antigens is sufficient to induce proliferation and antibody secretion by B cells in the absence of specific antigen binding to surface immunoglobulin, so all B cells respond (bottom two panels).

8-9   B-cell responses to bacterial antigens with intrinsic B-cell activating ability do not require T-cell help.

Although antibody responses to protein antigens are dependent on helper T cells, people (and mice) with T-cell deficiencies nevertheless make antibodies to many bacteria. This is because the special properties of some bacterial polysaccharides, polymeric proteins, and lipopolysaccharides enables them to stimulate naive B cells in the absence of T-cell help; that is, they are thymus-independent antigens (TI antigens). In normal individuals, these bacterial products induce antibody responses in the absence of T-cell responses, which cannot be induced by these non-protein antigens since T cells recognize antigen only as peptides bound to MHC molecules.

Thymus-independent antigens fall into two classes, which activate B cells by different mechanisms. Antigens in the first class, the **TI-1 antigens**, contain an intrinsic activity that can directly induce the proliferation of B cells. At high concentration, these molecules cause the proliferation and differentiation of all B cells, regardless of their antigen specificity; this is known as **polyclonal activation** (Fig. 8.13, top two panels). As a result of their ability to stimulate all B cells to divide, TI-1 antigens are often called **B-cell mitogens**, a mitogen being a substance that induces cells to undergo mitosis. When B cells are exposed to concentrations of TI-1 antigens that are 10^3–10^5 times lower than those used for polyclonal activation, only those B cells whose immunoglobulin receptors bind these TI-1 molecules become activated, because only by binding to antigenic determinants on the molecule are they able to concentrate sufficient TI-1 molecules on the cell surface to be activated Fig. 8.13, bottom two panels). In the presence of large amounts of the TI-1 antigen, this concentrating effect is not required and all B cells can be stimulated.

As it is likely that during normal infections *in vivo* concentrations of TI-1 antigens are low, only antigen-specific B cells are likely to be activated and these will produce antibodies specific for TI-1 antigens. Such responses play an important role in specific defense against several extracellular pathogens, and they arise earlier than T-dependent responses because they do not require prior priming and clonal expansion of helper T cells. However, TI-1 antigens are inefficient inducers of isotype switching, affinity maturation, or memory B cells, all of which require specific T-cell help.

8-10   B-cell responses to bacterial polysaccharides do not require specific T-cell help.

The second class of thymus-independent antigens consists of molecules such as bacterial cell wall polysaccharides that have highly repetitive structures. These thymus-independent antigens, called **TI-2 antigens**, contain no intrinsic B-cell stimulating activity. Whereas TI-1 antigens can activate both immature and mature B cells, TI-2 antigens can only activate mature B cells; immature B cells, as we saw in Chapter 5, are inactivated by repetitive epitopes. This may be why infants do not make antibodies to polysaccharide antigens efficiently; most of their B cells are immature. Responses to several TI-2 antigens have been shown to be dominated by CD5 B cells that comprise a minor subpopulation of B cells (see Chapter 5). Indeed, a major function of CD5 B cells in host defense may be the production of anti-polysaccharide antibody.

TI-2 antigens most probably act by extensively crosslinking the cell-surface immunoglobulin of specific mature B cells (Fig. 8.14, left panels). Too extensive crosslinking of receptors, however, renders mature B cells unresponsive, just as it does immature B cells. Thus epitope

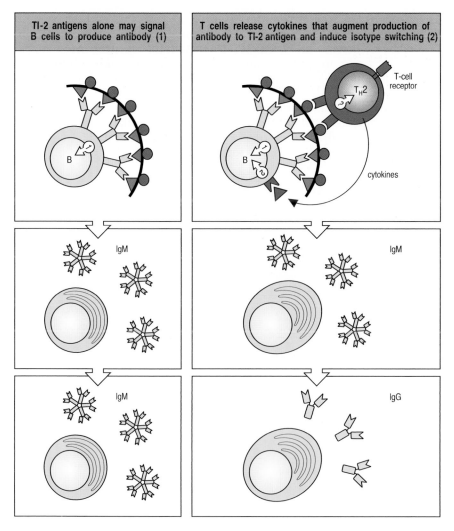

| TI-2 antigens alone may signal B cells to produce antibody (1) | T cells release cytokines that augment production of antibody to TI-2 antigen and induce isotype switching (2) |

Fig. 8.14 B-cell activation by TI-2 antigens requires, or is greatly enhanced by cytokines. Multiple crosslinking of the B-cell receptor by TI-2 antigens can lead to antibody production (left panels), but there is evidence that helper T cells (T$_H$2) greatly augment these responses and lead to isotype switching as well (right panels). It is not clear how T cells are activated in this case, since polysaccharide antigens cannot produce peptide fragments that might be recognized by T cells on the B-cell surface. One possibility is that a component of the antigen binds to a cell-surface molecule common to T cells of all specificities as shown in the figure; an alternative is that some minor population, such as γ:δ or double negative α:β T cells, can recognize polysaccharide antigens bound to unconventional MHC class I or class I-like molecules. However, these mechanisms are speculative.

density seems to be critical in the activation of B cells by TI-2 antigens: too low a density and the level of receptor crosslinking is insufficient to activate the cell; too high a density and the cell becomes anergic.

Although responses to TI-2 antigens can be seen in *nude* mice that are genetically T-cell deficient, depletion of all T cells eliminates responses to TI-2 antigens in culture. Moreover, responses to TI-2 antigens can be augmented *in vivo* by transferring small numbers of T cells to T-cell deficient mice. How T cells contribute to TI-2 responses is not clear. One possibility is that T cells can recognize TI-2 antigens through cell-surface triggering molecules shared by all T cells that stimulate the helper T cells (Fig. 8.14, right panels). Alternatively, some γ:δ or CD4, CD8 double-negative α:β T cells can recognize certain polysaccharides bound to CD1.

B-cell responses to TI-2 antigens provide an early and specific response to an important class of pathogens. Most extracellular bacterial pathogens have cell-wall polysaccharides that allow them to resist ingestion by phagocytes. This allows them not only to escape direct destruction by phagocytes but also to avoid stimulating T-cell responses through the presentation of bacterial peptides by macrophages. T-cell independent antibody to this polysaccharide capsule can coat such **encapsulated bacteria**, promoting their ingestion and hence destruction, and is likely to be an important part of the humoral immune response in many bacterial infections. We mentioned earlier the importance of antibodies to the capsular polysaccharide of *Haemophilus influenzae* B, a

TI-2 antigen, in protective immunity to this bacillus. A further example of the importance of TI responses can be seen in patients with an immunodeficiency disease known as **Wiskott-Aldrich syndrome**, who respond normally to protein antigens but fail to make antibody to polysaccharide antigens and are highly susceptible to infection with extracellular bacteria that have polysaccharide capsules. Thus, the TI responses are important components of the humoral immune response to non-protein antigens that are unable to recruit antigen-specific T-cell help; the distinguishing features of thymus-dependent, TI-1 and TI-2 antibody responses are summarized in Fig. 8.15.

Fig. 8.15 Properties of different classes of antigens that elicit antibody responses.

	TD antigen	TI-1 antigen	TI-2 antigen
Antibody production in normal animal	Yes	Yes	Yes
Antibody production in T-cell depleted animal	No	Yes	Yes
Primes T cells	Yes	No	No
Polyclonal B-cell activation	No	Yes	No
Requires repeating epitopes	No	No	Yes
Examples of antigen	Diphtheria toxin Viral hemagglutinin Purified protein derivative (PPD) of *Mycobacterium tuberculosis*	Bacterial lipopolysaccharide *Brucella abortus*	Pneumococcal polysaccharide Salmonella-polymerized flagellin Dextran Hapten-conjugated ficoll (polysucrose)

Summary.

B-cell activation by many antigens, especially monomeric proteins, requires binding of the antigen by the B-cell surface immunoglobulin and interaction of the B cell with antigen-specific helper T cells. These helper T cells induce a phase of vigorous B-cell proliferation, after which the clonally-expanded progeny of the naive B cells differentiate into either antibody-secreting cells or memory B cells. During the differentiation of activated B cells, several changes can occur in the antibody molecule. First, the antibody isotype may change. Second, the antigen-binding properties of the antibody may change by somatic hypermutation of variable-region genes. Somatic hypermutation can lead to the loss of antigen binding and the death of the B cell, or to increased affinity of the antibody for the eliciting antigen and further selective expansion. Somatic hypermutation and selection for high-affinity binding occur in germinal centers formed by proliferating B cells in the lymphoid follicles, where antigen is displayed on follicular dendritic cells. Helper T cells control these processes by selectively activating cells displaying antigenic peptides, by secreting cytokines that induce isotype switching, and by inducing differentiation into memory B cells. Some antigens stimulate B cells in the absence of specific helper T cells, and these T-independent antigens do not induce either isotype switching or memory B cells but play an important role in host defense to pathogens whose surface antigens cannot elicit T-cell responses.

The distribution and functions of isotypes.

Extracellular pathogens may find their way to most sites in the body, and antibodies must be equally widely distributed to combat them. Most are distributed by diffusion from their site of synthesis but specialized transport mechanisms are required to deliver them to internal epithelial surfaces, such as those of the lung and intestine. The location of antibodies is determined by their isotype, which can limit their diffusion or enable them to engage specific transporters that deliver them across various epithelia. In this part of the chapter, we shall describe the mechanisms whereby antibodies of different isotypes are directed to the compartments of the body in which their distinct effector functions are appropriate, and discuss the protective functions of antibodies that result solely from their binding to pathogens. In the last two parts of the chapter, we shall discuss the effector cells and molecules that are specifically engaged by antibodies of the different isotypes.

8-11 | Antibodies of different isotypes operate in distinct places and have distinct effector functions.

Pathogens most commonly enter the body across epithelial barriers presented by the mucosa of the respiratory, digestive, and urogenital tracts, or damaged skin. Pathogens entering in this way can then establish infections in the tissues. Less often, insects, wounds, or hypodermic needles introduce microbes directly into the blood. The body's mucosal surfaces, tissues, and blood all need to be protected from such infections by antibodies, and antibodies of different isotypes are adapted to function in different compartments. Since a given variable region can become associated with any constant region through isotype switching, B cells can produce antibodies, all specific for the same eliciting antigen, that provide all of the protective functions appropriate for each body compartment.

The first antibodies to be produced in a humoral immune response are always IgM, because VDJ joining occurs just 5′ to the Cμ gene exons (see Fig. 8.8 and Fig. 3.20). These early IgM antibodies are produced before B cells have undergone somatic hypermutation and therefore tend to be of low affinity. IgM molecules, however, form pentamers whose 10 antigen-binding sites can bind simultaneously to multivalent antigens, such as bacterial cell-wall polysaccharides, compensating for the relatively low affinity of the monomers by multipoint binding that confers high avidity. As a result of the large size of the pentamers, IgM is usually thought to be confined to the blood, although some studies in rats show it can enter tissues rapidly as well. Their pentameric structure also makes IgM antibodies especially potent in activating the complement system, as we shall see later. Infection of the bloodstream has serious consequences unless it is controlled quickly, and the rapid production of IgM and its efficient activation of the complement system are important in controlling such infections.

Antibodies of the other isotypes, IgG, IgA, and IgE, are smaller and easily diffuse out of the blood into the tissues. Although most IgA, as we saw in Chapter 3, forms dimers, IgG and IgE are always monomeric, as is some percentage of IgA. The affinity of the individual antigen-binding sites for antigen is therefore critical for the effectiveness of antibodies of all three of these isotypes, and B cells are selected for increased affinity in the germinal centers, mainly after they have undergone switching to these isotypes. IgG is the principal isotype in the blood and extracellular fluid, while IgA is the principal isotype in secretions, the most important being those of the mucous epithelium of the intestinal and respiratory tracts. While IgG efficiently opsonizes pathogens for engulfment by phagocytes and activates the complement system, IgA is a poor opsonin and a weak activator of complement. This distinction is not surprising, as IgG operates mainly in the body tissues where accessory cells and molecules are available, while IgA operates mainly on body surfaces where complement and phagocytes are not normally present, and therefore functions chiefly as a neutralizing antibody. Finally, IgE antibody is present only at very low levels in blood or extracellular fluid, but is bound avidly by receptors on mast cells that are found just beneath the skin and mucosa and along blood vessels in connective tissue. Antigen binding to this IgE triggers mast cells to release powerful chemical mediators that induce reactions, such as coughing, sneezing, and vomiting, that can expel infectious agents. The distribution and main functions of antibodies of the different isotypes are summarized in Fig. 8.16.

Fig. 8.16 Each human Ig isotype has specialized functions and a unique distribution. The dominant effector functions of each isotype (++++) are shaded in dark red, the major functions (+++) are shown in light red, while lesser functions (++) are shown in dark pink, and very minor functions (+) in pale pink. The distributions are similarly marked, with actual levels in serum shown in the bottom row.

Functional activity	IgM	IgD	IgG1	IgG2	IgG3	IgG4	IgA	IgE
Neutralization	+	–	++	++	++	++	++	–
Opsonizaton	–	–	+++	–	++	+	+	–
Sensitization for killing by natural killer cells	–	–	++	–	++	–	–	–
Sensitization of mast cells	–	–	–	–	–	–	–	++++
Activates complement system	++++	–	++	+	++	–	+	–

Distribution	IgM	IgD	IgG1	IgG2	IgG3	IgG4	IgA	IgE
Transport across epithelium	+	–	–	–	–	–	+++ (dimer)	–
Transport across placenta	–	–	+++	+++	+++	+++	–	–
Diffusion into extravascular sites	+/–	–	+++	+++	+++	+++	++ (monomer)	++
Serum level (mg ml^{-1})	1.5	0.04	9	3	1	0.5	2.1	0.00003

8-12   Transport proteins that bind to the Fc domain of antibodies carry specific isotypes across epithelial barriers.

The primary site of synthesis of IgA antibodies, and their main locus of action, is at the epithelial surfaces of the body. IgA-secreting plasma cells are found predominantly in the connective tissue called lamina propria that lies immediately below the basement membrane of many surface epithelia. From there, the IgA antibodies must be transported across the epithelium to its external surface, for example to the lumen of the gut or the bronchi. The IgA antibody synthesized in the lamina propria is secreted as an IgA dimeric molecule associated with a single J chain (see Fig. 3.31). This polymeric form of IgA binds specifically to a molecule called the **poly-Ig receptor** expressed on the basolateral surfaces of the overlying epithelial cells (Fig. 8.17). When the poly-Ig receptor has

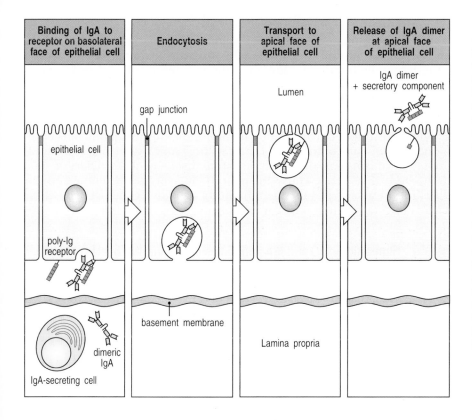

| Binding of IgA to receptor on basolateral face of epithelial cell | Endocytosis | Transport to apical face of epithelial cell | Release of IgA dimer at apical face of epithelial cell |

Fig. 8.17 Transcytosis of IgA antibody across epithelia is mediated by the poly-Ig receptor, a specialized transport protein. Most IgA antibody is synthesized in plasma cells lying just beneath epithelial basement membranes of the gut, respiratory epithelia, tear and salivary glands, and the lactating mammary gland. The IgA dimer bound to a J chain diffuses across the basement membrane and is bound by the poly-Ig receptor on the basolateral surface of the epithelial cell. The bound complex undergoes transcytosis in which it is transported in a vesicle across the cell to the apical surface, where the poly-Ig receptor is cleaved to leave the extracellular, IgA-binding component bound to the IgA molecule as the so-called secretory component. The residual piece of the poly-Ig receptor is non-functional and is degraded. In this way, IgA is transported across epithelia into the lumen of several organs that are in contact with the external environment.

bound a molecule of dimeric IgA, the complex is internalized and carried through the cytoplasm of the epithelial cell in a transport vesicle to its apical surface. This process is called **transcytosis**. At the apical surface of the epithelial cell, the poly-Ig receptor is cleaved enzymatically, releasing the extracellular portion of the receptor still attached to the Fc piece of the dimeric IgA. This fragment of the receptor, called **secretory component**, may help to protect the dimeric IgA from proteolytic cleavage.

The principal sites of IgA synthesis and secretion are the gut, the respiratory epithelium, the lactating breast, and various other exocrine glands such as the salivary and tear glands. It is believed that the primary functional role of IgA antibodies is to protect epithelial surfaces from infectious agents, much as IgG antibodies protect the extracellular spaces of the internal milieu. IgA antibodies prevent the attachment of bacteria or toxins to epithelial cells or the absorption of foreign substances, and provide the first line of defense against a wide variety of pathogens. Newborn infants are especially vulnerable to infection, having had no prior exposure to the microbes in the environment they enter at birth. IgA antibodies are secreted in breast milk and thereby transferred to the gut of the newborn infant where they provide protection from newly encountered bacteria until the infant can synthesize its own protective antibody.

IgA is not the only protective antibody conferred on the infant by its mother. Maternal IgG is transported across the placenta directly into the bloodstream of the fetus during intra-uterine life; human babies at birth have as high a level of plasma IgG as their mothers, and with the same range of specificities. The selective transport of IgG from mother to fetus is due to a specific IgG transport protein in the placenta, FcRn, which is closely related in structure to MHC class I molecules. Despite this similarity, FcRn binds IgG quite differently, as its peptide binding groove is occluded. Instead, two molecules of FcRn bind one molecule of IgG, bearing it across the placenta (Fig. 8.18).

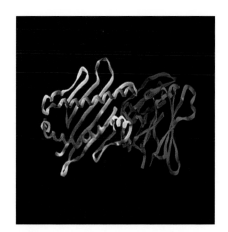

Fig. 8.18 FcRn binds to the Fc piece of IgG. The structure of a molecule of FcRn (white) bound to the Fc piece of IgG (blue) is shown. FcRn transports IgG molecules across the placenta in humans and across the gut in rats and mice. Photograph courtesy of P Bjorkman.

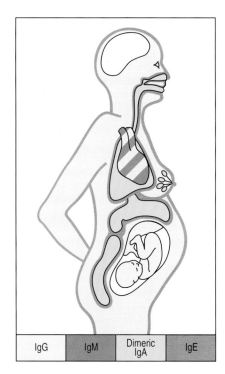

| IgG | IgM | Dimeric IgA | IgE |

Fig. 8.19 Immunoglobulin isotypes are selectively distributed in the body. IgG and IgM predominate in plasma, while IgG along with some IgM and monomeric IgA are the major isotypes in extracellular fluid within the body. Polymeric IgA predominates in secretions across epithelia, including breast milk. The fetus receives IgG from the mother by transplacental transport. IgE is found mainly as mast-cell-associated antibody just beneath epithelial surfaces (respiratory tract, gastrointestinal tract, and skin especially). The brain is normally devoid of immunoglobulin.

In some rodents, FcRn also delivers IgG to the circulation of the neonate from the gut lumen. Maternal IgG is ingested by the newborn animals in colostrum, the protein-rich fluid in the postnatal mammary gland. In this case, transport is from the lumen of the gut into the blood and tissues. This receptor is found only in fetal and early postnatal life and seems to have as its counterpart in humans the transplacental FcRn.

By means of these specialized transport systems, mammals of various species are supplied from birth with antibodies against pathogens common in their environments. As they mature and make their own antibodies of all isotypes, these are distributed selectively to different sites in the body (Fig. 8.19). Thus, throughout life, isotype switching and the distribution of isotypes through the body provides effective protection against infection in extracellular spaces.

8-13   High-affinity IgG and IgA antibodies can neutralize bacterial toxins.

Many bacteria cause pathology by secreting molecules, called bacterial toxins, that damage or disrupt the function of somatic cells (Fig. 8.20). To mediate these effects, the toxins must interact with a specific molecule that serves as a receptor on the surface of the target cell. In many toxins, the receptor-binding domain is carried on one polypeptide chain, while the toxic function is carried by a second chain. Antibodies that bind to the receptor-binding site on the toxin molecule can prevent the toxin from binding to the cell and thus protect the cell from toxic attack (Fig. 8.21). This protective effect of antibodies, as we have already mentioned, is called **neutralization**, and antibodies acting in this way are referred to as **neutralizing antibodies**.

Most toxins are active at nanomolar concentrations: a single molecule of diphtheria toxin can kill a cell. To neutralize toxins, therefore, antibodies must be able to diffuse into the tissues and bind the toxin rapidly and with high affinity. The diffusability of IgG antibodies in the extracellular fluids and their high affinity make these the principal neutralizing antibodies for toxins found at this site. IgA antibodies similarly neutralize toxins at the mucosal surfaces of the body.

Diphtheria and tetanus toxins are among the bacterial toxins in which the toxic and the receptor-binding functions of the molecule are on two separate chains. It is therefore possible to immunize individuals, usually infants, with modified toxin molecules in which the toxic chain has been denatured. These modified toxin molecules, which are called **toxoids**, lack toxic activity but retain the receptor-binding site, so that immunization with the toxoid induces neutralizing antibodies effective in protecting against the native toxin.

In the case of some insect or animal venoms, where toxicity is such that a single exposure is capable of causing severe tissue damage or death, the adaptive immune response is too slow to generate neutralizing antibodies. For these toxins, neutralizing antibodies are generated by immunizing other species, such as horses, with insect and snake venoms for use in protecting humans. Transfer of antibodies in this way is known as **passive immunization** (see Section 2-29).

8-14   High-affinity IgG and IgA antibodies can inhibit the infectivity of viruses.

When animal viruses infect cells, they must first bind to a specific cell-surface protein, often a cell-type-specific protein that determines which cells they can infect. For example, the influenza virus has a surface protein called **influenza hemagglutinin** that binds to terminal sialic acid

Disease	Organism	Toxin	Effects *in vivo*
Tetanus	*Clostridium tetani*	Tetanus toxin	Blocks inhibitory neuron action leading to chronic muscle contraction
Diphtheria	*Corynebacterium diphtheriae*	Diphtheria toxin	Inhibits protein synthesis leading to epithelial-cell damage, and myocarditis
Gas gangrene	*Clostridium perfringens*	Clostridial-α toxin	Phospholipase leading to cell death
Cholera	*Vibrio cholerae*	Cholera toxin	Activates adenylate cyclase, elevates cAMP in cells, leading to changes in intestinal epithelial cells that cause loss of water and electrolytes
Anthrax	*Bacillus anthracis*	Anthrax toxic complex	Increases vascular permeability leading to edema, hemorrhage and circulatory collapse
Botulism	*Clostridium botulinum*	Botulinus toxin	Blocks release of acetylcholine leading to paralysis
Whooping cough	*Bordetella pertussis*	Pertussis toxin	ADP-ribosylation of G proteins leading to lymphocytosis
		Tracheal cytotoxin	Inhibits cilia and causes epithelial-cell loss
Scarlet fever	*Streptococcus pyogenes*	Erythrogenic toxin	Vasodilation leading to scarlet-fever rash
		Leukocidin Streptolysins	Kills phagocytes, allowing bacterial survival
Food poisoning	*Staphylococcus aureus*	Staphylococcal enterotoxin	Acts on intestinal neurons to induce vomiting. Also a potent T-cell mitogen (SE superantigen)
Toxic shock syndrome	*Staphylococcus aureus*	Toxic-shock syndrome toxin	Causes hypotension and skin loss. Also a potent T-cell mitogen (TSST 1 superantigen)

Fig. 8.20 Many common diseases are caused by bacterial toxins. Several examples are shown here. These are all exotoxins, or secreted proteins of bacteria. Bacteria also have endotoxins, or non-secreted toxins that are released when the bacterium dies. The endotoxins are also important in the pathogenesis of disease but here the host response is more complex (see Chapter 9).

residues of the carbohydrate moieties found on certain glycoproteins expressed by epithelial cells of the respiratory tract. It is known as hemagglutinin because it recognizes similar sialic acid residues on chicken red blood cells and can agglutinate these cells by binding to

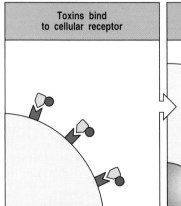

Toxins bind to cellular receptor

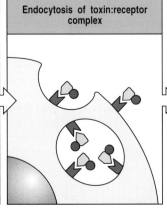

Endocytosis of toxin:receptor complex

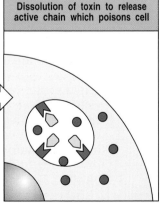

Dissolution of toxin to release active chain which poisons cell

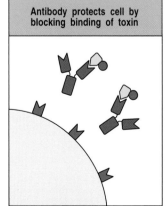

Antibody protects cell by blocking binding of toxin

Fig. 8.21 Neutralization by IgG antibodies protects cells from toxin action. Many bacteria (as well as venomous insects and snakes) mediate their effects by elaborating cellular poisons or toxins (see Fig. 8.20). These toxins usually contain several distinct moieties. One piece of the toxin must bind a cellular receptor, which allows the molecule to be internalized. A second part of the toxin molecule then enters the cytoplasm and poisons the cell. In some cases, a single molecule of toxin can kill a cell. Antibodies that inhibit toxin binding can prevent, or neutralize, these effects.

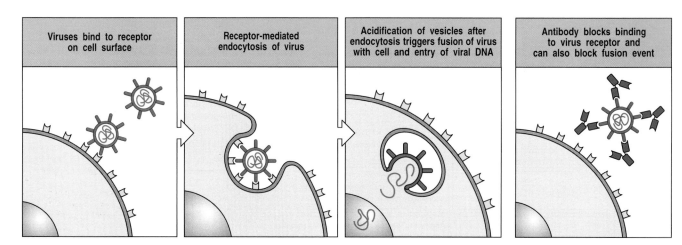

| Viruses bind to receptor on cell surface | Receptor-mediated endocytosis of virus | Acidification of vesicles after endocytosis triggers fusion of virus with cell and entry of viral DNA | Antibody blocks binding to virus receptor and can also block fusion event |

Fig. 8.22 Viral infection of cells can be blocked by neutralizing antibodies. For a virus to infect a cell, it must insert its genes into the cytoplasm. For enveloped viruses, as shown in the figure, this requires viral binding to the cell and fusion of the viral and cell membranes. For some viruses this fusion event takes place on the cell surface, for others it can only occur within the more acidic environment of endosomes. Non-enveloped viruses must also bind to receptors on cell surfaces but enter they the cell by disrupting endosomes. Antibodies can bind to viral surface proteins to inhibit either initial virus binding or the subsequent entry into the cell.

them. Antibodies to the hemagglutinin can inhibit infection by the influenza virus. Such antibodies are called viral-neutralizing antibodies and as with the neutralization of toxins, and for the same reasons, high-affinity IgA and IgG antibodies are particularly important in virus neutralization.

Many antibodies that neutralize viruses do so by inhibiting viral binding to surface receptors (Fig. 8.22). However, viruses are sometimes successfully neutralized when only a single molecule of antibody is bound to a virus particle that has many receptor-binding proteins on its surface. In these cases, the antibody must cause some change in the virus that disrupts its structure and either prevents it from interacting with its receptors or interferes with the fusion of the virus membrane with the cell surface after the virus has engaged its surface receptor, so that the viral nucleic acids cannot enter the cell and replicate there.

8-15   Antibodies can block the adherence of bacteria to host cells.

Many bacteria have specific cell-surface molecules called adhesins that allow them to bind to the surface of host cells. This adherence reaction is critical to the infectivity of these bacteria, whether they enter the cell, as occurs with some pathogens such as *Salmonella* spp, or remain attached to the cell surface as extracellular pathogens. For example, the bacterium *Neisseria gonorrhoeae*, the causative agent of the sexually transmitted disease gonorrhea, has a cell-surface protein known as pilin. Pilin allows the bacterium to adhere to the epithelial cells of the urinary and reproductive tracts and is essential to its infectivity. Antibodies to pilin can inhibit this adhesive reaction and prevent infection (Fig. 8.23).

IgA antibodies secreted onto the mucosal body surfaces of the intestinal, respiratory, and reproductive tracts are particularly important in preventing the adhesion of bacteria, viruses, or other pathogens to the epithelial cells that usually precedes infection by this route. The adhesion of bacteria to cells within the body can also contribute to pathogenesis, and IgG antibodies to adhesins can protect from damage in this way.

Summary.

The antibody response that begins with antigen binding to IgM-expressing B cells and can then lead to the production of antibody of the same specificity in all different isotypes. Each isotype is specialized both in its localization in the body and in the functions it can perform. IgM antibodies are synthesized early in a response and are found in blood and sometimes in extracellular fluids. They are specialized to activate complement efficiently upon binding antigen. IgG antibodies are synthesized later in the response, are usually of higher affinity, and are found in blood and in extracellular fluid, where they can neutralize toxins, viruses, and bacteria, opsonize them for phagocytosis, and activate the complement system. IgA antibodies are synthesized as monomers, which enter blood and extracellular fluids, or in lamina propria as dimeric molecules that are selectively transported across epithelia into sites such as the lumen of the gut, where they neutralize toxins and viruses and block the entry of bacteria across the intestinal epithelium. Most IgE antibody is bound to the surfaces of mast cells that reside mainly just below body surfaces; antigen binding to this IgE triggers local defense reactions. Thus, each of these isotypes occupies a specific site in the body and has a specific role to play in defending the body against extracellular pathogens and their toxic products.

Fc receptor-bearing accessory cells in humoral immunity.

The ability of high-affinity antibodies to neutralize toxins, viruses, or bacteria can protect against infection but does not, on its own, solve the problem of how to remove the pathogens and their products from the body. Moreover, many pathogens are not neutralized by antibody and must be destroyed by other means. To dispose of neutralized microorganisms and to attack resistant extracellular pathogens, antibodies can activate a variety of **accessory effector cells** bearing **Fc receptors** specific for the Fc piece of antibodies of a particular isotype. These accessory cells include the phagocytic cells (macrophages and polymorphonuclear neutrophilic leukocytes), which ingest antibody-coated bacteria and kill them, and other cells — natural killer cells, eosinophils, and mast cells (see Fig. 1.4) — which are triggered to secrete stored mediators when their Fc receptors are engaged. All of these accessory cells are activated when their Fc receptors are aggregated by binding to the multimerized Ig Fc pieces of antibody molecules bound to a pathogen.

8-16 　**The Fc receptors of accessory cells are signaling molecules specific for immunoglobulins of different isotypes.**

The Fc receptors comprise a family of molecules that bind to the Fc portion of immunoglobulin molecules, each member of the family recognizing immunoglobulin of one or a few closely related isotypes through a recognition domain on the α chain of the Fc receptors, itself a member of the immunoglobulin superfamily of proteins. Different accessory cells bear Fc receptors for antibodies of different isotypes, and the isotype of the antibody thus determines which accessory cell will be engaged in a given response. The different Fc receptors and the cells that express them are shown in Fig. 8.24.

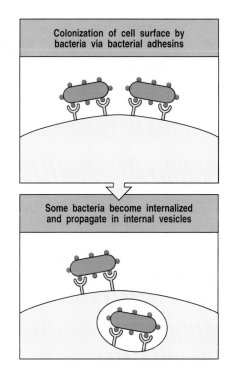

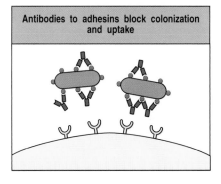

Fig. 8.23 Antibodies can prevent attachment of bacteria to cell surfaces. Many bacterial infections require an interaction between the bacterium and a cell surface. This is particularly true for infections of mucosal surfaces. The attachment process involves very specific molecular interactions between bacterial adhesins and their ligands on host cells; antibodies to bacterial adhesins can block such infections.

Fig. 8.24   Distinct receptors for the Fc region of the different immunoglobulin isotypes are expressed on different accessory cells. The subunit structure, binding properties and cell type expressing these receptors are shown. The complete multimolecular structure of most receptors is not yet known but they may all be multichain molecular complexes similar to the Fcε receptor I (FcεRI). The exact chain composition of any receptor may vary from one cell type to another. For example, FcγRIII in neutrophils is expressed as a molecule with a glycophosphoinositol membrane anchor, without γ chains, while in NK cells it is a transmembrane molecule associated with γ chains as shown. The binding affinities are taken from data on human receptors.

Receptor	FcγRI (CD64)	FcγRII-A (CD32)	FcγRII-B2	FcγRII-B1	FcγRIII (CD16)	FcεRI
Structure 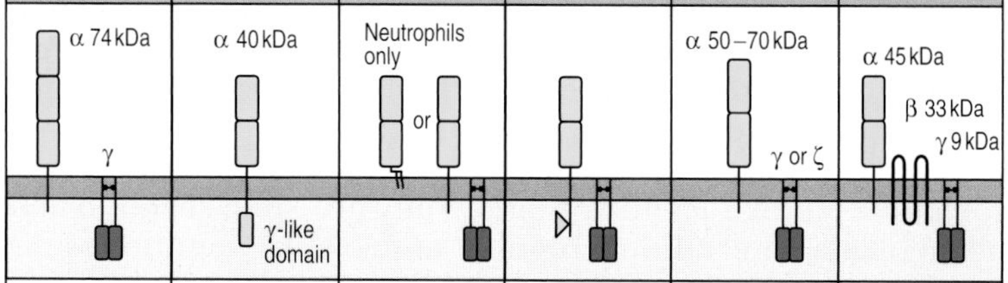	α 74 kDa / γ	α 40 kDa / γ-like domain	Neutrophils only / or		α 50–70 kDa / γ or ζ	α 45 kDa / β 33 kDa / γ 9 kDa
Binding / Order of affinity	IgG1 10^8 M^{-1} 1) IgG1 2) IgG3=IgG4 3) IgG2	IgG1 2×10^6 M^{-1} 1) IgG1 2) IgG3=IgG4 3) IgG2	IgG1 2×10^6 M^{-1} 1) IgG1 2) IgG3=IgG4 3) IgG2	IgG1 2×10^6 M^{-1} 1) IgG1 2) IgG3=IgG4 3) IgG2	IgG1 5×10^5 M^{-1} IgG1=IgG3	IgE 10^{10} M^{-1}
Cell type	Macrophages Neutrophils Eosinophils	Macrophages Neutrophils Eosinophils Platelets	Macrophages Neutrophils Eosinophils Platelets	B cells	NK cells Eosinophils Macrophages	Mast cells Eosinophils Basophils Monocytes
Effect of ligation	Uptake	Uptake	Uptake	Inhibition of stimulation —no uptake	Induction of killing (NK cells)	Secretion of granules

Fc receptors, like T-cell receptors, are multi-subunit proteins in which only the α chain is required for specific recognition. The other chains are required for transport to the cell surface and for signal transduction when Fc is bound. Indeed, most signal transduction by Fc receptors is mediated by a chain called the γ chain that is closely related to the T-cell receptor ζ chain (an exception is human FcγRII-A, in which the cytoplasmic domain of the α chain replaces the function of the γ chain). In the case of the FcγRII-B receptor, alternative splicing of the α chain in different cell types produces two isoforms, which differ in their ability to cause endocytosis of bound immune complexes.

The isoform found in macrophages, called FcγRII-B2, is endocytosed very efficiently. In B cells, alternative splicing gives rise to the B1 isoform, which has an insertion in its cytoplasmic tail that blocks endocytosis; instead, FcγRII-B1 is part of a regulatory mechanism that inhibits the activation of naive B cells (see Section 12-1), mediated by the binding of a phosphatase, PTP1C, to the cytoplasmic tail of FcγRII-B1.

Although the most prominent function of Fc receptors is the activation of accessory cells against pathogens, they may also contribute in other ways to immune responses. For example, the FcR on B cells regulates some B-cell responses, as we shall see in Chapter 12, while those of Langerhans' cells of the skin enable them to ingest antigen–antibody complexes and present peptides to T cells, and binding of such complexes to follicular dendritic cells enables them to drive the maturation of humoral immune responses.

8-17   Fc receptors on phagocytes are activated by antibodies bound to the surface of pathogens.

Phagocytes are activated by IgG antibodies, especially IgG1 and IgG2, which bind to specific Fcγ receptors on the phagocyte surface (see Fig. 8.24). IgG antibodies specific for a given antigen make up only a very small proportion of the total immunoglobulin in plasma. It is essential, therefore, that the Fc receptors on phagocytes be able to distinguish antibody molecules bound to a pathogen from the vast majority of free antibody molecules that are not bound to anything. This condition is met by the aggregation or multimerization of antibodies that occurs when antibodies bind to multimeric antigens or antigenic particles, such as viruses and bacteria.

If Fc receptors on the surface of an accessory cell bind each Ig monomer with low affinity, they will bind such antibody-coated particles with high avidity, and this is probably the principal mechanism by which bound antibodies are distinguished from free immunoglobulin. However, mutations in the hinge region of some antibodies affect the ability of aggregates to bind to the Fc receptor, although they have no effect on monomer binding. This suggests that subtle conformational changes in antibody molecules that accompany binding to antigen may also be important in allowing Fc receptors to distinguish bound from free antibody (Fig. 8.25).

The net result is that Fc receptors allow accessory cells to detect pathogens through bound antibody molecules. Thus, specific antibody and Fc receptors provide the means by which accessory cells that lack intrinsic specificity can identify and remove pathogens and their products from the extracellular spaces of the body.

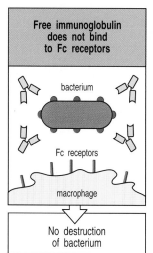
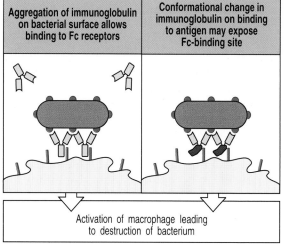

Free immunoglobulin does not bind to Fc receptors	Aggregation of immunoglobulin on bacterial surface allows binding to Fc receptors	Conformational change in immunoglobulin on binding to antigen may expose Fc-binding site
bacterium Fc receptors macrophage		
No destruction of bacterium	Activation of macrophage leading to destruction of bacterium	

Fig. 8.25 Bound antibody is distinguishable from free immunoglobulin by its state of aggregation and/or by conformational change. Free immunoglobulin molecules cannot bind Fc receptors. Antigen-bound immunoglobulin, however, can bind because several antibody molecules bound to the same surface bind to Fc receptors with high avidity. Some studies also suggest that antigen binding and aggregation induce a conformational change in the Fc portion of the immunoglobulin molecule, increasing its affinity for the Fc receptor. Both effects probably contribute to discrimination by Fc receptors between free and bound antibody.

| 8-18 | **Fc receptors on phagocytes allow them to ingest and destroy opsonized extracellular pathogens.** |

The most important accessory cells in humoral immune responses are the phagocytic cells of the monocytic and myelocytic lineages, particularly the macrophages and neutrophilic polymorphonuclear leukocytes or **neutrophils**. Phagocytosis is the ingestion of particles by cells and involves the binding of the particle to the surface of the phagocyte, followed by its internalization and destruction.

Many bacteria are directly recognized, ingested and destroyed by phagocytes, and these bacteria are not pathogenic in normal individuals. Bacterial pathogens, however, usually have polysaccharide capsules that allow them to resist direct engulfment by phagocytes. These bacteria become susceptible to phagocytosis only when they are coated with antibody that engages the Fcγ receptors on phagocytic cells, triggering the engulfment and destruction of the bacterium (Fig. 8.26). The coating

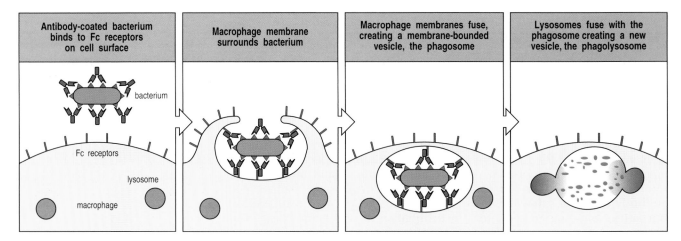

| Antibody-coated bacterium binds to Fc receptors on cell surface | Macrophage membrane surrounds bacterium | Macrophage membranes fuse, creating a membrane-bounded vesicle, the phagosome | Lysosomes fuse with the phagosome creating a new vesicle, the phagolysosome |

Fig. 8.26 A major function of Fc receptors on phagocytes is to trigger the uptake and degradation of antibody-coated bacteria. Many bacteria resist phagocytosis by macrophages and polymorphonuclear leukocytes. Antibodies binding to these bacteria, however, allow them to be ingested and degraded through interaction of the multiple Fc domains arrayed on the bacterial surface with Fc receptors on the phagocyte surface. Fc-receptor binding also signals the phagocyte to increase the rate of phagocytosis, fuse lysosomes with phagosomes, and increase its bacteriocidal activity (see Fig. 8.30).

of a microorganism with molecules that allow its destruction by phagocytes is known as **opsonization**. Bacterial polysaccharides, as we have seen, belong to the TI-2 class of T-cell independent antigens, and opsonization by thymus-independent antibodies produced in response to bacterial polysaccharides early in an immune response is important in ensuring the prompt destruction of many encapsulated bacteria.

Both the internalization and the destruction of microorganisms are greatly enhanced by interactions between the molecules coating an opsonized microorganism and specific receptors for them on the phagocyte surface. When an antibody-coated pathogen binds to Fcγ receptors on the surface of the phagocytic cell, for example, the phagocytic cell surface extends around the surface of the particle through successive binding of Fcγ receptors to bound antibody Fc domains on the pathogen surface. This is an active process that is triggered by the binding of Fcγ receptors. Engulfment of the particle leads to its enclosure in an acidified cytoplasmic vesicle called a phagosome. The phagosome then fuses with one or more lysosomes to generate a phagolysosome, releasing the lysosomal enzymes into the phagosome where they destroy the bacterium (see Fig. 8.26).

Phagocytes can also damage bacteria through the generation of a variety of toxic products. The most important of these are hydrogen peroxide (H_2O_2), the superoxide anion (O_2^-), and nitric oxide (NO), which are directly toxic to the bacterium. Production of these metabolites is induced by the binding of aggregated antibodies to Fcγ receptors. The bacteriocidal products of activated phagocytes can also damage host cells, and a series of enzymes, including catalase (which degrades hydrogen peroxide) and superoxide dismutase (which converts the superoxide anion into hydrogen peroxide) are also produced during phagocytosis to control the action of these products so that they act primarily on pathogens within phagolysosomes. The agents whereby phagocytic cells damage and destroy ingested bacteria are summarized in Fig. 8.27.

Some particles are too large for a phagocyte to ingest: helminthic parasitic worms are one example. In this case, the phagocyte attaches to the surface of the parasite via its Fcγ or Fcε receptors, and the lysosomes fuse with the attached surface membrane. This reaction discharges the

Class of mechanism	Specific products
Acidification	pH=~3.5 – 4.0, bacteriostatic or bacteriocidal
Toxic oxygen-derived products	Superoxide O_2^-, hydrogen peroxide H_2O_2, singlet oxygen $^1O_2$, hydroxyl radical OH·, hypohalite OCl^-
Toxic nitrogen oxides	Nitric oxide NO
Antimicrobial peptides	Defensins, cationic proteins
Enzymes	Lysozyme — dissolves cell walls of some Gram-positive bacteria. Acid hydrolases — further digest bacteria
Competitors	Lactoferrin — binds Fe, vitamin B12 binding protein

Fig. 8.27 Ingestion of antibody-coated bacteria triggers production or release of many bacteriocidal agents in phagocytic cells. Most of these agents are found in both macrophages and neutrophilic polymorphonuclear leukocytes. Some of them are toxic; others, such as lactoferrin, work by binding essential nutrients and preventing their uptake by the bacteria. The same agents can be released by phagocytes interacting with large, antibody-coated surfaces such as parasitic worms or host tissues. As these mediators are also toxic to host cells, phagocyte activation can cause extensive tissue damage in infection.

contents of the lysosome onto the surface of the antibody-coated parasite, damaging it directly in the extracellular space (Fig. 8.28). Whereas the principal phagocytes in the destruction of bacteria are macrophages and neutrophils, large parasites such as helminths are more usually attacked by eosinophils. Thus, Fcγ receptors can trigger the internalization of external particles by phagocytosis, or the externalization of internal vesicles by exocytosis. The latter process usually mediated by IgE binding to the high-affinity FcεI receptor. We shall see in the next three sections that natural killer cells and mast cells also release mediators stored in their vesicles when their Fc receptors are aggregated.

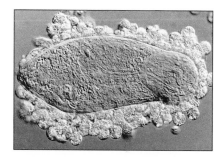

Fig. 8.28 Eosinophils attack a schistosome larva in the presence of serum from an infected patient. Large parasites, such as worms, cannot be ingested; however, when the worm is coated with antibody, especially IgE, eosinophils can attack it via the high-affinity Fcε receptor I. Similar attacks can be mounted by other Fc receptor-bearing cells on various larger targets. Photograph courtesy of A Butterworth.

| 8-19 | **Fc receptors activate natural killer cells to destroy antibody-coated targets.** |

Infected cells are usually destroyed by T cells alerted by foreign peptides bound to cell-surface MHC molecules. However, virus-infected cells may also signal the presence of intracellular infection by expressing on their surfaces viral proteins that can be recognized by antibodies. Cells bound by such antibodies can then be killed by a specialized non-T, non-B lymphoid cell called a **natural killer (NK) cell**.

Natural killer cells are large lymphoid cells with prominent cellular granules that make up a small fraction of peripheral blood lymphoid cells. These cells bear no known antigen-specific receptors but are able to recognize and kill a limited range of abnormal cells. They were first discovered because of their ability to kill some tumor cells but are now known to play an important part in innate immunity, as will be discussed in Chapter 9.

The destruction of antibody-coated target cells by natural killer cells is called **antibody-dependent cell-mediated cytotoxicity (ADCC)** and is triggered when antibody bound to the surface of a cell interacts with Fc receptors on the natural killer cell (Fig. 8.29). NK cells express the FcγRIII (CD16). FcγRIII recognizes the IgG1 and IgG3 subclasses and triggers cytotoxic attack by the NK cell on antibody-coated target cells by mechanisms exactly analogous to those we have encountered in cytotoxic T cells, involving the release of cytoplasmic granules containing perforin and granzymes. The importance of ADCC in defense against

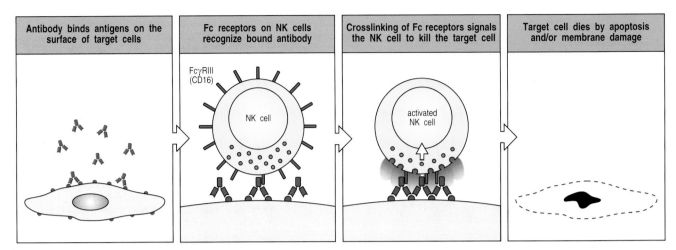

| Antibody binds antigens on the surface of target cells | Fc receptors on NK cells recognize bound antibody | Crosslinking of Fc receptors signals the NK cell to kill the target cell | Target cell dies by apoptosis and/or membrane damage |

Fig. 8.29 Antibody-coated target cells can be killed by natural killer (NK) cells in antibody-dependent cell-mediated cytotoxicity (ADCC). NK cells are large granular non-T, non-B cells that have FcγRIII receptors (CD16) on their surface. When these cells encounter cells coated with IgG antibody, they rapidly kill the target cell. The importance of ADCC in host defense or tissue damage is still controversial.

infection with bacteria or viruses has not yet been fully established. However, ADCC does represent yet another mechanism by which antibodies can direct an antigen-specific attack by an effector cell lacking specificity for antigen, through engaging its Fc receptor.

<h2>8-20   Mast cells bind IgE antibody with high affinity.</h2>

When pathogens cross the epithelial barriers and establish a local infection, the host defenses must be mobilized and directed to the site of pathogen growth. One mechanism by which this is achieved is through the activation of a specialized cell type known as a **mast cell**. Mast cells are large cells with distinctive cytoplasmic granules containing the vasoactive amines histamine and, in some species, such as rabbits and mice, serotonin. They have a distinct appearance after staining with the dye toluidine blue, which makes them readily identifiable in tissues (see Fig. 1.4), and they are seen in particularly high concentration in the submucosal tissues lying just beneath body surfaces, including those of the gastrointestinal and respiratory tracts, and in connective tissues along blood vessels, especially those layers known as the dermis that lie just below the skin. Local activation of mast cells causes increased blood flow and an increased leakage of fluid into the surrounding tissues, bringing with it proteins and cells that can attack the pathogen.

Mast cells are activated via antibody bound to Fc receptors specific for IgE. Unlike the other Fc receptors, however, which bind the Fc region of antibodies only when they are bound to antigen, these receptors, which are designated Fcε receptor I, bind monomeric IgE antibodies with a very high affinity, measured at approximately 10^{10} M^{-1}. Thus, even at the low levels of IgE found circulating in normal individuals, a substantial portion of the total IgE is bound to the Fcε receptors on mast cells and their circulating counterparts, the basophils. Although mast cells are thus usually stably associated with bound IgE, they are not activated by IgE in its monomeric form. Mast-cell activation occurs when the bound IgE is crosslinked by binding to multivalent antigen. Signaling in this way activates the mast cell to release the contents of its prominent granules and initiates a local inflammatory response.

8-21 **Mast-cell activation by antigen binding to IgE triggers a local inflammatory response.**

The immediate consequence of antigen crosslinking of IgE displayed on the mast-cell surface is degranulation, which occurs within seconds. This releases the stored vasoactive amines **histamine** and **serotonin** (Fig. 8.30), causing a local increase in blood flow and vascular permeability that quickly leads to fluid accumulation in the surrounding tissue and an influx of blood-borne cells, such as polymorphonuclear leukocytes. In the skin, this response is readily visualized as a 'wheal and flare' response and such local inflammatory responses serve to bring increased antibody and increased numbers of phagocytes to a site of infection within a few minutes. The same response directed at innocuous antigens is responsible for some of the symptoms of allergic reactions, which we shall consider in detail in Chapter 11.

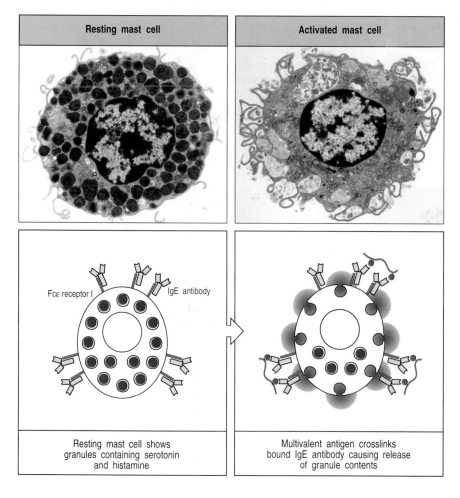

Resting mast cell	Activated mast cell

Resting mast cell shows granules containing serotonin and histamine

Multivalent antigen crosslinks bound IgE antibody causing release of granule contents

Fcε receptor I　IgE antibody

Fig. 8.30　IgE antibody crosslinking on mast cell surfaces leads to rapid mast cell release of inflammatory mediators. Mast cells are large cells found in connective tissue that can be distinguished by secretory granules containing many inflammatory mediators. They bind stably to monomeric IgE antibodies through the very high-affinity Fcε receptor I. Antigen crosslinking of the bound IgE antibody molecules triggers rapid degranulation, releasing inflammatory mediators into the surrounding tissue. These mediators trigger local inflammation, which recruits cells and proteins required for host defense to sites of infection. It is also the basis of the acute phase of the allergic reaction causing asthma, hay fever and the life-threatening response known as systemic anaphylaxis (see Chapter 11). Photographs courtesy of A M Dvorak.

Histamine and serotonin are small, short-lived mediators, and their effect is rapidly lost after mast-cell degranulation. However, the local inflammatory response is sustained by the subsequent production of other molecules. For example, mast-cell activation turns on an enzymatic pathway leading to the generation of metabolites of arachidonic acid known as leukotrienes (Fig. 8.31). These compounds are also vasoactive and generate a more sustained vascular response. Finally, mast cells synthesize and secrete a variety of cytokines upon activation, including IL-4 and TNF-α, the latter contributing to a prolonged local inflammatory reaction, which also acts to contain local infection.

Fig. 8.31 Lipid mediators of inflammation synthesized by mast cells upon stimulation by antigen binding to IgE. These mediators derive from phospholipids by release of the precursor molecule arachidonic acid. This molecule can be modified by two pathways, as shown, to give rise to prostaglandins, thromboxanes, and leukotrienes. The main products of mast cells are the leukotrienes, which sustain inflammatory responses in the tissue. This is especially true of the leukotriene molecules C4, D4, and E4. Many anti-inflammatory drugs are inhibitors of arachidonic acid metabolism. Aspirin, for example, is an inhibitor of cyclooxygenase and blocks the production of prostaglandins.

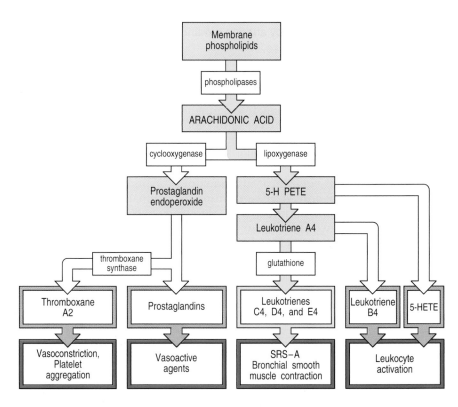

Although people in industrialized societies are familiar with IgE antibodies and mast-cell activation chiefly in the context of allergic responses, it is believed that mast cells serve at least two important functions in host defense. First, their location near body surfaces allows them to recruit both specific and non-specific effector elements to the sites where infectious agents are most likely to enter the internal milieu and they also increase the flow of lymph from sites of antigen deposition to the regional lymph nodes, where naive lymphocytes are first activated. The second effect occurs when IgE bound to mast cells encounters antigen in the submucosal tissue of the gut or the airway. The released mediators histamine, serotonin, and the leukotrienes induce smooth muscle contraction that allows the body to expel the contents of hollow organs, thereby discharging the infectious agent. Thus, mast-cell degranulation in the gut leads to diarrhea or vomiting, while mast-cell degranulation in the lungs leads to increased mucus secretion and bronchial contraction, making coughing more effective and recruiting antibodies and polymorphonuclear leukocytes to sites of antigen deposition in the airways. IgE antibody and mast cells appear to play a particularly important role in immunity to intestinal worms, and it is interesting to note that worm infestation leads to high levels of specific IgE-antibody production, further suggesting that IgE-antibody responses are specialized for responses to this class of pathogens.

Summary.

Antibody-coated pathogens are recognized by Fc receptors on the surfaces of various cells that bind to the constant-region domains of the bound antibodies and trigger the destruction of the pathogen. Fc receptors comprise a family of molecules each of which recognizes immunoglobulin of a specific isotype. Fc receptors on macrophages and neutrophils recognize the constant regions of IgG antibodies and trigger the engulfment and destruction of IgG-coated bacteria by these phagocytic cells. Binding to the Fc receptor also induces the production of bacteriocidal agents in the intracellular vesicles of the phagocyte. Eosinophils are important in the elimination of parasites too large to be engulfed; they bear Fc receptors specific for the constant region of IgG, as well as high affinity receptors for IgE, and binding of these receptors by antibody triggers the release of toxic substances onto the surface of the parasite. Natural killer cells and mast cells also release their granule contents when their Fc receptors are engaged. Mast cells act as accessory cells in humoral immune responses but their Fc receptors, which recognize IgE, are unlike those of other accessory cells in that they bind free monomeric antibody. When the IgE on the surface of a mast cell is aggregated by binding to antigen, it triggers the mast cell to release vasoactive amines that increase the blood flow to sites of infection and thereby recruit antibodies and effector cells. Mast cells are found principally below epithelial surfaces of the skin and the digestive and respiratory tracts and their activation by innocuous substances is responsible for many of the symptoms of acute allergic reactions.

The complement system in humoral immunity.

Complement was discovered many years ago as a heat-labile component of normal plasma that augments opsonization of bacteria by antibodies and allows some antibodies to kill bacteria. This activity was said to complement the antibacterial activity of antibody, hence the name complement. The complement system is made up of a large number of distinct plasma proteins; one is directly activated by bound antibody to trigger a cascade of reactions each of which results in the activation of another complement component. Some activated complement proteins bind covalently to the bacteria, opsonizing them for engulfment by phagocytes bearing **complement receptors**, while small fragments of complement proteins recruit phagocytes to the site of complement activation. The **terminal complement components** damage certain bacteria by creating pores in the bacterial membrane.

There are three pathways by which the effector functions of complement can be activated (Fig. 8.32). The **classical pathway** is activated by antibody binding to antigen and is thus part of the adaptive humoral immune response. The **lectin pathway** is initiated by binding of a serum lectin, the mannose binding protein, to mannose-containing

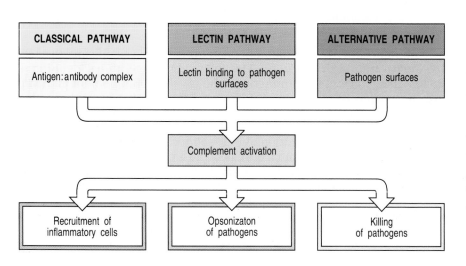

Fig. 8.32 Schematic overview of the complement cascade. There are three pathways of complement activation, the classical pathway, which is triggered by antibody, the lectin-mediated pathway, which is triggered by normal serum proteins that bind some encapsulated bacteria, and the alternative pathway that is triggered directly on pathogen surfaces. They generate a crucial enzymatic activity that, in turn, generates the effector activities of complement. The three main consequences of complement activation are opsonization of pathogens, the recruitment of inflammatory cells, and direct killing of pathogens.

proteins or to carbohydrates on bacteria or viruses; and the **alternative pathway** can be initiated when a spontaneously activated complement component binds to the surface of a pathogen. The alternative pathway and the lectin pathway are thus part of the innate immune system. The alternative pathway also provides an amplification loop for the classical pathway of complement activation because one of the activated components of the classical pathway can also initiate the alternative pathway. We shall focus here on the classical pathway, touching on the alternative pathway in its role in amplifying the classical pathway but leaving the details of how the lectin and the alternative pathways are initiated for Chapter 9 where we discuss innate mechanisms of immunity.

| 8-22 | **Complement is a system of plasma proteins that interacts with bound antibodies to aid in the elimination of pathogens.** |

In the humoral immune response, binding of either IgM or most classes of IgG to a pathogen activates the complement cascade. The events of the complement cascade can be divided into two sequences of reactions, which we shall call 'early' and 'late' events. The early events consist of a series of proteolytic steps in which an inactive precursor protein is cleaved to yield a large active fragment, which binds to the surface of a pathogen and contributes to the next cleavage, and a small peptide fragment that is released from the cell and often mediates inflammatory responses. The early events end with the production of a protease called a **C3 convertase** that is covalently bound to the pathogen surface. Here it generates the two main effector molecules of the complement system: an opsonin that bind covalently to pathogen surfaces, and a small peptide mediator of inflammation. The C3 convertase also generates a C5 convertase that initiates the late events of complement activation, which comprise a sequence of polymerization reactions in which the terminal complement components interact to form a **membrane-attack complex**, which creates a pore in membranes of certain pathogens that can lead to their death. The C3 convertase thus occupies a central position in the cascade (see Fig. 8.33). The reactions triggered by bound antibody molecules are called the **classical pathway** of complement activation because this pathway was discovered first. However, the **alternative pathway** of complement activation, in which the early events are triggered in the absence of antibody, probably arose first in evolution. The related lectin-dependent pathway may be an evolutionary intermediate (see Chapter 9). Each pathway generates a C3 convertase by a different route but two of the three convertases are identical, and all are homologous and have the same activity, so the principal effector molecules and the late events are the same for all three pathways.

The nomenclature of complement proteins is often a significant obstacle to understanding this system. The following conventional definitions will be used here. All components of the classical complement pathway are designated by the letter C followed by a number, and the native components have a simple number designation, for example C1 and C2. Unfortunately, the components were numbered in the order of their discovery, and not the sequence of reactions, which is C1, C4, C2, C3, C5, C6, C7, C8, and C9. The products of the cleavage reactions are designated by added lower-case letters, the larger fragment being designated b and the smaller a; thus for example C4 is cleaved to C4b and C4a. The components of the alternative pathway, instead of being numbered, are designated by different upper case letters, for example B and D. As with the classical pathway, their cleavage products are designated by the addition of lower-case a and b: thus, the large fragment of B is called Bb and the small fragment Ba. Activated complement components are often designated by a horizontal line, for example $\overline{C2b}$; however, we shall not use this convention. It is also useful to be aware that the large active fragment of C2 was originally designated C2a, and is still called that in some texts and research papers. Here, for consistency, we will call all large fragments of complement b, so the large active fragment of C2 will be designated C2b.

An overview of the complement system is shown in Fig. 8.33. The generation of the C3 convertase, so called because it is specific for the cleavage of complement component C3, results in the rapid cleavage of many molecules of C3 to produce C3b, which binds covalently to the pathogen surface. The cleavage of C3 and the binding of large numbers of C3b molecules to the surface of the pathogen is a pivotal event in complement activation. At this point the pathways of complement activation converge, the main effector activities of complement are generated, and the late events begin, with C3b playing a central part. The bound C3b is the major opsonin of the complement system, binding to **complement receptors** on phagocytes and facilitating engulfment of the pathogen. C3b also binds C5, allowing it to be cleaved by the C2b component of the C4b,2b,3b C5 convertase to initiate the assembly of the membrane-attack complex. C5a and C3a mediate local inflammatory responses, recruiting fluid, cells, and proteins to the site of infection. Finally, the binding of C3b initiates the alternative pathway, thereby amplifying complement activation.

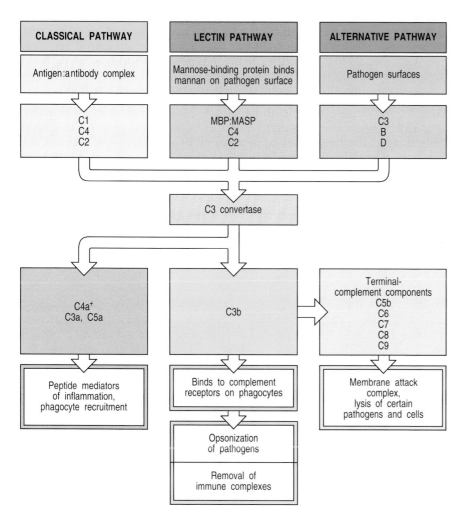

Fig. 8.33 Overview of the main components and effector actions of complement. The early events of all three pathways of complement activation involve a series of cleavage reactions culminating in the formation of an enzymatic activity called a C3 convertase, which cleaves complement component C3. This is the point at which the three pathways converge and the effector functions of complement are generated. The larger cleavage fragment of C3 (C3b) binds to the membrane and opsonizes bacteria, allowing phagocytes to internalize them. The small fragments of C5 and C3, called C5a and C3a, are peptide mediators of local inflammation. C4a, generated by cleavage of C4 during the early events of the classical pathway (and not by the action of C3 or C5 convertase), is also a peptide mediator of inflammation but its effects are relatively weak (+). Similarly, the large cleavage fragment of C4, C4b, is a weak opsonin (not shown). Finally, the C3b bound to the C3 convertase binds C5, allowing the C3 convertase to generate C5b, which associates with the bacterial membrane and triggers the late events, in which the terminal components of complement assemble into a membrane-attack complex that can damage the membrane of certain pathogens.

Functional protein classes in the complement system	
Binding to antigen: antibody complexes	C1q
Activating enzymes	C1r C1s C2b Bb D
Membrane-binding proteins and opsonins	C4b C3b
Peptide mediators of inflammation	C5a C3a C4a
Membrane-attack proteins	C5b C6 C7 C8 C9
Complement receptors	CR1 CR2 CR3 CR4 C1qR
Complement-regulatory proteins	C1INH C4bp CR1 MCP DAF H I P CD59

Fig. 8.34 Functional protein classes in the complement system.

It is clear that a pathway that leads to such potent inflammatory and destructive effects, and which, moreover, has a built-in amplification step, is potentially dangerous and must be subject to tight regulation. One important safeguard is that key activated complement components are rapidly inactivated unless they bind the pathogen surface on which their activation is initiated. There are also several points on the pathway where regulatory proteins act on complement components to prevent the inadvertent activation of complement on host cells and hence accidental damage to them. We shall return to these regulatory mechanisms at the end of this part of the chapter.

We have now met all the relevant components of complement, albeit in a superficial manner, and we are ready for a more detailed account of their functions. To help distinguish the different components according to their functions, we shall use a color code in figures in this section that list the various components and their activities: this is introduced in Fig. 8.34, where all the components of complement are grouped by function.

8-23   **The C1q molecule binds to antibody molecules to trigger the classical pathway of complement activation.**

The first component of the classical pathway of complement activation is C1, which is a complex of three proteins called C1q, C1r, and C1s, two molecules each of C1r and C1s being bound to each molecule of C1q (Fig. 8.35). Complement activation is initiated when antibodies attached to the surface of a pathogen bind C1q. C1q can be bound by either IgM or IgG antibodies (see Fig. 8.16) but because of the structural requirements of binding to C1q neither of these types of antibodies can activate complement in solution, and the cascade is initiated only when they are bound to multiple sites on a cell surface, normally that of a pathogen.

The C1q molecule has six globular heads joined to a common stem by long, filamentous domains that resemble collagen molecules; the whole C1q complex has been likened to a bunch of six tulips held together by the stems. Each globular head can bind to one Fc domain, and binding of two or more globular heads activates the C1q molecule. In plasma, the pentameric IgM molecule has a planar conformation that does not bind C1q (Fig. 8.36, left panel); however, binding to the surface of a pathogen deforms the IgM pentamer so that it looks like a staple (Fig. 8.36, right panel), and this distortion exposes binding sites for the C1q heads. C1q does bind with low affinity to some subclasses of IgG in solution but the binding energy required for C1q activation is achieved only when

Fig. 8.35 The first protein in the classical pathway of complement activation is C1, which is a complex of C1q, C1r, and C1s. C1q is composed of six identical subunits with globular heads and long, collagen-like tails. The tails bind to two molecules each of C1r and C1s; the heads bind to the Fc domains of immunoglobulin molecules. Photograph (x 500 000) courtesy of K B M Reid.

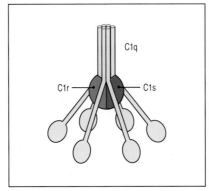

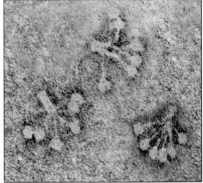

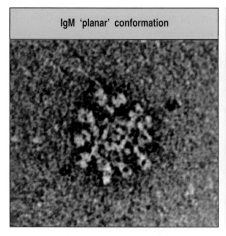
IgM 'planar' conformation

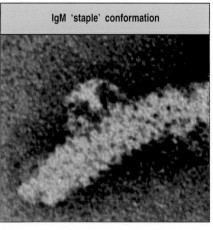
IgM 'staple' conformation

Fig. 8.36 The two conformations of IgM. The left panel shows the planar conformation of soluble IgM while the right panel shows the staple conformation of IgM bound to a bacterial flagellum. Photographs (x 760 000) courtesy of K H Roux.

C1q can bind two or more IgG molecules aggregated on a 30–40 nm of each other to bind the heads of a single C1q molecule, and this requires the random binding of many IgG molecules to a single pathogen. For this reason, IgM is much more efficient in activating complement than IgG.

The binding of C1q to a single bound IgM molecule, or to two or more bound IgG molecules, leads to the activation of an enzymatic activity in C1r, and the active form of C1r then cleaves its associated C1s to generate an active serine protease (Fig. 8.37). The activation of C1s completes the first step in the classical pathway of complement activation.

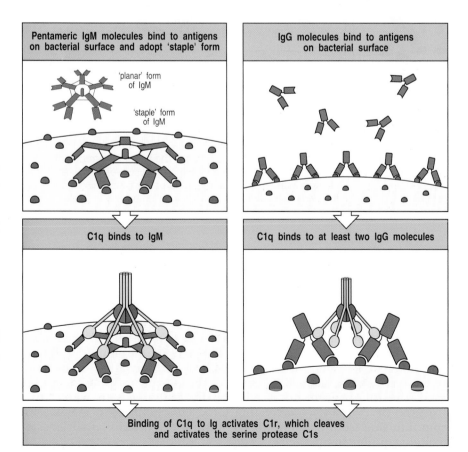

Pentameric IgM molecules bind to antigens on bacterial surface and adopt 'staple' form

'planar' form of IgM

'staple' form of IgM

IgG molecules bind to antigens on bacterial surface

C1q binds to IgM

C1q binds to at least two IgG molecules

Binding of C1q to Ig activates C1r, which cleaves and activates the serine protease C1s

Fig. 8.37 The classical pathway of complement activation is initiated by binding of C1q to antibody on a bacterial surface. In the left panel, one molecule of IgM, bent into the 'staple' conformation by binding several identical epitopes on a pathogen surface, allows binding by the globular heads of C1q to its Fc pieces on the surface of the pathogen. In the right panel, multiple molecules of IgG bound on the surface of a pathogen allow binding by C1q to two or more Fc pieces. In both cases, binding of C1q activates the associated C1r, which becomes an active enzyme that cleaves the proenzyme C1s, a serine protease that initiates the classical complement cascade.

8-24 | **The classical pathway of complement activation generates a C3 convertase bound to the pathogen surface.**

Once bound antibody has activated C1s, the C1s enzyme acts on the next two components of the classical pathway, cleaving C4 and then C2 to generate two large fragments, C4b and C2b, which together form the C3 convertase of the classical pathway. In the first step, C1s cleaves the plasma protein C4 to produce C4b, which binds covalently to the surface of the pathogen. The covalently attached C4b then binds one molecule of C2, making it susceptible, in turn, to cleavage by C1s. C1s cleaves C2 to produce the large fragment C2b, which is itself a serine protease. The complex of C4b with the active serine protease C2b remains on the surface of the pathogen as the C3 convertase of the classical pathway. Its most important activity is to cleave large numbers of C3 molecules to C3b, which bind to the pathogen surface, and C3a, which initiates a local inflammatory response. These reactions, which comprise the classical pathway of complement activation, are shown in schematic form in Fig. 8.38.

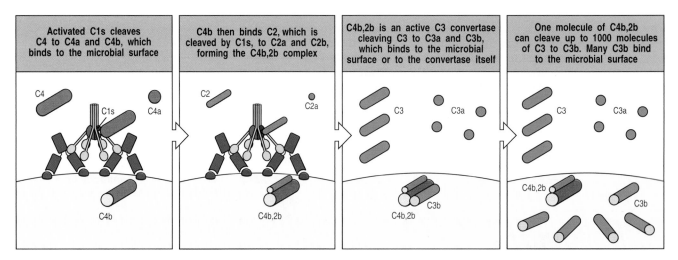

| Activated C1s cleaves C4 to C4a and C4b, which binds to the microbial surface | C4b then binds C2, which is cleaved by C1s, to C2a and C2b, forming the C4b,2b complex | C4b,2b is an active C3 convertase cleaving C3 to C3a and C3b, which binds to the microbial surface or to the convertase itself | One molecule of C4b,2b can cleave up to 1000 molecules of C3 to C3b. Many C3b bind to the microbial surface |

Fig. 8.38 The classical pathway of complement activation generates a C3 convertase that deposits large numbers of C3b molecules on the pathogen. The steps in the reaction are outlined here and detailed in the text. The cleavage of C4 by C1s exposes a reactive group on C4b that allows it to bind covalently to the pathogen surface. C4b then binds C2, making it susceptible to cleavage by C1s. The larger C2b fragment is the active protease component of the C3 convertase, which cleaves many molecules of C3 to produce C3b, which binds to the pathogen surface, and C3a, an inflammatory mediator.

It is important that the C3 convertase is firmly attached to the pathogen so that C3 activation occurs there and not on host-cell surfaces. This is achieved principally by the covalent binding of C4b to the pathogen surface. Cleavage of C4 exposes a highly reactive thioester bond on the C4b molecule that allows it to bind covalently to molecules in the immediate vicinity of its site of activation: this may be the bound antibody molecule that activated the classical pathway, or any adjacent protein on the pathogen surface (Fig. 8.39). If C4b does not rapidly form this bond, the thioester bond is cleaved by reacting with water (hydrolysis), irreversibly inactivating C4b. This helps to prevent C4b from diffusing from its site of activation on the microbial surface to become coupled to host cells.

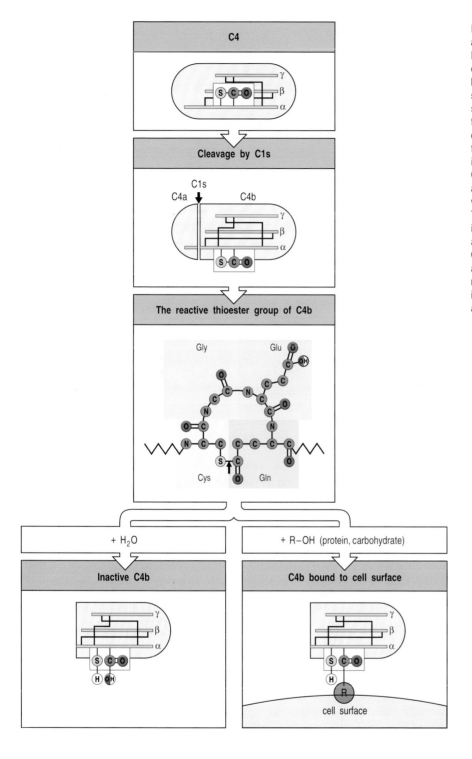

Fig. 8.39 Cleavage of C4 exposes an active thioester bond that causes the large fragment, C4b, to bind covalently to nearby molecules on the bacterial cell surface. Intact C4 consists of an α, a β and a γ chain with a shielded thioester bond on the α chain that is exposed when the α chain is cleaved by C1s to produce C4b. The thioester bond (arrowed in the third panel) is rapidly hydrolyzed by water, inactivating C4b unless it reacts with hydroxyl or amino groups to form a covalent linkage with molecules on the pathogen surface. The homologous protein C3 has an identical reactive thioester bond that is also exposed on the C3b fragment when C3 is cleaved by C2b. The covalent attachment of C3b and C4b enables these molecules to act as opsonins and is important in confining complement activation to the pathogen surface.

C2 becomes susceptible to cleavage by C1s only when it is bound by C4b, and the C2b serine protease is thereby also confined to the pathogen surface where it remains associated with C4b, providing the enzymatic activity of the C3 convertase of the classical pathway. The activation of C3 molecules thus also occurs at the surface of the pathogen, and the C3b cleavage product of C3 binds covalently by the same mechanism as C4b, as we shall see below. The proteins of the classical pathway of complement activation and their active forms are listed in Fig. 8.40.

Fig. 8.40 The proteins of the classical pathway of complement activation.

Proteins of the classical pathway of complement activation		
Native component	Active form	Function of the active form
C1 (C1q: C1r$_2$:C1s$_2$)	C1q	Binds to antibody that has bound antigen, activates C1r
	C1r	Cleaves C1s to active protease
	C1s	Cleaves C4 and C2
C4	C4b	Covalently binds to pathogen and opsonizes it. Binds C2 for cleavage by C1s
	C4a	Peptide mediator of inflammation (weak)
C2	C2b	Active enzyme of classical pathway C3/C5 convertase: cleaves C3 and C5
	C2a	Unknown
C3	C3b	Many molecules bind pathogen surface and act as opsonin. Initiates amplification via the alternative pathway. Binds C5 for cleavage by C2b
	C3a	Peptide mediator of inflammation (intermediate)

8-25   **The cell-bound C3 convertase deposits large numbers of C3b molecules on the pathogen surface.**

The C3 convertase of the classical pathway, consisting of the complex C4b,2b, cleaves C3 into C3b and C3a. C3 is structurally and functionally homologous to C4, and C3b, like C4b, has a reactive thioester bond that is exposed by cleavage. This allows C3b to bind covalently to adjacent molecules on the pathogen surface; otherwise it is inactivated by hydrolysis. Complement component C3 is the most abundant complement protein in plasma, and up to 1000 molecules of C3b can bind in the vicinity of a single active C3 convertase (see Fig. 8.38). Thus, the main effect of complement activation is to deposit large quantities of C3b on the surface of the initiating pathogen where it forms a covalently-bonded coat that, as we shall see, can signal the ultimate destruction of the pathogen by phagocytes.

The next step in the cascade is the generation of the C5 convertase by the binding of C3b to C4b,2b to yield C4b,2b,3b. This complex binds C5 and makes it C5 susceptible to cleavage by the serine protease activity of C2b: this initiates the generation of the membrane attack complex. This reaction is much more limited than cleavage of C3, as C5 can be cleaved only if it binds C3b that is part of the C4b,2b,3b C5 convertase complex. Thus, the end result of the early events of complement activation by the classical pathway is the binding of large numbers of C3b molecules on the surface of the pathogen, with the generation of a more limited number of C5b molecules, and the release of C3a and C5a.

The many C3b molecules deposited on the pathogen surface can be recognized by **complement receptors** on phagocytic cells, which are thereby stimulated to engulf the pathogen. The peptides C4a, C3a and especially C5a, which are generated by the cleavage of C4, C3 and C5, are potent local inflammatory mediators. Finally, as already mentioned, the generation of C5b leads to the formation of the membrane-attack complex. Before discussing these effector functions of complement in greater detail, we will see how bound C3b can amplify the effects of the classical pathway by initiating activation of the alternative pathway.

8-26 | Bound C3b initiates the alternative pathway of complement activation to amplify the effects of the classical pathway.

Apart from the initiating step, the events of the alternative pathway of complement activation are exactly analogous to those of the classical pathway and involve homologous activated components. Thus in each case, a large active fragment is deposited on the surface of the pathogen where it binds a second component and renders it susceptible to cleavage by an activating protease to generate the active protease component of the resulting C3 convertase (Fig. 8.41).

In the classical pathway, the covalently bound fragment is C4b generated by the cleavage of C4 by activated C1s. In the alternative pathway, the covalently bound fragment is C3b, and the alternative pathway can be activated by the covalent binding of C3b to the pathogen surface.

We have already seen that C3b is structurally and functionally homologous to C4b, the first active fragment to bind to the pathogen surface in the classical pathway. In the second step of the alternative pathway, C3b binds to factor B, which is structurally and functionally homologous to C2.

Binding of factor B to C3b makes it susceptible to cleavage by the plasma protease factor D. This cleavage yields a small fragment Ba and an active protease Bb, which remains bound to C3b to make the complex C3b,Bb, which is the C3 convertase of the alternative pathway of complement activation. Note that C3b,Bb is the exact structural and functional homolog of C4b,2b, the C3 convertase of the classical pathway, and that the homologous components C2 of the classical and factor B of the alternative pathways are encoded in adjacent genes in the class III region of the MHC (see Fig. 4.18). The components of the alternative pathway of complement activation are summarized in Fig. 8.42.

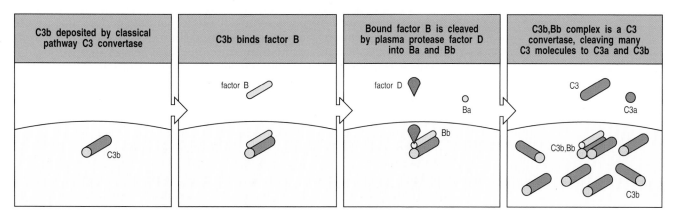

C3b deposited by classical pathway C3 convertase	C3b binds factor B	Bound factor B is cleaved by plasma protease factor D into Ba and Bb	C3b,Bb complex is a C3 convertase, cleaving many C3 molecules to C3a and C3b

Fig. 8.41 The alternative pathway of complement activation can amplify the classical pathway by depositing more C3b molecules on the pathogen. C3b deposited by the classical pathway can bind factor B, making it susceptible to cleavage by factor D. The C3b,Bb complex is the C3 convertase of the alternative pathway of complement activation and its action, like that of C4b,2b, results in the deposition of many molecules of C3b on the pathogen surface.

The C3 convertase of the alternative pathway, like that of the classical pathway, can cleave many molecules of C3 to generate yet more active C3b on the surface of the pathogen (see Fig. 8.41). The net result of activation of the classical pathway and its amplification via the alternative pathway is the rapid saturation of the surface of a pathogen with C3b, with the release of the small inflammatory mediator C3a. Some of the bound C3b binds to pre-existing C3 convertase, yielding C3b$_2$Bb, the alternative pathway C5 convertase. C3b$_2$Bb can cleave C5 into C5b, which initiates the generation of the membrane attack complex, and C5a, a potent inflammatory mediator (see Fig. 8.49). We now return to the effector actions initiated by C3b.

Fig. 8.42 The proteins of the alternative pathway of complement activation.

Proteins of the alternative pathway of complement activation		
Native component	**Active fragments**	**Function**
C3	C3b	Binds to pathogen surface, binds B for cleavage by D, C3b,Bb is C3 convertase and C3b$_2$,Bb is C5 convertase
Factor B (B)	Ba	Small fragment of B, unknown function
	Bb	Bb is active enzyme of the C3 convertase C3b,Bb and C5 convertase C3B$_2$,Bb
Factor D (D)	D	Plasma serine protease, cleaves B when it is bound to C3b to Ba and Bb

8-27   Some complement components bind to specific receptors on phagocytes and help to stimulate their activation.

The most important action of complement is to facilitate the uptake and destruction of pathogens by phagocytic cells. This occurs by specific recognition of bound complement components by **complement receptors (CR)** on phagocytes. Similar receptors on red blood cells play a role in the clearance of soluble antigen:antibody complexes from the circulation, as we shall see in the next section. The complement receptors expressed on phagocytic cells bind pathogens opsonized with bound complement components: opsonization of pathogens is a major function of C3b. C4b, its functional homolog, also acts as an opsonin but plays a relatively minor role, largely because so much more C3b is generated than C4b.

The five known types of receptors for bound complement components are listed, with their functions and distribution, in Fig. 8.43. The best-characterized of these receptors is the C3b receptor CR1, which is expressed on both macrophages and polymorphonuclear leukocytes. C3b alone cannot stimulate phagocytosis via CR1 but enhances phagocytosis and microbicidal activity induced either by the binding of IgG to the Fcγ receptor (Fig. 8.44) or by other immune mediators, such as the T cell-derived cytokine interferon-γ. The small complement fragment C5a can also activate macrophages to ingest bacteria coated with complement alone by binding to a specific receptor, the **C5a receptor**, which has seven membrane-spanning domains. Receptors of this type typically couple with three-chain guanine nucleotide binding proteins, called

Receptor	Specificity	Functions	Cell types
CR1	C3b, C4b	Promotes C3b and C4b decay, Stimulates phagocytosis. Erythrocyte transport of immune complexes	Erythrocytes, macrophages, monocytes, polymorphonuclear leukocytes, B cells
CR2	C3d, C3dg, iC3b Epstein-Barr virus	Part of B-cell co-receptor, Epstein-Barr virus receptor	B cells
CR3 (CD11b/ CD18)	iC3b	Stimulates phagocytosis	Macrophages, monocytes, polymorphonuclear leukocytes
CR4 (gp150,95) (CD11c/ CD18)	iC3b	Stimulates phagocytosis	Macrophages, monocytes, polymorphonuclear leukocytes
C1q receptor	C1q (collagen region)	Binding of immune complexes to phagocytes	B cells, macrophages, monocytes, platelets, endothelial cells

Fig. 8.43　Distribution and function of receptors on the surface of accessory cells specific for bound complement fragments. There are several different receptors specific for different bound complement components. CR1 and CR3 are especially important in inducing phagocytosis of bacteria with complement components bound to their surface. CR1 on erythrocytes also plays an important role in clearing immune complexes from the circulation. CR2 is found mainly on B cells, where it is also part of the B cell co-receptor complex and the receptor by which the Epstein-Barr virus selectively infects B cells, causing infectious mononucleosis.

G proteins, and it is known that the C5a receptor signals cells in this way. This is particularly important in the destruction of pathogens coated with complement and IgM, since phagocytes do not have Fc receptors for IgM (Fig. 8.45). A further contribution to activation can be made by binding of the phagocyte to extracellular matrix- associated proteins like fibronectin, encountered when phagocytes are recruited to connective tissue and activated there.

Three other complement receptors, CR2, CR3 and CR4, bind to inactivated forms of C3b that remain attached to the pathogen surface. Like several other key components of complement, C3b is subject to the action of regulatory mechanisms that can cleave C3b into inactive derivatives (discussed later). One of the inactive derivatives of C3b, known as iC3b, remains attached to the pathogen and acts as an opsonin in its

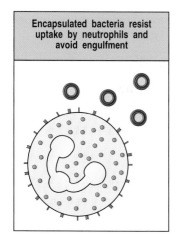

Encapsulated bacteria resist uptake by neutrophils and avoid engulfment

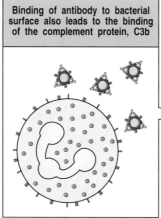

Binding of antibody to bacterial surface also leads to the binding of the complement protein, C3b

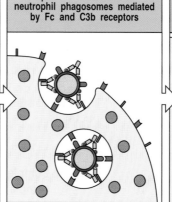

Uptake of bacteria into neutrophil phagosomes mediated by Fc and C3b receptors

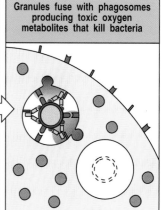

Granules fuse with phagosomes producing toxic oxygen metabolites that kill bacteria

Fig. 8.44　Encapsulated bacteria are more efficiently engulfed by phagocytes when they are also coated with complement. The phagocytes shown here are polymorphonuclear neutrophilic leukocytes (neutrophils); macrophages also bear complement receptors that act in the same way. Here, the neutrophil binds the bacterium by both Fc receptors and complement receptors, which synergize in inducing pathogen uptake and neutrophil activation.

Fig. 8.45 Complement receptors require ancillary activating signals to participate in phagocytosis. Fc receptors and complement receptors synergize in inducing phagocytosis, and bacteria coated with IgG antibody and complement are therefore more readily ingested than those coated with IgG alone (upper panels). When bacteria are coated with IgM antibody and complement, however, they cannot be ingested unless the phagocyte is pre-activated, for example by T cells or by C5a, as phagocytes do not have Fc-receptors for IgM (lower panels).

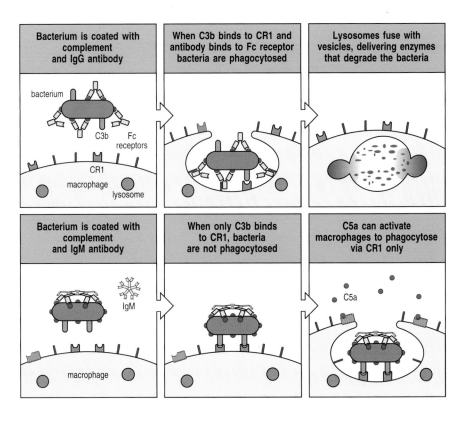

own right when bound by the complement receptors CR2 or CR3. Unlike the binding of C3b to CR1, binding of iC3b to CR3 is sufficient on its own to stimulate phagocytosis. A second breakdown product of C3b, called C3dg, binds only to CR2.

The complement receptor CR2, which recognizes iC3b and C3dg, is an important part of the B-cell co-receptor complex. It is believed that binding of iC3b and/or C3dg to CR2 plays a critical role in B-cell responses by providing a link between the B-cell antigen receptor and its co-receptor, making the B cell 100-fold more sensitive to antigen. CR2 also makes B cells susceptible to the **Epstein-Barr virus (EBV)**, which binds specifically to CR2 and is the cause of **infectious mononucleosis**. CR3 and CR4 are members of the CD11/CD18 leukocyte integrin family, of which LFA-1 is the third member. Their roles as complement receptors are less well understood, as is the role of the C1q receptor.

The central role of opsonization by C3b and its inactive fragments in the destruction of extracellular pathogens can be seen in the effects of various complement deficiency diseases. Whereas individuals deficient in any of the late components of complement are relatively little affected, individuals deficient in C3 or in molecules that catalyze C3b deposition show increased susceptibility to infection by a wide range of extracellular bacteria, as we shall see in Chapter 10.

8-28   Complement receptors are important in the removal of immune complexes from the circulation.

Many small soluble antigens form antibody:antigen complexes that contain too few molecules of IgG to be readily bound to Fcγ receptors. These include toxins bound by neutralizing antibodies and debris from dead microorganisms. Such **immune complexes** are found following most antibody responses, and they are removed from the circulation through the action of complement. The soluble immune complexes trigger their own removal by directly activating complement, so that the activated components C4b and C3b bind covalently to the complex which is then cleared from the circulation by the binding of C4b and C3b to CR1 on the surface of erythrocytes. The erythrocytes transport the bound complexes of antigen, antibody and complement to the liver and spleen. Here, macrophages remove the complexes from the erythrocyte surface without destroying the erythrocyte, and then degrade the immune complexes (Fig. 8.46). Even larger aggregates of particulate antigen and antibody can be solubilized by activation of the classical complement pathway, and then removed by binding to complement receptors.

Immune complexes that are not removed tend to deposit in the basement membranes of small blood vessels, most notably those of the renal glomerulus where the blood is filtered to form urine. Immune complexes that pass through the basement membrane of the glomerulus bind to CR1 on the renal podocytes that lie beneath the basement membrane. The functional significance of these receptors is unknown; however, they play an important part in the pathology that can arise in some autoimmune diseases.

In the autoimmune disease systemic lupus erythematosus, which we describe in Chapter 11, excessive levels of circulating immune complexes cause huge deposits of antigen, antibody, and complement on the podocytes, damaging the glomerulus; kidney failure is the principal danger in this disease. Immune complexes can also be a cause of pathology in patients with deficiencies in the early components of complement. Such patients do not clear immune complexes effectively and they also suffer tissue and especially kidney damage in a similar way.

8-29 Small peptide fragments released during complement activation trigger a local response to infection.

Many molecules released during immune responses induce a local inflammatory response. We have seen earlier in this chapter how mast cells can be triggered to release local inflammatory mediators, and we shall see in Chapter 9 that similar reactions can be produced by activated macrophages.

The small complement fragments C3a, C4a, and C5a act on specific receptors to produce similar local inflammatory responses and are therefore often referred to as **anaphylatoxins** (anaphylaxis is an acute systemic inflammatory response). Of the three, C5a is the most stable, has the highest specific biological activity, and acts on the best defined receptor. All three induce smooth muscle contraction and increase vascular permeability, and C3a and C5a can activate mast cells to release mediators that cause similar effects. These changes recruit antibody, complement, and phagocytic cells to the site of an infection, and the increased fluid in the tissues hastens the movement of pathogens to the local lymph nodes, contributing to the prompt initiation of the adaptive immune response.

C5a also acts directly on neutrophils and monocytes to increase their adherence to vessel walls, their migration toward sites of antigen deposition, and their ability to ingest particles, as well as increasing the expression of CR1 and CR3 on the surfaces of these cells. In this way C5a and, to a lesser extent, C3a and C4a, act in concert with other complement components to hasten the destruction of pathogens by phagocytes (Fig. 8.47).

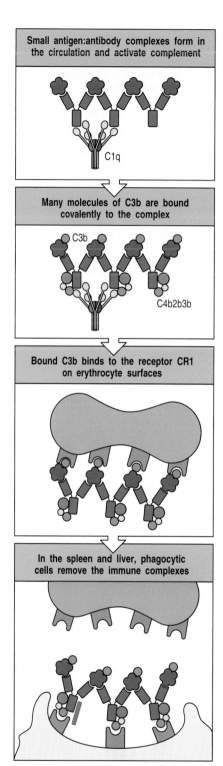

Fig. 8.46 Erythrocyte CR1 helps to clear immune complexes from the circulation. CR1 on the erythrocyte surface plays an important role in the clearance of immune complexes from the circulation. Immune complexes bind to CR1 on erythrocytes, which transport them to the liver and spleen, where they are removed by macrophages.

Fig. 8.47 Local inflammatory responses can be induced by small complement fragments, especially C5a. The small complement fragments are differentially active, C5a being more active than C3a, which is more active than C4a. They cause local inflammatory responses by acting directly on local blood vessels and C5a also acts indirectly by activating mast cells. Like mast-cell activation by IgE, these small complement fragments stimulate local increases in blood flow, increased binding of phagocytes to local endothelial cells, and increased local vascular permeability leading to fluid, protein and cell accumulation in the local tissues. The fluid increases lymphatic drainage, bringing antigen to local lymph nodes. The antibodies, complement and cells thus recruited participate in pathogen clearance by enhancing phagocytosis. The small complement fragments also directly increase the activity of the phagocytes.

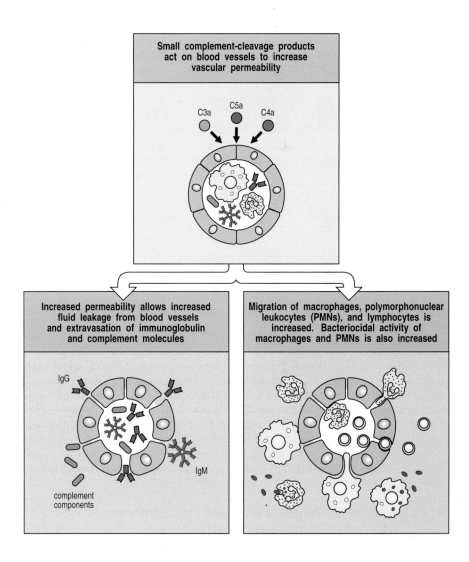

8-30 | **The terminal complement proteins polymerize to form pores in membranes that can kill pathogens.**

The most dramatic effect of complement activation is the assembly of the terminal components of complement (Fig. 8.48) to form a membrane-attack complex. The reactions leading to the formation of this complex are shown schematically in Fig. 8.49 and Fig. 8.50. The end result is a pore in lipid bilayer membrane that destroys its integrity. This is thought to kill the pathogen by destroying the proton gradient across the pathogen membrane.

The first step in the formation of the membrane-attack complex is the cleavage of C5 by a C5 convertase (sections 8-25 and 8-26). One molecule of C5b binds one molecule of C6, and the C5b,6 complex then binds one molecule of C7. This reaction leads to a conformational change in the constituent molecules, with the exposure of a hydrophobic site on C7. This hydrophobic domain of C7 inserts into the lipid bilayer. Hydrophobic sites are similarly exposed on the later components C8 and C9 when they are bound to the complex, allowing these proteins also to insert into the lipid bilayer. The next step is the binding of one molecule of C8 to the membrane-associated C5b,6,7 complex. C8 is a complex of two proteins, called C8β, which binds to C5b, and C8α-γ, which inserts into the lipid bilayer. The binding of C8β allows the binding of the α-γ component. Finally, C8α-γ induces the polymerization

The terminal complement components that form the membrane-attack complex		
Native protein	Active component	Function
C5	C5a	Small peptide mediator of inflammation
	C5b	Initiates assembly of the membrane-attack system
C6	C6	Binds C5b, forms acceptor for C7
C7	C7	Binds C5b,C6, amphiphilic complex inserts in lipid bilayer
C8	C8	Binds C5b,6,7, initiates C9 polymerization
C9	C9n	Polymerizes to C5b,6,7,8 to form a membrane-spanning channel, lysing membrane

Fig. 8.48 The terminal complement components that assemble to form the membrane-attack complex.

of 10 to 16 molecules of C9 into the annular or ring structure called the membrane-attack complex. The membrane-attack complex, shown schematically and by electron microscopy in Fig. 8.50, has a hydrophobic external face, allowing it to associate with the lipid bilayer, but a hydrophilic internal channel. The diameter of this channel is about 100 Å, allowing free passage of solute and water across the lipid bilayer. The disruption of the lipid bilayer leads to the loss of cellular homeostasis, the disruption of the proton gradient across the membrane, the penetration of enzymes such as lysozyme into the cell, and the eventual destruction of the pathogen.

The membrane-attack complex is strikingly similar to the perforin pores generated by cytotoxic T cells and natural killer cells, and the main components of these two structures, C9 and perforin 1, are products of closely related genes. The diameter of the membrane-attack complex inner channel is smaller than that of the perforin ring, which has an inner diameter of about 160 Å. The larger perforin pore may be required to allow ready access of granzymes to the interior of the target cell to initiate apoptosis.

Although the effect of the membrane-attack complex is very dramatic (see Fig. 8.50, lower panels), particularly in experimental demonstrations when antibodies to red blood cell membranes are used to trigger the complement cascade, the significance of these components in host defense seems to be quite limited. To date, deficiencies in complement components C5–C8 have been associated with susceptibility only to *Neisseria* spp., the bacteria that cause the sexually transmitted disease gonorrhea and a common form of bacterial meningitis, while C9 deficiency is not associated with detectable susceptibility to infection. The opsonizing and inflammatory actions of the earlier components of the complement cascade thus appear to be most important for host defense against infection.

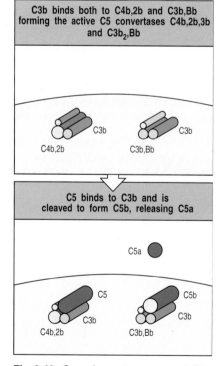

Fig. 8.49 Complement component C5 is activated by a C5 convertase when C5 is complexed to C3b. Top panel: C5 convertases are formed when C3b binds either the classical pathway C3 convertase C4b, 2b to form C4b, 2b, C3b or the alternative pathway C3 convertase to form C3b₂, Bb. Bottom Panel: C5 binds to the C3b in these complexes and is cleaved by the active enzyme C2b or Bb to form C5b and the inflammatory mediator C5a. The production of C5b initiates the assembly of the terminal complement components.

8-31	**Complement regulatory proteins serve to protect host cells from the effects of complement activation.**

When the components of complement are activated, as we have seen, they usually bind immediately to molecules on the pathogen surface and are thereby confined to the microbe on which their activation was initiated. However, activated complement components can sometimes

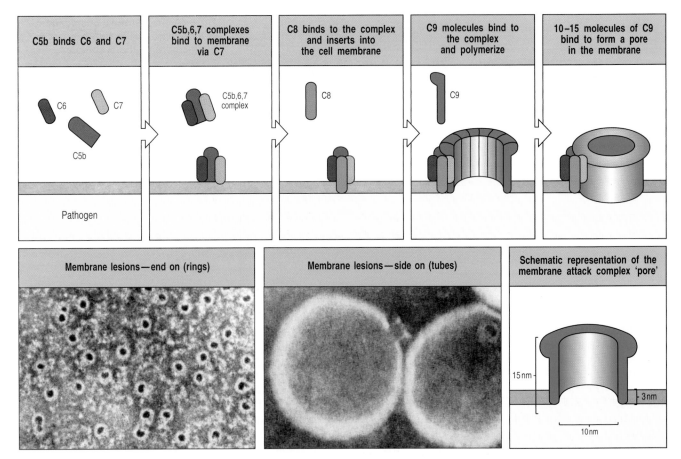

Fig. 8.50. The membrane-attack complex assembles to generate a pore in the lipid bilayer membrane. The sequence of steps and their approximate appearance is shown here in schematic form. C5b, generated by cleavage of C5 bound to C3b by the convertase C4b,2b,3b (or, in the alternative pathway, C3b$_2$,Bb), triggers the assembly of one molecule each of C6, C7 and C8, in that order. C7 and C8 undergo conformational changes that expose hydrophobic domains that insert into the membrane. This complex causes moderate membrane damage in its own right, and also serves to induce polymerization of C9, again with exposure of a hydrophobic site. Up to 16 molecules of C9 are then added to the assembly to generate a channel of 100 Å diameter in the membrane. This channel disrupts the bacterial outer membrane, killing the bacterium. The electron micrographs show erythrocyte membranes with membrane-attack complexes in two orientations, end on and side on. Note the resemblance of these complexes to pores caused by perforin. C9 and perforin 1, the major components of these two membrane lesions, are products of related genes. Photographs courtesy of S Bhakdi and J Tranum-Jensen.

escape to bind proteins on host cells; and all components of complement are activated spontaneously at a low rate in plasma. These activated complement components have the potential to destroy any cells to which they bind. Host cells are protected from such inadvertent damage by a series of complement regulatory proteins, summarized in Fig. 8.51. Some of these proteins are associated with the host cell surface, and similar proteins protect host cells from accidental triggering of the alternative pathway of complement activation, thereby confining these reactions to the surfaces of pathogens.

The activation of C1 is controlled by a plasma protein, the **C1 inhibitor (C1INH)**, which binds its the active enzyme moiety, C1r:C1s, and causes it to dissociate from C1q, which remains bound to antibody on the pathogen. In this way, C1INH limits to a few minutes the time during which active C1s is able to cleave C4 and C2. In the same way, C1INH serves to prevent the activation of complement by C1 that is spontaneously activated in plasma. Its importance can be seen in the C1INH deficiency disease **hereditary angioneurotic edema**, in which chronic spontaneous complement activation leads to the production of excess

Control proteins of the classical and alternative pathways	
Name (symbol)	**Role in the regulation of the complement activation**
C1 inhibitor (C1INH)	Binds to activated C1r, C1s, removing it from C1q
C4-binding protein (C4BP)	Binds to C4b displacing C2b; co-factor for C4b cleavage by I
Complement-receptor 1 (CR1)	Binds C4b displacing C2b, or C3b displacing Bb; co-factor for I
Factor H (H)	Binds C3b displacing Bb; co-factor for I
Factor I (I)	Serine protease that cleaves C3b and C4b; aided by H, MCP, C4BP or CR1
Decay-accelerating factor (DAF)	Membrane protein that displaces Bb from C3b and C2b from C4b
Membrane co-factor protein (MCP)	Membrane protein that promotes C3b and C4b inactivation by I
CD59 (protectin)	Prevents formation of MAC on homologous cells. Widely expressed on membranes

Fig. 8.51 The proteins that regulate the activity of complement.

cleaved fragments of C4 and C2. The small fragment of C2 is further cleaved into a vasoactive peptide that causes extensive swelling, the most dangerous being local swelling in the trachea, which can lead to suffocation. This disease is fully corrected by replacing C1INH. The large activated fragments of C4 and C2, which normally combine to form the C3 convertase, do not damage host cells in such patients because C4b is rapidly inactivated in plasma (see Fig. 8.39) and the convertase does not form. Any convertase that does accidentally form on a host cell, however, is inactivated by further control mechanisms.

First, C2b can be displaced from the complex by either of two proteins — a serum protein called C4-binding protein (C4bp), or a cell-surface protein called decay-accelerating factor (DAF). These compete with C2b for binding to C4b. When C4bp binds to C4b, C4b becomes highly susceptible to cleavage by a plasma protein called factor I. Factor I inactivates C4b by cleaving it into the subfragments C4c and C4d. An essentially analogous mechanism operates to inactivate C3b. In this case, either the complement receptor CR1 or a plasma protein called factor H bind to C3b, displacing C2b and making C3b susceptible to cleavage by factor I. A second membrane-associated protein, called membrane co-factor protein (MCP) can bind to membrane-associated C3b and catalyze its destruction by factor I. These regulatory reactions are shown in Fig. 8.52. All of the proteins that bind the homologous C4b and C3b molecules share one or more copies of a structural element called the short consensus repeat (SCR), complement control protein (CCP) repeat or (especially in Japan) Sushi domains.

The activity of the terminal complement components is also regulated by cell-surface proteins; the best known is protectin or CD59. CD59 and DAF are both linked to the cell surface by a phosphoinositol glycolipid tail, like many other membrane proteins. The disease **paroxysmal nocturnal hemoglobinuria**, characterized by episodes of intravascular red blood cell lysis by complement, is most often caused by deficiencies of both CD59 and DAF in patients who fail to generate the glycophosphoinositol linkage. Cells that lack CD59 only are also susceptible to destruction from spontaneous activation of the complement cascade.

Fig. 8.52 Complement activation is regulated by a series of proteins that serve to protect host cells from accidental damage. These act on different stages of the complement cascade, dissociating complexes or catalyzing the enzymatic degradation of covalently bound complement proteins. The complement cascade is shown schematically down the left side of the figure, with the control reactions shown on the right.

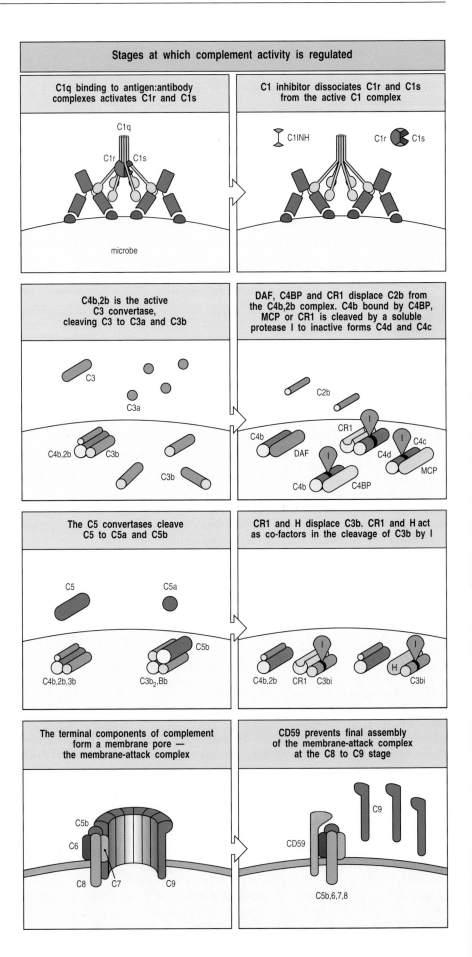

Summary.

The complement system is one of the major mechanisms whereby antigen recognition is converted into an effective defense against infection and is particularly important in defense against extracellular bacteria. Complement is a system of plasma proteins that can be activated by antibody, leading to a cascade of reactions that occurs on the surface of pathogens and generates active components with various effector functions. There are three pathways of complement activation, the classical pathway, which is triggered by antibody, the lectin-activated pathway, and the alternative pathway, which provides an amplification loop for the classical pathway. Both the lectin-activated pathway and the alternative pathway can be initiated independently of antibody as part of innate immunity. The early events in all pathways consist of a sequence of cleavage reactions in which the larger cleavage product contributes to the activation of the next component. The pathways converge with the formation of a C3 convertase enzyme, which is different but homologous for all pathways and cleaves C3 to produce the active complement component C3b. The binding of large numbers of C3b molecules to the pathogen is the central event in complement activation. Bound complement components, especially bound C3b and its inactive fragments, are recognized by specific complement receptors on phagocytic cells, which engulf pathogens opsonized by C3b, and which, on erythrocytes, bind soluble immune complexes, leading to their clearance. The small cleavage fragments of C3, C4, and especially C5 recruit phagocytes to sites of infection and activate them by binding to specific receptors having seven membrane-spanning domains. Together, these activities promote the uptake and destruction of pathogens by phagocytes. The molecules of C3b that bind the C3 convertase itself initate the late events, binding C5 to make it susceptible to cleavage by C2b or Bb. The larger C5b fragment triggers the assembly of a membrane-attack complex, which can result in the lysis of certain pathogens. These effects seem to be important only for killing of a few pathogens but play a major role in immunopathology. The activity of complement components is modulated by a system of regulatory proteins that prevent tissue damage as a result of inadvertent binding of activated complement components to host cells or spontaneous activation of complement components in plasma.

Summary to Chapter 8.

The humoral immune response to infection involves the production of antibody by B lymphocytes, the binding of this antibody to the pathogen, and the elimination of the pathogen by accessory cells and molecules of the humoral immune system. The production of antibody usually requires the action of helper T cells specific for a peptide fragment of the antigen recognized by the B cell. The B cell then proliferates and differentiates in the specialized microenvironment of lymphoid tissues, where somatic hypermutation generates diversity in the surface immunobglobulin of the B cell, and the B cells that bind antigen most avidly are selected for further differentiation by contact with antigen on the surface of follicular dendritic cells. These events allow the affinity of antibodies to increase over the course of an antibody response, and especially in repeated responses to the same antigen. Helper T cells also direct isotype switching, leading to the production of antibody of various isotypes that can be distributed to various body compartments. IgM is produced early in the response and plays a major role in protecting against infection in the bloodstream, while more mature isotypes such as IgG diffuse into the tissues. Multimeric IgA is produced below and transported across epithelial surfaces, while IgE is made in small amounts and binds avidly to the surface of mast cells. Antibodies that bind with high affinity to critical sites on toxins, viruses, and bacteria can neutralize them. However, pathogens and their products are destroyed and removed from the body largely through uptake into phagocytes and degradation inside these cells. Antibodies that coat pathogens bind to Fc receptors on phagocytes, which are thereby triggered to engulf and destroy them. Fc receptors on other cells lead to exocytosis of stored mediators, and this is particularly important in allergic reactions, where mast cells are triggered by antigen binding to IgE antibody to release inflammatory mediator molecules, as we shall learn in Chapter 11. Antibodies can also initiate pathogen destruction by activating the complement system of plasma proteins. Components of complement can opsonize pathogens for uptake by phagocytes, can recruit phagocytes to sites of infection, and can directly destroy pathogens by creating membrane pores in their surfaces. Thus, the humoral immune response is targeted to specific pathogens through production of specific antibody, but the effector actions of that antibody are determined by the isotype of the antibody and are the same for all pathogens bound by antibody of a particular isotype.

General references.

Gallin, J.I., Goldstein, I.M., and Snyderman, R. (eds): *Inflammation — basic principles and clinical correlates*, 2nd edn. New York, Raven Press, 1992.

Law, S.K.A. and Reid, K.B.M.: *Complement.*, 1st edn. Oxford, IRL Press, 1988.

MacLennan, I.C.M.: **Germinal centres**. *Annu. Rev. Immunol. 1994,* **12**: 117-139.

Metzger, H. (ed.): *Fc receptors and the action of antibodies*, 1st edn. Washington, DC, American Society for Microbiology, 1990.

Moller, G. (ed.): **The B-cell antigen receptor complex**. *Immunol. Rev.* 1993, **132**:1-206.

Ross, G.D. (ed.): *Immunobiology of the complement system*, 1st edn. Orlando, Academic Press, 1986.

Underdown, B.J. and Schoff, J.M.: **Immunoglobulin A: strategic defense initiative at the mucosal surface**. *Ann. Rev. Immunol.* 1993, **4**: 389-417.

Cambien, J.C., Pleissen, C.M. and Clack M.E.: **Signal transduction by B-cell antigen receptors and its conceptions**. *Ann. Rev. Immunol.* 1994. **12**: 458-486.

Section references.

8-1 The antibody response is initiated when B cells bind antigen and are signaled by helper T cells or by certain microbial antigens.

DeFranco, A.L.: **Molecular aspects of B-lymphocyte activation**. *Ann. Rev. Cell Biol.* 1987, **3**:143-178.

Mond, J.J., Lees, A, and Snapper, C.M. **T cell independent antigens type 2**. *Ann. Rev. Immunol.* 1995, **13**: 655.

8-2 Armed helper T cells activate B cells that recognize the same antigen.

Parker, D.C.: **T cell-dependent B-cell activation**. *Ann. Rev. Immunol.* 1993, **11**:331-340.

8-3 Peptide:MHC class II complexes on a B cell trigger armed helper T cells to make membrane and secreted molecules that activate the B cell.

Noelle, R.J., Roy, M., Shepherd, D.M., Stamekovic, I., Ledbetter, J.A., and Aruffo, A.: **A 39-kDa protein in activated helper T cells binds CD40 and transduces the signal for cognate activation of B cells**. *Proc. Natl. Acad. Sci. USA* 1992, **89**:6550-6554.

Banchereau, J., Bazan, F., Blanchard, D., Briere, F., Galizzi, J.P., Vankooten, C., Liu, Y.J., Rousset, F., and Saeland, S. **The CD40 antigen and its ligand**. *Ann. Rev. Immunol.* 1994, **12**: 881-922.

8-4 Isotype switching requires expression of CD40 ligand by the helper T cell and is directed by cytokines.

Aruffo, A., Farrington, M., Hollenbaugh, D., Li, X., Milatovich, A., Nonoyama, S., Bajorath, J., Grosmaire, L.S., Stenkamp, R., Neubauer, M, Roberts, R.L., Noelle, R.J., Ledbetter, J.A., Francke, U., and Ochs, H.D.: **The CD40 ligand, gp39, is defective in activated T cells from patients with X-linked hyper-IgM syndrome**. *Cell* 1993, **72**:291-300.

Harriman, W., Volk, H., Defranoux, N., and Wabl. M.: **Immunoglobulin class switch recombination**. *Ann. Rev. Immunol.* 1993, **11**:361-384.

Rothman, P., Chen, Y.-Y., Lutzker, S., Li, S.C., Stewart, V., Coffman, R., and Alt, F.W.: **Structure and expression of germline immunoglobulin heavy-chain ε transcripts: interleukin-4 plus lipopolysaccharide-directed switching to Cε**. *Mol. Cell. Biol.* 1990, **10**:1672-1679.

8-5 Activated B cells proliferate extensively in the specialized microenvironment of the germinal center.

Kelsoe, G. and Zheng, B.: **Sites of B-cell activation *in vivo***. *Curr. Opin. Immunol.* 1993, **5**:418-422.

MacLennan, I.C., Liu, Y.J., and Johnson, G.D.: **Maturation and dispersal of B-cell clones during T cell-dependent antibody responses**. *Immunol. Rev.* 1992, **126**:143.

8-6 Somatic hypermutation occurs in the rapidly dividing centroblasts in the germinal center.

Jacob, J. and Kelsoe, G.: *In situ* studies of the primary immune response to (4-hydroxy-3-nitrophenyl) acetyl II. A common clonal origin for periarteriolar lymphoid sheath-associated foci and germinal centers. *J. Exper. Med.* 1992, **176**:679-687.

Jacob, J., Kelsoe, G., Rajewsky, K., and Weiss, U.: Intraclonal generation of antibody mutants in germinal centres. *Nature* 1991, **354**:389-392.

8-7 Non-dividing centrocytes with the best antigen-binding receptors are selected for survival by binding antigen on a follicular dendritic cell.

Berek, C.: The development of B cells and the B-cell repertoire in the microenvironment of the germinal center. *Immunol. Rev.* 1992, **126**:5.

Humphrey, J.H., Grennan, D., and Sundaram, V.: The origin of follicular dendritic cells in the mouse and the mechanism of trapping of immune complexes on them. *Eur. J. Immunol.* 1984, **14**:1859.

8-8 B cells leaving the germinal center differentiate into antibody-secreting plasma cells or memory B cells.

Liu, Y.J., Cairns, J.A., Hoder, M.J., Abbot, S.D., Jansen, K.U., Bonnefoy, J.Y., Gordon, J., and MacLennan, I.C.M: Recombinant 25-kDa CD23 and interleukin 1 alpha promote the survival of germinal center B cells: evidence for bifurcation in the development of centrocytes rescued from apoptosis. *Eur. J. Immunol.* 1991, **21**:1107.

8-9 B-cell responses to bacterial antigens with intrinsic B-cell activating ability do not require T-cell help.

Anderson, J., Coutinho, A., Lernhardt, W., and Melchers, F.: Clonal growth and maturation to immunoglobulin secretion *in vitro* of every growth-inducible B lymphocyte. *Cell* 1977, **10**:27-34.

Coutinho, A.: The theory of the one non-specific model for B-cell activation. *Transplant. Rev.* 1975, **23**:49.

8-10 B-cell responses to bacterial polysaccharides do not require specific T-cell help.

Dintzis, H.M., Dintzis, R.Z., and Vogelstein, B.: Molecular determinants of immunogenicity: the immunon model of immune response. *Proc. Natl. Acad. Sci. USA* 1976, **73**:3671-3675.

Pecanha, L., Snapper, C., Finkelman, F., and Mond, J.: Dextran-conjugated anti-Ig antibodies as a model for T-cell-independent type 2 antigen-mediated stimulation of Ig secretion *in vitro*. I. Lymphokine dependence. *J. Immunol.* 1991, **146**:833-839.

8-11 Antibodies of different isotypes operate in distinct places and have distinct effector functions.

Janeway, C.A., Rosen, F.S., Merler, E., and Alper, C.A.: *The gamma globulins*, 2nd edn. Boston, Little Brown and Co., 1967.

8-12 Transport proteins that bind to the Fc domain of antibodies carry specific isotypes across epithelial barriers.

Simister, N.E. and Mostov, K.E.: An Fc receptor structurally related to MHC class I antigens. *Nature* 1989, **337**:184-187.

Mostov, K.E.: Transepithelial transport of Immunoglobulins. *Ann. Rev. Immunol.* 1994. **12**: 63-84.

Burmeister, W.P., Gastinel, L.N., Simister, N.E., Blum, M.L., Bjorkman, P.J.: Crystal structure at 2.2 Å resolution of the MHC-related neonatal Fc receptor. *Nature.* 1994. **372**: 336-343.

8-14 High-affinity IgG and IgA antibodies can inhibit the infectivity of viruses.

Mandel, B.: Neutralization of polio virus: a hypothesis to explain the mechanism and the one hit character of the neutralization reaction. *Virology* 1976, **69**:500-510.

Possee, R.D., Schild, G.C., and Dimmock, N.J.: Studies on the mechanism of neutralization of influenza virus by antibody: evidence that neutralizing antibody (anti-hemaglutanin) inactivates influenza virus *in vivo* by inhibiting virion transcriptase activity. *J. Gen. Virol.* 1982, **58**:373-386.

8-15 Antibodies can block the adherence of bacteria to host cells.

Fischetti, V.A. and Bessen, D.: Effect of mucosal antibodies to M protein in colonization by group A streptococci. In Switalski L., Hook, M., and Beachery, E. (eds.): *Molecular mechanisms of microbial adhesion.* New York, Springer, 1989, pp.128-142.

8-16 The Fc receptors of accessory cells are signaling molecules specific for immunoglobulins of different isotypes.

Ravetch, J.V. and Kinet, J.: Fc receptors. *Ann. Rev. Immunol.* 1993, **9**:457-492.

Takai, T., Li, M., Sylvestre, D., Clynes, R., and Ravetch, J.V.: FcRγ chain deletion results in pleiotrophic effector-cell defects. *Cell* 1994, **76**:519-529.

8-17 Fc receptors on phagocytes are activated by antibodies bound to the surface of pathogens.

Burton, D.R.: The conformation of antibodies. In Metzger, H. (ed.): *Fc receptors and the action of antibodies*, 1st edn. Washington, DC, Raven Press, 1990, 3154.

8-18 Fc receptors on phagocytes allow them to ingest and destroy opsonized extracellular pathogens.

Gounni, A.S., Lamkhioued, B., Ochiai, K., Tanaka, Y., Delaporte, E., Capron A., Kinet, J-P. and Capron, M.: High-affinity IgE receptor on eosinophils is involved in defence against parasites. *Nature*, 1994 **367**:183-186.

Karakawa, W.W., Sutton, A., Schneerson, R., Karpas, A., and Vann, W.F.: Capsular antibodies induce type-specific phagocytosis of capsulated *Staphylococcus aureus* by human polymorphonuclear leukocytes. *Infect. Immun.* 1986, **56**:1090-1095.

8-19 Fc receptors activate natural killer cells to destroy antibody-coated targets.

Lanier, L.L. and Phillips, J.H.: Evidence for three types of human cytotoxic lymphocyte. *Immunol. Today* 1986, **7**:132.

Lanier, L.L., Ruitenberg, J.J., and Phillips, J.H.: Functional and biochemical analysis of CD16 antigen on natural killer cells and granulocytes. *J. Immunol.* 1988, **141**:3487-3485.

8-20 Mast cells bind IgE antibody with high affinity.

Beaven, M.A. and Metzger, H.: Signal transduction by Fc receptors: the FcεRI case. *Immunol. Today* 1993, **14**:222-226.

Paolini, R., Numerof, R., and Kinet, J.P.: Phosphorylation/ dephosphorylation of high-affinity IgE receptors: a mechanism for coupling/uncoupling a large signaling complex. *Proc. Natl. Acad. Sci. USA* 1992, **89**:10733-10737.

Sutton, B.J. and Gould, H.J.: **The human IgE network**. *Nature* 1993, **366**:421-428.

8-21	**Mast-cell activation by antigen binding to IgE triggers a local inflammatory response.**

Bradding, P., Feather, J.H., Howarth, P.H., Mueller, R., Roberts, J.A., Britten, K., Bews, J.P.A., Hunt, T.C., Okayama, Y., Huesser, C.H., Bullock, G.R., Church, M.K., and Holgate, S.T.: **Interleulkin-4 is localized to and released by human mast cells**. *J. Exper. Med.* 1992, **176**:1381-1386.

Schleimer, R.P., MacGlashan, D.W. Jr, Peters, S.P., Pinchard, R.N., Adkinson, N.F. Jr, and Lichtenstein, L.M.: **Characterization of inflammatory mediator release from purified human lung mast cells**. *Ann. Rev. Resp. Dis.* 1986, **133**:614-617.

Walsh, L., Trinchieri, G., Waldorf, H.A., Whitaker, D.A., and Murphy, G.F.: **Human dermal mast cells contain and release TNF-alpha, which induces endothelial-leukocyte adhesion molecule-1**. *Proc. Natl. Acad. Sci. USA* 1991, **88**:4220-4224.

Zweiman, B.: **The late-phase reaction of IgE, its receptor and cytokines**. *Curr. Opin. Immunol.* 1993, **5**:950-955.

8-22	**Complement is a system of plasma proteins, that interacts with bound antibodies to aid in the elimination of pathogens.**

Tomlinson, S.: **Complement defense mechanisms**. *Curr. Opin. Immunol.* 1993, **5**:83-89.

8-23	**The C1q molecule binds to antibody molecules to trigger the classical pathway of complement activation.**

Cooper, N.R.: **The classical complement pathway. Activation and regulation of the first complement component**. *Adv. Immunol.* 1985, **37**:151-216.

Feinstein, A., Munn, E.A., and Richardson, N.E.: **The three-dimensional conformation of gamma-M and gamma-A globulin molecules**. *Ann. N.Y. Acad. Sci.* 1971, **190**:104-107.

Perkins, S.J. and Nealis, A.S.: **The quaternary structure in solution of human complement subcomponent C1r2Cls2**. *Biochem. J.* 1989, **263**:463-469.

8-24	**The classical pathway of complement activation generates a C3 convertase bound to the pathogen surface.**

Chan, A.R., Karp, D.R., Shreffler, D.C., and Atkinson, J.P.: **The 20 faces of the fourth component of complement**. *Immunol. Today* 1984, **5**:200-203.

Levine, R.P. and Dodds, A.W.: **The thioester bond of C3**. *Curr. Top. Microbiol. Immunol.* 1989, **153**:73-82.

Oglesby, T.J., Accavitti, M.A., and Volanakis, J.E.: **Evidence for a C4b binding site on the C2b domain of C2**. *J. Immunol.* 1988, **141**:926-931.

8-25	**The cell-bound C3 convertase deposits large numbers of C3b molecules on the pathogen surface.**

deBruijn, M.H.L. and Fey, G.M.: **Human complement component C3: cDNA coding sequence and derived primary structure**. *Proc. Natl. Acad. Sci. USA* 1985, **82**:708-712.

Volanakis, J.E.: **Participation of C3 and its ligand in complement activation**. *Curr. Top. Microbiol. Immunol.* 1989, **153**: 1-21.

8-26	**Bound C3b initiates the alternative pathway of complement activation to amplify the effects of the classical pathway.**

Kolb, W.P., Morrow, P.R., and Tamerius, J.D.: **Ba and Bb fragments of Factor B activation: fragment production, biological activities, neoepitope expression and quantitation in clinical samples**. *Complement Inflamm.* 1989, **6**:175-204.

8-27	**Some complement components bind to specific receptors on phagocytes and help to stimulate their activation.**

Ahearn, J.M. and Fearon, D.T.: **Structure and function of the complement receptors of CR1 (CD35) and CR2 (CD21)**. *Adv. Immunol.* 1989, **46**:183-219.

Krych, M., Atkinson, J.P., and Holers, V.M.: **Complement receptors**. *Curr. Opin. Immunol.* 1992, **4**:8-13.

8-28	**Complement receptors are important in the removal of immune complexes from the circulation.**

Schifferli, J.A. and Taylor, J.P.: **Physiologic and pathologic aspects of circulating immune complexes**. *Kidney Intl.* 1989, **35**:993-1003.

Schifferli, J.A., Ng, Y.C., and Peters, D.K.: **The role of complement and its receptor in the elimination of immune complexes**. *N. Engl. J. Med.* 1986, **315**:488-495.

8-29	**Small peptide fragments released during complement activation trigger a local response to infection.**

Frank, M.M. and Fries, L.F.: **The role of complement in inflammation and phagocytosis**. *Immunol. Today* 1991, **12**:322-326.

Gerald, C., and Berand, N.P. **CSA anaphylotoxin and its seven transmembrane segment scripts**. *Ann. Rev. Immunol.* 1994. **12**: 775-808.

8-30	**The terminal complement proteins polymerize to form pores in membranes that can kill pathogens.**

Bhakdi, S. and Tranum-Jensen, J.: **Complement lysis: a hole is a hole**. *Immunol. Today* 1991, **12**:318-320.

Esser, A.F.: **Big MAC attack: complement proteins cause leaky patches**. *Immunol. Today* 1991, **12**:316-318.

Morgan, B.P.: **Effects of the membrane attack complex of complement on nucleated cells**. *Curr. Top. Microbiol. Immunol.* 1992, **178**:115-140.

8-31	**Complement regulatory proteins serve to protect host cells from the effects of complement activation.**

Davies, A., Simmons, D.I., Hale, G., Harrison, R.A., Tighe, H., Lachmann, P.J., and Waldmann, H.: **CD59, an Ly-6-like protein expressed in human lymphoid cells, regulates the action of the complement membrane attack complex on homologous cells**. *J. Exper. Med.* 1989, **170**:637-654.

Mollnes, T.E. and Lachmann, P.J.: **Regulation of complement**. *Scand. J. Immunol.* 1988, **27**:127-142.

PART V

THE IMMUNE SYSTEM IN HEALTH AND DISEASE

Host Defense Against Infection

9

Throughout this book we have examined the individual mechanisms by which the adaptive immune response acts to protect the host from pathogenic infectious agents. In the remaining four chapters, we will consider how the cells and molecules of the immune system work as an integrated host defense system to eliminate the infectious agent and to provide long-lasting protective immunity. In this chapter we shall examine the role of the immune system as a whole in host defense, including those innate, non-adaptive defenses that are the earliest barrier to infectious disease.

The microorganisms that are encountered daily in the life of a normal healthy individual only occasionally cause perceptible disease. Most are detected and destroyed within hours by defense mechanisms that are not antigen-specific and do not require a prolonged period of induction: these are the mechanisms of **innate immunity**. Only if an infectious organism can breach these early lines of defense will an **adaptive immune response** ensue, with the generation of antigen-specific effector cells that specifically target the pathogen, and memory cells that prevent subsequent infection with the same microorganism.

In the preceding two chapters of this book, we have discussed how an adaptive immune response is induced, and how pathogens are eliminated by the effector cells generated in such a response. Here these mechanisms will be set in the broader context of the entire array of mammalian host defenses against infection, beginning with the innate immune mechanisms that successfully prevent most infections from becoming established. This type of immunity also plays an essential part in inducing the subsequent adaptive response to those infections that do overcome the first lines of defense.

The time course of the different phases of an immune response is summarized in Fig. 9.1. The innate immune mechanisms act immediately, and are followed some hours later by **early induced responses**, which can be activated by infection but do not generate lasting protective immunity. These early phases help to keep infection under control while the antigen-specific lymphocytes of the adaptive immune response are activated. Moreover, cytokines produced during these early phases play an important part in shaping the subsequent development of the adaptive immune response, and can determine whether the response is predominantly T-cell mediated or humoral. Several days are required for the clonal expansion and differentiation of naive lymphocytes into the effector T cells and antibody-secreting cells that defend the infected host. During this period, specific immunological memory is established, providing long-lasting protection against re-infection with the same pathogen. In this chapter, we shall learn how the different phases of

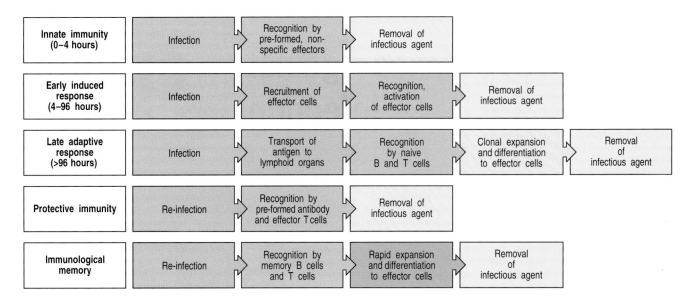

Fig. 9.1   The response to an initial infection occurs in three phases. The effector mechanisms that remove the infectious agent (eg phagocytes, NK cells, complement) are similar or identical in each phase but the recognition mechanisms differ. Adaptive immunity occurs late, because rare, antigen-specific cells must undergo clonal expansion before they can differentiate into effector cells. The response to re-infection is much more rapid; pre-formed antibodies and effector cells act immediately on the pathogen, and immunological memory speeds a renewed adaptive response.

host defense are orchestrated in space and time, and how changes in specialized cell-surface molecules guide lymphocytes to the appropriate site of action at different stages of the immune response.

Infection and innate immunity.

Microorganisms that cause pathology in humans and animals enter the body at different sites and produce disease by a variety of mechanisms. The most effective means of countering such invasions in vertebrates is by innate defense mechanisms that pre-exist in all individuals and act within minutes of infection. Only when the innate host defenses are by-passed or overwhelmed is an induced or adaptive immune response required. In this section, we shall describe briefly the infectious strategies of microorganisms, before examining the innate host defenses that, in most cases, prevent infection becoming established.

9-1   The infectious process can be divided into several distinct phases.

The process of infection can be broken down into stages, each of which can be blocked by different defense mechanisms. The infection is established initially by infectious particles shed by an infected individual. The number, route, mode of transmission, and stability of an infectious agent outside the host determine its infectivity. Some pathogens, such as anthrax, are spread by spores that are highly resistant to heat and drying, while others, such as the human immunodeficiency virus, are spread only by the exchange of tissues because they are unable to survive as isolated infectious agents.

Although the body is constantly exposed to infectious agents, infectious disease is fortunately quite rare. The epithelial surfaces of the body serve as an efficient barrier to most microorganisms. Only when a microorganism has crossed an epithelial barrier does infection occur, and little pathology will be caused unless the agent is able to spread. Extracellular pathogens spread by direct extension of the infectious center, via the lymphatics, or via the bloodstream. Usually, spread via the bloodstream occurs only after the lymphatic system has been overwhelmed by the burden of infectious agent. Obligate intracellular pathogens must spread from cell to cell; they do so either by direct transmission from one cell to the next or by release into the extracellular fluid and re-infection of both adjacent and distant cells.

Most infectious agents show a significant degree of host specificity, causing disease only in one or a few related species. What determines host specificity for each agent is not known, but the requirement for attachment to a particular cell-surface molecule is one factor. As other interactions with host cells are also commonly needed to support replication, most pathogens have a limited host range. The molecular mechanism of host specificity is an area of intense research interest known as molecular pathogenesis.

While most microorganisms are repelled by innate host defenses, an initial infection, once established, generally leads to perceptible disease followed by an effective host immune response. A cure involves the clearance of both extracellular infectious particles and intracellular residues of infection. In many infections, there is little or no residual pathology after an effective primary response. In some cases, however, the infection or the response to it cause significant tissue damage.

In addition to clearance of the infectious agent, an effective adaptive immune response prevents re-infection. For some infectious agents, this protection is essentially absolute, while for others infection is reduced or attenuated upon re-exposure. The progress of an infection is illustrated in Fig. 9.2, which summarizes the defense mechanisms activated at each stage, each of which will be described in detail in the course of this chapter.

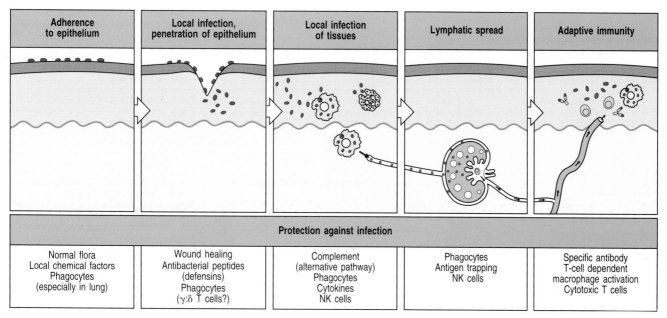

Fig. 9.2 Infections and the responses to them can be divided into a series of stages. These are illustrated here for an infectious organism entering through the epithelium, the commonest route of entry. The infectious organism must first adhere to the epithelial cells and then cross the epithelium. A local non-adaptive response helps contain the infection and delivers antigen to local lymph nodes, leading to adaptive immunity and clearance of the infection.

Fig. 9.3 A variety of microorganisms can cause disease. Pathogenic organisms are of five main types: viruses; bacteria; fungi; protozoa; and worms. Some common pathogens in each group are listed in the right-hand column.

Some common causes of disease in humans			
Viruses	DNA viruses	Adenoviruses	Human adenoviruses (eg types 3, 4, and 7)
		Herpesviruses	Herpes simplex, varicella-zoster, Epstein-Barr virus, cytomegalovirus
		Poxviruses	Vaccinia virus
		Parvoviruses	Human parvovirus
		Papovaviruses	Papilloma virus
		Hepadnaviruses	Hepatitis B virus
	RNA viruses	Orthomyxoviruses	Influenza virus
		Paramyxoviruses	Mumps, measles, respiratory syncytial virus
		Coronaviruses	Common cold viruses
		Picornaviruses	Polio, coxsackie, hepatitis A, rhinovirus
		Reoviruses	Rotavirus, reovirus
		Togaviruses	Rubella, arthropod-borne encephalitis
		Flaviviruses	Arthropod-borne viruses, (yellow fever, dengue fever)
		Arenaviruses	Lymphocytic choriomeningitis, Lassa fever
		Rhabdoviruses	Rabies
		Retroviruses	Human T-cell leukemia virus, HIV
Bacteria	Gram (+) cocci	Staphylococci	*Staphylococcus aureus*
		Streptococci	*Streptococcus pneumoniae, S. pyogenes*
	Gram (-) cocci	Neisseriae	*Neisseria gonorrhoeae, N. meningitidis*
	Gram (+) bacilli		*Corynebacteria, Bacillus anthracis, Listeria monocytogenes*
	Gram (-) bacilli		*Salmonella, Shigella, Campylobacter, Vibrio, Yersinia, Pasteurella, Pseudomonas, Brucella, Haemophilus, Legionella, Bordetella*
	Anaerobic bacteria	Clostridia	*Clostridium tetani, C. botulinum, C. perfringens*
	Spirochetes		*Treponema pallidum, Borrelia burgdorferi, Leptospira interrogans*
	Mycobacteria		*Mycobacterium tuberculosis, M. leprae*
	Rickettsias		*Rickettsia prowazeki*
	Chlamydias		*Chlamydia trachomatis*
	Mycoplasmas		*Mycoplasma pneumoniae*
Fungi			*Candida albicans, Cryptococcus neoformans, Aspergillus, Histoplasma capsulatum, Coccidioides immitis, Pneumocystis carinii*
Protozoa			*Entamoeba histolytica, Giardia, Leishmania, Plasmodium, Trypanosoma, Toxoplasma gondii, Cryptosporidium*
Worms	Intestinal		*Trichturis trichiura, Trichinella spiralis, Enterobius vermicularis, Ascaris lumbricoides, Ancylostoma, Strongyloides*
	Tissues		*Filaria, Onchocerca volvulus, Loa loa, Dracuncula medinensis*
	Blood, liver		*Schistosoma, Clonorchis sinensis*

<table>
<tr><td>9-2</td><td>Infectious diseases are caused by diverse living agents that replicate in their hosts.</td></tr>
</table>

The agents that cause disease fall into five groups: viruses, bacteria, fungi, protozoa, and helminths (worms). Protozoa and worms are usually grouped together as parasites, and are the subject of the discipline of parasitology, whereas viruses, bacteria, and fungi are the subject of microbiology. In Fig. 9.3, the common classes of microorganisms and parasites are listed with typical examples of each. The remarkable variety of these pathogens has required potential hosts to develop two crucial features of adaptive immunity. First, the need to recognize a wide range of different pathogens has driven the development of receptors of equal or greater diversity. Second, the distinct habitats and life cycles of pathogens have to be countered by a range of distinct effector mechanisms. The characteristic features of each pathogen are its mode of transmission, its mechanism of replication, and its pathogenesis, or the means by which it causes disease, and the response it elicits. We will focus here on the immune responses to these pathogens.

Infectious agents can grow in various body compartments, as shown schematically in Fig. 9.4. We have already seen that two major compartments can be defined, intracellular and extracellular. Intracellular pathogens must invade host cells in order to replicate, and must either be prevented from entering cells or detected and eliminated once they have. Such pathogens can be subdivided further into those that replicate free in the cell, such as viruses and certain bacteria (species of *Chlamydia* and *Rickettsia*), and those, such as the mycobacteria, that replicate in cellular vesicles. Many microorganisms replicate in extracellular spaces, either within the body or on the surface of epithelia. Extracellular bacteria are usually susceptible to phagocytosis and have developed means to resist engulfment. The encapsulated Gram-positive cocci, for instance, grow in extracellular spaces and resist phagocytosis by means of their polysaccharide capsule; if this mechanism of resistance is overcome by opsonization they are readily killed after ingestion by phagocytic cells.

Site of infection	Intracellular		Extracellular	
	Cytoplasmic	Vesicular	Interstitial spaces blood, lymph	Epithelial surfaces
Organisms	Viruses *Chlamydia* spp. *Rickettsia* spp. *Listeria monocytogenes* Protozoa	Mycobacteria *Salmonella typhimurium* *Leishmania* spp. *Listeria* spp. *Trypanosoma* spp. *Legionella pneumophila* *Cryptoccccus neoformans* *Histoplasma* *Yersinia pestis*	Viruses Bacteria Protozoa Fungi Worms	*Neisseria gonorrhoeae* Worms Mycoplasma *Streptococcus pneumoniae* *Vibrio cholerae* *Escherichia coli* *Candida albicans* *Helicobacter pylori*
Protective immunity	Cytotoxic T cells ADCC NK cells	T-cell dependent macrophage activation	Antibodies Complement Phagocytosis Neutralization	Antibodies, especially IgA Inflammatory cells

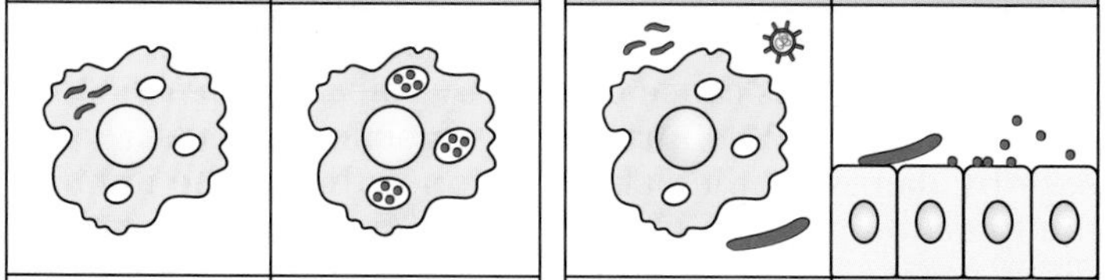

Fig. 9.4 Pathogens can be found in various compartments in the body, where they must be combated by different host defense mechanisms. Virtually all pathogens have an extracellular phase where they are vulnerable to antibody-mediated effector mechanisms. However, intracellular phases are not accessible to antibody, and these are attacked by T cells. ADCC, antibody-dependent cell-mediated cytotoxicity (see Section 8-19).

	Direct mechanisms of tissue damage by pathogens			Indirect mechanisms of tissue damage by pathogens		
	Exotoxin production	Endotoxin	Direct cytopathic effect	Immune complexes	Anti-host antibody	Cell-mediated immunity
Pathogenic mechanism	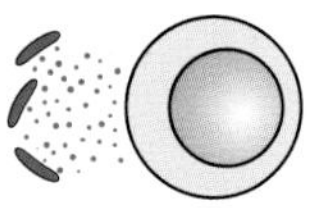	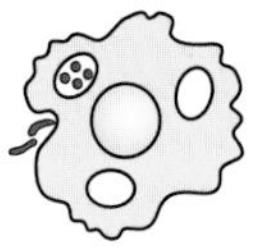	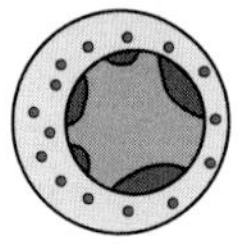	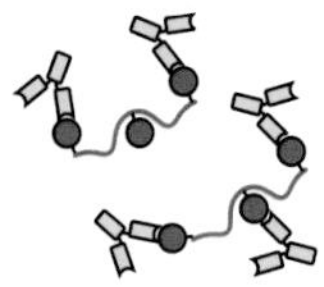	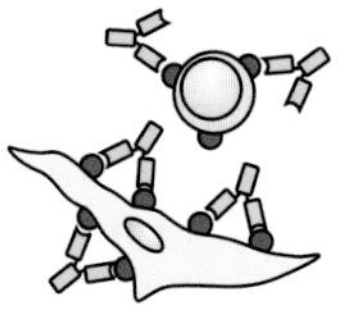	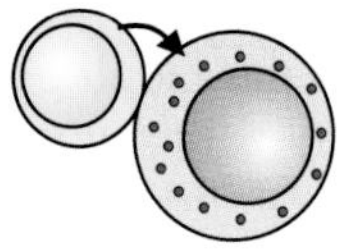
Infectious agent	*Streptococcus pyogenes* *Staphylococcus aureus* *Corynebacterium diphtheriae* *Clostridium tetani* *Vibrio cholerae*	*Escherichia coli* *Haemophilus influenzae* *Salmonella typhi* *Shigella* *Pseudomonas aeruginosa* *Yersinia pestis*	Variola Varicella-zoster Hepatitis B virus Polio virus Measles virus Influenza virus Herpes simplex virus	Hepatitis B virus Malaria *Streptococcus pyogenes* *Treponema pallidum* Most acute infections	*Streptococcus pyogenes* *Mycoplasma pneumoniae*	*Mycobacterium tuberculosis* *Mycobacterium leprae* Lymphocytic choriomeningitis virus Human immunodeficiency virus *Borrelia burgdorferi* *Schistosoma mansoni* Herpes simplex virus
Disease	Tonsilitis, scarlet fever Boils, toxic shock syndrome Food poisoning Diphtheria Tetanus Cholera	Gram-negative sepsis Meningitis, pneumonia Typhoid Bacillary dysentery Wound infection Plague	Smallpox Chickenpox, shingles Hepatitis Poliomyelitis Measles, subacute sclerosing panencephalitis Influenza Cold sores	Kidney disease Vascular deposits Glomerulonephritis Kidney damage in secondary syphilis Transient renal deposits	Rheumatic fever Anemia	Tuberculosis Tuberculoid leprosy Aseptic meningitis AIDS Lyme arthritis Schistosomiasis Herpes stromal keratitis

Fig. 9.5 Pathogens can damage tissues in a variety of different ways. The mechanisms of damage, representative infectious agents, and the common name of the disease associated with each are shown. Exotoxins are released by microorganisms and act at the surface of host cells, for example by binding receptors and entering specific cells (see Fig. 8.21). Endotoxins trigger macrophages to release cytokines that produce local or systemic symptoms. Many pathogens directly damage cells they infect. Finally, adaptive immune responses to the pathogen can generate antigen:antibody complexes, antibodies that cross-react with host tissues, or T cells that kill infected cells, all of which damage the host's tissues as well as removing the pathogen.

Different infectious agents cause markedly different diseases, reflecting the diverse processes by which they damage tissues (Fig. 9.5). Many extracellular pathogens cause disease by releasing specific toxic products or toxins (see Fig. 8.20). Intracellular infectious agents frequently cause disease by damaging the cells that house them. The immune response to the infectious agent can itself be a major cause of pathology in several diseases (see Fig. 9.5). The pathology caused by a particular infectious agent also depends on the site in which it grows, so that *Streptococcus pneumoniae* in the lung causes pneumonia, whereas in the blood it causes a rapidly fatal systemic illness.

9-3   Surface epithelia make up a natural barrier to infection.

Our body surfaces are defended by epithelia, which provide a physical barrier between the internal milieu and the external world containing pathogens. These epithelia comprise the skin and the linings of the body's tubular structures, such as the gastrointestinal, respiratory and genito-urinary tracts. Infections occur only when the pathogen can colonize or cross over these barriers. The importance of epithelia in protection against infection is obvious where the barrier is breached, as in the tendency of wounds to get infected, and in patients with burns, where infection is the major cause of mortality and morbidity. In the absence of wounding or disruption, pathogens normally cross epithelial barriers by adhering to molecules on mucosal epithelial cells. This specific attachment allows the pathogen to infect the epithelial cell, or to damage it so that the epithelium can be crossed.

Our surface epithelia are more than mere physical barriers to infection; they also produce chemical substances that are microbicidal or inhibit microbial growth (Fig. 9.6). For instance, the acid pH of the stomach and the digestive enzymes of the upper gastrointestinal tract make a substantial chemical barrier to infection, and anti-bacterial peptides called cryptidins are made by Paneth cells, which are resident in the base of the crypts in the small intestine beneath the epithelial stem cells. Furthermore, most epithelia are associated with a normal flora of non-pathogenic bacteria that compete with pathogenic microorganisms for nutrients and for attachment sites on cells. The normal flora can also produce anti-microbial substances, such as the colicins (anti-bacterial proteins made by *Escherichia coli*) that prevent colonization by other bacteria. When the non-pathogenic bacteria are killed by antibiotic treatment, pathogenic microorganisms frequently replace them and cause disease.

When a pathogen crosses an epithelial barrier and begins to replicate in the tissues of the host, the host's defense mechanisms are required to remove the pathogen. The first phase of host defense depends upon the cells and molecules that mediate innate immunity.

Epithelial barriers to infection	
Mechanical	Epithelial cells joined by tight junctions Longitudinal flow of air or fluid across epithelium
Chemical	Fatty acids (skin) Enzymes: lysozyme (saliva, sweat, tears), pepsin (gut) Low pH (stomach) Antibacterial peptides (defensins) (intestine)
Microbiological	Normal flora compete for nutrients and attachment to epithelium and can produce antibacterial substances

Fig. 9.6 Surface epithelia comprise a mechanical, chemical and micro-biological barrier to infection. Infectious agents must pass across this barrier to cause systemic infection. Normal, non-pathogenic micro-organisms (the normal body flora) attach to epithelia and compete with pathogens for attachment sites and nutrients, helping to prevent infection. Antibiotic treatments that kill the normal flora can make an individual susceptible to infection with a pathogen.

9-4 | **The alternative pathway of complement activation provides a non-adaptive first line of defense against many microorganisms.**

The alternative pathway of complement activation can proceed on many microbial surfaces in the absence of specific antibody (see Fig. 8.41). In this way, it triggers the same antimicrobial actions as the classical pathway without the delay of five to seven days required for antibody production.

The reaction cascade is shown schematically in Fig. 9.7. C3 is abundant in plasma, and C3b is produced at a significant rate by spontaneous cleavage (known as 'tickover'); although much of this C3b is inactivated

Fig. 9.7   Complement activated by the alternative pathway attacks pathogens while sparing host cells, which are protected by complement regulatory proteins. The complement component C3b is cleaved spontaneously in serum and can attach to host or pathogen where it binds factor B. Factor B, in turn, is rapidly cleaved by a serum protease, factor D, to Bb, which remains bound to C3b, and Ba, which is released (top panels). Host cells are unaffected by the binding of C3b,Bb (bottom left panels) as they express the membrane proteins complement receptor 1 (CR1), decay-accelerating factor (DAF) and membrane cofactor of proteolysis (MCP) and also favor binding of factor H from serum. CR1, DAF, and factor H displace Bb from C3b, while CR1, MCP, and factor H catalyze the cleavage of bound C3b by factor I to produce inactive C3b (known as iC3b). Bacterial surfaces (bottom right panels) do not express complement regulatory proteins and favor binding of factor P (properdin), which stabilizes the C3b,Bb convertase activity. This convertase is the equivalent of C4b,C2b of the classical pathway (see Fig. 9.8) and initiates the cleavage of further molecules of C3 leading to opsonization by C3b, the generation of C3b$_2$Bb, the alternative pathway C5 convertase, and activation of the terminal complement components.

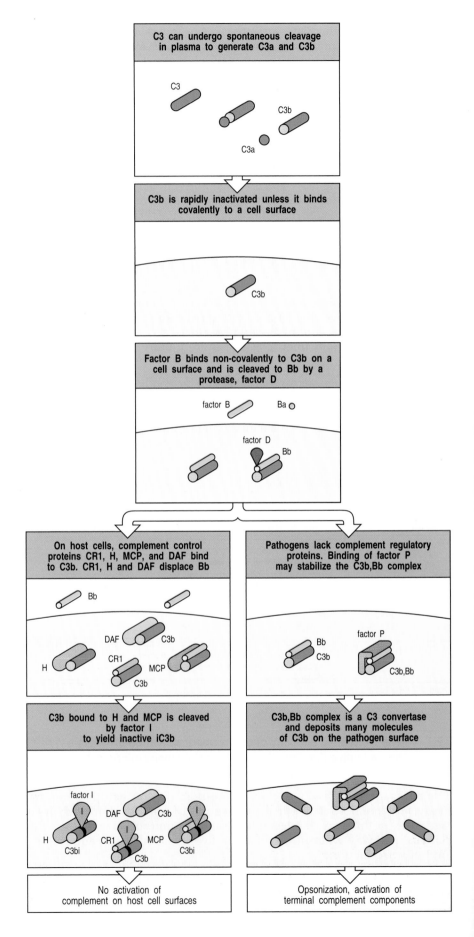

by hydrolysis, some C3b attaches covalently, through its reactive thioester group, to the surfaces of host cells or to pathogens. C3b bound in this way is able to bind factor B, inducing its cleavage by the serum protease factor D, to yield Bb and Ba. When this occurs on the surface of a host cell, as we learned in Chapter 8, the C3b,Bb complex is prevented from initiating further activation steps by the cell-surface proteins CR1 (complement receptor 1), DAF (delay-accelerating factor), and MCP (membrane cofactor of proteolysis), and by the plasma protein factor H. CR1, DAF, and factor H bind to C3b, displacing Bb and thus preventing the next step in the activation pathway. In addition, factor H and the cell-surface proteins CR1 and MCP render C3b susceptible to cleavage by factor I, a serine protease that circulates in active form and cleaves C3b first into iC3b and then further to C3dg, thus permanently inactivating it (see Fig. 9.7).

Microbial cells lack the protective proteins CR1, MCP, and DAF, and factor H binds preferentially to C3b on the surface of host cells. Consequently, the C3b,Bb complexes formed on the surface of a microorganism are not dissociated and function as active C3 convertases. It appears that microbial cells also favor the binding of a positive regulatory component of the alternative pathway known as **properdin**, or **factor P**, which augments activation by binding to C3b,Bb complexes and stabilizing them, preventing their dissociation by factor H and subsequent cleavage by factor I. The stabilized C3 convertase then acts in the same way as the C3 convertase of the classical pathway (see Section 8-25) and converts large numbers of free C3 molecules to C3b, which coat the adjacent surface, and C3a, which mediates local inflammation.

Some molecules of C3b bind to the existing C3b,Bb complex to form C3b$_2$,Bb, the alternative pathway C5 convertase. This binds and cleaves C5, initiating the lytic pathway and releasing the potent inflammatory peptide C5a. Once initiated, the alternative pathway can promote its own feedback amplification, with bound C3b binding more molecules of factor B, increasing C3 and C5 convertase activity on the pathogen surface.

Not all microbial surfaces allow activation of the alternative pathway, and it is not clear what distinguishes surfaces that allow the cascade to proceed from those that do not. Some bacterial surfaces have high levels of sialic acid residues, like the surfaces of vertebrate cells, and are therefore more resistant to attack by the alternative pathway than most bacteria, which do not have surface sialic acid. Other bacteria appear to favor binding of factor H, which displaces factor B from the bound C3b and makes C3b susceptible to inactivation by factor I.

Only two events in the classical pathway of complement activation are not exactly homologous to the equivalent steps in the alternative pathway: the first is the initial cleavage that, in the classical pathway, deposits C4b on the bacterial surface; the second is the cleavage that generates C2b, the active protease of the classical pathway, C3 convertase. Both of these steps are mediated in the classical pathway by activation of C1s by bound antibody; in the alternative pathway, C3 is activated spontaneously, while factor B is activated by the plasma protein factor D.

The alternative pathway of complement activation thus illustrates the general principle that most of the immune effector mechanisms that can be activated by the adaptive immune response can also be induced in a non-clonal fashion as part of the early, non-adaptive host response against infection. It is almost certain that the adaptive response evolved by adding specific recognition to the original non-adaptive system. This is illustrated particularly clearly in the complement system, which can be activated in three different ways, because here the components are defined, and the functional homologs can be seen to be related in evolution (Fig. 9.8).

Fig. 9.8 There is a close relationship between the factors of the alternative, lectin-activated, and classical pathways of complement activation. Most of the factors operating at corresponding stages in the different pathways are either identical, or the product of genes that have duplicated and then diverged in sequence. The proteins C4 and C3 are homologous and contain the unstable thioester bond required for membrane binding. The genes for the proteins C2 and B are adjacent in the class III region of the MHC and arose by duplication. The regulatory proteins factor H, CR1, and C4 binding protein (C4bp) share a repeat sequence common to many complement regulatory proteins. The greatest divergence in the pathways is in their initiation: in the classical pathway C1 serves to convert antibody binding into enzyme activity on a specific surface; a mannose-binding protein (MBP)-associated serine esterase initiates the lectin-mediated pathway; in the alternative pathway the initiating enzyme activity is provided by factor D.

Step in pathway	Protein serving function in pathway			Relationship
	Alternative (innate)	Lectin	Classical	
Initiating serine protease	D	MBP-associated serine esterase	C1s	Unknown
Covalent binding to cell surface	C3b	C4b		Homologous
C3/C5 convertase	Bb	C2b		Homologous
Control of activation	CR1 H	CR1 C4bp		Identical Homologous
Opsonization	C3b			Identical
Initiation of effector pathway	C5b			Identical
Local inflammation	C5a, C3a			Identical

9-5   Macrophages provide innate cellular immunity in tissues and initiate host defense responses.

Macrophages mature continuously from circulating monocytes (see Fig. 1.3) and leave the circulation to migrate into tissues throughout the body. They are found in especially large numbers in connective tissue and along certain blood vessels in the liver and spleen. These large phagocytic cells play a key part in all phases of host defense. In addition to the Fc and complement receptors by which they engulf opsonized particles, tissue macrophages have, on their surface, receptors for various microbial constituents. These receptors include the macrophage mannose receptor, which is not found on monocytes, the scavenger receptor, and CD14, a molecule that binds bacterial lipopolysaccharide (LPS) (Fig. 9.9). The leukocyte integrin CD11b/CD18, also known as CR3 or Mac-1, is also able to recognize a number of microbial substances, including lipopolysaccharide, the lipophosphoglycan of *Leishmania*, the filamentous hemagglutinin of *Bordetella*, and structures on yeasts such as *Candida* and *Histoplasma*. When pathogens cross an epithelial barrier they are recognized by phagocytes in the subepithelial connective tissues, with three important consequences.

The first is the trapping, engulfment, and destruction of the pathogen by tissue macrophages, thereby providing an immediate innate cellular immune response. This process may be sufficient to prevent an infection from becoming established, even after a microbe has crossed an epithelial barrier. Indeed, the great cellular immunologist Elie Metchnikoff believed that the innate response of macrophages encompassed all host defense. For a microbe to become pathogenic, it must devise strategies to avoid engulfment by phagocytes, or, like the mycobacteria, devise ways to grow inside the phagosome. As an alternative strategy, many extracellular bacteria coat themselves with a thick polysaccharide capsule that is not recognized by any phagocyte receptor. Alternatively, if sufficient bacteria enter the body to simply overwhelm this innate system of host defense, they can establish a focus of infection.

The second important effect of the interaction of macrophages with pathogens is the secretion of cytokines by the phagocyte. It is thought that the pathogen induces cytokine secretion by binding to the same receptors used for engulfment. Cytokines are an important component of the next phase of host defense, which comprises a series of induced but non-adaptive responses, as discussed in the next section.

Finally, as we learned in Chapter 7, receptors on macrophages are likely to play an important role in antigen uptake and processing as well as in the induction of co-stimulatory activity. Thus, macrophages are important in the induction of the adaptive immune response, and their released cytokines play an additional role in determining the form of the adaptive immune response, as we shall see in the third part of this chapter.

Summary.

The mammalian body is susceptible to infection by a diverse array of pathogens, which must first make contact with the host and then establish a focus of infection in order to cause disease. These pathogens differ greatly in their lifestyles and means of pathogenesis, requiring a functionally diverse response from the host defenses that make up the immune system. The first phase of host defense is called innate immunity, those mechanisms that are present and ready to attack an invader at any time. The epithelial surfaces of the body keep pathogens out as a first line of defense, and many viruses and bacteria can enter only through specialized cell-surface interactions. Bacteria that overcome this barrier are faced with two immediate lines of defense. First, they are subject to humoral attack by the alternative pathway of complement activation, which is spontaneously active in plasma and can opsonize or destroy bacteria while sparing host cells, which are protected by complement regulatory proteins. Second, they may be engulfed by macrophages with receptors for common bacterial components. Innate immunity involves the direct engagement of an effector mechanism by the pathogen, acts immediately on contact with it, and is unaltered in its ability to resist a subsequent challenge. This distinguishes innate immunity from the induced responses we shall consider next and from the adaptive immune response that provides long-lasting protection against re-infection.

Non-adaptive host responses to infection.

The activation of complement by the alternative pathway and the engulfment of microorganisms by tissue macrophages occur in the early hours of local infection. If the microorganism evades or overwhelms these innate defenses, the infection may still be contained by a second wave of responses involving the activation of a variety of humoral and cell-mediated effector mechanisms that are strikingly similar to those discussed in Chapters 7 and 8. These are the early induced responses. Unlike the adaptive response, these responses to pathogens involve recognition mechanisms that are based on relatively invariant receptors, and they do not lead to the lasting protective immunity against the inducing pathogen that is the hallmark of adaptive immunity. Instead, the same response is usually made to all pathogens.

The early induced but non-adaptive responses are important for two main reasons. First, they can repel a pathogen or, more often, hold it in check until an adaptive immune response can be mounted. The early

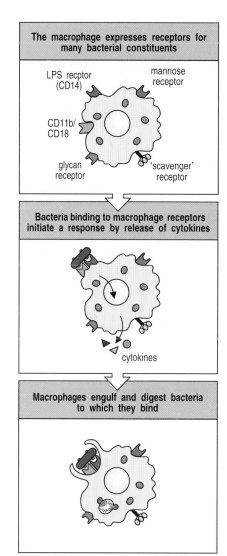

Fig. 9.9 Macrophages bear several different receptors that recognize microbial components and induce phagocytosis and the release of cytokines. The figure illustrates this for two macrophage receptors, CD14 and CR3, both specific for bacterial lipopolysaccharide (LPS).

responses occur rapidly, because they do not require clonal expansion, whereas adaptive responses have a latent period of clonal expansion before the proliferating lymphocytes mature into effector cells capable of eliminating an infection. Second, these early responses influence the adaptive response in several ways, as we shall see when we consider this later phase of host defense in the next part of this chapter.

| 9-6 | **The innate immune response produces inflammatory mediators that recruit new phagocytic cells to local sites of infection.** |

One important function of the innate immune response is to recruit more phagocytic cells and effector molecules to the site of the infection through the release of a battery of cytokines and other inflammatory mediators that have profound effects on subsequent events. Cytokines whose synthesis is stimulated when macrophages recognize microbial constituents are often called **monokines**, because they are produced mainly by cells of the monocyte — macrophage lineage; they comprise a structurally diverse group of molecules and include interleukin-1 (IL-1), interleukin-6 (IL-6), interleukin-8 (IL-8), interleukin-12 (IL-12), and tumor necrosis factor-α (TNF-α). All have important local and systemic effects, which are summarized in Fig. 9.10.

The other mediators released by macrophages in response to infectious agents comprise a mixed bag of molecules, including prostaglandins, nitrous oxide (NO), leukotrienes, particularly leukotriene B4 (LTB4), and platelet-activating factor (PAF) (see section 8-21 for the effects of prostaglandins, leukotrienes and other lipid mediators of inflammation). In addition to these products of macrophages, the activation of complement by infectious agents contributes the inflammatory mediators C5a (the most potent), C3a, and, to a lesser extent, C4a. As well as being an inflammatory mediator in its own right, C5a is also able to activate mast cells, causing them to release their granule contents, which include histamine, serotonin (in mice) and LTB4. These contribute to the changes in endothelial cells that occur in sites of infection.

We have already discussed the activation of mast cells and the actions of the inflammatory mediators they release in Sections 8-20 and 8-21; however, when an individual first encounters a new pathogen there is unlikely to be any IgE of an appropriate specificity bound to the mast cells, so this route of activation is only likely to occur on re-infection. We will return to the role of mast cells in inflammatory responses in Chapter 11, when we discuss allergic responses mediated by IgE.

The combined local effects of these mediators contribute to local reactions to infection in the form of an **inflammatory response**. Inflammatory responses, which are operationally characterized by pain, redness, heat and swelling at the site of an infection, reflect two types of changes in the local blood vessels. The first of these is an increase in vascular diameter, leading to increased local blood volume — hence the heat and redness — and a reduction in the velocity of the blood flow.

Under normal conditions, leukocytes are restricted to the center of blood vessels, where the flow is fastest. In inflammatory sites, where the vessels are dilated, the slower blood flow allows the leukocytes to move out of the center of the blood vessel and interact with the vascular endothelium. In addition to these changes, there is an increase in vascular permeability, leading to the local accumulation of fluid — hence the swelling and pain — as well as the accumulation of immunoglobulins, complement, and other blood proteins in the tissue.

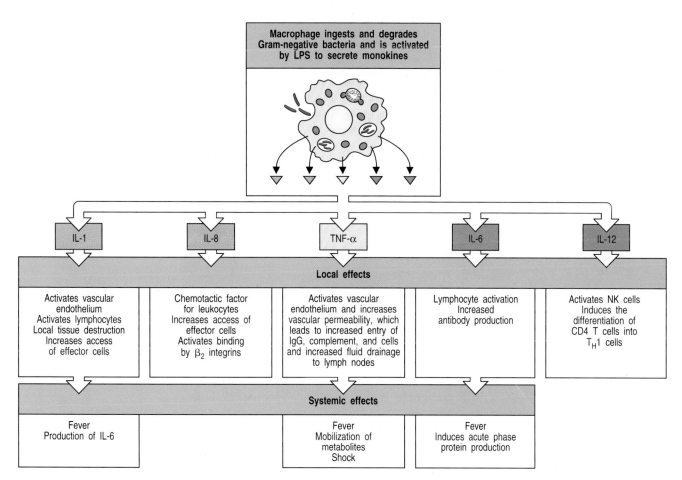

Fig. 9.10 Important monokines secreted by macrophages in response to bacterial products include IL-1, IL-6, IL-8, IL-12, and TNF-α. In particular, TNF-α is an inducer of a local inflammatory response that helps to contain infections (see Fig. 9.12). It also has systemic effects, many of which are harmful. IL-1, IL-6, and TNF-α play a critical role in inducing the acute phase response in the liver (see Fig. 9.15) and IL-1 and IL-6 induce fever, which favors effective host defense in several ways. IL-8 is particularly important in directing neutrophil migration to sites of infection. IL-12 is a two-chain cytokine that is crucial in activating NK cells and in diverting a CD4 T-cell response towards differentiation of inflammatory T cells (T_H1).

The second effect of these mediators on endothelium is to induce the expression of adhesion molecules that bind to the surface of circulating monocytes and polymorphonuclear leukocytes and greatly enhance the rate at which these phagocytic cells migrate across local small blood vessel walls into the tissues. We have seen earlier that monocytes migrate continuously into the tissues where they differentiate into macrophages. During an inflammatory response, the induction of adhesion molecules on the local blood vessels, as well as induced changes in the adhesion molecules expressed on the leukocytes, recruit large numbers of circulating phagocytic cells, mainly neutrophils and monocytes, into the site of an infection.

The migration of leukocytes out of blood vessels, a process known as **extravasation**, is thought to occur in four steps (Fig. 9.11). The first of these is mediated by selectins (see Fig. 7.5). The adhesive molecule P-selectin, which is carried inside granules in endothelial cells known as **Weibel-Palade bodies**, appears on endothelial cell surfaces within a few minutes of exposure to LTB4, C5a, or histamine. A second selectin, E-selectin, appears a few hours after exposure to lipopolysaccharide or TNF-α. These selectins recognize carbohydrate epitopes, in this case

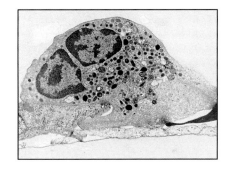

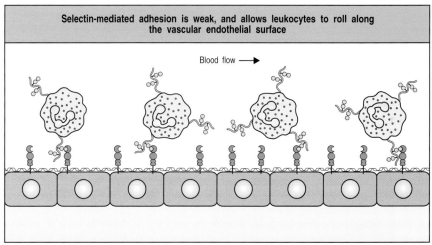

Selectin-mediated adhesion is weak, and allows leukocytes to roll along the vascular endothelial surface

Blood flow →

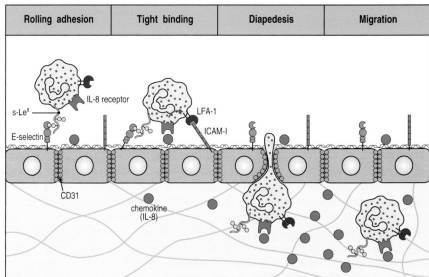

| Rolling adhesion | Tight binding | Diapedesis | Migration |

IL-8 receptor
s-Le^x
LFA-1
ICAM-I
E-selectin
CD31
chemokine (IL-8)

Fig. 9.11 Phagocytic leukocytes are directed to sites of infection through interactions between adhesion molecules induced by monokines. The first step (top panel) involves reversible binding of leukocytes to vascular endothelium through interactions between selectins induced on the endothelium and their carbohydrate ligands on the leukocyte, shown here for E-selectin and its ligand the sialyl-Lewis x moiety (s-Le^x). This binding cannot anchor the cells against the shearing force of the flow of blood and instead they roll along the endothelium, continually making and breaking contact. The binding does, however, allow stronger interactions, which occur as a result of the induction of ICAM-1 on the endothelium and the activation of its counter receptors LFA-1 and Mac-1 (not shown) on the leukocyte. Tight binding between these molecules arrests the rolling and allows the leukocyte to squeeze between the endothelial cells forming the wall of the blood vessel (extravasate). The leukocyte integrins LFA-1 and Mac-1 are required for extravasation, and for migration toward chemoattractants. Adhesion between molecules of CD31, expressed on both the leukocyte and the junction of the endothelial cells, is also thought to contribute to diapedesis. Finally, the leukocyte migrates along a concentration gradient of chemokines (here shown as IL-8) secreted by cells at the site of infection. The electron micrograph shows a neutrophil that has just started to migrate between two endothelial cells (bottom of photo). Note the pseudopod that the neutrophil has inserted between adjacent endothelial cells. The dark mass at the bottom right is an erythrocyte that has become trapped underneath the neutrophil. Photograph (x 5 500) courtesy of I Bird and J Spragg.

the sialyl-Lewis x moiety of certain leukocyte glycoproteins. The interaction of P-selectin and E-selectin with these surface glycoproteins allows polymorphonuclear leukocytes to adhere reversibly to the vessel wall, so that circulating leukocytes can be seen to 'roll' along endothelium that has been treated with inflammatory cytokines (Fig. 9.11, upper panel). This adhesive interaction permits the stronger interactions of the second step in leukocyte migration.

The second step depends upon interactions between the leukocyte integrins known as LFA-1 (CD11a:CD18) and CR3 (CD11b:CD18 — also called Mac-1) with molecules on endothelium such as the immuno-globulin-related molecule ICAM-1, which is also induced on endothelial cells by TNF-α (Fig. 9.11, bottom panel). LFA-1 and CR3 normally have a relatively low capacity to mediate adhesion, but IL-8 or other chemo-attractants trigger a conformational change in LFA-1 and CR3 on the rolling leukocyte, which greatly increases its adhesive capacity. In consequence, the leukocyte attaches firmly to the endothelium and the rolling is arrested.

In the third step, the leukocyte crosses the endothelial wall, or extra-vasates. This step also involves the leukocyte integrins LFA-1 and Mac-1, as well as a further adhesive interaction, this time involving an immuno-globulin-related molecule, called PECAM or CD31, which is expressed both on the leukocyte and at the junctions of endothelial cells. These interactions between leukocytes and the endothelial cells finally enable the phagocyte to cross the vascular endothelial wall, a process known as **diapedesis**, and enter the site of infection.

The fourth step is the migration of the leukocytes through the tissues under the influence of chemoattractant molecules, discussed in more detail later in this chapter. Similar processes are thought to account for the homing of naive T lymphocytes to peripheral lymphoid organs and the delivery of effector T cells to sites of infection, again as we shall see later.

The molecular changes at the endothelial cell surface induced by the inflammatory mediators also induce expression of molecules on endo-thelial cells that trigger blood clotting in these local small vessels, occluding them and cutting off blood flow. This may be important in preventing the pathogen from entering the bloodstream and spreading via the blood to organs all over the body. Instead, the fluid that has leaked into the tissue from the plasma early on carries the pathogen, either directly or enclosed in phagocytic cells, via the lymph to the regional lymph nodes, where an adaptive immune response can be initiated. The importance of TNF-α in this process is illustrated by experiments in which rabbits are infected locally with a bacterium. Normally, the infection will be contained at the site of the inoculation; if, however, an injection of anti-TNF-α antibody is also given, the infection spreads via the blood to other organs.

Once an infection spreads to the bloodstream, however, the same mechanisms whereby TNF-α so effectively contains local infection instead become catastrophic (Fig. 9.12). This condition, known as **sepsis**, is accompanied by the release of TNF-α by macrophages in the liver, spleen, and other sites. The systemic release of TNF-α causes vaso-dilation and loss of plasma volume owing to increased vascular perme-ability, leading to shock. In septic shock, disseminated intravascular coagulation is also triggered by TNF-α, leading to the generation of microthrombi and the consumption of clotting proteins, so that the patient's ability to clot blood appropriately is lost. This condition frequently leads to failure of vital organs such as the kidneys, liver, heart, and lungs, which are quickly compromised by failure of normal perfusion; consequently, septic shock has a high mortality rate.

Mice with a mutant TNF-α receptor gene are resistant to septic shock; however, such mutants are also unable to control local infec-tion. Although the features of TNF-α that make it so valuable in containing local infection are precisely those that allow it to play a central role in the pathogenesis of septic shock, it is clear from the evolutionary con-servation of TNF-α that its benefits in the former arena outweigh the devastating con- sequences of its systemic release.

Fig. 9.12   The release of TNF-α by macrophages induces local protective effects, but TNF-α can have damaging effects when released systemically. The left-hand panels show the causes and consequences of local release of TNF-α, the right-hand panels show the causes and consequences of systemic release. The central panels illustrate the common effects of TNF-α, which acts on blood vessels, especially venules, to increase blood flow, vascular permeability to fluid, proteins, and cells, and increased adhesiveness for white blood cells and platelets. Local release thus allows an influx into the infected tissue of fluid, cells, and proteins that participate in host defense. The small vessels later clot, preventing spread of the infection to the blood, and the fluid drains to regional lymph nodes where the adaptive immune response is initiated. When there is a systemic infection, or sepsis, with bacteria that elicit TNF-α production, then TNF-α acts in similar ways on all small blood vessels. The result is shock, disseminated intravascular coagulation with depletion of clotting factors and consequent bleeding, multiple organ failure, and death.

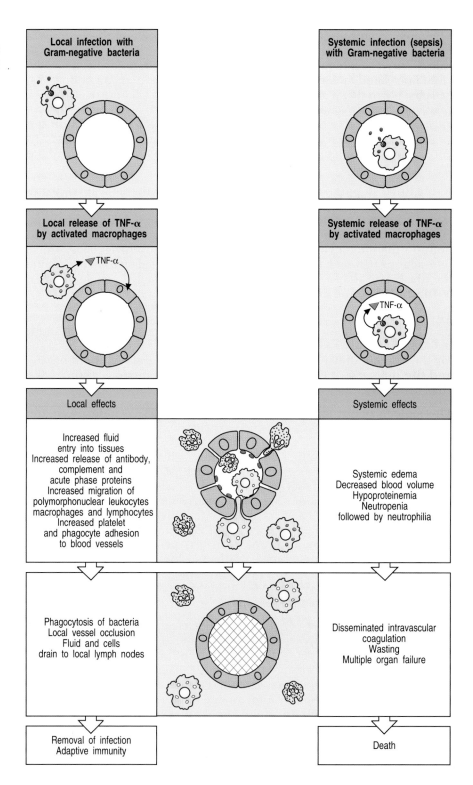

| Local infection with Gram-negative bacteria | Systemic infection (sepsis) with Gram-negative bacteria |

Local release of TNF-α by activated macrophages

Systemic release of TNF-α by activated macrophages

Local effects

Systemic effects

Increased fluid entry into tissues
Increased release of antibody, complement and acute phase proteins
Increased migration of polymorphonuclear leukocytes macrophages and lymphocytes
Increased platelet and phagocyte adhesion to blood vessels

Systemic edema
Decreased blood volume
Hypoproteinemia
Neutropenia followed by neutrophilia

Phagocytosis of bacteria
Local vessel occlusion
Fluid and cells drain to local lymph nodes

Disseminated intravascular coagulation
Wasting
Multiple organ failure

Removal of infection
Adaptive immunity

Death

9-7   **Small proteins called chemokines recruit new phagocytic cells to local infectious sites.**

Some of the monokines released in response to infection belong to a family of closely related proteins called **chemokines**, small polypeptides that are synthesized not only by macrophages but also by endothelial cells, the keratinocytes of the skin, and the fibroblasts and smooth muscle cells of connective tissue. IL-8, whose contribution to extravasation we have just discussed, belongs to this subset of monokines. All the chemokines are related in amino acid sequence. The chemokines function mainly as chemoattractants for phagocytic cells, recruiting monocytes and neutrophils from the blood to sites of infection.

Members of the chemokine family fall into two broad groups: CC chemokines with two adjacent cysteines; and CXC chemokines, in which the same two cysteine residues are separated by another amino acid. The two groups of chemokines act on different cell types; in general, the CXC chemokines promote migration of neutrophils, while the CC chemokines promote the migration of monocytes. IL-8 is an example of a CXC chemokine; a representative CC chemokine is the so-called human macrophage chemoattractant and activating factor (MCAF or MCP-1). IL-8 and MCAF have similar, although complementary, functions. IL-8 induces neutrophils to leave the bloodstream and migrate into the surrounding tissues. MCAF, on the other hand, acts on monocytes, inducing their migration from the bloodstream to become tissue macrophages. Other chemokines may promote the infiltration into tissues of other cell types including effector T cells (see Section 9-17), with individual chemokines acting on different subsets of cells (Fig. 9.13).

The role of chemokines such as IL-8 and MCAF in cell recruitment is two-fold: firstly to convert the initial rolling interaction of the leukocyte and endothelial cells into stable binding; and secondly to direct its migration along a gradient of the chemokine that increases in concentration towards the site of infection. It was initially puzzling how the small, soluble chemokines could perform the first of these functions without being swept away in the bloodstream. It is now thought that they bind to proteoglycan molecules, both in the extracellular matrix and on endothelial cells, which thus display the chemokines on a solid substrate along which the leukocytes can migrate. Once the leukocytes have crossed the endothelium into the tissues, their migration to the focus of infection is directed by the gradient of matrix-associated chemokine molecules.

Chemokines can be produced by a wide variety of cell types in response to bacterial products, viruses, and agents that cause physical damage, such as silica or the urate crystals that occur in gout. Thus,

Chemokine	Subclass	Produced by	Effects on		
			T cells	Monocytes	Neutrophils
IL-8	CXC	Monocytes Macrophages Fibroblasts Keratinocytes	Chemoattractant for naive T cells		Chemoattractant Acivation
PBP/β-TG/ NAP-2	CXC	Platelets			Chemoattractant, Induction of degranulation
MIP-1β	CC	Monocytes Macrophages Neutrophils Endothelium	Chemoattractant for CD8 T cells		
MCP-1 or MCAF	CC	Monocytes Macrophages Fibroblasts Keratinocytes	Chemoattractant for memory T cells	Chemoattractant Acivation	
RANTES	CC	T cells	Chemoattractant for memory CD4 T cells	Chemoattractant	

Fig. 9.13 Properties of selected chemokines. Chemokines fall into two related but distinct groups. The CC chemokines have two adjacent cysteines, and in humans are all encoded in one region of chromosome 4. The CXC chemokines have an extra amino acid residue between the two invariant cysteines, and are encoded in a cluster of genes on chromosome 17. The table lists the actions of some chemokines in each group.

either infection or physical damage to tissues sets in motion processes that recruit phagocytic cells to the site of damage. Both IL-8 and MCAF also activate their respective target cells, so that not only are neutrophils and macrophages brought to potential sites of infection but, in the process, they are armed to deal with any pathogens they may encounter. Just as all of the chemokines have similar structures, all of the receptors for chemokines are similar in structure (see Fig. 7.33); all are integral membrane proteins that have seven membrane-spanning helices. This structure is characteristic of receptors such as rhodopsin and the muscarinic acetylcholine receptor, which are coupled to guanine nucleotide binding or G proteins, and the chemokines also activate G proteins.

Thus, tissue macrophages initiate host responses in tissues, and their numbers are soon augmented through the action of chemokines, which recruit large numbers of phagocytic cells to sites of infection and tissue damage. Why there are so many chemokines, and the exact role of each one in host defense and in pathological responses is not known.

| 9-8 | **Neutrophils predominate in the early cellular infiltrate into inflammatory sites.** |

Neutrophils are abundant in the blood but are absent from normal tissues. They are short-lived, surviving only three to four days. The innate immune response produces a variety of factors that are chemotactic for neutrophils and they rapidly emigrate fom the blood to enter sites of infection, where they are the earliest phagocytic cells to be recruited. Once in an inflammatory site, the neutrophils are able to eliminate many pathogens by phagocytosis.

The role of neutrophils in the phagocytosis of antibody-coated pathogens was discussed in Chapter 8, and where the individual has had a previous encounter with the pathogen this is likely to be the dominant mechanism by which microorganisms are removed. However, neutrophils are able to phagocytose bacteria even in the absence of specific antibodies and can thus provide a protective response in the first encounter with a pathogen. Bacterial cell wall components can be bound directly by neutrophils, or indirectly in the case of LPS, which is first bound by a serum protein, lipopolysaccharide-binding protein (LBP). The complex of LPS and LBP is then bound by CD14 on the surface of the neutrophil. Neutrophils can also phagocytose microorganisms coated with the complement components C3b and its inactive derivative iC3b, which are deposited on the surface of the pathogen by the alternative pathway of complement activation (see Sections 8-27 and 9-4).

Neutrophils express a number of bacteriostatic and toxic products and phagocytosed pathogens are rapidly killed (see Section 8-18). The combination of toxic oxygen metabolites, proteases, phospholipases and defensins is able to eliminate Gram-positive and Gram-negative bacteria, fungi, and even some enveloped viruses. The importance of neutrophils in host defense is best illustrated by considering inherited defects in neutrophil maturation or antibacterial functions; patients with such deficiencies suffer recurrent infections, often of bacteria and fungi that form part of the normal flora. In patients with no neutrophils such infections frequently escape from the local site to produce a life-threatening septicemia. Neutrophils themselves are short-lived and the pus formed at sites of inflammation contains many dead and dying neutrophils. Any microorganisms that have been phagocytosed but not killed are released at this point and can be re-phagocytosed by other neutrophils or by macrophages that accumulate later in the inflammatory response. Even this sequestration of microorganisms can be important in host defence;

in individuals whose neutrophils are unable to kill phagocytosed organisms, in contrast to those with absent neutrophils, infections only rarely spread beyond the local inflammatory site.

| 9-9 | **Cytokines released by macrophages also activate the acute phase response.** |

As well as their important local effects, the monokines produced by macrophages have long-range effects that contribute to host defense. One of these is the elevation of body temperature, which is mediated by TNF-α, IL-1, and IL-6. These are termed 'endogenous pyrogens' because they cause fever and derive from an endogenous source. Fever is generally beneficial to host defense; most pathogens grow better at lower temperatures and adaptive immune responses are more intense at elevated temperatures. Host cells are also protected from deleterious effects of TNF-α at elevated temperatures.

The effects of TNF-α, IL-1, and IL-6 are summarized in Fig. 9.14. One of the most important of these is the initiation of a response known as the **acute phase response** (Fig. 9.15). This involves a shift in the proteins secreted by the liver into the blood plasma and results from the action of IL-1, IL-6, and TNF-α on hepatocytes. In the acute phase response, levels of some plasma proteins go down, while levels of others increase markedly. The proteins whose synthesis is induced by TNF-α, IL-1, and IL-6 are called **acute phase proteins**. Of the acute phase proteins, two are of particular interest because they mimic the action of antibodies.

One of these proteins, **C-reactive protein**, is a member of the **pentraxin** protein family, so called because they are formed from five identical subunits. C-reactive protein binds to the phosphoryl choline portion of certain bacterial and fungal cell wall polysaccharides. Phosphoryl choline is also found in mammalian cell membrane phospholipids but in a form that cannot react with C-reactive protein. When C-reactive protein binds to a bacterium, it is not only able to opsonize it but can also activate the complement cascade.

The **mannose-binding protein** (**MBP**) is found in normal serum at low levels, but is also produced in increased amounts during the acute phase response. It is a calcium-dependent sugar-binding protein or lectin, a member of a structurally related family of proteins known as the **collectins**. It binds to mannose residues, which are accessible on many bacteria but are covered by other sugar groups

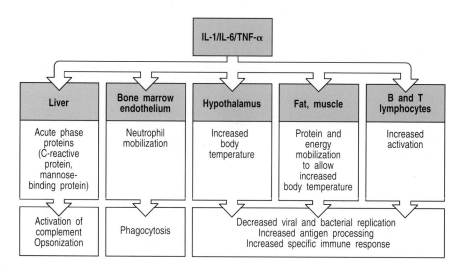

Fig. 9.14   The monokines IL-1, IL-6, and TNF-α have a wide spectrum of biological activities that help coordinate the body's responses to infection. They are endogenous pyrogens, raising body temperature by resetting the hypothalamic thermostat, which is believed to help eliminate infections. IL-1, IL-6, and TNF-α activate hepatocytes to synthesize acute phase proteins. The acute phase proteins act as opsonins, and this activity is augmented by enhanced recruitment of neutrophils from the bone marrow. Finally, they help to initiate the adaptive immune response.

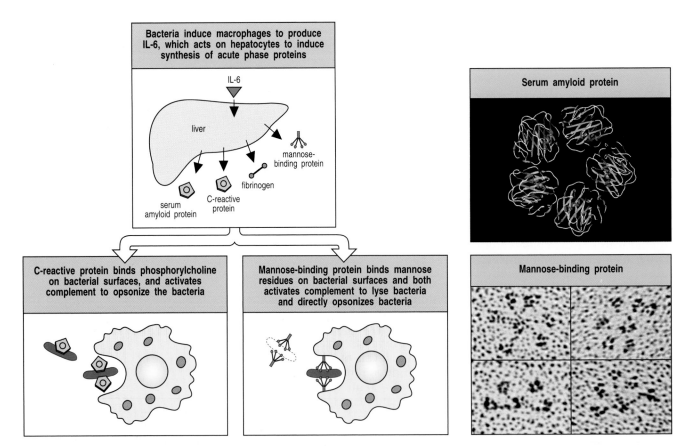

Fig. 9.15 The acute phase response produces molecules that bind bacteria but not host cells. Acute phase proteins are produced by liver cells in response to IL-6 released by macrophages in the presence of bacteria. They include serum amyloid protein (SAP), C-reactive protein (CRP), fibrinogen and mannose-binding protein (MBP). SAP and CRP are homologous in structure; both are pentraxins, forming five-membered disks, as shown for SAP below (upper photograph). CRP binds phosphorylcholine on bacterial surfaces, but does not recognize it in the form in which it is found in host cell membranes, and can both act as an opsonin in its own right and activate the classical complement pathway to lyse bacteria. MBP resembles C1q in its structure, as shown in the lower photograph below, and binds mannose residues on bacterial cell surfaces. Like CRP, MBP is an opsonin and can also activate the classical complement pathway; MBP binds and activates a serine esterase, resembling C1rs, that in turn activates C4 and C2. Thus, CRP and MBP can lead to bacterial clearance in the same way as an IgM antibody. Photographs courtesy of J Emsley (SAP) and K Reid (MBP).

in the carbohydrates on vertebrate cells. Mannose-binding protein also acts as an opsonin for monocytes, which, unlike tissue macrophages, do not express the macrophage mannose receptor. The structure of mannose-binding protein resembles that of the C1q component of complement, although the two proteins do not share sequence homology. When it binds to bacteria, mannose-binding protein can, like C1q, activate a proteolytic enzyme complex that cleaves C4 and C2 to initiate the classical pathway of complement activation (see Fig. 9.8). Thus, within a day or two, the acute phase response provides the host with two molecules with the functional properties of antibodies that can bind a broad range of bacteria. However, unlike antibodies, they have no structural diversity, and are made in response to any stimulus that triggers TNF-α, IL-1, and IL-6 release, so their synthesis is not specifically induced and targeted.

A final distant effect of the cytokines produced by macrophages is to induce a leukocytosis, an increase in circulating polymorphonuclear leukocytes. These cells, the neutrophils and eosinophils, are important phagocytes in both innate and adaptive immunity. The leukocytes come from two sources: the bone marrow, from which mature leukocytes are released in increased numbers; and sites in blood vessels where the leukocytes are attached loosely to endothelial cells. All these effects of monokines produced in response to infection contribute to the control of infection while the adaptive immune response is being developed.

9-10 | **Interferons inhibit viral replication and activate certain host defense responses.**

Infection of cells with viruses induces the production of proteins known as interferons because they were found to interfere with viral replication in previously uninfected tissue culture cells; they are believed to play a similar role *in vivo*, blocking the spread of viruses to uninfected cells. These interferons, called **interferon-α (IFN-α)** and **interferon-β (IFN-β)**, are quite distinct from interferon-γ (IFN-γ), which is produced chiefly by effector T cells and appears mainly after the induction of the adaptive immune response. IFN-α, actually a family of several closely related proteins, and IFN-β, the product of a single gene, are synthesized by many cell types after viral infection. Double-stranded RNA is not found in mammalian cells, but is a constituent of some viruses and is apparently made as part of the infectious cycle of all viruses. It is a potent inducer of interferon synthesis and may be the common element in interferon induction. These proteins make several contributions to host defense against viral infection (Fig. 9.16).

An obvious and important effect of interferons is the inhibition of viral replication in uninfected host cells. IFN-α and IFN-β bind to a common receptor on cells. The interferon receptor is coupled to a tyrosine kinase called Jak, which in turn phosphorylates signal-transducing transcriptional activators known as STATs. The binding of phosphorylated STATs to the promoters of several genes induces the synthesis of host-cell proteins that contribute to the inhibition of viral replication. One of these is the enzyme oligo-adenylate synthetase, which polymerizes ATP into a series of 2′-5′-linked oligomers that activate an endoribonuclease that then degrades viral RNA. A second protein activated by IFN-α and IFN-β is a serine/threonine kinase called P1 kinase. This enzyme phosphorylates the eukaryotic protein synthesis initiation factor eIF-2, thereby inhibiting translation and thus contributing to the inhibition of viral replication. The importance of interferon-induced inhibition of viral replication can be seen in mice that lack an interferon-inducible protein called Mx, which is required for cellular resistance to influenza virus replication. These animals are highly susceptible to infection with the influenza virus, while genetically normal mice are resistant to influenza virus infection.

The second effect of interferons in host defense is to increase expression of MHC class I molecules, TAP transporter proteins, and the Lmp2 and Lmp7 components of the proteasome, enhancing the ability of virus-infected cells to present viral peptides to CD8 T cells (see Section 4-8). At the same time, this increase in MHC class I expression protects uninfected host cells against attack by natural killer cells (NK cells), which are strongly activated by IFN-α and IFN-β, and make several important contributions to early host responses to viral infections, as we shall see in the next section.

9-11 | **Natural killer cells serve as an early defense against certain intracellular infections.**

Natural killer cells or **NK cells**, which we introduced in Chapter 8 as the effectors in antibody-dependent cell-mediated cytotoxicity, are identified by their ability to kill certain lymphoid tumor cell lines *in vitro*

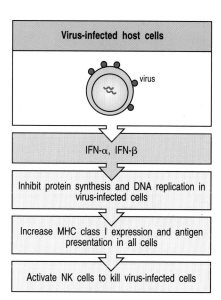

Fig. 9.16 Interferons are anti-viral proteins produced by cells in response to viral infection. The α and β interferons have two major functions. First, they inhibit viral replication by activating cellular genes that destroy mRNA and inhibit protein translation. Second, they induce MHC class I expression by most cells in the body except virus-infected cells, enhancing resistance to natural killer (NK) cells and increasing susceptibility to CD8 cytotoxic T cells. Third, they activate NK cells, which then kill virus-infected cells selectively (see Figs 9.17 and 9.18).

Figure content:
Virus-infected host cells — virus

IFN-α, IFN-β

Inhibit protein synthesis and DNA replication in virus-infected cells

Increase MHC class I expression and antigen presentation in all cells

Activate NK cells to kill virus-infected cells

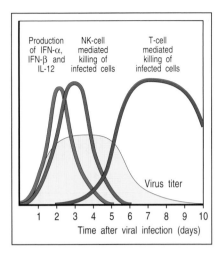

Fig. 9.17 NK cells are an early component of the host response to virus infection. Interferons α and β and the monokine IL-12 appear first, followed by a wave of NK cells, which together control virus replication but do not eliminate the virus. Viral elimination is accomplished when specific CD8 T cells are produced. Without NK cells, levels of certain viruses such as herpes simplex, Epstein-Barr virus, and cytomegalovirus are much higher in the early days of the infection.

without the need for prior immunization or activation. However, their known function in host defense is in the early phases of infection with several intracellular pathogens, particularly herpes viruses and *Listeria monocytogenes*, and we shall consider them here from that point of view.

Although NK cells that can kill sensitive targets can be isolated from uninfected individuals, this activity is increased by between 20- and 100-fold when NK cells are exposed to IFN-α and IFN-β or to the NK cell-activating factor IL-12, which is one of the monokines produced early in many infections (Fig. 9.17). IL-12, in synergy with TNF-α, can also elicit production of large amounts of IFN-γ by NK cells, and this secreted IFN-γ is crucial in controlling some infections before T cells have been activated to produce this cytokine. One example is the response to the intracellular bacterium *Listeria monocytogenes*. Mice that lack T or B lymphocytes are quite resistant to this pathogen; however, depletion of NK cells or mutations in the genes encoding TNF-α or IFN-γ or their receptors renders them highly susceptible, so that they die a few days after infection, before adaptive immunity can be induced.

If NK cells are to mediate host defense against infection with viruses, they must have some mechanism for distinguishing infected from uninfected cells. Exactly how this is achieved is not yet worked out; the observation, however, that NK cells selectively kill target cells bearing low levels of MHC class I molecules suggests one possible mechanism (Fig. 9.18).

NK cells have two types of surface receptor. One, which triggers killing by NK cells, is known as NKR-P1. This receptor has the characteristics of a calcium-binding or C-type lectin, like the macrophage mannose receptor, and recognizes a wide variety of carbohydrate ligands, especially sulfated proteoglycans, which are an important constituent of extracellular matrix and are probably found on many cells. The activation of NK cells to kill normal cells through this receptor is prevented by a second receptor, also a C-type lectin, which recognizes self (and some non-self) MHC class I molecules. These second, inhibitory receptors, are encoded by a multigene family called Ly49 whose members recognize specific HLA-B alleles or, in mice, H-2D alleles; in humans there are additional receptors with a similar function to the Ly49 family but with distinct structural features and which recognize distinct HLA-B and HLA-C alleles. The binding of the Ly49 receptors to these MHC class I molecules inhibits NK activity, and normal syngeneic cells are therefore not susceptible to cytotoxic attack by NK cells. Both NKR-P1 and Ly49 are encoded by members of a small family of related genes that are differentially expressed on different subsets of NK cells and thus allow some variability in the structures that can be recognized by NK cells. Other NK receptors, specific for the products of other MHC class I loci, are being defined at a rapid rate.

Virus-infected cells, by contrast, may be made susceptible to killing by NK cells by either of two mechanisms. First, some viruses inhibit all host protein synthesis, so the augmented synthesis of MHC class I proteins induced by interferon would be blocked selectively in infected cells, and NK cells would no longer be inhibited through their MHC-specific receptor. Second, some viruses can selectively prevent export of MHC class I molecules, which might allow the infected cell to evade recognition by CD8 T cells but would make it sensitive to NK cell killing.

There is also evidence that introduction of new peptides into self MHC class I is detectable by NK cells. Whether these peptides are recognized directly, or whether they displace protective host peptides that prevent attack by the NK cell, is not known. Nevertheless, this would allow infected cells to be detected even when MHC expression itself is not altered by infection.

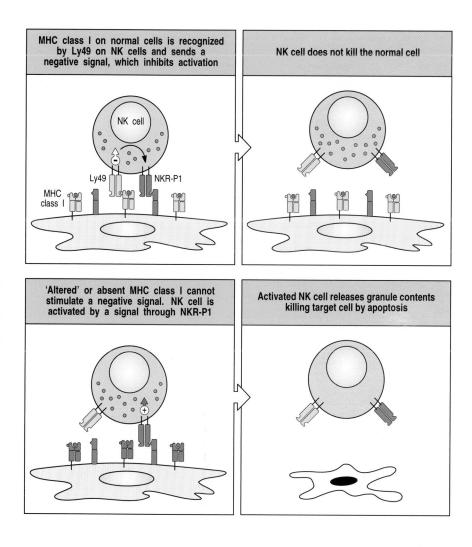

MHC class I on normal cells is recognized by Ly49 on NK cells and sends a negative signal, which inhibits activation

NK cell

Ly49   NKR-P1

MHC class I

NK cell does not kill the normal cell

'Altered' or absent MHC class I cannot stimulate a negative signal. NK cell is activated by a signal through NKR-P1

Activated NK cell releases granule contents killing target cell by apoptosis

Fig. 9.18 Possible mechanisms whereby NK cells distinguish infected from uninfected cells. A proposed mechanism of NK cell recognition is shown. NK cells have lectin-like receptors, called NKR-P1, that recognize carbohydrate on self cells. This recognition event triggers NK cells to kill. However, a second receptor, called Ly49, recognizes MHC class I molecules and inhibits killing by NK cells, overriding any signal through NKR-P1. This inhibitory signal is lost when host cells do not express MHC class I molecules and perhaps also in cells infected with virus, which may inhibit MHC class I expression or alter its conformation. Normal cells respond to interferons α and β by increasing levels of MHC class I expression, making them resistant to activated NK killing. Infected cells may fail to increase MHC class I expression, making them targets for activated NK cells.

Clearly much remains to be learned about this innate mechanism of cytotoxic attack; we shall see in Chapter 10 that a rare human patient deficient in NK cells proved highly susceptible to early phases of herpes virus infection, presently the only clue to the function of NK cells in humans. These cells, which operate early in host defense by mechanisms that involve recognition of self MHC molecules, may foreshadow the evolution of T cells. Two other 'primitive' lymphocyte types, γ:δ T cells and CD5 B cells, may also participate in the pre-adaptive immune response: of these, the γ:δ T cells, which we discuss first, are the more enigmatic.

9-12 | **T cells bearing γ:δ T-cell receptors are found in most epithelia and may contribute to host defense at the body surface.**

One of the most striking features of γ:δ T cells, whose discovery was accidental and whose function remains unclear, is the relative lack of diversity in their receptors (see Section 4-30). This is particularly striking in the γ:δ T cells found in surface epithelia, whose receptors are essentially homogeneous in any one epithelium. Moreover, although gut intraepithelial lymphocytes appear to have diverse receptor sequences, they all respond to the same antigen, and are thus functionally if not absolutely homogeneous. For most intraepithelial lymphocytes the ligand is unknown. What might cells with such invariant receptors be able to recognize, and why are these homogeneous lymphocytes found at the body surfaces?

A possible explanation is that γ:δ T cells, although expressing receptors encoded in rearranging genes, are really part of a non-adaptive, early acting line of host defense. It has been proposed that because epithelial γ:δ T cells express but a single receptor within any epithelium, and also because they do not recirculate, they must recognize alterations on the surfaces of epithelial cells infected with any agent, rather than specific features of the pathogen. For instance, infected cells could make stress or heat-shock proteins in response to infection, and indeed, many γ:δ T cells do respond to such ligands. Equally, they may recognize the aberrant expression of MHC class IB genes that occurs when epithelial cells are infected. As intraepithelial lymphocytes have been shown *in vitro* to kill targets to which their receptors bind, they may act *in vivo* by killing infected epithelial cells and preventing further propagation of the pathogen. These ideas are, however, highly speculative and the function of γ:δ T cells remains to be established definitively.

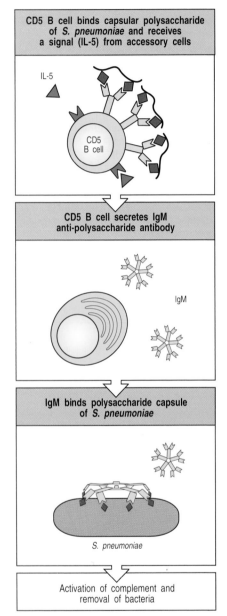

| 9-13 | CD5 B cells form a separate population of B cells producing antibodies to common bacterial polysaccharides. |

The production of antibody by conventional B cells plays a major part in the adaptive immune response. However, there is a separate lineage of B cells marked by the cell-surface protein CD5 that have properties quite distinct from those of conventional B cells (see Section 5-13). These so-called CD5 B cells are in many ways analogous to epithelial γ:δ T cells: they arise early in ontogeny, they use a distinctive and limited set of V genes to make their receptors, they are self renewing in the periphery, and they are the predominant lymphocyte in a distinctive microenvironment, the peritoneal cavity.

CD5 B cells appear to make antibody responses mainly to polysaccharide antigens of the TI-2 type. These T-cell independent responses do not induce significant class switching or somatic hypermutation of immunoglobulin variable regions; as a consequence, the predominant antibody isotype produced is IgM (Fig. 9.19). Although these responses can be augmented by T cells, with IL-5 playing an important part (see Section 8-10), this interaction is not antigen specific and does not generate immunological memory: repeated exposures to the same TI-2 antigen elicit similar responses each time. Moreover, these responses appear within 48 hours of exposure to antigen, which is too soon for the generation of antigen-specific T cells. Thus, these responses, although generated by lymphocytes with rearranging receptors, resemble innate rather than adaptive immune responses.

Fig. 9.19 CD5 B cells may be important in the response to carbohydrate antigens such as bacterial polysaccharides. These TI-2 responses may require IL-5 provided by T cells but this help is not antigen-specific and its mechanism is not clear. These responses are rapid, with antibody appearing in 48 hours, presumably because there is a high precursor frequency so that little clonal expansion of B cells is required. In the absence of antigen-specific T-cell help, only IgM is produced and these responses therefore work through the activation of complement.

As with γ:δ T cells, the precise role of CD5 B cells in host defense is uncertain. Mice that are deficient in CD5 B cells are more susceptible to infection with *Streptococcus pneumoniae*; this is because they fail to produce an antibody to phosphatidylcholine that effectively protects against this organism. A significant fraction of the CD5 B cells can make antibodies of this specificity, and since no T-cell help is required, a potent response can be produced early in infection with this pathogen. Whether human CD5 B cells play the same role is uncertain.

In terms of evolution, it is interesting to note that γ:δ T cells appear to defend the body surfaces, while CD5 B cells defend the body cavity. Both cell types are relatively limited in their range of specificities and in the efficiency of their responses. It is possible that these two cell types represent a transitional phase in the evolution of the adaptive immune response, guarding the two main compartments of primitive organisms, the epithelial surfaces and the body cavity. Whether they are still critical to host defense, or whether they represent an evolutionary relic, is not yet clear. Nevertheless, as each cell type is prominent in certain sites in the body and contributes to certain responses, they must be incorporated into our thinking about host defense.

Summary.

The early induced but non-adaptive responses to infection involve a wide variety of effector mechanisms directed at distinct classes of pathogen. These responses are triggered by receptors that are either non-clonal or of very limited diversity, and are distinguished from adaptive immunity by their failure to provide lasting immunity or immunological memory. Some are induced by monokines released by macrophages in response to bacterial infection, and these have three major effects. First, they induce the production of acute phase proteins by the liver; these can bind to bacterial surface molecules and activate complement or phagocytes. Second, they can elevate body temperature, which is thought to be deleterious to the microorganism but to enhance the immune response. Third, they induce inflammation, in which the surface properties and permeability of blood vessels are changed, recruiting phagocytes, immune cells, and molecules to the site of infection. Interferons are produced by cells infected with viruses, and these also protect uninfected cells from replicating viruses, as well as activating natural killer cells (NK cells), which can distinguish infected from uninfected host cells. NK cells, CD5 B cells, and γ:δ T cells are lymphocytes with receptors of limited diversity that seem to provide early protection from a limited range of pathogens but do not generate lasting immunity. All these mechanisms play an important role both on their own in holding infection in check during its early phases while the adaptive immune response is being developed, and also because of their impact on the adaptive immune response that develops subsequently.

Adaptive immunity to infection.

It is not known how many infections are dealt with solely by non-adaptive mechanisms of host defense; because they are eliminated early, such infections produce little in the way of symptoms or pathology. Moreover, deficiencies in non-adaptive defenses are rare, so it has seldom been possible to study their consequences. Adaptive immunity is triggered when an infection eludes the innate defense mechanisms and generates a threshold dose of antigen (Fig. 9.20). This antigen then initiates an adaptive immune response, which becomes effective only after several days, the time required for antigen-specific T and B cells to proliferate and differentiate into effector cells. Meanwhile, the pathogen continues to grow in the host, held in check mainly by innate and non-adaptive mechanisms. In the earlier chapters of this book we have discussed the cells and molecules that mediate the adaptive immune response, and the interactions between cells that stimulate individual steps in its development. We are now ready to see how each cell type is recruited in turn in

Fig. 9.20 The course of a typical acute infection. 1. The level of infectious agent increases with pathogen replication. 2. When the pathogen level exceeds the threshold dose of antigen required for an adaptive response, the response is initiated; the pathogen continues to grow, retarded only by the innate and early, non-adaptive responses. 3. After 4–5 days, effector cells and molecules of the adaptive response start to clear the infection. 4. When the infection is cleared, and the dose of antigen falls below the response threshold, the response ceases but antibody, residual effector cells, and also immunological memory provide lasting protection against re-infection.

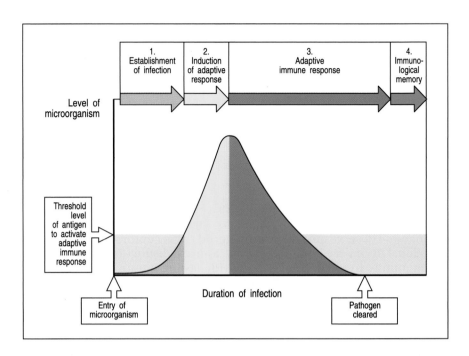

the course of a primary immune response to a pathogen, and how the effector cells and molecules that are generated in response to antigen are dispersed to their sites of action, leading to clearance of the infection and the establishment of a state of protective immunity.

9-14   T-cell activation is initiated when recirculating T cells encounter specific antigen in draining lymphoid tissues.

The first step in any adaptive immune response leading to protective immunity is the activation of T cells in the draining lymphoid organs. The importance of the peripheral lymphoid organs was first shown by ingenious experiments in which a skin flap was isolated from the body wall so that it had a blood circulation but no lymphatic drainage. Antigen placed in this site did not elicit a T-cell response, showing that T cells do not become sensitized in peripheral tissues. We now know that T lymphocytes generally become sensitized in lymphoid organs: antigens in tissues are trapped in draining lymph nodes through which T cells circulate, while antigens introduced directly into the bloodstream, or that reach the bloodstream from an infected lymph node, are picked up by antigen-presenting cells in the spleen, and lymphoid cell sensitization then occurs in the splenic white pulp (see Fig. 1.8). The trapping of antigen by antigen-presenting cells in the lymphoid tissues and the continuous recirculation of T cells through them ensures that rare antigen-specific T cells will encounter their specific antigen on a professional antigen-presenting cell.

The recirculation of naive T cells through the lymphoid organs is orchestrated by adhesive interactions between lymphocytes and endothelial cells. The mechanism whereby naive T cells enter the lymphoid organs is essentially similar to that described earlier for the entry of phagocytes into sites of infection (see Fig. 9.11), except that in this case the selectin is expressed on the T cell rather than the endothelium. L-selectin on naive T cells binds to sulfated carbohydrates on the vascular addressins GlyCAM-1 and CD34 (see Fig. 7.5). CD34 is expressed

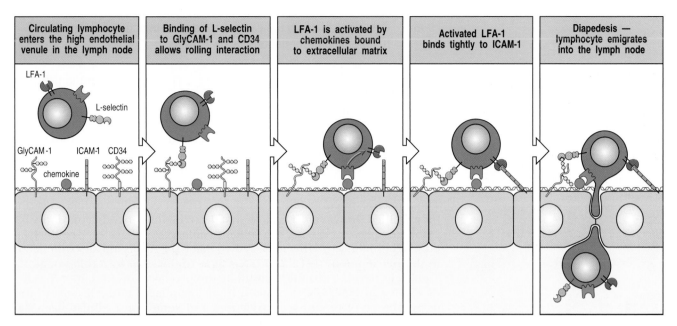

Circulating lymphocyte enters the high endothelial venule in the lymph node	Binding of L-selectin to GlyCAM-1 and CD34 allows rolling interaction	LFA-1 is activated by chemokines bound to extracellular matrix	Activated LFA-1 binds tightly to ICAM-1	Diapedesis — lymphocyte emigrates into the lymph node

Fig. 9.21 Lymphocytes in the blood enter lymphoid tissue by crossing high endothelial venules. The first step in lymphocyte entry is the binding of L-selectin on the lymphocyte to sulfated carbohydrates on GlyCAM-1 and CD34 on the high endothelial venule cell. Local chemokines activate LFA-1 on the lymphocyte and cause it to bind tightly to ICAM-1 on the endothelial cell, allowing transendothelial migration.

on endothelial cells in many tissues but is properly glycosylated for L-selectin binding only on the high endothelial venule cells of lymph nodes. L-selectin binding promotes a rolling interaction like that mediated by P- and E-selectin when they bind to the surface of phagocytes. This interaction is critical to the selectivity of naive lymphocyte homing. Although this interaction is too weak to promote extravasation, it is essential for the initiation of the stronger interactions that then follow between the T cell and the high endothelium, mediated by molecules with a relatively broad tissue distribution.

Stimulation by locally bound chemokines activates the adhesion molecule LFA-1, increasing its affinity for ICAM-2, which is expressed constitutively on all endothelial cells, and ICAM-1, which, in the absence of inflammation, is expressed only on high endothelial venule cells. The binding of LFA-1 on the T cell to its ligands ICAM-1 and ICAM-2 on the high endothelial cell plays a major role in T-cell adhesion to and migration through the wall of the blood vessel into the lymph node (Fig. 9.21).

After leaving the high endothelial venule, most of the naive T cells pass through the lymph node cortex to the medulla and are carried by the efferent lymphatics back to the blood to recirculate through other lymph nodes. Rarely, a naive T cell recognizes its specific peptide:MHC complex on the surface of a professional antigen-presenting cell, which signals the activation of LFA-1, causing the T cell to adhere strongly to the antigen-presenting cell and cease migrating. Binding to the peptide:MHC complex also activates the cell and results in the production of armed, antigen-specific effector T cells (see Fig. 7.2). The number of T cells that interact with each antigen-presenting cell in lymph nodes is very high, as can be seen by the rapid trapping of antigen-specific T cells in a single lymph node containing antigen: all antigen-specific T cells can be trapped in a lymph node within 48 hours of antigen deposition there (Fig. 9.22).

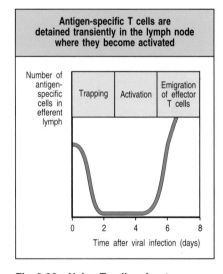

Antigen-specific T cells are detained transiently in the lymph node where they become activated

Fig. 9.22 Naive T cells migrate continually from blood through lymphoid tissue. In the cortex of the lymph node, T cells encounter many antigen-presenting cells. T cells that do not recognize their specific antigen in the lymph node cortex leave through the medulla and re-enter the lymph. T cells that do recognize their specific antigen bind in a stable manner to the antigen-presenting cell and are activated through the T-cell receptor, resulting in the production of armed effector T cells. Lymphocyte recirculation is so active that all specific T cells can be trapped by antigen in one node within two days. By five days after antigen arrives, activated effector T cells are leaving the lymph node in large numbers via the afferent lymphatics.

9-15　Cytokines made in the early phases of an infection influence the functional differentiation of CD4 T cells.

It is during the initial response of naive CD4 T cells to antigen in the peripheral lymphoid tissues that the differentiation of these cells into the two major classes of CD4 effector T cells occurs. This step, at which a CD4 T cell becomes either an inflammatory T cell (T_H1 cell) or a helper T cell (T_H2 cell), has a critical impact on the outcome of an adaptive immune response, determining whether it will be dominated by antibody production or by macrophage activation. This is one of the most important events in the induction of adaptive immune responses.

The mechanism controlling this step in CD4 T-cell differentiation is not fully defined; however, it is clear that it can be influenced profoundly by cytokines present during the initial proliferative phase of T-cell activation. Experiments *in vitro* have shown that CD4 T cells initially stimulated in the presence of IL-12 and IFN-γ tend to develop into inflammatory T cells, in part because IFN-γ inhibits the proliferation of helper T cells. As IL-12 and IFN-γ are produced by macrophages and NK cells in the early phases of responses to viruses and some intracellular bacteria, such as *Listeria* spp., T-cell responses in viral and *Listeria* infections tend to be dominated by inflammatory T cells. By contrast, CD4 T cells activated in the presence of IL-4 tend to differentiate into helper T cells (Fig. 9.23), as IL-4 promotes differentiation of helper T cells, while IL-4 and IL-10 inhibit the generation of inflammatory T cells.

It is not clear where IL-4 would come from early in an adaptive immune response, before IL-4-secreting helper T cells have developed. One possible source of IL-4 is mast cells, and their circulating counterparts, basophils. Mast cells are present beneath the skin and mucosal epithelia

Fig. 9.23　The differentiation of naive CD4 T cells into armed effector cell types is influenced by cytokines elicited by the pathogen. Many pathogens, especially intracellular bacteria and viruses, activate macrophages and NK cells to produce IL-12 and interferon γ, which act on proliferating CD4 T cells, causing them to differentiate into inflammatory T cells (T_H1). IL-4 can inhibit these responses. IL-4, perhaps produced by an unidentified cell type in response to some parasitic worms, acts on proliferating CD4 T cells to cause them to become helper T cells (T_H2). The mechanism of factor production is not known for sure, however, nor is the mechanism by which these cytokines produce selective differentiation of the CD4 T cells: they could act either when the CD4 T cell is first activated by an antigen-presenting cell (second panel), or during the proliferative phase that ensues.

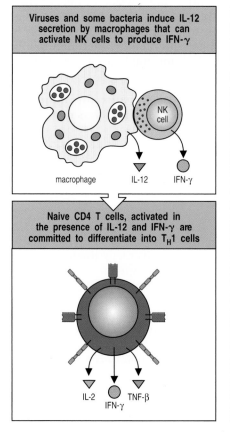
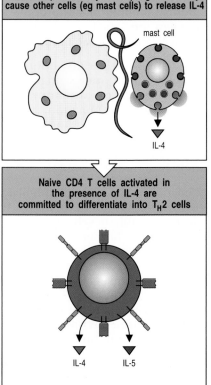

Viruses and some bacteria induce IL-12 secretion by macrophages that can activate NK cells to produce IFN-γ

macrophage　IL-12　IFN-γ

Other pathogens (eg worms) do not induce IL-12 expression by macrophages but may cause other cells (eg mast cells) to release IL-4

mast cell

IL-4

Naive CD4 T cells, activated in the presence of IL-12 and IFN-γ are committed to differentiate into T_H1 cells

IL-2　IFN-γ　TNF-β

Naive CD4 T cells activated in the presence of IL-4 are committed to differentiate into T_H2 cells

IL-4　IL-5

as well as in peripheral lymphoid tissue and can secrete IL-4 along with several other cytokines when stimulated through their Fcε receptors or by C5a. A second possibility, which has received much attention lately, is that the IL-4 is produced by a specialized subset of CD4 T cells that express the NK1.1 marker associated with NK cells. These T cells have a nearly invariant T-cell receptor; in fact essentially the same receptor appears to be used in the NK1.1-positive cells of mice and their counterparts in humans. Unlike other CD4 T cells, the development of the NK1.1 CD4 T cells does not depend on the expression of MHC class II molecules. Instead, these T cells recognize an MHC class Ib molecule, CD1, which is not encoded within the MHC. In mice there are two CD1 genes (CD1.1 and CD1.2), while in humans there are 5 (CD1a–e); CD1 molecules are expressed by thymocytes, antigen-presenting cells, and intestinal epithelium. Although the exact function of CD1 molecules is not well defined, CD1b is known to present a bacterial lipid, mycolic acid, to α:β T cells, while other CD1 molecules are recognized by γ:δ T cells. The nature of the antigen recognized by the NK1.1 CD4 T cells is unknown but, on activation, these cells secrete very large amounts of IL-4 and can therefore enhance the development of helper T cells and a subsequent humoral immune response.

The differential capacity of pathogens to interact with macrophages, mast cells, NK cells, and NK1.1 CD4 T cells may therefore influence the overall balance of cytokines present early in the immune response and determine whether the adaptive immune response is biased towards a cellular or a humoral response, in other words, towards the development of inflammatory T cells or helper T cells. Since the cytokines produced by inflammatory T cells promote the differentiation of naive CD4 T cells into inflammatory T cells, and those produced by helper T cells promote differentiation into helper T cells, any initial bias may thus be amplified by the subsequent adaptive response. For some pathogens, such as *Mycobacterium* or *Leishmania*, a humoral response is ineffective in eliminating the pathogen, while a cell-mediated, inflammatory response is protective. The initial interaction of pathogens with the innate immune system may thus determine whether the pathogen is eliminated or survives within the host, and some pathogens may have evolved to interact with the immune system so as to generate responses that are beneficial to them, rather than to the host.

| 9-16 | **The nature and amount of antigenic peptide can also affect the differentiation of CD4 T cells.** |

Another factor that influences the differentiation of CD4 T cells into distinct effector subsets is the amount and exact sequence of the specific peptide used to initiate the response. Large amounts of peptides that achieve a high density on the surface of antigen-presenting cells tend to stimulate a inflammatory T cell response, while low-density presentation tends to elicit helper T-cell responses. Moreover, peptides that interact strongly with the T-cell receptor tend to stimulate inflammatory T cell-like responses, while peptides that bind weakly tend to stimulate helper T-cell responses (Fig. 9.24).

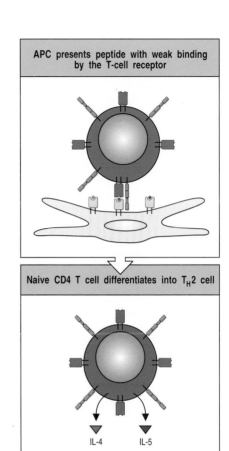

APC presents peptide with weak binding by the T-cell receptor

Naive CD4 T cell differentiates into T$_H$2 cell

IL-4   IL-5

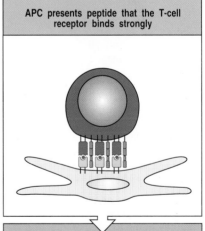

APC presents peptide that the T-cell receptor binds strongly

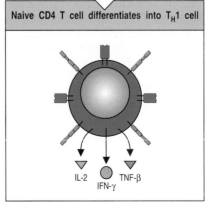

Naive CD4 T cell differentiates into T$_H$1 cell

IL-2   TNF-β
IFN-γ

Fig. 9.24 The nature and amount of ligand presented to a CD4 T cell during primary stimulation can determine its functional phenotype. Naive CD4 T cells presented with ligands that bind the T-cell receptor weakly differentiate preferentially into helper T cells (T$_H$2) making IL-4 and IL-5, which are active in helping B cells make antibody. Naive CD4 T cells presented with ligands that bind strongly differentiate into inflammatory T cells (T$_H$1) that secrete IL-2, TNF-β and IFN-γ, and are effective in activating macrophages.

This may be very important in several circumstances. For instance, allergy is caused by the production of IgE antibody, which, as we learned in Chapter 8, requires high levels of IL-4 but does not occur in the presence of IFN-γ, a potent inhibitor of IL-4-driven class switching to IgE. We shall see in Chapter 11 that antigens that elicit IgE-mediated allergy are generally delivered in minute doses, and they elicit helper T cells that make IL-4 and no IFN-γ. It is also relevant that allergens do not elicit any of the known innate immune responses, which produce cytokines that tend to bias CD4 T-cell differentiation toward inflammatory T cells. Whether the type of antigen-presenting cell that activates the CD4 T cell has any role in directing its differentiation is not known.

Most protein antigens that elicit CD4 T-cell responses stimulate both inflammatory and helper T cells. This reflects the presence in most proteins of several different peptide sequences that can bind to MHC class II molecules and be presented to the T-cell receptor with distinct affinities. As these peptides are likely to bind the same MHC class II molecule with a broad range of affinities, T cells responding to a given protein antigen will probably encounter several different densities of ligand, depending on their specificity. Some of these peptides are likely to bind to MHC class II molecules with high affinity and consequently may be present at high density on the antigen presenting cell, while others may bind with low affinity and be present only at low density. T cells specific for peptide antigens that have high affinity for MHC molecules are likely therefore to encounter a high density of their ligand, while others may only encounter a low density, and these differences in ligand density may affect the subsequent response of the T cell. Indeed, it can be demonstrated experimentally that some peptides in a protein tend to elicit helper T cells, while others tend to elicit inflammatory T cells.

The difference in ligand density required to prime inflammatory or helper T cells may be an adaptation to differences in the behavior of the infectious agents against which the two types of CD4 T cell are directed. Helper T cells are required for effective immunity to extracellular forms of pathogens; they must mount a rapid response to combat these rapidly proliferating microorganisms. Thus, it would be advantageous if they could respond to low levels of foreign peptide. Inflammatory T cells are required primarily to combat intracellular pathogens that initially infect single cells, proliferate more slowly, and cause little damage early in the course of an infection. Thus, responses required for the control of such infectious agents can afford a higher threshold of antigen for activation. The high level of antigen required would be achieved through the growth of many bacteria or viruses within a single infected cell, providing a large endogenous source of antigenic peptides for shipment to the cell surface by MHC class II molecules.

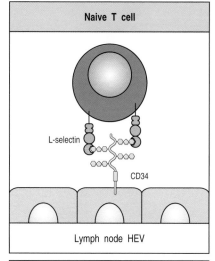

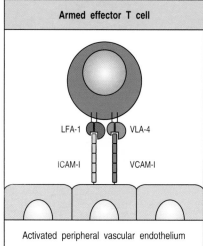

Fig. 9.25 Armed effector T cells change their surface molecules so that they home to sites of infection via the blood. Naive T cells home to lymph nodes through L-selectin binding to sulfated carbohydrates displayed by CD34 (upper panel) and GlyCAM-1 (not shown). If they encounter antigen and differentiate into effector cells, they may lose expression of L-selectin, leave the lymph node about 4–5 days later, and now express VLA-4 and increased levels of LFA-1, which bind to VCAM-1 and ICAM-1 respectively on peripheral vascular endothelium at sites of inflammation (lower panel). HEV = high endothelial venule.

9-17 | **Armed effector T cells are guided to sites of infection by newly expressed surface molecules.**

The full activation of naive T cells takes 4–5 days and is accompanied by changes in cell-surface adhesion molecules that direct the newly differentiated armed effector T cells to the site of infection in the peripheral tissues. Thus, some armed effector T cells lose expression of the L-selectin molecule that mediates homing to the lymph nodes, while the expression of other adhesion molecules is increased (Fig. 9.25). One important change is a marked increase in the expression of the integrin VLA-4 (see Section 7-2), which binds to vascular cell adhesion molecule-1 (VCAM-1); monokines induce expression of VCAM-1 on endothelial cells at sites of infection in peripheral tissues.

Differential expression of adhesion molecules may also direct different subsets of armed effector T cells to specific sites. Some, for example, migrate to Peyer's patches, where they are thought to contribute to mucosal immunity. Homing to Peyer's patches and to the lamina propria of the gut involves both L-selectin and α_4 integrins expressed on the T cell, which bind separate sites on MadCAM-1. T cells that home to the epithelium of the gut express a novel integrin, called $\alpha_e\beta_7$, and bind to E-cadherin expressed on epithelial cells. Cells that home to the skin, by contrast, express the cutaneous lymphocyte antigen (CLA) and may bind E-selectin.

Not all infections trigger innate immune responses that activate local endothelial cells, and it is not so clear how T cells are guided to the sites of infection in these cases. Armed effector T cells appear to enter all tissues in very small numbers, perhaps via adhesive interactions such as the binding of LFA-1 to ICAM-2, which is constitutively expressed on all endothelial cells. If these T cells then recognize specific antigen in the tissue they enter, they produce cytokines, such as TNF-α, which activates endothelial cells to express E-selectin, VCAM-1, and ICAM-1, and chemokines such as RANTES, which can then act on effector T cells to activate their adhesion molecules. The increased levels of VCAM-1 and ICAM-1 on endothelial cells bind VLA-4 and LFA-1, respectively, on armed effector T cells, recruiting more of these cells into tissues that contain antigen. At the same time, monocytes and polymorphonuclear leukocytes are recruited to these sites by adhesion to E-selectin. The TNF-α and IFN-γ released by the activated T cells also act synergistically to change the shape of endothelial cells, allowing increased blood flow, increased vascular permeability, and increased emigration of leukocytes, fluid, and protein into a site of infection.

Thus, one or a few specific effector T cells encountering antigen in a tissue can initiate a potent local inflammatory response that recruits both more specific effector cells and many accessory cells to that site. Most of the armed effector T cells that migrate at random into tissues will of course not encounter specific antigen, and these cells either enter afferent lymph and return to the bloodstream, or undergo apoptotic death in the tissues. Many of the T cells in afferent lymph draining peripheral tissues are memory or effector T cells that express CD45R0. They appear to be committed to migration through potential sites of infection.

| 9-18 | **Antibody responses develop in lymphoid tissues under the direction of armed helper T cells.** |

Migration into the periphery is clearly important for the effector actions of CD8 cytotoxic T cells, and for inflammatory T cells, which must activate macrophages at the site of an infection. The most important functions of helper T cells, however, depend upon their interactions with B cells, and these interactions occur in the lymphoid tissues. B cells specific for protein antigens cannot be activated until they encounter an armed helper T cell that is specific for one of the peptides derived from that antigen or antigenic complex, and it therefore follows that humoral immune responses to protein antigens cannot occur until after antigen-specific helper T cells have been generated.

One of the most interesting unsolved questions in immunology is how two antigen-specific lymphocytes, the naive antigen-binding B cell and the antigen-specific armed helper T cell, find one another to initiate a

T-cell dependent antibody response. The likely answer lies in the migratory path of B cells through the lymphoid tissues and the presence of armed helper T cells on that path (Fig. 9.26).

B cells migrate through peripheral lymphoid organs in much the same way that T cells do, and it is thought that the trapping and activation of naive CD4 T cells in the T-cell areas of lymphoid tissues provides a concentration of antigen-specific armed helper T cells capable of activating those rare B cells that are specific for the same antigen. Antigen-specific B cells may also be enriched in lymph nodes draining an infection by being trapped by antigen that accumulates there.

The initial phase of B-cell proliferation occurs in the T-cell areas of lymphoid tissues (see Fig. 9.26, first panel), usually near to the lymphoid follicles, where a primary focus of B-cell clonal expansion forms (see Fig. 9.26, second panel). These foci appear about five days after primary immunization, correlating with the time needed for helper T cells to differentiate. Some of the B cells in the primary focus may secrete specific antibody after a few days (see Fig. 9.26, third panel), while others migrate to the follicle, where they enter a further phase of proliferation, forming a germinal center in which they undergo somatic hypermutation (see Chapter 8). The antibodies secreted by B cells differentiating early in the response not only provide early protection; they may also be important in trapping antigen, in the form of antigen:antibody complexes, on the surface of the local follicular dendritic cells, and thereby contribute to the selection of B cells by antigen that underlies the maturation of the antibody response (see Fig. 9.26, last panel). The antigen is held by a non-phagocytic Fc receptor on the follicular dendritic cells in the form of antigen:antibody complexes. Antigen can be retained in lymphoid follicles in this form for very long periods.

The proliferation, somatic hypermutation, and selection that occur in the germinal centers during a primary antibody response have been

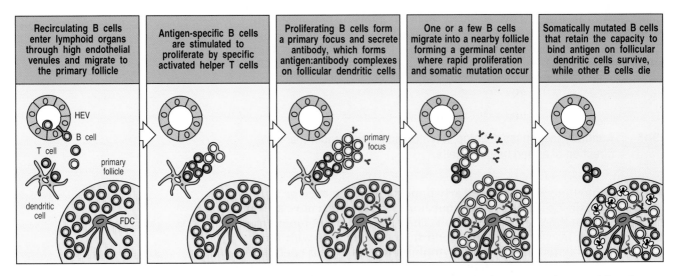

Fig. 9.26 The specialized regions of lymphoid tissue provide an environment where antigen-specific B cells can interact with armed helper T cells specific for the same antigen. The initial encounter of antigen-specific B cells with the appropriate helper T cells occurs at the margin of the T- and B-cell areas in lymphoid tissue and stimulates proliferation of B cells in contact with the helper T cell (T$_H$2), resulting in some isotype switching. The activated B-cell blasts then migrate to primary lymphoid follicles where they proliferate rapidly to form a germinal center under the influence of trapped antigen on follicular dendritic cells and helper T cells. The germinal center is the site of somatic hypermutation and selection of high-affinity B cells on the follicular dendritic cell network. In the primary response, antigen trapping occurs only after initial production of antibody by B cells in the primary focus.

described in Chapter 8. The adhesion molecules that govern the migratory behavior of B cells are likely to be very important to this process but, as yet, little is known of their nature or of the ligands to which they bind.

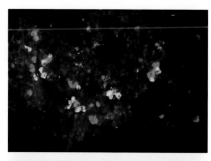

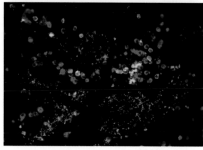

9-19   Antibody responses are sustained in medullary cords and bone marrow.

The antibody-secreting plasma cells that differentiate in the lymphoid tissues remain in the medullary cords of lymph nodes and in the red pulp of spleen, both areas that also contain numerous macrophages that may help confine infectious agents to the lymphoid tissues. Other B cells, leaving the germinal center as **plasmablasts** (pre-plasma cells), migrate to the bone marrow to complete their differentiation into plasma cells, and about 90% of all antibody produced *in vivo* after hyper-immunization is secreted by these bone marrow-resident plasma cells (Fig. 9.27). The tendency of plasma cells to home and persist in bone marrow may explain why tumors of plasma cells occur as multiple foci in the bone marrow, giving this tumor its name of multiple myeloma (tumor of bone marrow cells). The molecular changes on the surface of these differentiating cells that lead them to migrate to bone marrow are again not known.

IgA-secreting plasmablasts have a different migratory pathway, usually beginning in Peyer's patches, and travelling via efferent lymphatics to mesenteric lymph nodes and into the blood. The blood distributes them to the lamina propria of the intestine, the sweat, tear, and salivary glands, and the breast in lactating women. In this way, IgA is synthesized in the site where it is needed for export across epithelial layers.

Fig. 9.27 Plasma cells are dispersed in medullary cords and bone marrow. In these sites, they secrete antibody at high rates directly into the blood for distribution to the rest of the body. In the upper micrograph, plasma cells in lymph node medullary cords are stained green (with fluorescein anti-IgM) if they are secreting IgM, and red (with rhodamine anti-IgG) if they are secreting IgG. In the lower micrograph, plasma cells in the bone marrow are revealed with light-chain specific antibodies (fluorescein anti-λ and rhodamine anti-κ stain). Plasma cells secreting immunoglobulins containing λ light chains are stained green, while those secreting immunoglobulins containing κ chains stain red. Photographs courtesy of P Brandtzaeg.

9-20   The effector mechanisms used to clear an infection depend on the infectious agent.

The function of a primary adaptive immune response to an infection is to clear the primary infection from the body and to provide protection against re-infection with the same pathogen. Fig. 9.28 summarizes the different types of infection and the ways in which they can be eliminated effectively by an initial adaptive immune response.

Immunity to re-infection is called **protective immunity**, and inducing protective immunity is the goal of vaccine developers. Protective immunity consists of two components, immune reactants generated in the initial infection or by vaccination, and long-lived immunological memory, which we shall consider in the last part of this chapter (Fig. 9.29). Protective immunity may require the presence of pre-formed reactants such as antibody molecules or armed effector T cells. For instance, effective protection against polio virus requires pre-existing antibody, because the virus will rapidly infect motor neurons and lead to their destruction unless it is neutralized by antibody when it enters the body. Specific IgA may also neutralize the virus before it enters the body. Thus, protective immunity may involve effector mechanisms that do not operate in the elimination of a primary infection (see Fig. 9.28). Pre-formed reactants may also allow the immune system to respond more rapidly and more efficiently to a second exposure to a pathogen. Thus, when antibody is present, opsonization and phagocytosis of pathogens will be more efficient. If specific IgE is present, then pathogens will also be able to activate mast cells, rapidly initiating an inflammatory response through the release of histamine and leukotrienes.

	Infectious agent	Disease	Humoral immunity				Cell-mediated Immunity	
			IgM	IgG	IgE	IgA	CD4 T cells (macrophages)	CD8 killer T cells
Viruses	Variola	Smallpox						
	Varicella-zoster	Chickenpox						
	Epstein-Barr virus	Mononucleosis						
	Influenza virus	Influenza						
	Mumps virus	Mumps						
	Measles virus	Measles						
	Polio virus	Poliomyelitis						
	Human immunodeficiency virus	AIDS						
Bacteria	*Staphylococcus aureus*	Boils						
	Streptococcus pyogenes	Tonsilitis						
	Streptococcus pneumoniae	Pneumonia						
	Neisseria gonorrhoeae	Gonorrhea						
	Neisseria meningitidis	Meningitis						
	Corynebacterium diphtheriae	Diphtheria						
	Clostridium tetani	Tetanus						
	Treponema pallidum	Syphilis			Transient			
	Borrelia burgdorferi	Lyme disease			Transient			
	Salmonella typhi	Typhoid						
	Vibrio cholerae	Cholera						
	Legionella pneumophila	Legionnaire's disease						
	Rickettsia prowazeki	Typhus						
	Chlamydia trachomatis	Trachoma						
	Mycobacteria	Tuberculosis, leprosy						
Fungi	*Candida albicans*	Candidiasis						
Protozoa	*Plasmodium*	Malaria						
	Toxoplasma gondii	Toxoplasmosis						
	Trypanosoma spp.	Trypanosomiasis						
	Leishmania spp.	Leishmaniasis						
Worms	Schistosome	Schistosomiasis						

Fig. 9.28 Different effector mechanisms are used to clear primary infections with different pathogens and to protect against subsequent re-infection. The pathogens are listed in order of increasing complexity, and the defense mechanisms clearing a primary infection are identified by the red shading of the boxes where these are known. Yellow shading indicates a role in protective immunity. Paler shades indicate less well-established mechanisms. Much has to be learned about such host–pathogen interactions. It is clear that classes of pathogens elicit similar protective immune responses, reflecting similarities in their lifestyles.

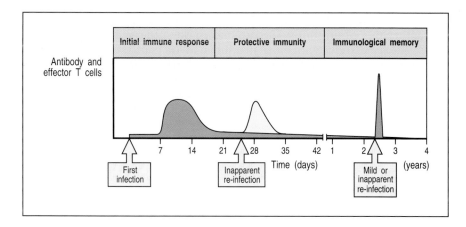

Fig. 9.29 Protective immunity consists of pre-formed immune reactants and immunological memory. Antibody levels and armed effector T-cell activity (dark blue) gradually decline after an infection is cleared. An early re-infection is rapidly cleared by these immune reactants, with few symptoms, but levels of immune reactants (light blue) increase. Re-infection at later times leads to rapid increases in antibody and armed effector T cells owing to immunological memory, and infection may be mild or even inapparent.

Summary.

The adaptive immune response is required for effective protection of the host against pathogenic microorganisms. Adaptive immunity occurs when pathogens have overwhelmed or evaded non-adaptive mechanisms of host defense and established a focus of infection. The antigens of the pathogen are transported to local lymphoid organs by migrating antigen-presenting cells, or trapped there by resident cells. This trapped antigen is processed and presented to antigen-specific naive T cells that continuously recirculate through the lymphoid organs. T-cell priming and the differentiation of armed effector T cells occurs here, and the armed effector T cells either leave the lymphoid organ to effect cell-mediated immunity in sites of infection in the tissues, or remain in the lymphoid organ to participate in humoral immunity by activating antigen-binding B cells. Which response occurs is determined by non-adaptive cellular production of cytokines, which in turn influences CD4 T-cell differentiation into inflammatory or helper T cells. CD4 T-cell differentiation is also affected by ill-defined characteristics of the priming antigen and by its overall abundance. Humoral immunity is mediated by antibodies produced by B cells that are activated initially in lymphoid organs but which migrate to remote sites, especially bone marrow and the lamina propria of epithelia, where the antibody is secreted into the blood or transported across the epithelium. Thus, primary sensitization of B and T lymphocytes occurs in specialized lymphoid organs, but their effector functions are distributed all over the body by the bloodstream. This response ideally eliminates the infectious agent and provides the host with a state of protective immunity against re-infection with the same pathogen.

Immunological memory.

One of the most important consequences of an adaptive immune response is the establishment of a state of **immunological memory**. Immunological memory is the ability of the immune system to respond more rapidly and effectively to pathogens that have been encountered previously, and reflects the pre-existence of a clonally expanded population of antigen-specific lymphocytes. Memory responses, which are called secondary, tertiary, and so on, depending on the number of exposures to antigen, also differ qualitatively from primary responses.

This is particularly clear in the case of the antibody response, where the characteristics of antibodies produced in secondary and subsequent responses are distinct from those produced in the primary response to the same antigen. How immunological memory is maintained, however, is still poorly understood. The principal focus of this section will therefore be the altered character of memory responses, although we shall also outline the mechanisms that have been suggested to explain the persistence of immunological memory after exposure to antigen.

9-21   Immunological memory is long-lived following infection.

Most children in the United States are now vaccinated against measles virus; before vaccination was widespread, most were naturally exposed to this virus and suffered from an acute, unpleasant, and potentially dangerous viral illness. Whether through vaccination or through infection, children exposed to the virus acquire long-term protection from measles. The same is true of many other acute infectious diseases: this is the consequence of immunological memory.

The basis for immunological memory has been hard to explore experimentally; although the phenomenon was first recorded by the ancient Greeks and has been routinely exploited in vaccination programs for more than 200 years, it is still not clearly established whether memory reflects a long-lived population of specialized memory cells or depends upon the persistence of undetectable levels of antigen that continuously restimulate antigen-specific lymphocytes.

It can be demonstrated, however, that only individuals who were themselves previously exposed to a given infectious agent are immune, and that memory is not maintained through continuous re-infection by other individuals. This is established by observations on remote island populations, where a virus such as measles can cause an epidemic, infecting all people living on the island at that time, and then disappear for many years. On re-introduction from outside the island, the virus does not affect the original population but causes disease in those people born since the initial epidemic. This means that immunological memory cannot be caused by repeated exposure to infectious virus and leaves two alternative explanations. The first is that memory is sustained by long-lived lymphocytes induced by the original exposure that persist in a resting state until a second encounter with the pathogen. The second is that the lymphocytes activated by the original exposure to antigen are restimulated continuously. This could occur either by the persistence in each individual of small amounts of the pathogen sufficient to restimulate the activated cells but not to spread the infection to others, or by the existence of other, cross-reactive, antigens that would not be able to activate naive cells but which could stimulate previously activated cells.

The experimental measurement of immunological memory has depended upon quantitative adoptive transfer assays of lymphocytes from animals immunized with simple, non-living antigens. When an animal is immunized with a protein antigen, helper T cells appear abruptly after five days or so, while antigen-specific B cells appear some days later, because B-cell activation cannot begin until armed helper T cells are available and must then enter a further phase of proliferation and selection in germinal centers. By one month after immunization, both memory B cells and memory helper T cells can be detected at what will be their maximal levels. These levels are then maintained with little alteration for the lifetime of the animal. In these experiments, the existence of memory cells is measured purely in terms of the transfer of specific responsiveness from an immunized or 'primed' animal to an irradiated, immune-incompetent host (see Section 2-29 and 2-32). In succeeding sections, we shall look in more detail at the changes that occur in lymphocytes after antigen priming and discuss the mechanisms that may account for these changes.

| 9-22 | **Both clonal expansion and clonal differentiation contribute to immunological memory in B cells.** |

Immunological memory in B cells can be examined by isolating B cells from primed mice and restimulating them with antigen in the presence of armed helper T cells specific for the same antigen. In this way, it is possible to show that antigen-specific memory B cells differ both quantitatively and qualitatively from naive B cells. B cells that can respond to antigen increase in frequency after priming by about 5- to 10-fold (Fig. 9.30) and produce antibody of higher average affinity than unprimed B lymphocytes; the affinity of that antibody continues to increase during ongoing secondary and subsequent antibody responses (Fig. 9.31). Unlike the primary antibody response, which is characterized in its early phases by abundant production of IgM antibody, the dominant antibody isotypes produced early in secondary and subsequent responses are usually IgG, with some IgA and IgE. These antibodies are produced by memory B cells that have already switched from IgM to these more mature isotypes and express IgG, IgA, or IgE on their surface, as well as a somewhat higher level of MHC class II molecules than is characteristic of naive B cells. All of these changes facilitate antigen uptake and presentation and allow memory B cells to initiate their critical interactions with armed helper T cells at lower doses of antigen.

The distinction between primary and secondary antibody responses is most clearly seen in those cases where the primary response is dominated by antibodies that are closely related and show few if any somatic hypermutations. This occurs in responses to selected haptens that may by chance activate a pre-existing set of naive B cells poised to respond to such antigens. Such antibodies are encoded by the same V_H and V_L genes in all animals of an inbred mouse strain, suggesting that these variable regions may have been selected by evolution for recognition of determinants on pathogens that happen to cross-react with some haptens. As a result of the uniformity of these primary responses, changes in the antibody molecules produced in secondary responses to the same antigens are easy to see. These differences include not only numerous somatic mutations in antibodies containing the dominant variable regions, but also the addition of antibodies containing V_H and V_L gene segments not detected in the primary response because of their

Fig. 9.30 The generation of secondary antibody responses from memory B cells is distinct from the generation of the primary antibody response. The primary response usually consists of antibody molecules from a relatively large number of different precursors of relatively low affinity with few somatic mutations, while the secondary response comes from far fewer, high-affinity precursors whose receptors show extensive somatic mutation and which have undergone significant clonal expansion. Thus, there is usually only a 4- to 10-fold increase in the frequency of activatable B cells after priming; however, the quality of the antibody response is radically altered, such that these precursors induce a far more intense and effective response.

	Source of B cells	
	Unimmunized donor Primary response	Immunized donor Secondary response
Frequency of specific B cells	$1:10^4$	$1:10^3$
Isotype of antibody produced	IgM > IgG	IgG, IgA
Affinity of antibody	Low	High
Somatic hypermutation	Low	High

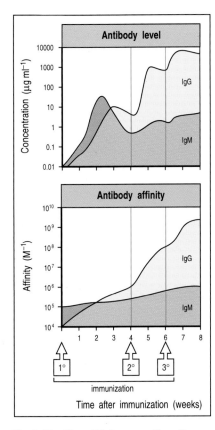

Fig. 9.31 The affinity as well as the amount of antibody increases with repeated immunization. (Note that these graphs are on a logarithmic scale.) The upper panel shows the increase in the level of antibody with time after primary, followed by secondary and tertiary, immunization; the lower panel shows the increase in the affinity of each antibody. The increase in affinity (affinity maturation) is seen largely in IgG antibody (as well as IgA and IgE, which are not shown), coming from mature B cells that have undergone isotype switching and somatic hypermutation to yield higher-affinity antibodies. Although some affinity maturation occurs in the primary antibody response, most arises in later responses to repeated antigen injections.

relatively low frequency. These are thought to derive from B cells that were activated during the primary response and which differentiated into memory B cells. The distinctive character of secondary antibody responses is caused, in part, by changes in the specialized micro-environment in which memory B cells are activated and which are a direct consequence of the original primary response, as we now discuss.

9-23 | Repeated cycles of immunization lead to increasing affinity in antibody owing to somatic hypermutation and selection by antigen in germinal centers.

In a primary antibody response, B cells stimulated by armed helper T cells form a primary focus in the T-cell areas of lymphoid tissues. Some of these activated B cells differentiate and secrete antibody that is thought to help localize antigen on the surface of follicular dendritic cells (Fig. 9.32). The follicular dendritic cells then stimulate the establishment of germinal centers where B cells that have not undergone terminal differentiation in the primary focus enter a second phase of proliferation. During this second proliferative phase, the DNA encoding the immunoglobulin variable domains of these cells undergoes somatic hypermutation before the B cells differentiate into antibody-secreting plasma cells. The antibodies produced by these plasma cells play an important part in driving the secondary response. In secondary and subsequent immune responses, any persisting antibodies produced by the B cells that differentiated in the primary response are immediately available to bind to the newly introduced antigen. Some of these antibodies divert antigen to phagocytes for degradation and disposal; however, some seem to be trapped by special antigen-transporting cells in the marginal sinuses of lymphoid organs. These cells bind antigen:antibody complexes and, instead of ingesting them, transport them to the lymphoid follicles, where they are subsequently found on the surface of follicular dendritic cells. It is possible that the antigen-transporting cells are either B cells or the precursors of follicular dendritic cells, whose origins are otherwise obscure.

The follicular dendritic cells then package the antigen into bundles of membrane coated with antigen:antibody or immune complexes that bud off the follicular dendritic cell surface; these structures are called **iccosomes** (Fig. 9.33). It is believed that B cells whose receptors bind the antigen with sufficient avidity to compete with existing circulating antibody take up these iccosomes, process the antigen, and present it to armed helper T cells. These helper T cells are thereby stimulated to induce vigorous proliferation of the B cells, which undergo clonal expansion in the germinal centers. By five days after secondary immunization, the number of new antigen-specific germinal centers reaches its maximum, and large numbers of antibody-secreting cells are produced from them.

As in a primary immune response, proliferation of the B cells as centroblasts in the germinal centers is accompanied by somatic hypermutation of rearranged variable-region genes followed by selection of the resulting centrocytes for binding to antigen trapped on the surface of follicular dendritic cells. The germinal center events in secondary responses, however, differ in two important ways from those of primary responses. First, the prior availability of antibody greatly increases the efficiency of antigen trapping on follicular dendritic cells, strongly amplifying the signal to the B cells; and second, by competing with centrocytes for binding to antigen on the surface of follicular dendritic cells, the pre-existing antibody prevents selection of B cells bearing surface immunoglobulin of lower affinity than the existing antibody. Thus, the

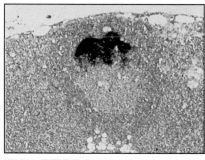

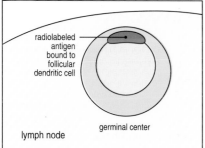

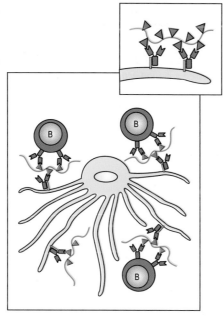

Fig. 9.32 **B cells recognize antigen as immune complexes bound to the surface of follicular dendritic cells.** Radiolabeled antigen localizes to, and persists in, lymphoid follicles of draining lymph nodes (see light micrograph and schematic representation, showing a germinal center in a lymph node. Radiolabeled antigen has been injected three days previously and its localization in the germinal center is shown by the intense dark staining). The antigen is displayed in the form of antigen: antibody:complement complexes bound to Fc and complement receptors on the surface of the follicular dendritic cell. These complexes are not internalized, as depicted schematically for antigen: antibody complexes bound to the Fc receptor in the right-hand panel and insert. Antigen can persist in this form for long periods. Photograph courtesy of J Tew.

pre-existence of antibody both greatly amplifies the secondary humoral immune response and ensures that only those B cells with high-affinity receptors will contribute to secondary and subsequent antibody responses, leading to a striking maturation in the affinity of antibodies produced upon repeated restimulation (Fig. 9.34).

The higher the affinity of an antibody, the more effective its action at low concentrations, and the greater its ability to bind to soluble antigens like toxins that may be active at very low concentrations. One reason for booster injections in immunization regimes is to induce secondary antibody responses, not only to increase the numbers of memory B cells but also to elicit memory B cells making high-affinity antibody. Affinity maturation is also exploited in experimental immunizations designed to produce antibodies for use in serological assays; the higher the affinity

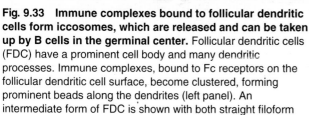

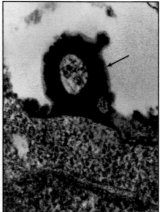

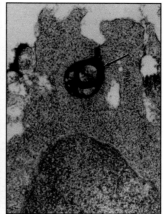

Fig. 9.33 **Immune complexes bound to follicular dendritic cells form iccosomes, which are released and can be taken up by B cells in the germinal center.** Follicular dendritic cells (FDC) have a prominent cell body and many dendritic processes. Immune complexes, bound to Fc receptors on the follicular dendritic cell surface, become clustered, forming prominent beads along the dendrites (left panel). An intermediate form of FDC is shown with both straight filiform dendrites and those that are becoming beaded. These beads are shed from the cell as iccosomes (immune complex coated bodies) and can bind (center panel) and be taken up by B cells in the germinal center (right panel). In the left and center panels the iccosome has been formed with immune complexes containing horseradish peroxidase, which is electron dense and thus appears dark in the transmission electron micrographs. Photographs courtesy of A Szakal.

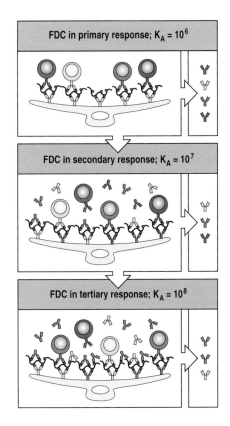

FDC in primary response; $K_A = 10^6$

FDC in secondary response; $K_A = 10^7$

FDC in tertiary response; $K_A = 10^8$

Fig. 9.34   The mechanism of affinity maturation in an antibody response. High concentrations of antigen in the absence of antibody can interact with B cells of a wide variety of affinities, most of which will bind with low affinity. In a primary response, those B cells with receptors of the highest affinity are signaled most efficiently by follicular dendritic cells (FDCs) in germinal centers, and these are selected to survive, even if the cells are actually quite infrequent. On re-introduction of antigen, antibody produced in the primary response competes with B-cell receptors for binding, and in the secondary response, only B cells with receptors that bind well enough to compete with existing antibodies can bind antigen and contribute to the response. In the tertiary response, the same mechanism selects for antibodies with still higher affinity.

of an antibody, the more efficient it is in reacting with antigen and the more sensitive the assay. For this reason, animals are often hyper-immunized to obtain high-affinity antibodies.

9-24   Memory T cells are increased in frequency and have distinct activation requirements and cell-surface proteins distinguishing them from armed effector cells.

Because the T-cell receptor does not undergo isotype switching or affinity maturation, memory T cells have been more difficult to characterize than memory B cells. The number of T cells reactive to an antigen increases markedly after immunization, and the cell-surface proteins that these cells carry are more characteristic of activated rather than naive T cells. However, it is not easy to establish whether these are long-lived armed effector T cells, or whether they are cells with distinct properties that should be specifically designated memory T cells. Note that this issue does not arise with B cells because effector B cells, as we saw in Chapter 8, are terminally differentiated and die in a few weeks.

A major problem in experiments aimed at establishing the existence of memory T cells is that most assays for T-cell effector function take several days, during which the putative memory T cells could be re-induced to armed effector cell status, so that the assays do not distinguish pre-existing effector from memory T-cell populations. This problem does not apply in the case of cytotoxic T cells, however, which can program a target cell for lysis in five minutes; and experiments with CD8 T cells from primed animals show that exposure to antigen generates a population of CD8 T cells that cannot kill in short term assays but can be induced to kill after one to two days' exposure to antigen provided in a form that is not able to arm a naive CD8 T cell for killing. Thus, it is clear that for CD8 T cells, long term protective immunity is not mediated by long-lived effector T cells but that a distinct population of memory CD8 T cells can be defined.

The issue is more difficult to address for CD4 T-cell responses, and the identification of memory CD4 T cells rests largely on the existence of a population of cells with the surface characteristics of activated T cells (Fig. 9.35) that cannot act immediately on target cells. Changes in three cell-surface proteins — L-selectin, CD44, and CD45 — are particularly significant after exposure to antigen. L-selectin is lost on a subset of cells, while CD44 levels increase after priming; and the isoform of CD45 changes because of alternative splicing of exons that encode the extracellular domain of CD45 (Fig. 9.36), leading to isoforms that bind to the T-cell receptor and CD4 and facilitate antigen recognition. However, some of the cells on which these changes have occurred have many characteristics of resting CD4 T cells, suggesting that they are not simply

Molecule	Other names	Relative expression on cells of indicated subset		Comments
		Naive	Memory	
LFA-3	CD58	1	>8	Ligand for CD2, involved in adhesion and signaling
CD2	T11	1	3	Mediates T-cell adhesion and activation
LFA-1	CD11a/CD18	1	3	Mediates leukocyte adhesion and signaling
α_4 integrin	VLA4	1	4	Involved in T-cell homing to tissues
CD44	Ly24 Pgp-1	1	2	Lymphocyte homing to tissues
CD45RO		1	30	Lowest molecular weight isoform of CD45
CD45RA		10	1	Highest molecular weight form of CD45
L-selectin		High	Some high, some low	Lymph node homing receptor
CD3		1.0	1.0	Part of antigen-specific receptor complex

Fig. 9.35 Many cell-surface molecules alter their expression on memory T cells. This is seen most clearly with CD45, where there is a change in the isoforms expressed. These changes are also seen on activated effector T cells. The changes increase the adhesion of the T cell to antigen-presenting cells and to endothelial cells. They also increase the sensitivity of the memory T cell to antigen stimulation.

armed effector T cells. Only after re-exposure to antigen do they achieve armed effector T cell status, and now they have the characterisitcs of helper or inflammatory CD4 T cells, secreting IL-4 and IL-5, or IFN-γ and TNF-β, respectively. It thus seems reasonable to designate these cells as memory CD4 T cells. These observations together suggest that naive

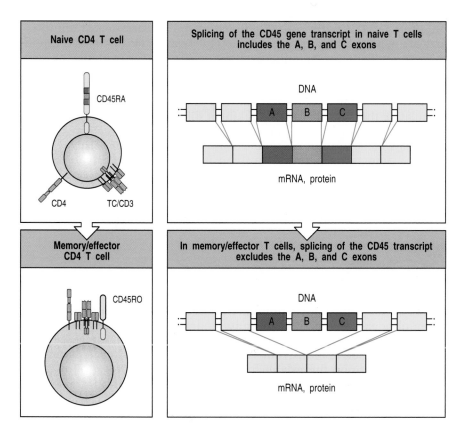

Fig. 9.36 Memory CD4 and CD8 T cells express altered CD45 isoforms that regulate the interaction of the T-cell receptor with its co-receptors. CD45 is a transmembrane tyrosine phosphatase with three variable exons (A, B, C) that encode part of its external domain. In naive T cells, high molecular weight isoforms (CD45RA) are found that do not associate with either the T-cell receptor or co-receptors. In memory T cells, the variable exons are removed by alternative splicing of CD45 RNA, and this isoform, known as CD45R0, associates with both the T-cell receptor and the co-receptor. This assembled receptor appears to transduce signals more effectively than the receptor on naive T cells.

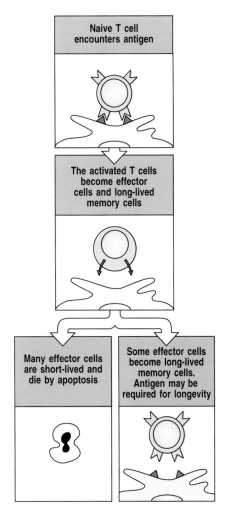

Fig. 9.37 Encounter with antigen generates effector T cells and long-lived memory T cells. Most of the effector T cells that are derived from antigen-stimulated naive T cells are relatively short-lived, dying either from antigen overload or the absence of antigenic stimulus. Some may become long-lived memory T cells, which may also differentiate directly from activated T cells; antigenic stimulation may be required for these cells to persist.

CD4 T cells can differentiate into armed effector T cells or into memory T cells; whether armed effector T cells can persist *in vivo*, and whether they can differentiate into memory T cells is not clear.

| 9-25 | **Retained antigen may play a role in immunological memory.** |

A successful adaptive immune response clears antigen from the body, halting further activation of naive lymphocytes. Antibody levels gradually decline, and effector T cells can no longer be detected. Residual antigen is difficult to detect, either in the form of surviving infectious agents or as antigens derived from them. Nevertheless, some antigen is probably retained for long periods as immune complexes bound to follicular dendritic cells in lymphoid follicles. Some intact virions may persist in this site as well, and a few infected cells may escape immune elimination. It has been proposed that this residual antigen is crucial for sustaining the cells that mediate immunological memory.

The long-lived cells that mediate memory may be derived in one of two ways from naive T cells that have been activated by antigen. One possibility is that the activated naive T cells differentiate directly into memory T cells. The other is that the activated naive T cells first differentiate into effector T cells, which then either become long-lived memory T cells or are short-lived and die by apoptosis (Fig. 9.37). Antigen plays a critical role in determining the fate of the activated T cells, in a fashion reminiscent of positive selection in the thymus (see Chapter 6). Thus, high doses of antigen can trigger apoptosis of the effector T cells, in much the same way as happens in clonal deletion; however, the absence of antigen can also lead to their apoptosis, just as developing T cells die if they are not positively selected. Memory T cells persist either because antigen has programmed them for a longer life span or because a low level of residual antigen preserves them by repetitive sub threshold signaling.

Attempts to clarify the role of antigen in the persistence of immunological memory are fraught with difficulty. Transferring primed lymphocytes to irradiated recipients does not produce clear evidence of long-term immunological memory, while administering antigen along with the cells prolongs responsiveness to the priming antigen. However, the antigen treatment also increases the number of specific cells by stimulating their proliferation, making it difficult to determine whether there are simply more precursors in the mice that received antigen, or whether the life span of individual cells is also increased. Although it is hard to determine whether antigen is absolutely required for the persistence of immunological memory, persistent antigen can clearly help to maintain a population of lymphocytes able to respond rapidly to the priming antigen. Thus, antigen retention in specialized sites, such as germinal centers, may be very important in immunological memory.

| | **Summary.** |

Protective immunity against re-infection is one of the most important consequences of adaptive immunity operating through clonal selection of lymphocytes. Protective immunity depends not only on pre-formed antibody and armed effector T cells, but also on immunological memory, an increased responsiveness to previously encountered pathogens that depends upon the establishment of a new population of memory lymphocytes. The capacity of these cells to respond rapidly to antigen can be transferred to naive recipients with primed B and T cells. The precise changes that distinguish naive, effector, and memory lymphocytes are not well characterized, and in the case of T cells, the relative contributions of clonal expansion and differentiation to the memory phenotype are not yet clear. Memory B cells, however, can be distinguished by changes in their immunoglobulin genes because of isotype switching and somatic hypermutation, and secondary and subsequent immune responses are characterized by antibodies of increasing affinity for antigen because of the effects of pre-existing antibody on the activation and selection of B cells in the lymphoid tissues. It seems likely that residual antigen or infection is important in sustaining memory lymphocytes, although it may not be essential.

Summary to Chapter 9.

Vertebrates resist infection by pathogenic microorganisms in several ways. First, innate defenses against infection exclude infectious agents or kill them on first contact. For those pathogens that establish an infection, several early, non-adaptive responses are crucial to control infections and hold them in check until an adaptive immune response can be generated. Adaptive immunity takes several days to develop, as T and B lymphocytes must encounter their specific antigen, proliferate, and differentiate into effector cells. T-cell dependent B-cell responses cannot be initiated until antigen-specific T cells have had a chance to proliferate and differentiate. The same final effector mechanisms are used in all three phases of immunity, only the recognition mechanism changes (Fig. 9.38). Once an adaptive immune response has occurred, the infection is usually controlled and the pathogen eliminated, and a state of protective immunity ensues. This state consists of the presence of effector cells and molecules produced in the initial response, and immunological memory. Immunological memory is manifest as a heightened ability to respond to pathogens that have been encountered previously and successfully eliminated. It is a property of memory T and B lymphocytes, which can transfer memory to naive recipients.

Phase of the immune response		
Immediate (0–4 hours)	Early (4–96 hours)	Late (after 96 hours)
Non-specific Innate No memory No specific T cells	Non-specific + specific Inducible No memory No specific T cells	Specific Inducible Memory Specific T cells

	Immediate (0–4 hours)	Early (4–96 hours)	Late (after 96 hours)
Barrier functions	Skin, epithelia	Local inflammation (C5a) Local TNF-α	IgA antibody in luminal spaces IgE antibody on mast cells
Response to extracellular pathogens	Phagocytes Alternative complement pathway	Mannose-binding protein C-reactive protein T-cell independent B-cell antibody plus complement	IgG antibody and Fc receptor-bearing cells IgG, IgM antibody + classical complement pathway
Response to intracellular bacteria	Macrophages	T-cell independent macrophage activation IL-1, IL-6, TNF-α, IL-12	T-cell activation of macrophages by interferon-γ
Response to virus-infected cells	Natural killer (NK) cells	Interferon-α and -β IL-12-activated NK cells	Cytotoxic T cells Interferon-γ

Fig. 9.38 The components of the three phases of the immune response involved in defense against different classes of microorganisms. There are striking similarities in the effector mechanisms at each phase of the response; the main difference is in the recognition structures used.

However, the precise mechanism of immunological memory, which is a crucial feature of adaptive immunity, remains obscure. The artificial induction of protective immunity including immunological memory by vaccines is the most outstanding accomplishment of immunology in the field of medicine. Understanding how this is accomplished still lags behind its practical success.

General references.

Gallin, J.I., Goldstein, I.M., and Snyderman, R. (eds): *Inflammation — Basic Principles and Clinical Correlates,* 2nd edn. New York, Raven Press, 1992.

Gorbach, S.L., Bartlett, J.G., and Blacklow, N.R. (eds): In: *Infectious Diseases,* 1st edn. Philadelphia, W.B. Saunders, 1992.

Gray, D.: **Immunological memory**. *Annu. Rev. Immunol.* 1993, **11**:49-77.

Mims, C.A.: *The Pathogenesis of Infectious Disease,* 3rd edn. London, Academic Press, 1987.

Moller, G. (ed.): **T helper cell subpopulations**. *Immunol. Rev.* 1991, **123**:1-229.

Picker, L.J. and Butcher, E.C.: **Physiological and molecular mechanisms of lymphocyte homing**. *Annu. Rev. Immunol.* 1993, **10**:561-591.

Section references.

9-1   The infectious process can be divided into several distinct phases.

&

9-2   Infectious diseases are caused by diverse living agents that replicate in their hosts.

Gibbons, R.J.: **How microorganisms cause disease**. In: Gorbach, S.L., Bartlett, J.G., and Blacklow, N.R. (eds): *Infectious Diseases*, 1st edn. 1992, 7-106.

9-3   Surface epithelia make up a natural barrier to infection.

Isberg, R.R.: **Discrimination between intracellular uptake and surface adhesion of bacterial pathogens**. *Science* 1991, **252**:934-938.

Lehrer, R.I., Lichtenstein, A.K., Ganz, T.: **Defensins: antimicrobial and cytotoxic peptides of mammalian cells**. *Ann. Rev. Immunol.* 1993, **11**:105-128.

Mackowiak, P.A.: **The normal microbial flora**. *N. Engl. J. Med.* 1982, **307**:83.

9-4   The alternative pathway of complement activation provides a non-adaptive first line of defense against many microorganisms.

Liszewski, M.K., Post, T.W., and Atkinson, J.P.: **Membrane co-factor protein (MCP or CD46): newest member of the regulators of complement activation gene cluster**. *Ann. Rev. Immunol.* 1993, **9**:431-455.

Lublin, D.M. and Atkinson, J.P.: **Decay-accelerating factor: biochemistry, molecular biology and function**. *Ann. Rev. Immunol.* 1991, **7**:35-58.

Pangburn, M.K.: **The alternative pathway**. In: Ross, G.D. (ed.): *Immunobiology of the Complement System*. Orlando, Academic Press, 1986, pp. 45-62.

9-5   Macrophages provide innate cellular immunity in tissues and initiate host defense responses.

Ezekowitz, R.A.B., Williams, D.J., Koziel, H., Armstrong, M.Y.K., Warner, A., Richards, F.F., and Rose, R.M.: **Uptake of *Pneumocystis carinii* mediated by the macrophage mannose receptor**. *Nature* 1991, **351**:155-158.

Stahl, P.D.: **The mannose receptor and other macrophage lectins**. *Curr. Opin. Immunol.* 1992, **4**:49-52.

Ulevitch, R.J., and Tobias, P.S.: **Receptor-dependent mechanism of cell stimulation by bacterial endotoxin**. *Ann. Rev. Immunol.* 1995, **13**:437-457.

Wright, S.D.: **Multiple receptors for endotoxin**. *Curr. Opin. Immunol.* 1991, **3**:83-90.

Wright, S.D., Ramos, R.A., Tobias, P.S., Ulevitch, R.J., and Mathison, J.C.: **CD14, a receptor for complexes of lipopolysaccharide (LPS) and LPS-binding protein**. *Science* 1990, **249**:1431-1433.

9-6   The innate immune response produces inflammatory mediators that recruit new phagocytic cells to local sites of infection.

Bevilacqua, M.P.: **Endothelial leukocyte adhesion molecules**. *Ann. Rev. Immunol.* 1993, **11**:767-804.

Dinarello, C.A.: **Role of interleukin-1 and tumor necrosis factor in systemic responses to infection and inflammation**. In: Gallin, J.I., Goldstein, I.M., and Snyderman, R. (eds): *Inflammation — basic principles and clinical correlates*. New York, Raven Press, 1992, pp. 211-232.

Downey, G.P.: **Mechanisms of leukocyte motility and chemotaxis**. *Curr. Opin. Immunol.* 1994, **6**:113–124.

Springer, T.A.: **Traffic signals for lymphocyte recirculation and leukocyte emigration: the multi-step paradigm**. *Cell* 1994, **76**:301-304.

Pfieffer, K., Matsuyama, T., Kundig, T.M., Wakeham, A., Kishihara, K., Shahinian, A., Wiegmann, K., Ohashi, P.S., Kromke, M., and Mak, T.W.: **Mice deficient for the 55kd tumor necrosis factor receptor are resistant to endotoxic shock, yet succumb to *L. monocytogenes* infection**. *Cell* 1993, **73**:457-467.

Van Snik, J.: **Interleukin-6: An overview**. *Ann. Rev. Immunol.* 1993, **8**:253-278.

Vassalli, P.: **The pathophysiology of tumor necrosis factors**. *Ann. Rev. Immunol.* 1992, **10**:411-452.

9-7   Small proteins called chemokines recruit new phagocytic cells to local infectious sites.

Baggiolini, M., Dewald, B., and Waltz, A.: **Interleukin-8 and related chemotactic cytokines**. In: Gallin, J.I., Goldstein, I.M., and Snyderman, R. (eds): *Inflammation — basic principles and clinical correlates*. New York, Raven Press, 1992, pp. 247-263.

Gerard, C., and Gerard, N.P: **The pro-inflammatory seven transmembrane spanning receptors of the leukocyte**. *Curr. Opin. Immunol.* 1994, **6**:140.

Miller, M.D. and Krangel, M.S.: **Biology and biochemistry of the chemokines: a family of chemotactic and inflammatory cytokines**. *CRC Crit. Rev. Immunol.* 1992, **12**:30.

Murphy, P.M.: **The molecular biology of leukocyte chemoattractant receptors**. *Ann. Rev. Immunol.* **12**:593-633.

Oppenheim, J.J., Zachariae, C.O.C., Mukaida, N., and Matsushima, K.: **Properties of the novel proinflammatory supergene intercrine cytokine family**. *Ann. Rev. Immunol.* 1993, **9**:817-848.

9-8 Neutrophils predominate in the early cellular infiltrate into inflammatory sites.

Rosales, C., and Brown, E.J.: **Neutrophil receptors and modulation of the immune response.** In: Abramson, J.S., and Wheeler, J.G. (eds): *The Natural Immune System*, New York, IRL Press, 1993, pp. 24-62.

9-9 Cytokines released by macrophages also activate the acute phase response.

Emsley, J., White, H.E., O'Hara, B.P., Oliva, G., Srinivasan, N., Tickle, I.J., Blundell, T.L., Pepys, M.B., and Wood, S.P.: **Structure of pentameric human serum amyloid P component.** *Nature* 1994, **367**:338.

Ezekowitz, R.A.B.: **Ante-antibody immunity.** *Curr. Biol.* 1991, **1**:60-62.

MacLeod, C.M., Avery, O.T.: **The occurrence during acute infections of a protein not normally present in blood. Isolation and properties of the reactive protein.** *J. Exper. Med.* 1941, **73**:183-190.

Sastry, K. and Ezekowitz, R.A.: **Collectins: pattern-recognition molecules involved in first-line host defense.** *Curr. Opin. Immunol.* 1993, **5**:59-66.

Weiss, W.I., Drickamer, K., Hendrickson, W.A.: **Structure of a C-type mannose-binding protein complexed with an oligosaccharide.** *Nature* 1992, **360**:127-134.

9-10 Interferons inhibit viral replication and activate certain host defense responses.

Friedman, R.M.: **Interferons.** In: Oppenheim, J.J. and Shevach, E.M. (eds): *Textbook of Immunophysiology.* New York, Oxford University Press, 1988, p. 94.

Ortaldo, J.R. and Herberman, R.B.: **Augmentation of natural killer activity** In: *Immunobiology of Natural Killer Cells, vol. II.* Boca Raton, FL, CRC Press, 1986, p. 145.

Vilcek, J. and De Maeyer, E. (eds): *Interferons and the Immune System,* 1st edn. Amsterdam, Elsevier Press, 1984.

9-11 Natural killer cells serve as an early defense against certain intracellular infections.

Bezouska, K., Yued, C.T., O'Brien, J., Childs, R.A., Chai, W., Lawson, A.M., Drbal, K., Fiserova, A., Pospisil, M., and Feizi, T.: **Oligosaccharide ligands for NKR-P1 protein activate NK cells and cytotoxicity.** *Nature* **372**:150-157.

Ciccone, E., Pende, D., Viale, O., Di Donato, C., Tripodi, G., Oriengo, A.M., Guardiola, J., Moretta, A., and Moretta, L.: **Evidence of a natural killer (NK) cell repertoire for (allo) antigen recognition: definition of five distinct NK-determined allospecificities in humans.** *J. Exper. Med.* 1992, **175**:709-718.

Karlhofer, F.M., Ribaudo, R.K., and Yokoyama, W.M.: **MHC class I alloantigen specificity of Ly-49+ IL-2 activated natural killer cells.** *Nature* 1992, **358**:66-70.

Malnati, M.S., Peruzzi, M., Parker, K. C., Biddison, W.E., Ciccone, E., Moretta, A., and Long, E.O.: **Peptide specificity in the recognition of MHC class I by natural killer cell clones.** *Science* 1995, **267**:1016-1018.

Raulet, D.H., and Held, W.: **Natural killer cell receptors: The offs and ons of NK cell recognition.** *Cell* 1995, **82**:697-700.

Wolf, S.F., Temple, P.A., Kobayashi, M., Young, D., Dicig, M., Lowe, L., Dzialo, R., Fitz, L., Ferenz, C., Hewick, R.M., Kelleher, K., Hermann, S.H., Clark, S.C., Azzoni, L., Chan, S.H., Trinchieri, G., and Perussia, B.: **Cloning of cDNA for natural killer cell stimulatory factor, a heterodimeric cytokine with multiple biologic effects on T and natural killer cells.** *J. Immunol.* 1991, **146**:3074.

9-12 T cells bearing γ:δ T-cell receptors are found in most epithelia and may contribute to host defense at the body surface.

Davis, M.M., and Chien, Y-h.: **Issues concerning the nature of antigen recognition by αβ and γδ T cell receptors.** *Immunol. Today.* 1995, **16**:316-318.

Haas, W., Pereira, P., and Tonegawa, S.: **γ:δ cells.** *Ann. Rev. Immunol.* 1993, **11**:637-685.

Janeway, C.A. Jr, Jones, B., and Hayday, A.: **Specificity and function of T cells bearing γ:δ receptors.** *Immunol. Today* 1988, **9**:73-76.

Raulet, D.H.: **The structure, function, and molecular genetics of the γ:δ T-cell receptor.** *Ann. Rev. Immunol.* 1993, **7**:175-207.

Schild, H., Mavaddat, N., Litzenberger, C., Ehrich, E.W., Davis, M.M., Bluestone, J.A., Matis, L., Draper, R.K., and Chein, Y-h.: **The nature of major histocompatibility complex recognition by γδ T cells.** *Cell* 1994, **76**:29-37.

9-13 CD5 B cells form a separate population of B cells producing antibodies to common bacterial polysaccharides.

Hayakawa, K. and Hardy, R.R.: **Normal, autoimmune, and malignant CD5+ B cells: The LY-1 B lineage.** *Ann. Rev. Immunol.* 1993, **6**:197-218.

Kantor, A.B. and Herzenberg, L.A.: **Origin of murine B-cell lineages.** *Ann. Rev. Immunol.* 1993, **11**:501-538.

9-14 T-cell activation is initiated when recirculating T cells encounter specific antigen in draining lymphoid tissues.

Bergstresser, P.R.: **Sensitization and elicitation of inflammation in contact dermatitis.** In: Norms, D. (ed.): *Immunologic Mechanisms in Cutaneous Disease.* New York, Marcel Dekker, 1988, p. 20.

Cumberbatch, M. and Kimber, I.: **Phenotypic characteristics of antigen-bearing cells in the draining lymph nodes of contact sensitized mice.** *Immunology* 1990, **71**:404.

Ford, W.L.: **Lymphocyte migration and immune responses.** *Prog. Allergy* 1975, **19**:1-59.

Macatonia, S.E., Knight, S.C., Edwards, A.J., Griffith, S., and Fryer, P.: **Localization of antigen on lymph node dendritic cells after exposure to the contact sensitizer fluorescein isothyiocyanate. Functional and morphological studies.** *J. Exper. Med.* 1987, **166**:1654.

Shunizu, Y. and Shaw, S.: **Mucins in the mainstream.** *Nature* 1993, **366**:630-631.

Tanaka, Y., Adams, D.H., Hubscher, S., Hirano, H., Siebenlist, U., and Shaw, S.: **T cell adhesion induced by proteoglycan-immobilized cytokine MIP-1β.** *Nature* 1993, **361**:79-82.

9-15 Cytokines made in the early phases of an infection influence the functional differentiation of CD4 T cells.

Bendelac, A., Lantz, O., Quimby, M.E., Yewdell, J.W., Bennick, J.R., and Brutkiewicz, R.R.: **CD1 recognition by mouse NK1.1+ T lymphocytes.** *Science* 1995, **268**:863-865.

Hsieh, C.S., Heimberger, A.B., Gold, J., O'Garra, A., and Murphy, K.: **Differential regulation of T-helper phenotype development by interleukins 4 and 10 in an α:β T-cell receptor transgenic system.** *Proc. Natl. Acad. Sci. USA* 1992, **89**:6065-6069.

Hsieh, C.-S., Macatonia, S.E., Tripp, C.S., Wolf, S.F., O'Garra, A., and Murphy, K.M.: **Development of Th1 CD4+ T cells through IL-12 produced by *Listeria*-induced macrophages.** *Science* 1993, **260**:547-549.

Lantz, O., and Bendelac, A.: **An invariant T cell receptor α chain is used by a unique subset of major histocompatibility complex class I specific CD4+ and CD4-8- T cells in mice and humans.** *J.Exp. Med.* 1994, **180**:1097-2010.

Manetti, R., Parronchi, P., Guidizi, M.G., Piccini, M.-P., Maggi, E., Trinchieri, G., and Romagnani, S.: **Natural killer cell stimulatory factor (NKSF/IL-12) induces Th1-type specific immune responses and inhibits the development of IL-4 producing Th cells.** *J. Exper. Med.* 1993, **177**:1199-1204.

Scott, P.: **Selective differentiation of CD4+ T-helper cell subsets.** *Curr. Opin. Immunol.* 1993, **5**:391-397.

Seder, R.A., and Paul, W.E.: **Acquisition of lymphokine-producing phenotype by CD4 T cells.** *Ann. Rev. Immunol.* 1994, **12**:635-673.

Seder, R.A., Paul, W.E., Davis, M.M., and Fasekas De St. Groth, B.: **The presence of interleukin-4 during *in vitro* priming determines the lymphokine-producing potential of CD4$^+$ T cells from T-cell receptor transgenic mice.** *J. Exper. Med.* 1992, **176**:1091-1098.

Sher, A. and Coffman, R.L.: **Regulation of immunity to parasites by T cells and T cell-derived cytokines.** *Ann. Rev. Immunol.* 1992, **10**:385-409.

9-16   **The nature and amount of antigenic peptide can also effect the differentiation of CD4 T cells.**

Constant, S., Pfeiffer, C., Woodard, A., Pasqualini, T., and Bottomly, K.: **Extent of T cell receptor ligation can determine the functional differentiation of naive CD4 T cells.** *J.Exp. Med.* 1995, In press.

Pfeiffer, C., Stein, J., Southwood, S., Ketelaar, H., Sette, A., and Bottomly, K.: **Altered peptide ligands can control CD4 T lymphocyte differentiation *in vivo*.** *J.Exp. Med.* 1995, **181**:1569-1574.

9-17   **Armed effector T cells are guided to sites of infection by newly expressed surface molecules.**

Baron, J.L., Madri, J.A., Ruddle, N.H., Hashim, G., and Janeway, C.A. Jr: **Surface expression of α4 integrin by CD4 T cells is required for their entry into brain parenchyma.** *J. Exper. Med.* 1993, **177**:57-68.

MacKay, C.R., Marston, W., and Dudler, L.: **Altered patterns of T-cell migration through lymph nodes and skin following antigen challenge.** *Eur. J. Immunol.* 1992, **22**:2205-2210.

MacKay, C.R.: **Homing of naive, memory and effector lymphocytes.** *Curr. Opin. Immunol.* 1993, **5**:423-427.

9-18   **Antibody responses develop in lymphoid tissues under the direction of armed helper T cells.**

Jacob, J. and Kelsoe, G.: ***In situ* studies of the primary immune response to (4-hydroxy-3-nitrophenyl)acetyl II. A common clonal origin for periarteriolar lymphoid sheath-associated foci and germinal centers.** *J. Exp. Med.* 1992, **176**:679-687.

Kelsoe, G. and Zheng, B.: **Sites of B-cell activation *in vivo*.** *Curr. Opin. Immunol.* 1993, **5**:418-422.

Liu, Y.J., Johnson, G.D., Gordon, J., and MacLennan, I.C.M.: **Germinal centres in T cell-dependent antibody responses.** *Immunol. Today* 1992, **13**:17-21.

MacLennan, I.C.M.: **Germinal centres.** *Ann. Rev. Immunol.* 1994, **12**:117-139.

Moller, G. (ed.): *Immunological Reviews* 1993, **126**:1-178.

9-19   **Antibody responses are sustained in medullary cords and bone marrow.**

Benner, R., Hijmans, W., and Haaijman, J.J.: **The bone marrow: the major source of serum immunoglobulins, but still a neglected site of antibody formation.** *Clin. Exper. Immunol.* 1981, **46**:1-8.

MacLennan, I.C.M. and Gray, D.: **Antigen-driven selection of virgin and memory B cells.** *Immunol. Rev.* 1986, **91**:61.

9-21   **Immunological memory is long-lived following infection.**

Black, F.L. and Rosen, L.: **Patterns of measles antibodies in residents of Tahiti and their stability in the absence of re-exposure.** *J. Immunol.* 1962, **88**:725-731.

Vitetta, E.S., Berton, M.S., Burger, C., Kepron, M., Lee, W.T., and Yin, X.-M.: **Memory B and T cells.** *Annu. Rev. Immunol.* 1991, **9**:193-217.

9-22   **Both clonal expansion and clonal differentiation contribute to immunological memory in B cells.**

Jacob, J., Kelsoe, G., Rajewsky, K., and Weiss, U.: **Intraclonal generation of antibody mutants in germinal centres.** *Nature* 1991, **354**:389-392.

Kraal, G., Weissman, I.L., and Butcher, E.C.: **Memory B cells express a phenotype consistent with migratory competence after secondary but not short-term primary immunization.** *Cell. Immunol.* 1988, **115**:78.

Linton, P.J., Lai, L., Lo, D., Thorbecke, G.R., and Klinman, N.R.: **Among naive precursor cell subpopulations only progenitors of memory B cells originate germinal centers.** *Eur. J. Immunol.* 1992, **22**:1293-1297.

Shittek, B. and Rajewsky, K.: **Natural occurrence and origin of somatically mutated memory in mice.** *J. Exper. Med.* 1992, **176**:427.

9-24   **Memory T cells are increased in frequency and have distinct activation requirements and cell-surface proteins distinguishing them from armed effector cells.**

MacKay, C.R.: **Immunological memory.** *Adv. Immunol.* 1993, **53**:217-265.

Michie, C.A., McLean, A., Alcock, C., Beverly, P.C.L.: **Lifespan of human lymphocyte subsets defined by CD45 isoforms.** *Nature* 1992, **360**:264-265.

Novak. T.J., Farber, D., Leitenberg, D., Hong, S., Johnson, P., and Bottomly, K.: **Isoforms of the transmembrane tyrosine phosphatase CD45 differentially affect T-cell recognition.** *Immunity* 1994,**1**:81-92.

9-25   **Retained antigen may play a role in immunological memory.**

Gray, D.: **The dynamics of immunological memory.** *Semin. Immunol.* 1992, **4**:29-34.

Gray, D. and Skarvall, H.: **B-cell memory is shortlived in the absence of antigen.** *Nature* 1988, **336**:70-72.

Gray, D. and Matzinger, P.: **T-cell memory is shortlived in the absence of antigen.** *J. Exper. Med.* 1991, **174**:969-974.

Sprent, J.: **Lifespan of naive, memory and effector lymphocytes.** *Curr. Opin. Immunol.* 1993, **5**:433-438.

Failures of Host Defense Mechanisms

10

In the normal course of an infection, disease is followed by an adaptive immune response that clears the infection and establishes a state of protective immunity. This does not always happen, however, and in this chapter we will examine three examples of the failure of host defense against infection: resistance of the pathogen; inherited failures of defense because of gene defects; and the acquired immune deficiency syndrome (AIDS), a generalized susceptibility to infection which is itself due to the failure of the host to control and eliminate the human immunodeficiency virus (HIV).

The propagation of a pathogen depends upon its ability to replicate in a host and to spread to new hosts. Common pathogens must therefore grow without activating too vigorous an immune response, and conversely, must not kill the host too quickly. The most successful pathogens persist either because they do not elicit a response, or by evading the response once it has occurred.

Over millions of years of co-evolution with their hosts, pathogens have evolved various strategies for avoiding destruction by the immune system, and we have encountered some of them in earlier chapters. In the first part of this chapter, we shall examine these in more detail, and discuss some that have not yet been mentioned. In the second part of the chapter, we turn to the **immunodeficiency diseases**, in which host defense fails. In most of these diseases, a defective gene eliminates one or more components of the immune system, leading to heightened susceptibility to infection with specific classes of pathogen. Immunodeficiency diseases caused by defects in T- or B-lymphocyte development, phagocyte function, and components of the complement system have all been described.

The acquired immune deficiency syndrome, AIDS, is caused by infection with the human immunodeficiency virus, HIV, and causes failure of host defense by inactivating and depleting CD4 T cells. The analysis of these diseases has already made an important contribution to our understanding of host defense mechanisms and in the longer term may help to provide new methods for controlling or preventing infections, including AIDS.

Persistent infection in normal individuals.

Just as vertebrates have developed many different defenses against pathogens, so pathogens have devised elaborate strategies to evade these defenses. Many pathogens use one or more of these strategies to evade the immune system but we shall see that HIV may succeed in defeating the immune response by using several of them in combination.

10-1 | Antigenic variation can allow pathogens to escape from immunity.

One way in which an infectious agent can evade immune surveillance is by altering its antigens; this is particularly important for extracellular pathogens, the principal defense against which is production of antibody to their surface structures. There are three ways in which **antigenic variation** can occur. First, many infectious agents exist in a wide variety of antigenic types. There are, for example, 84 known types of *Streptococcus pneumoniae*, the cause of bacterial pneumonia. Each type differs from the others in the structure of its polysaccharide capsule. The different types are distinguished by serological tests and so are often known as serotypes. Infection with one serotype of such an organism can lead to type-specific immunity, which protects against re-infection with that type but not against a different serotype. Thus, from the point of view of the immune system, each serotype of *S. pneumoniae* represents a distinct organism. The result is that essentially the same pathogen can cause disease many times in the same individual (Fig. 10.1).

Fig. 10.1 Host defense against *Streptococcus pneumoniae* is type-specific. The different strains of *S. pneumoniae* have antigenically distinct capsular polysaccharides. The capsule prevents effective phagocytosis until the bacterium is opsonized by specific antibody and complement, allowing phagocytes to destroy it. Antibody to one type of *S. pneumoniae* does not cross-react with the other types, so an individual immune to one type has no protective immunity to a subsequent infection with a different type. An individual must generate a new immune response each time he or she is infected with a different type of *S. pneumoniae*.

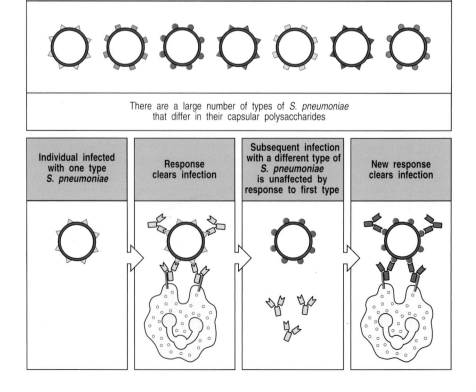

A second, more dynamic mechanism of antigenic variation is seen in the influenza virus. At any one time, a single virus type is responsible for infection throughout the world. The human population gradually develops protective immunity to this virus type, mostly in the form of neutralizing antibody directed against the major surface protein of the influenza virus, the hemagglutinin. Influenza spreads very readily, and the virus might be in danger of running out of potential hosts, if it had not evolved two distinct ways of changing its antigenic type (Fig. 10.2).

The first of these, **antigenic drift**, is caused by point mutations in the genes encoding hemagglutinin and a second surface protein, neuraminidase. Every two to three years, a variant arises with mutations that allow the virus to evade neutralization by antibodies in the population; other mutations affect epitopes that are recognized by T cells, and in particular CD8 T cells, so that cells infected with the mutant virus also escape destruction. Individuals who were previously infected with, and hence immune to, the old variant are thus susceptible to the new variant. This causes an epidemic that is relatively mild, because there is still some cross-reaction with antibodies and T cells produced against the previous variant of the virus, and therefore most of the population have some level of immunity.

Major influenza pandemics with widespread and often fatal disease occur as the result of the second process, which is termed **antigenic shift**. This happens when there is reassortment of the segmented RNA genome of the influenza virus and related viruses in an animal host, leading to major changes in the hemagglutinin protein on the viral surface. The resulting virus is recognized poorly, if at all, by antibodies and T cells directed at the previous variant, so that most people are highly susceptible to the new virus, and severe infection results.

The third mechanism of antigenic variation involves programmed rearrangements in the DNA of the pathogen. The most striking example occurs in African trypanosomes, where changes in the major surface antigen occur repeatedly within a single infected host. Trypanosomes are insect-borne protozoa that replicate in the extracellular tissue spaces of the body and cause sleeping sickness in humans. The trypanosome is coated with a single type of glycoprotein, the variant-specific glycoprotein (VSG), which elicits a potent protective antibody response that rapidly clears most of the parasites. The trypanosome genome, however, contains about 1 000 VSG genes, each with distinct antigenic properties. To escape surveillance by a system capable of generating many distinct antibodies by gene rearrangment, the trypanosome has developed its own system of gene rearrangement that causes a change

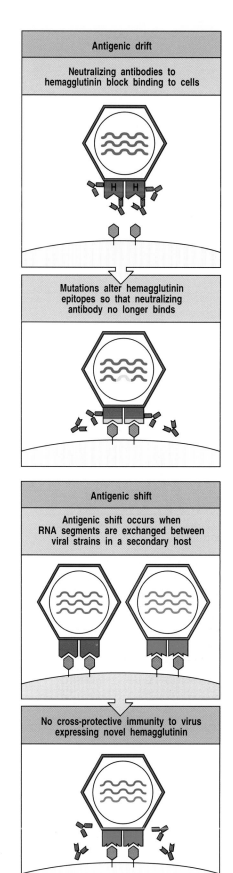

Fig. 10.2 Two types of variation allow repetitive infection with type A influenza virus. Neutralizing antibody that mediates protective immunity is directed at the surface protein hemagglutinin (H), which mediates viral binding to and entry into cells. Antigenic drift (upper two panels) involves the emergence of point mutants that alter the binding sites of protective antibodies on the hemagglutinin. When this happens, the new virus can grow in a host that is immune to the previous strain of virus. However, as T cells and some antibodies can still recognize epitopes that have not been altered, the new variants cause only mild disease in previously infected individuals. Antigenic shift (lower two panels) is a rare event involving reassortment of the segmented RNA viral genome between two influenza viruses, probably in avian hosts. These antigen-shifted viruses have large changes in their hemagglutinin molecule and therefore T cells and antibodies produced in earlier infections are not protective. For this reason, these shifted strains cause severe infection that spreads widely, causing the influenza pandemics that occur every 10–20 years.

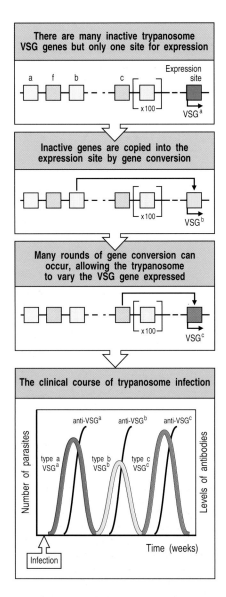

Fig. 10.3 Antigenic variation in trypanosomes allows them to escape immune surveillance. The surface of a trypanosome is covered with a variant-specific glycoprotein (VSG). Each trypanosome has about 1 000 genes encoding different VSGs but only the gene in a specific telomeric expression site is active. Although several genetic mechanisms have been observed for changing the VSG gene expressed, the usual mechanism is gene duplication. Here an inactive gene, which is not at the telomere, is copied and transposed into the telomeric expression site, becoming active. When an individual is first infected, antibodies are raised against the VSG initially expressed by the trypanosome population. A small number of trypanosomes spontaneously switch their VSG gene to a new type, and while the host antibody eliminates the initial variant, the new variant is unaffected. As the new variant grows, the whole sequence of events is repeated.

in which VSG genes are expressed. A few trypanosomes with such changed surface glycoproteins escape the antibodies, and these soon grow and cause a recurrence of disease (Fig. 10.3). Antibodies are then made to the new VSG, and the whole cycle repeats. This chronic cycle of antigen clearance leads to immune complex damage and inflammation, and eventually to neurological damage, finally resulting in coma. This gives the disease, sleeping sickness, its name. These cycles of evasive action make trypanosome infections very difficult for the immune system to defeat and they are a major health problem in Africa.

DNA rearrangements also help to account for the success of two important bacterial pathogens, *Salmonella typhimurium*, a common cause of salmonella food poisoning and *Neisseria gonorrhoeae*, which causes gonorrhea, a major sexually transmitted disease and an increasing public health problem in the USA. *S. typhimurium* regularly changes its surface flagellin protein by inverting a segment of its DNA containing the flagellin promoter so that the gene is turned on or off. *N. gonorrhoeae* has several variable antigens, the most dramatic of which is the pilin protein, which, like the variable surface glycoproteins of the African trypanosome, is encoded by several variant genes only one of which is active at any given time. Silent versions of the gene from time to time replace the active version downstream of the pilin promoter.

10-2   Some viruses persist *in vivo* by ceasing to replicate until immunity wanes.

Viruses usually betray their presence to the immune system once they have entered cells, by directing the synthesis of viral proteins, fragments of which are displayed on the surface MHC molecules of the infected cell where they are detected by T lymphocytes. To replicate, a virus must make viral proteins, and rapidly replicating viruses, which produce acute viral illnesses, are therefore readily detected by T cells, which normally control them. Some viruses, however, can enter a state known as **latency** in which the virus is not transcriptionally active. In the latent state, the virus does not cause disease but, because there are no viral peptides to flag its presence, it cannot be eliminated. Such latent infections can later be reactivated, and this results in recurrent illness.

Herpes viruses often enter latency. Herpes simplex virus, the cause of cold sores, infects epithelia and spreads to sensory neurons serving the area of infection. After an effective immune response controls the epithelial infection, the virus persists in a latent state in the sensory neurons. Factors such as sunlight, bacterial infection, or hormonal changes reactivate the virus, which then travels down the axons of the sensory neuron and re-infects the epithelial tissues (Fig. 10.4). At this point, the immune response again becomes active and controls the local infection by killing the epithelial cells, producing a new sore. This cycle can be repeated many times. There are two reasons why the sensory neuron remains infected: first, the virus is quiescent in the nerve and therefore few viral proteins are produced, generating few virus-derived peptides to present on MHC class I; and second, neurons carry very low levels of MHC class I molecules, which makes it harder for CD8 T cells to recognize infected cells and attack them. This low level of MHC class I expression may be beneficial, as it reduces the risk that neurons, which cannot regenerate, will be attacked inappropriately by CD8 T cells. It also makes neurons unusually vulnerable to persistent infections. Similarly, herpes zoster (or varicella zoster), which causes chickenpox, is latent in one or a few dorsal root ganglia after the acute illness is over. Stress or immunosuppression can reactivate the virus, which spreads down the nerve and infects the skin. This re-infection causes the reappearance of the classic rash of varicella in the area of skin served by the infected dorsal root, a disease commonly called shingles. Herpes simplex reactivation is frequent but herpes zoster usually reactivates only once in a lifetime in an immunocompetent host.

The Epstein-Barr virus (EBV), yet another herpes virus, causes infectious mononucleosis (glandular fever), an acute infection of B lymphocytes. EBV infects B cells by binding to CR2, a component of the B cell CD19 co-receptor complex, and causes most of the infected cells to proliferate, leading to the excess of mononuclear white cells in the blood that gives the disease its name. The infection is controlled eventually by specific CD8 T cells, which kill the infected proliferating B cells. A fraction of B lymphocytes is latently infected, however, and EBV remains quiescent in these cells. They can be detected by taking B cells from individuals who have apparently cleared their EBV infection and placing them in tissue culture: the latently infected cells have retained the EBV genome and will transform into continuously growing cell lines. *In vivo*, EBV-infected B cells sometimes undergo malignant transformation, giving rise to a B-cell lymphoma called Burkitt's lymphoma (see Section 5-18). This is a rare event and it seems likely that a crucial part of this process is a failure of T-cell surveillance. Recent evidence suggests that EBV may also infect dendritic cells and transform them into the malignant cell in Hodgkin's disease (see Section 6-21).

10-3 | Some pathogens resist destruction by host defense mechanisms or exploit them for their own purposes.

Some pathogens induce a normal immune response but have evolved specialized mechanisms for resisting its effects. For instance, some bacteria that are engulfed in the normal way by macrophages have evolved ways of avoiding destruction by these phagocytes; indeed they use macrophages as their primary host. *Mycobacterium tuberculosis*, for example, is taken up by macrophages but prevents the fusion of the phagosome with the lysosome, protecting itself from the bacteriocidal actions of the lysosomal contents. Other microorganisms, such as *Listeria monocytogenes*, escape from the phagosome into the cytoplasm of the macrophage, where they can multiply readily, and then spread to adjacent cells in tissues without emerging from the cell into the extracellular medium, and hence resist antibody-mediated killing. However, cells infected with *L. monocytogenes* are susceptible to killing by cytotoxic T cells.

The protozoan parasite *Toxoplasma gondii* can apparently generate its own vesicle that isolates it from the rest of the cell because it does not fuse with any cellular vesicle. This may actually enable *T. gondii* to

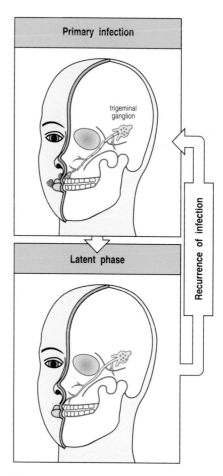

Fig. 10.4 Persistence and reactivation of herpes simplex virus infection. The initial infection in the skin is cleared by an effective immune response, but residual infection persists in sensory neurons such as those of the trigeminal ganglion, whose axons innervate the lips. When the virus is reactivated, usually by some environmental stress and/or alteration in immune status, the skin in the area served by the nerve is re-infected and a new cold sore results. This process can be repeated many times.

avoid making peptides derived from its proteins accessible for loading onto MHC molecules, and thereby to remain invisible to the immune system.

Two prominent spirochetal infections, **Lyme disease** and syphilis, avoid elimination by antibodies through less well understood mechanisms, and establish a persistent and extremely damaging infection in tissues. Lyme disease is caused by the spirochete *Borrelia burgdorferi*, while syphilis is caused by *Treponema pallidum*. Syphilis is the more widespread and much the better understood of the two diseases, and the bacterium is believed to avoid recognition by antibodies by coating its surface with host molecules until it has invaded the tissues, where it is less easily reached by antibodies.

Finally, many viruses have evolved mechanisms to subvert various arms of the immune system. These range from capturing cellular genes for cytokines or cytokine receptors, to synthesizing complement regulatory molecules or inhibition of MHC class I synthesis or assembly. This area is one of the most rapidly expanding areas in the field of host–pathogen relationships.

10-4 | Immunosuppression or inappropriate immune responses can contribute to persistent disease.

Many pathogens suppress immune responses in general. For example, staphylococcal bacteria produce toxins, such as the **staphylococcal enterotoxins** and **toxic shock syndrome toxin-1**, that act as **superantigens**. Superantigens are proteins that bind the antigen receptor of very large numbers of T cells (see Section 4-25), stimulating them to produce cytokines that cause significant suppression of all immune responses. The details of this suppression are not understood. The stimulated T cells proliferate and then disappear rapidly, apparently because they undergo apoptosis, leaving a generalized suppression together with peripheral deletion of many T cells.

Many other pathogens cause mild or transient immunosuppression during acute infection. These forms of suppressed immunity are poorly understood but important, as they often make the host susceptible to secondary infections by common environmental organisms. A crucially important example of immune depression follows trauma, burns, or even major surgery. The burned patient has a clearly diminished capability to respond to infection, and generalized infection is a common cause of death in these patients. The reasons for this are not fully understood.

The most extreme case of immune suppression caused by a pathogen is infection with HIV. The ultimate cause of death in AIDS is usually infection with an **opportunistic pathogen**, a term used to describe a microorganism that is present in the environment but does not usually cause disease because it is well controlled by the normal immune response. HIV infection leads to gradual loss of immune competence, allowing infection with organisms that are not normally pathogenic.

Leprosy, which we discussed in Section 7-12, is a more complex case, in which the causal bacterium, *Mycobacterium leprae*, may suppress either cell-mediated immunity or humoral immunity, leading to two major forms of the disease: lepromatous and tuberculoid leprosy. In **lepromatous leprosy**, cell-mediated immunity is profoundly depressed, *M. leprae* are present in great profusion, and immune responses to many antigens are suppressed, leading to a phenotypic state in such patients called **anergy**, here meaning the absence of delayed-type hypersensitivity to a wide range of antigens unrelated to *M. leprae*. In

tuberculoid leprosy, by contrast, there is potent cell-mediated immunity with macrophage activation, which controls but does not eradicate infection. Few viable microorganisms are found in tissues, the patients usually survive, and most of the symptoms and pathology are caused by the inflammatory response to these persistent microorganisms. The difference between the two forms of disease may lie in a difference in the ratio of inflammatory CD4 T cells (T$_H$1) to helper CD4 T cells (T$_H$2) (Fig. 10.5), although it is not known why these differences arise. We shall discuss this further in Chapter 12.

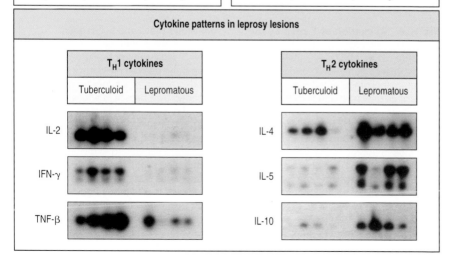

Leprosy — infection with *Mycobacterium leprae* shows a number of clinical forms	
There are two polar forms, tuberculoid and lepromatous leprosy, but several intermediate forms also exist	
Tuberculoid leprosy	**Lepromatous leprosy**
Organisms present at low to undetectable levels	Organisms show florid growth in macrophages
Low infectivity	High infectivity
Granulomas and local inflammation. Peripheral nerve damage	Disseminated infection. Bone, cartilage, and diffuse nerve damage
Normal serum immunoglobulin levels	Hypergammaglobulinemia
Normal T-cell responsiveness. Specific response to *M. leprae* antigens	Low or absent T-cell responsiveness. No response to *M. leprae* antigens

Cytokine patterns in leprosy lesions

T$_H$1 cytokines — Tuberculoid, Lepromatous: IL-2, IFN-γ, TNF-β

T$_H$2 cytokines — Tuberculoid, Lepromatous: IL-4, IL-5, IL-10

Fig. 10.5   T-cell and macrophage responses to *Mycobacterium leprae* are sharply different in the two polar forms of leprosy. Infection with *M. leprae*, which stain red in the photographs, can lead to two very different forms of disease. In tuberculoid leprosy, growth of the organism is well controlled by T$_H$1-like cells that activate infected macrophages. The tuberculoid lesion contains granulomas and is inflamed but the inflammation is local and causes only local effects, such as peripheral nerve damage. In lepromatous leprosy, infection is widely disseminated and the bacilli grow uncontrolled in macrophages; in the late stages of disease there is major damage to connective tissues and to the peripheral nervous system. There are several intermediate stages between these two polar forms. As shown by analysis of mRNA isolated from lesions of three patients with lepromatous leprosy, and three patients with tuberculoid leprosy (photographs of dot blots), the cytokine patterns in the two forms of the disease are sharply different. Cytokines typically produced by T$_H$2 cells (helper T cells) (IL-4, IL-5, and IL-10) dominate in the lepromatous form, while cytokines produced by T$_H$1 cells (inflammatory T cells) (IL-2, interferon-γ (IFN-γ), and tumor necrosis factor-β (TNF-β)) dominate in the tuberculoid form. It appears therefore that T$_H$1-like cells predominate in tuberculoid leprosy, and T$_H$2-like cells in lepromatous leprosy. Interferon-γ would be expected to activate macrophages, enhancing killing of *M. leprae*, whereas IL-4 can actually inhibit macrophage activation. High levels of IL-4 would also explain the hypergammaglobulinemia observed in lepromatous leprosy. The determining factors in the initial induction of T$_H$1- or T$_H$2-like cells are not known, and the mechanism for the anergy or generalized loss of effective cell-mediated immunity in lepromatous leprosy is also not understood. Photographs courtesy of G Kaplan; cytokine patterns courtesy of R Modlin.

Tuberculoid leprosy is just one example of an infection in which the pathology is largely caused by the immune response. This is true to some degree in most infections. For example, the fever that accompanies a bacterial infection is caused by the release of cytokines released by macrophages. In some cases, the immune response causes most or all of the pathology; immunosuppressed animals infected with the same organism are completely healthy. The classic example of this is the infection of mice with **lymphocytic choriomeningitis virus (LCMV)**. This virus can cause a chronic infection with no obvious symptoms when mice are infected neonatally, so that the immature immune system develops tolerance to the virus, or when the animal is prevented from mounting a T-cell mediated immune response by immunosuppression by neonatal thymectomy. Replacing the missing effector T cells causes a severe inflammatory response in the central nervous system, which leads to death.

Another example of a pathogenic immune response is the response to the eggs of the schistosome. Schistosomes are parasitic worms that lay eggs in the hepatic portal vein. Some of the eggs reach the intestine and are shed in the feces, spreading the infection; others lodge in the portal circulation of the liver, where they elicit a potent immune response leading to chronic inflammation, hepatic fibrosis, and eventually to liver failure. This process reflects the excessive activation of helper T cells, and can be modulated by inflammatory T cells, interferon-γ (IFN-γ), or CD8 T cells, which may act by producing IFN-γ.

In the case of the **mouse mammary tumor virus (MMTV)**, which causes mammary tumors in mice, the immune response is required for the infective cycle of the pathogen. MMTV is transferred from the mother's mammary gland to her pups in milk. The virus then enters the B lymphocytes of the new host where it must replicate in order to be transported in turn to the mammary epithelium and continue its life cycle. As it is a retrovirus, however, MMTV can only replicate in dividing cells. The virus ensures that infected B cells will proliferate by causing them to express on their surface a superantigen encoded within the MMTV genome. This superantigen enables the B cells to bypass the requirement for specific antigen and stimulate large numbers of CD4 T cells with the appropriate T-cell receptor Vβ domain (see Section 4-25), causing them to produce cytokines and express CD40 ligand, which in turn stimulate the B cells to divide (Fig. 10.6). The mouse

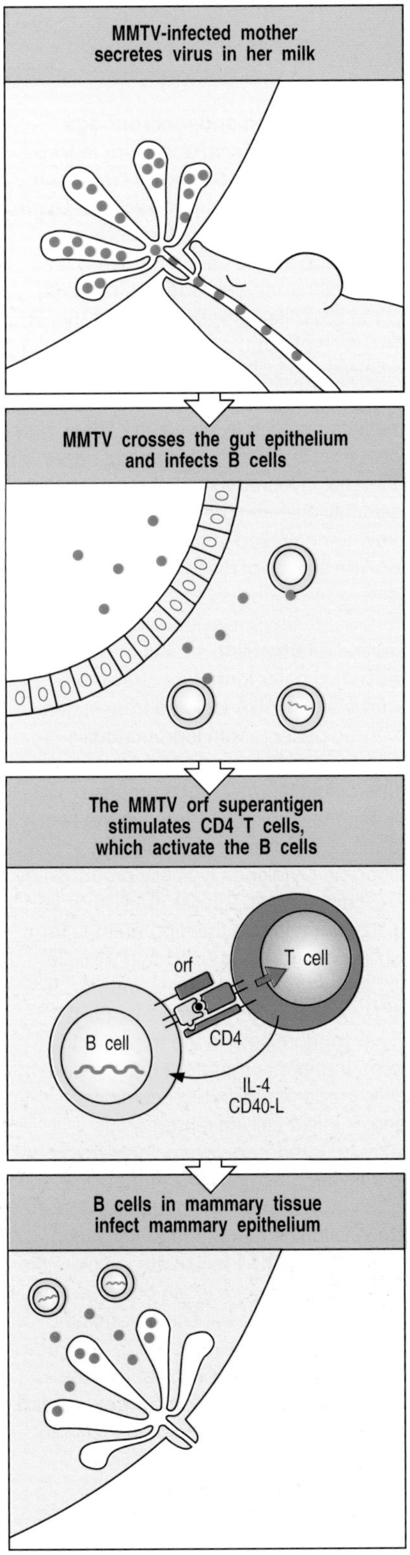

MMTV-infected mother secretes virus in her milk

MMTV crosses the gut epithelium and infects B cells

The MMTV orf superantigen stimulates CD4 T cells, which activate the B cells

B cells in mammary tissue infect mammary epithelium

Fig. 10.6 Activation of T cells by the MMTV superantigen is crucial for the virus life cycle. MMTV is transferred from mother to pup in milk, and crosses the gut epithelium to reach the lymphoid tissue of its new host and infect B lymphocytes. The superantigen encoded by MMTV, called orf, is expressed on the surface of the B cell and binds to appropriate T-cell receptor Vβ domains on CD4 T cells. The superantigen also has binding sites for MHC class II molecules, so that a complex between superantigen, MHC, T-cell receptor and CD4 is formed, activating the T cell. The T cell in turn activates the B cell to divide, allowing viral replication within the B cell and subsequent infection of the mammary epithelium. If the T cells with appropriate Vβ domains have been deleted previously because of the expression of a superantigen encoded by a defective endogenous MMTV genome (see Section 6-18), the infected B cell cannot activate any of the remaining T cells and therefore no B cells are stimulated to divide, blocking MMTV replication. Many different defective endogenous MMTV genomes are expressed in wild mouse populations, each deleting a characteristic Vβ subset. Thus, individual mice are resistant to different MMTV strains.

host can protect itself against the virus by deleting the particular subset of T cells carrying the V_β domain recognized by the viral superantigen.

There are several different strains of MMTV whose superantigens bind to different V_β domains. As we learned in Section 6-18, most mouse strains have MMTV genomes stably integrated into their DNA. These endogenous retroviruses have lost certain essential genes and are unable to produce virions but they have retained the genes encoding their superantigens, which are expressed on the cells of the host. Since these superantigens can induce clonal deletion in the thymus, the T cells carrying appropriate V_β domains are lost.

Why might it be beneficial to the mouse to lose a section of its repertoire? It has been proposed that removing the T cells that can be stimulated by a given superantigen might prevent infection with intact mouse mammary tumor viruses encoding the same superantigen. To test this, mice containing a transgenic MMTV genome were constructed. These mice express the MMTV superantigen and therefore delete T cells expressing V_β domains that bind to it. Since there are no T cells left that can be stimulated by the superantigen encoded by this strain of MMTV, B cells infected with the intact virus cannot be activated and this particular strain of MMTV, therefore, cannot be transmitted in these transgenic mice. Thus, in this example, the ability of a pathogen to elicit a response from the immune system is essential to its ability to cause disease. Mice containing different endogenous MMTV genomes delete different parts of their T-cell receptor repertoire, reducing the risk that whole mouse populations will be susceptible to a given mammary tumor virus. No human diseases dependent on such mechanisms have yet been described.

Summary.

Infectious agents can cause persistent disease by avoiding normal host defense mechanisms or by subverting them to promote their own replication. There are many different ways to evade or subvert the immune response. Antigenic variation, latency, resistance to immune effector mechanisms, and suppression of the immune response all contribute to persistent and medically important infections. In some cases, the immune response is part of the problem; some pathogens use immune activation to spread infection, others would not cause disease if it were not for the immune response. Each of these mechanisms teaches us something about the nature of the immune response and its weaknesses, and each requires a different medical approach to prevent or to treat persistent infection.

Inherited immunodeficiency diseases.

Immunodeficiency diseases occur when one or more components of the immune system is defective. The commonest cause of immune deficiency worldwide is malnutrition; but in developed countries, most immunodeficiency diseases are inherited, and these are usually seen in the clinic as recurrent or overwhelming infection in very young children. Less commonly acquired immunodeficiencies with causes other than malnutrition can manifest later in life. While the pathogenesis of many of these acquired disorders has remained obscure, some are caused by known agents such as drugs or irradiation that damage lymphocytes, or infection with HIV. By examining which infections accompany a particular inherited or acquired immunodeficiency, we can see the role of each component of the immune system in the response to particular infectious agents. The inherited immunodeficiency diseases also reveal the relationships between the various cellular components of the immune system and their place in the developmental sequence of T and B lymphocytes. Finally, these diseases can lead us to the defective gene, often revealing new information about the molecular basis of immune processes and providing the necessary information for diagnosis, genetic counseling and gene therapy.

10-6   Inherited immunodeficiency diseases are caused by recessive gene defects.

Before the advent of antibiotic therapy, it is likely that most individuals with inherited immune defects died in infancy or early childhood because of their susceptibility to particular classes of pathogens (Fig. 10.7). Such deaths would not have been easy to identify, since many normal infants also died of infection. Thus, the first immunodeficiency disease was not described until 1952; since that time many inherited immunodeficiency diseases have been identified. Most of the gene defects that cause these inherited immunodeficiencies are recessive, and several are caused by mutations of genes on the X chromosome. Recessive defects cause disease only when both chromosomes are defective. As males have only one X chromosome, however, all males who inherit an X chromosome carrying a defective gene will manifest disease, whereas female carriers, having two X chromosomes, are perfectly healthy. Immunodeficiency diseases that affect many steps in B- and T-lymphocyte development have been described, as have defects in surface molecules that are important for T- or B-cell function. Defects in phagocytic cells, in cytokines, in cytokine receptors, and in molecules that mediate effector responses also occur (see Fig. 10.7). Individual examples of these diseases will be described in later sections.

Most of the described immunodeficiency diseases involve the adaptive immune systems, but neutropenia and other deficiencies in innate immunity exist. It is possible that more such deficiencies will be identified as we learn more about the innate immune system and its function.

More recently, the use of gene knock-out techniques in mice has allowed the creation of many immunodeficient states that are rapidly adding to our knowledge. Nevertheless, human immunodeficiency disease is still the best source of insight into host defense in humans.

10-7   The main effect of low levels of antibody is an inability to clear extracellular bacteria.

Pyogenic or pus-forming bacteria have polysaccharide capsules that make them resistant to phagocytosis. Normal individuals can clear infections by such bacteria because antibody and complement opsonize the bacteria, making it possible for phagocytes to ingest and destroy them. The principal effect of deficiencies in antibody production is therefore failure to control this class of bacterial infections, although susceptibility to some viral infections is also increased because of the importance of antibodies in neutralizing infectious virus (see Chapter 8).

The first description of an immunodeficiency disease was Ogden C. Bruton's account in 1952 of the failure of a male child to produce antibody. As this defect is inherited in an X-linked fashion and is detected using electrophoresis by the absence of immunoglobulin in the serum (see Section 2-9), it was called **X-linked agammaglobulinemia (XLA)**.

Name of deficiency syndrome	Specific abnormality	Immune defect	Susceptibility
Severe combined immune deficiency	ADA deficiency	No T or B cells	General
	PNP deficiency	No T or B cells	General
	X-linked *scid*, γ_c chain deficiency	No T cells	General
	Autosomal *scid* DNA repair defect	No T or B cells	General
DiGeorge syndrome	Thymic aplasia	Variable numbers of T and B cells	General
MHC class II deficiency	Lack of expression of MHC class II	No CD4 T cells	General
MHC class I deficiency	TAP mutations	No CD8 T cells	Viruses
Wiskott-Aldrich syndrome	X-linked; defective WASP gene	Defective polysaccharide antibody responses	Encapsulated extracellular bacteria
Common variable immunodeficiency	Unknown; MHC-linked	Defective antibody production	Extracellular bacteria
X-linked agamma-globulinemia	Loss of Btk tyrosine kinase	No B cells	Extracellular bacteria, viruses
X-linked hyper IgM syndrome	Defective CD40 ligand	No isotype switching	Extracellular bacteria
Selective IgA and/or IgG deficiency	Unknown; MHC-linked	No IgA synthesis	Respiratory infections
Phagocyte deficiencies	Many different	Loss of phagocyte function	Extracellular bacteria
Complement deficiencies	Many different	Loss of specific complement components	Extracellular bacteria especially *Neisseria* spp.
Natural killer cell defect	Unknown	Loss of NK function	Herpes viruses
X-linked lympho-proliferative syndrome	Unknown; X-linked	EBV-triggered immunodeficiency	EBV
Ataxia telangiectasia	Gene with PI-3 kinase homology	T cells reduced	Respiratory infections
Autoimmune lympho-proliferative disease	Mutant *Fas*	Failure of T- and B-cell apoptosis	Autoimmune disorders

Fig. 10.7 Human immunodeficiency syndromes. The specific gene defect, the consequence for the immune system, and the resulting disease susceptibilities are listed for some common human immunodeficiency syndromes. ADA, adenosine deaminase; PNP, purine nucleotide phosphorylase; TAP, transporters associated with antigen processing; WASP, Wiskott-Aldrich syndrome protein; EBV, Epstein-Barr virus.

Since then, many more diseases of antibody production have been described, most of them the consequence of failures in the development or activation of B lymphocytes.

The defective gene in XLA is now known to encode a protein tyrosine kinase known as Btk (Bruton's tyrosine kinase). This protein is expressed in polymorphonuclear neutrophilic leukocytes as well as in B cells, although only B cells are defective in these patients, in whom B-cell maturation halts at the pre-B-cell stage. Thus it is likely that Btk is required to couple the pre-B-cell receptor (which consists of heavy chains, surrogate light chains, and Igα and Igβ) to nuclear events that lead to pre-B cell growth and differentiation. A homologous kinase, called Itk, has been found in T cells but its function is unknown. Defects in Btk are analogous to defects in Lck in T-cell development (see Section 6-8). In the mouse, Lck deficiency leads to the arrest of thymocyte development at the double-negative stage, after T-cell receptor β chain gene rearrangement and cell-surface expression but before the rearrangement of the α-chain genes. Thus, there may be a cascade of tyrosine kinases, involving Lck and Itk in double-negative thymocytes, and Blk and Btk in pre-B cells, that is important for lymphocyte development. In both of these deficiencies, some B or T cells mature despite the defect in the signaling molecule, suggesting that such signals promote rearrangement of light-chain or α-chain genes, respectively, but are not absolutely required.

Since the gene responsible for XLA is found on the X chromosome, it is possible to identify female carriers by analyzing X-chromosome inactivation in their B cells. During development, female cells randomly inactivate one of their two X chromosomes. Since the product of a normal *btk* gene is required for normal B-lymphocyte development, only cells in which the X chromosome carrying the normal allele of *btk* is active can develop into mature B cells (with a very few exceptions: see above). Thus, in female carriers of mutant *btk* genes, almost all B cells have the

Fig. 10.8 The product of the *btk* gene is important for B-cell development. In X-linked agammaglobulinemia (XLA), a protein tyrosine kinase called Btk, encoded on the X chromosome, is defective. In normal individuals, B-cell development proceeds through a stage in which the pre-B-cell receptor consisting of μ:λ5:Vpre-B transduces a signal via Btk, triggering further B-cell development. In males with XLA, no signal can be transduced and, although the pre-B-cell receptor is expressed, the B cells develop no further. In female mammals, including humans, one of the two X chromosomes in each cell is permanently inactivated early in development. Since the choice of which chromosome to inactivate is random, half of the pre-B cells in a carrier female express a wild-type *btk*, while half express the defective gene. None of the pre-B cells that express *btk* from the defective chromosome can develop into mature B cells. Therefore, in the carrier, mature B cells always have the non-defective X chromosome active. This is in sharp contrast to all other cell types, which express the non-defective chromosome in only half of the population. Non-random X chromosome inactivation in a particular cell lineage is a clear indication that the product of the X-linked gene is required for the development of cells of that lineage. It is also sometimes possible to identify the stage at which the gene product is required, by detecting the point in development at which X-chromosome inactivation develops bias. Using this kind of analysis, one can identify carriers of traits like XLA without needing to know the nature of the gene.

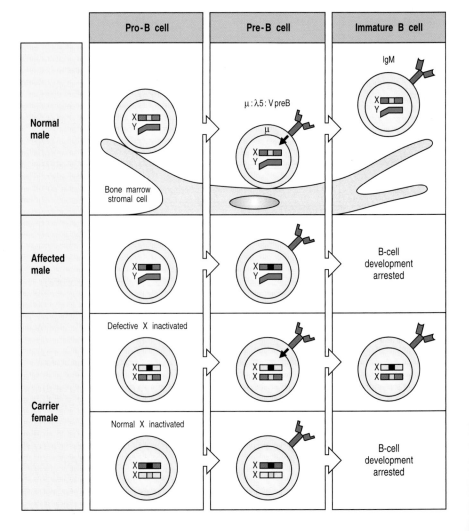

normal X chromosome as the active X. By contrast, the active X chromosomes in the T cells and macrophages of carriers are equally distributed between normal and *btk* mutant. This fact allowed female carriers of XLA to be identified even before the nature of *btk* was known. Non-random X inactivation only in B cells also demonstrates conclusively that the *btk* gene is required for normal B-cell development but not for the development of other cell types, and that Btk must act within B cells rather than on stromal cells or other cells required for B-cell development (Fig. 10.8).

The commonest humoral immune defect is the transient deficiency in immunoglobulin production that occurs in the first 6–12 months of life. The newborn infant has initial antibody levels comparable to those of the mother, thanks to the transplacental transport of maternal IgG (see Chapter 8). As the transferred IgG is catabolized, antibody levels gradually decrease until the infant begins to produce useful amounts of its own IgG at about six months of age (Fig. 10.9). Thus, IgG levels are quite low between the ages of three months and one year and active IgG antibody responses are poor. In some infants, this can lead to a period of heightened susceptibility to infection. This is especially true for premature babies, who begin with lower levels of maternal IgG and also reach immune competence longer after birth.

The most common inherited form of immunoglobulin deficiency is selective IgA deficiency, which is seen in about one person in 800. Although no obvious disease susceptibility is associated with selective IgA defects, they are commoner in people with chronic lung disease than in the general population. This suggests that lack of IgA may result in a predisposition to lung infections with various pathogens and is consistent with the role of IgA in defense at the body's surfaces. The genetic basis of this defect is unknown but some data suggest that a gene of unidentified function mapping in the class III region of the MHC may be involved. A related syndrome called common variable immunodeficiency, in which there is generally a deficiency in IgG and IgA, also maps to the class III region of the MHC.

Finally, some rare families have selective defects in the ability to produce one or more immunoglobulin isotypes owing to deletions of heavy-chain constant-region genes; these deletions are generally seen only in heterozygotes as homozygotes are rare. There have also been reports of two families that lack κ chain genes and make all of their immunoglobulin using λ chains. These deficiencies are not generally associated with any increased susceptibility to infection.

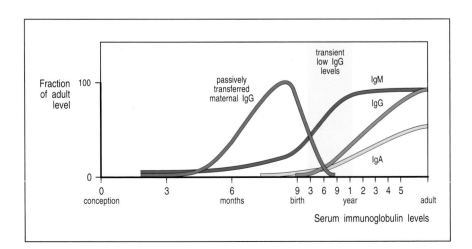

Fig. 10.9 Immunoglobulin levels in newborn infants fall to low levels around six months of age. Newborn babies have high levels of IgG, transported across the placenta from the mother during gestation. After birth, production of IgM starts almost immediately; production of IgG, however, does not begin for about six months, during which time the total level of IgG falls as the maternally acquired IgG is catabolized. Thus IgG levels are low from about the age of three months to one year, which may lead to susceptibility to disease. IgG levels fall further for longer in premature infants, resulting in a higher rate of infection because, at the time of birth, the level of transferred maternal IgG is lower. Furthermore, the premature infant's immune system is less developed so that antibody production by the infant occurs at a later time after birth.

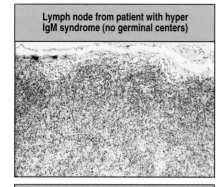

Lymph node from patient with hyper IgM syndrome (no germinal centers)

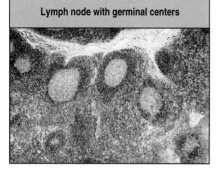

Lymph node with germinal centers

Fig. 10.10 Patients with X-linked hyper IgM syndrome are unable to activate their B cells fully. Lymphoid tissues in patients with hyper IgM syndrome are devoid of germinal centers (top panel), in comparison with a normal lymph node (bottom panel). B-cell activation by T cells is required both for isotype switching and for the formation of germinal centers, where extensive B-cell proliferation takes place. Patients with hyper IgM syndrome have a mutation in the CD40 ligand gene, which lies on the X chromosome, and thus their T cells cannot fully activate the B cells. Only weak IgM responses are made to T-cell dependent antigens and serum immunoglobulin is predominantly IgM. Photographs courtesy of R Geha and A Perez-Atayde.

Low levels of antibody production lead to a relatively defined susceptibility to infection. People with pure B-cell defects resist many pathogens successfully. They cannot control infection with extracellular bacteria but these infections can be suppressed with antibiotics and periodic infusions with human immunoglobulin collected from a large pool of donors. Since there are antibodies to most pathogens in the immunoglobulin pool, it serves as a fairly successful shield against infection.

| 10-8 | **T-cell defects can result in low antibody levels.** |

Patients with **X-linked hyper IgM syndrome** have normal B- and T-cell development and high serum levels of IgM but make only limited IgM antibody responses against T-cell dependent antigens and produce immunoglobulin isotypes other than IgM and IgD only in trace amounts. This makes them susceptible to infection with extracellular bacteria and certain opportunistic organisms such as *Pneumocystis carinii*. The defect is in the CD40 ligand on activated T cells, which cannot engage CD40; the B cells themselves are normal. We learned in Chapter 8 that CD40 ligand plays a critical role in the T-cell dependent activation of B-cell proliferation, and these patients show that CD40 ligand is also essential for induction of the isotype switch and the formation of germinal centers (Fig. 10.10). Moreover, such individuals often have defects in cell-mediated immunity, presumably because CD40 ligand plays an important role in macrophage or T-cell activation.

In XLA, the hunt for the cause of the disease led to a previously unidentified gene product. In the case of X-linked hyper IgM syndrome, the gene for CD40 ligand was cloned independently and only then identified as the defective gene in this disorder. Thus, inherited immunodeficiencies can either lead us to new genes or help us to determine the roles of known genes in normal immune system function.

| 10-9 | **Defects in complement components cause defective humoral immune function and persistence of immune complexes.** |

Not surprisingly, the spectrum of immune defects caused by complement deficiencies overlaps substantially with that seen in patients with deficiencies in antibody production. Defects in the early components of the alternative complement pathway, for example, are associated with pyogenic infections, especially with *Neisseria* spp., the cause of meningitis and gonorrhea (Fig. 10.11). Defects in the membrane attack components of complement (C5–C8) have more limited effects and result mainly in susceptibility to *Neisseria* spp., indicating that the membrane-attack complex is particularly important in immunity to these pathogens. Interestingly, patients with C9 deficiencies appear to be normal, perhaps because the C5–C8 complex has some level of lytic activity.

The early components of the classical complement pathway are particularly critical for the elimination of immune complexes, which can cause significant pathology in autoimmune diseases such as **systemic lupus erythematosus** (see Chapter 11) and, occasionally, in persistent infections. As we learned in Chapter 8, complement components attached to soluble immune complexes allow them to be transported, ingested, and degraded by cells bearing complement receptors. When this mechanism is inoperative, immune complexes are deposited in the tissues. Accumulating immune complexes activate phagocytes, causing inflammation and local tissue damage.

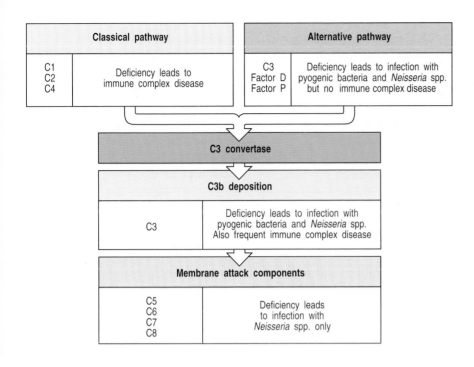

Fig. 10.11 Defects in complement components are associated with susceptibility to certain infections as well as accumulation of immune complexes. Defects in the early components of the alternative pathway lead to susceptibility to extracellular pathogens, and defects in the early components of the classical pathway affect removal of immune complexes via the complement receptor CR1, leading to immune complex disease. Finally, defects in the membrane attack components are associated only with susceptibility to different strains of *Neisseria*, the causative agents of meningitis and gonorrhea, implying that the effector pathway is chiefly important in defense against these organisms.

Deficiencies in control proteins that regulate complement activation can cause either immunodeficiency or autoimmune-like disease. People defective in properdin, which enhances the activity of the alternative pathway, have a heightened susceptibility to *Neisseria* spp. By contrast, patients lacking decay-accelerating factor and CD59, which protect host cell surfaces from alternative pathway activation, destroy their own red blood cells. This results in the disease paroxysmal nocturnal hemoglobinuria, as we learned in Chapter 8. More dramatically, patients with C1-inhibitor defects fail to control the activation of the classical pathway of complement activation, and the uncontrolled cleavage of C2 allows the generation of a vasoactive fragment of C2a, causing fluid accumulation in the tissues and epiglottal swelling that may lead to suffocation. This syndrome is called **hereditary angioneurotic edema**.

10-10   Phagocytic cell defects permit widespread bacterial infections.

The leukocyte integrins CD11a/CD18 (LFA-1), CD11b/CD18 (MAC-1/CR3), and CD11c/CD18 (CR4/gp150,95) are important for phagocytic cell adhesion, migration across blood vessel walls, and ingestion of bacteria opsonized with complement fragments. If these integrins are defective, phagocytes cannot get to sites of infection to ingest and destroy pathogens. Deficiencies have been identified in the leukocyte integrin common β_2 subunit — CD18 — and result in infections that are resistant to antibiotic treatment and persist despite an apparently effective cellular and humoral adaptive immune response.

Most of the other known defects in phagocytic cells affect their ability to kill intracellular and/or ingested extracellular bacteria (Fig. 10.12). In **chronic granulomatous disease**, phagocytes cannot produce the superoxide radical and their antibacterial activity is thereby seriously impaired. Several different genetic defects, affecting any one of the four constituent proteins of the NADPH oxidase system, can cause this. Patients with this disease have chronic bacterial infections, which in some cases lead to the formation of granulomas. Deficiencies in the enzymes glucose-6-phosphate dehydrogenase and myeloperoxidase also impair

Fig. 10.12 Defects in phagocytic cells are associated with persistence of bacterial infection. Defects in the leukocyte integrins with a common β subunit (CD18) prevent phagocytic cell adhesion and migration to sites of infection. The respiratory burst is defective in chronic granulomatous disease, glucose-6-phosphate dehydrogenase (G6-PD) deficiency and myeloperoxidase deficiency. In chronic granulomatous disease, infections persist because macrophage activation is defective, leading to chronic stimulation of CD4 T cells and hence to granulomas. Vesicle fusion in phagocytes is defective in Chediak-Higashi syndrome. These diseases illustrate the critical role of phagocytes in removing and killing pathogenic bacteria.

Type of defect / name of syndrome	Associated infectious or other diseases
Leukocyte adhesion (CD18) deficiency	Widespread pyogenic bacterial infections
Chronic granulomatous disease	Intra- and extracellular infection, granulomas
G6-PD deficiency	Defective respiratory burst, chronic infection
Myeloperoxidase deficiency	Defective intracellular killing, chronic infection
Chediak-Higashi syndrome	Intra- and extracellular infection, granulomas

intracellular killing and lead to a similar, although less severe, phenotype. Finally, in **Chediak-Higashi syndrome**, an unknown defect causes a failure to fuse lysosomes properly with phagosomes; the cells in these patients have enlarged granules and impaired intracellular killing.

10-11 Defects in T-cell function result in severe combined immunodeficiencies.

Although patients with B-cell defects can deal with most pathogens adequately, patients with defects in T-cell development are highly susceptible to a broad range of infectious agents. This demonstrates the central role of T cells in the adaptive immune response to virtually all antigens. As such patients make neither specific T-cell dependent antibody responses nor cell-mediated immune responses, and thus cannot develop protective immunity, such defects are called **severe combined immune deficiency (SCID)**.

There are several different defects that lead to the SCID phenotype. In X-linked severe combined immune deficiency, T cells fail to develop because of a mutation in the common γ chain of several cytokine receptors, including those for the interleukins IL-2, IL-4, IL-7, IL-13, and IL-15. We will examine this defect further in Section 10-12. Two defects in enzymes involved in purine degradation, **adenosine deaminase (ADA) deficiency** and **purine nucleotide phosphorylase (PNP) deficiency**, also give rise to T-cell deficiencies and a SCID phenotype. Both defects result in an accumulation of nucleotide metabolites that are particularly toxic to developing T cells. B cells are also somewhat compromised in these patients.

Recently, the molecular basis of **Wiskott-Aldrich syndrome (WAS)**, a disease that affects not only B and T lymphocytes but also platelets, has begun to emerge. It is caused by a defective gene on the X chromosome, encoding a protein called WAS protein (WASP). This protein is proline-rich, and has several features indicating that it may be a transcription factor. It is expressed in thymus, spleen, and certain tumors of hematopoietic origin. It is likely to be a key regulator of lymphocyte and platelet development and function.

One class of SCID individuals lack expression of all MHC class II gene products on their cells. This condition is also referred to as the **bare lymphocyte syndrome**. As the thymus also lacks MHC class II molecules, CD4 T cells cannot be positively selected and therefore few develop. The antigen-presenting cells in these individuals also lack MHC class II molecules, and so the few CD4 T cells that do develop cannot be stimulated by antigen. In these patients, MHC class I expression is normal and CD8 T cells develop normally. These patients suffer severe combined immunodeficiency, illustrating the central importance of CD4 T cells in adaptive immunity to most pathogens. The syndrome is caused by mutations in one of several different genes that regulate MHC class II gene expression rather than in the MHC genes themselves. At least four complementing gene defects have been defined in patients who fail to express MHC class II molecules, which implies that at least four different genes are required for normal MHC class II gene expression. One of these, named the class II transactivator, or CIITA, is known to be responsible for some cases, while a protein that binds to the MHC class II promoters, called RFX, is defective in others. An understanding of the other genes that cause this defect is still being sought.

A family showing almost complete absence of cell-surface MHC class I molecules has been described. These patients have normal levels of mRNA encoding MHC class I molecules and normal levels of production of MHC class I proteins. The defect was shown to be similar to that of the TAP mutant cells we learned about in Section 4-6, indeed affected members of this family had mutations in a TAP gene. These people are immunodeficient, owing to a lack of CD8 T cells.

A very interesting mutant mouse strain called *scid* (because it has a severe combined B- and T-cell immune deficiency) has a defect in the enzyme DNA-dependent kinase, which binds to the end of the double-stranded breaks that occur during the process of antigen receptor gene recombination. Many of the hairpins formed when DNA rearrangement is initiated are found in T-cell receptor δ-chain genes of immature thymocytes of *scid* mice. Thus, it seems likely that DNA-dependent kinase will be involved in resolving the hairpin structure (see Fig. 3.21). Only rare VJ or VDJ joints are seen in *scid* B and T cells, and most of these have abnormal features. These mice therefore produce very few mature B and T cells. Recently, similar abnormal DJ joints have been observed in pre-B cells of some patients with autosomal severe combined immunodeficiency, and cells of such patients, like those of *scid* mice, are abnormally sensitive to ionizing radiation.

In patients with **DiGeorge syndrome**, the thymic epithelium fails to develop normally. Without the proper inductive environment T cells cannot mature, and both T-cell dependent antibody production and cell-mediated immunity are absent. Such patients have some serum immunoglobulin and variable numbers of B and T cells.

The severe combined immunodeficiency diseases abundantly illustrate the central role of T cells in virtually all adaptive immune responses. In most cases B-cell development is normal, yet the response to nearly all pathogens is profoundly suppressed.

10-12 | Defective cytokine production or cytokine action can cause immunodeficiency.

Virtually all adaptive immune responses require the activation of T lymphocytes and their differentiation into cells that produce cytokines, which act on specific cytokine receptors. Several gene defects have been described that interfere with these processes. Thus, patients that lack CD3γ chains have low levels of surface T-cell receptors and defective T-cell responses. Patients making low levels of mutant CD3ε chains are also deficient in T-cell activation.

Another group of patients shows absence of IL-2 production upon receptor ligation, and these patients have a severe immunodeficiency; however,

T-cell development is normal in these individuals, as it is in mice that have mutations in their IL-2 genes from gene knock-out (see Section 2-38). These IL-2-negative patients have heterogeneous defects; some of them fail to activate the transcription factor NF-AT (see Section 4-28), which induces transcription of several cytokine genes in addition to the IL-2 gene, and therefore presumably have low levels of these cytokines as well. This may explain why their immunodeficiency is more profound than that of mice whose IL-2 gene has been disrupted; these mice can mount adaptive immune responses through an IL-2-independent pathway, possibly involving the cytokine IL-15, which shares many activities with IL-2.

Patients who make a defective form of the cytosolic protein tyrosine kinase ZAP-70 (see Section 4-28) have recently been described. Their CD4 T cells emerge from the thymus in normal numbers, whereas CD8 T cells are absent. However, the CD4 T cells that do mature fail to respond to stimuli that normally activate via the T-cell receptor, and the patients are thus very immunodeficient.

There is an interesting contrast between patients deficient in IL-2 and those with X-linked severe combined immunodeficiency (X-linked SCID), which is caused by a defect in the γ chain of the IL-2 receptor. T cells in X-linked SCID patients fail to develop, while B cells appear reasonably normal. As mice and humans that lack IL-2 have normal T-cell development, the γ chain of the IL-2 receptor must be important in T-cell development for reasons unrelated to IL-2 binding or IL-2 responses. The recent demonstration that the IL-2 receptor γ chain is also part of other cytokine receptors, including the IL-7 receptor, may explain its role in early T-cell development. Furthermore, although their B cells appear normal, X-linked SCID patients do not make effective antibody responses to most antigens.

As the gene defect is on the X chromosome, one can determine whether the lack of B-cell function is solely caused by the lack of T-cell help by examining X-chromosome inactivation (see Section 10-7) in B cells of unaffected carriers. Naive, IgM-positive B cells have an inactive defective X chromosome more often than an inactive normal one, showing that B-cell development is affected by, but not wholly dependent on, the common γ chain. Mature memory B cells that have switched to isotypes other than IgM, however, almost all carry an inactive defective X chromosome. This may reflect the fact that the IL-2 receptor γ chain is also part of the IL-4 receptor. Thus, B cells that lack this chain will have defective IL-4 receptors and will not proliferate in T-cell dependent antibody responses. The defect is so severe that children who inherit it can survive only in a completely pathogen-free environment. A famous case in Houston became known as the 'bubble baby' because of the plastic bubble in which he was enclosed to protect him from infection.

The production of defects in several cytokine and cytokine receptor genes in gene knock-out mice is rapidly increasing our understanding of the role of individual cytokines in immunity. Mice lacking tumor growth factor-β (TGF-β) die of overwhelming inflammatory disease, while mice lacking IFN-γ or the IFN-γ receptor succumb to infection with a range of intracellular pathogens, including *M. tuberculosis*.

10-13 | Transplantation or gene therapy may be useful to correct genetic defects.

It is frequently possible to correct the defects in lymphocyte development that lead to the SCID phenotype by replacing the defective component, generally by bone marrow transplantation. The major difficulties in these therapies result from MHC polymorphism. To be useful, the graft must share some MHC alleles with the host. As we learned in Section 6-14, the MHC alleles expressed by the thymic epithelium determine which T cells are positively selected. When bone marrow cells are used to restore immune function to individuals with a normal thymic stroma, both the T cells and the antigen-presenting cells are derived from the graft. Therefore, unless the graft shares at least some MHC alleles with the recipient, the T cells that are selected on host thymic epithelium cannot be activated by graft-derived antigen-presenting cells (Fig. 10.13). There is also a danger that mature, post-thymic T cells in donor bone marrow may recognize the host as foreign and attack it, causing **graft-versus-host (GVH) disease** (Fig. 10.14). This can be overcome by depleting the donor bone marrow of mature T cells. In patients with the SCID phenotype, there is little problem with the host response to the graft, since the patient is immunodeficient.

Now that specific gene defects are being identified, a different approach to correcting these inherited immune deficiencies can be attempted. The strategy would be to extract a sample of the patient's own bone marrow cells, insert a normal copy of the defective gene into them, and return them to the patient by transfusion. This treatment should correct the gene defect, and this approach is called **gene therapy**. Moreover, in immunodeficient patients, it may be possible to re-infuse the bone marrow into the patient without the usual irradiation to suppress the

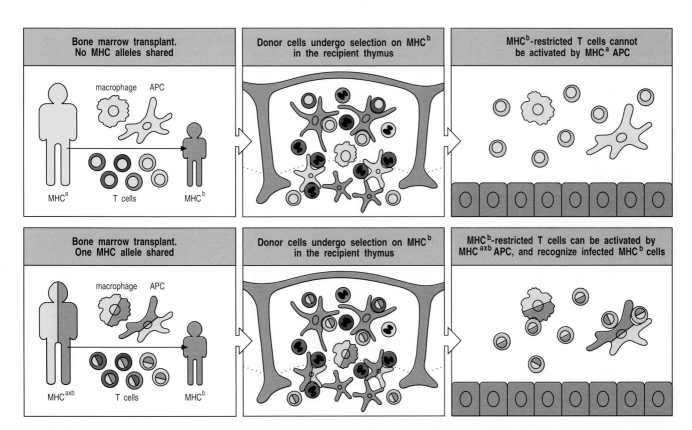

Fig. 10.13 Bone marrow donor and recipient must share at least some MHC molecules to restore immune function. If the bone marrow and the recipient thymus do not share any MHC alleles, T cells will mature in the thymus with receptors selected to recognize peptides presented by MHC molecules that are not expressed on the donor-derived antigen-presenting cells (APCs). These cells will not therefore be competent to mediate protective immunity (top panels). In the bottom panels, donor and recipient share the MHC^b allele, and cells recognizing MHC^b molecules are selected in the thymus. The antigen-presenting cells in the periphery can activate T cells that recognize MHC^b molecules; the activated T cells can then recognize infected MHC^b-bearing cells.

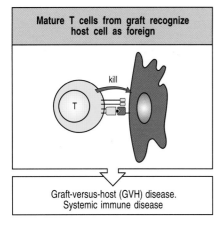

Mature T cells from graft recognize host cell as foreign

Graft-versus-host (GVH) disease. Systemic immune disease

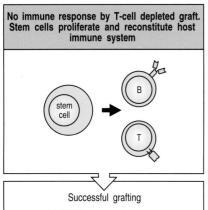

No immune response by T-cell depleted graft. Stem cells proliferate and reconstitute host immune system

Successful grafting

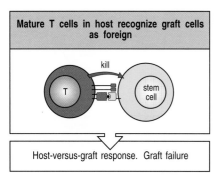

Mature T cells in host recognize graft cells as foreign

Host-versus-graft response. Graft failure

Fig. 10.14   Bone-marrow grafting can be used to correct immunodeficiencies caused by defects in lymphocyte maturation but two problems can arise. First, if there are mature T cells in the bone marrow, they can attack cells of the host by recognizing their MHC antigens, causing graft-versus-host disease (top panel). This can be prevented by T-cell depletion of the donor bone marrow (center panel). Second, if the recipient has competent T cells, these may reject the bone marrow stem cells (bottom panel). This causes failure of the graft.

recipient's bone marrow function. There is no risk of graft-versus-host immunity in this case, although it is possible that the host may respond to the replaced gene product and reject the engineered cells. Although this kind of approach is theoretically attractive, efficient transfer of genes into bone marrow stem cells is technically difficult and has been achieved only in mouse models.

The few trials of gene therapy for correcting immunodeficiency, such as the treatment of a child with ADA deficiency at NIH in 1990, have used the patient's lymphocytes as the vehicle for gene introduction. However, because most lymphocytes are short-lived, the treatment has to be repeated regularly.

Summary.

Genetic defects can occur in almost any molecule involved in the immune response. These defects give rise to characteristic deficiency diseases, which, although rare, provide a great deal of information about the normal development and function of the immune system. Inherited immunodeficiencies have provided information about the separate roles of B and T lymphocytes in humoral and cell-mediated immunity, the importance of innate immunity in host defense against viruses and bacteria, and the specific functions of several cell-surface or signaling molecules in the adaptive immune response. There are also some inherited immune disorders whose causes we still do not understand. The study of these diseases will undoubtedly teach us more about the normal immune response and its control.

Acquired immune deficiency syndrome.

The first cases of the **acquired immune deficiency syndrome** (**AIDS**) were reported in 1981 but it is now clear that the disease had been spreading silently for several years prior to its identification as a distinct entity. The disease is characterized by susceptibility to infection with opportunistic pathogens or the occurrence of an aggressive form of Kaposi's sarcoma or B-cell lymphoma, accompanied by a profound decrease in the number of CD4 T cells. As it appeared to be spread by contact with body fluids, it was early suspected to be caused by a new virus, and by 1983 the agent now known to be responsible for AIDS, called the **human immunodeficiency virus** (**HIV**), was isolated and identified. There are now known to be at least two types of HIV, HIV-1 and HIV-2, which share about 40% of their genome. HIV-2 is endemic in West Africa and now spreading in India. Most AIDS worldwide, however, is caused by HIV-1.

While the reason for the depletion of CD4 T cells in HIV and whether all infected patients will progress to overt disease remain controversial, nevertheless accumulating evidence clearly implicates the growth of the virus and the immune response to it as the central keys to the puzzle of AIDS. HIV is now clearly a world pandemic and, while great strides are being made in understanding the pathogenesis and epidemiology of the disease, the number of infected people worldwide continues to grow at an alarming rate, presaging the death of many people from AIDS for many years to come (Fig. 10.15).

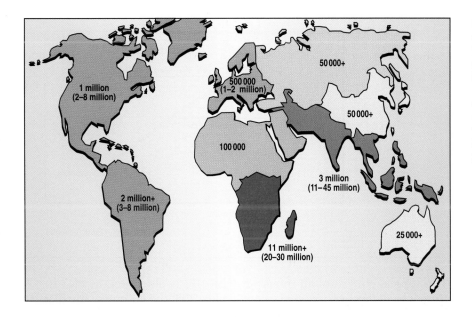

Fig. 10.15   HIV infection is spreading on all continents. The number of HIV-infected individuals is large (data are estimated total number of HIV infections by the end of 1994) and is increasing rapidly, especially in developing countries. Numbers in parentheses indicate the range of predictions for the total number of HIV infections from the beginning of the epidemic until the year 2 000, in the major areas of infection.

| 10-14 | **Most individuals infected with HIV progress over time to AIDS.** |

Many viruses cause an acute but limited infection inducing lasting protective immunity. Others, such as herpes viruses, set up a latent infection that is not eliminated but is controlled adequately by an adaptive immune response. However, infection with HIV seems rarely, if ever, to lead to an immune response that can eliminate the virus. While the initial acute infection does seem to be controlled by the immune system, HIV continues to replicate rapidly and is damaging existing CD4 T cells all the time.

The initial infection with HIV generally occurs after transfer of bodily fluids from an actively infected person. The virus is carried in infected CD4 T cells or as free virus in blood, semen, vaginal fluid, or milk. It is most commonly spread by sexual intercourse, contaminated needles used for intravenous drug delivery, and the therapeutic use of infected blood or blood products (although this last route of transmission has largely been eliminated in the developed world, where blood products are screened routinely for HIV). The virus can also be transmitted from an infected mother to her baby at birth or even through breast milk.

Acute infection with HIV causes a flu-like illness with abundant virus in the peripheral blood and a marked drop in the level of circulating CD4 T cells. This initial phase is followed in virtually all patients by antibody production, or **seroconversion**, and by the activation of CD8 T cells that kill HIV-infected syngeneic cells. This leads to a clearance of much of the viremia and a rebound of CD4 T cell counts to around 500 per microliter (the normal value is 1 200 cells μl^{-1}). The extent of this response is suspected to play a role in the future course of the disease but, like so much else about AIDS, this point has not been examined rigorously.

Most patients who are infected with HIV will eventually develop AIDS, after a period of apparent quiescence of the disease known as clinical latency or the asymptomatic period. This period is not silent, however, for there is a gradual decline in CD4 T-cell function and cell numbers until eventually patients have few CD4 T cells left. At this point, which can occur anywhere between 3 and 15 years or more after the primary infection (Fig. 10.16), the period of clinical latency ends and opportunistic infections appear.

Fig. 10.16 Most HIV-infected individuals progress to AIDS over a period of years. The incidence of AIDS increases progressively with time after infection, and is predicted to reach ~95% within 15 years, although data are only available for 12 years. Homosexuals and hemophiliacs are two of the groups at highest risk, homosexuals from sexually transmitted virus and hemophiliacs from infected human blood used to replace clotting factor VIII. Hemophiliacs are now protected by screening of blood products and the use of recombinant factor VIII. Hemophiliacs who were over the age of 20 years at the time of infection and homosexual males progress to AIDS at the same rate, while younger hemophiliacs in some cases progress more rapidly. Neither homosexuals nor hemophiliacs who have not been infected with HIV show any evidence of AIDS. There are few individuals who, while infected with HIV, appear not to have progressed to develop AIDS and may, in some way, be protected.

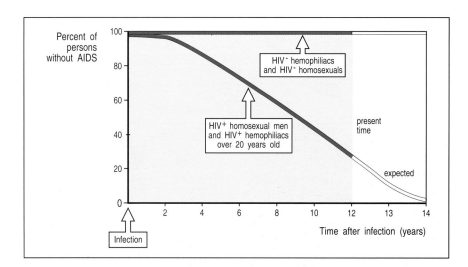

The typical course of an infection with HIV is illustrated in Fig. 10.17. However, it has become increasingly clear that the course of the disease can vary widely. Thus, while most people infected with HIV go on to develop AIDS and ultimately to die of opportunistic infection or cancer, this is not true of all individuals. One group comprises a small percentage of people who seroconvert, making antibodies to many HIV proteins but who do not appear to have progressive disease, in that their CD4 T-cell counts and other measures of immune competence are maintained. These long-term non-progressors are now being studied intensively to determine how they are able to control the infection with HIV. A second group consists of seronegative people who have been highly exposed to HIV, yet remain disease-free and virus-negative. These individuals have specific cytotoxic lymphocytes directed against infected cells and if these could be induced by vaccination with modified HIV or other strategies, it might be possible to prevent AIDS.

Fig. 10.17 The typical course of infection with HIV. The first few weeks are typified by an acute influenza-like viral illness, sometimes called seroconversion disease, with high titers of virus in the blood. An adaptive immune response follows, which controls the acute illness and largely restores CD4 T cell levels but does not eradicate the virus. Opportunistic infections and other symptoms become more frequent as the CD4 T-cell count falls, starting at around 500 cells μl^{-1}. The disease then enters the symptomatic phase. When CD4 T-cell counts fall below 200 cells μl^{-1} the patient is said to have AIDS.

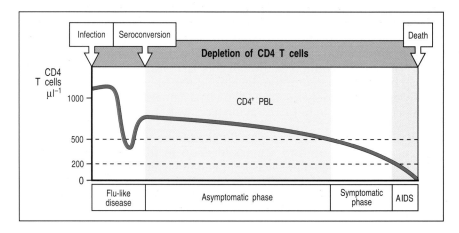

Before going on to discuss in more detail the interactions of the virus with the immune system and the prospects for manipulating them, we must first describe the viral life cycle and the proteins on which it depends. Some of these proteins are the targets of the most successful drugs in use at present for the treatment of AIDS.

10-15   HIV is a retrovirus that infects CD4 T cells and macrophages.

HIV is an enveloped retrovirus. Each virus particle has two copies of an RNA genome that is transcribed into DNA in the infected cell and integrated into the host cell chromosome. The RNA transcripts produced from the integrated viral DNA serve both as mRNA to direct the synthesis of the viral proteins, and later as the RNA genomes of new viral particles, which escape from the cell by budding from the plasma membrane, each in a membrane envelope. The structure of the viral particle, or virion, is shown in Fig. 10.18.

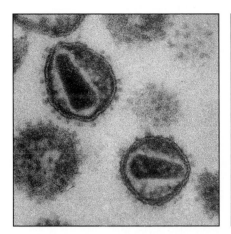
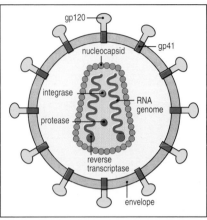

Fig. 10.18　The virion of human immunodeficiency virus (HIV) The virus illustrated is HIV-1, the leading cause of AIDS. HIV-2 is similar in general structure. The reverse transcriptase, integrase, and viral protease enzymes are packaged in the virion and are shown schematically in the viral capsid. In reality, many molecules of these enzymes are contained in the virion. Some structural proteins of the virus have been omitted for simplicity. Photograph courtesy of H Gelderblom.

As they escape from cells by budding, the enveloped viruses are less immediately destructive than viruses that lyse infected cells. Indeed, HIV belongs to a group of retroviruses called the **lentiviruses**, from the Latin *lentus*, meaning slow, because of the gradual course of the disease they cause. Although infected cells in AIDS patients are eventually destroyed, it is still not clear whether this is a direct effect of the virus on the infected cell, or an indirect effect caused by the immune response to the virus. We shall return to this question later.

HIV enters cells by means of a complex of two, noncovalently-associated viral glycoproteins, gp120 and gp41, in the viral envelope. The gp120 portion of the glycoprotein complex binds with high affinity to CD4 on the cell surface. This glycoprotein thereby draws the virus to CD4 T cells and to macrophages, which also express some CD4. The gp41 component then mediates fusion of the viral envelope with the plasma membrane of the cell, allowing the viral genome and associated viral proteins to enter the cytoplasm.

One of the proteins that enters the cell with the viral genome is the viral reverse transcriptase, which transcribes the viral RNA into a complementary DNA (cDNA) copy. The viral cDNA is then integrated into the host cell genome by the viral integrase, which also enters the cell with the viral RNA. The integrated cDNA copy of the viral RNA genome is known as the **provirus**. The infectious cycle up to the integration of the provirus is shown in Fig. 10.19.

The entire HIV genome consists of nine genes flanked by long terminal repeat sequences (LTR), which are required for integration of the provirus into the host cell DNA and contain binding sites for gene regulatory proteins that control the expression of the viral genes. HIV shares with all other retroviruses three major genes, *gag*, *pol*, and *env*. The *gag* gene encodes the structural proteins of the viral core, the *pol* gene encodes the enzymes involved in viral replication and integration, and the *env* gene encodes the viral envelope glycoproteins. The *gag* and *pol* mRNAs are translated to give polyproteins — long polypeptide chains that are then cleaved by the viral protease (also encoded by *pol*) into individual functional proteins. The product of the *env* gene, gp160, has to be cleaved by a host-cell protease into gp120 and gp41, which remain

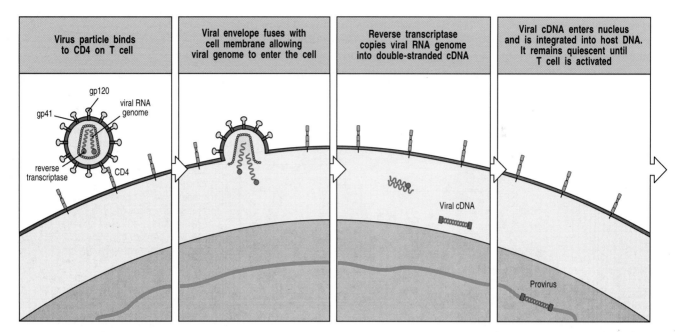

Fig. 10.19 The life cycle of HIV in CD4 T cells. The virus binds to CD4 using gp120; gp41 then mediates fusion with the target cell. Once in the cytoplasm, the RNA genome is reverse transcribed into double-stranded cDNA, which migrates to the nucleus and is integrated into the host cell genome, where it is called a provirus.

associated on the viral envelope. The other six genes encode proteins that affect viral replication and infectivity in various ways that we discuss in the next sections. The viral genes and the functions of their products are summarized in Fig. 10.20.

Fig. 10.20 The genes and proteins of HIV-1. Like all retroviruses, HIV-1 has an RNA genome flanked by long terminal repeats (LTR) involved in viral integration and in regulation of the viral genome. The genome can be read in three frames, and several of the viral genes overlap in different reading frames. This allows the virus to encode many proteins in a small genome. The three main protein products, Gag, Pol, and Env, are synthesized by all infectious retroviruses. The known functions of the different genes and their products are listed. The products of *gag*, *pol* and *env* are known to be present in the mature viral particle, together with the viral RNA. The other gene products affect the infectivity of the virus in various ways that are not fully understood.

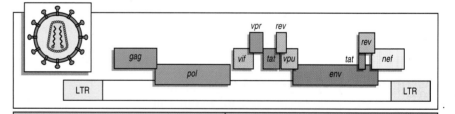

Gene		Gene product/function
gag	Group-specific antigen	Core protein
pol	Polymerase	Reverse transcriptase, protease, and integrase enzymes
env	Envelope	Transmembrane glycoproteins. gp120 binds CD4; gp41 required for virus internalization
tat	Transactivator	Positive regulator of transcription
rev	Regulator of viral expression	Allows export of unspliced transcripts from nucleus
vif	Viral infectivity	Affects particle infectivity; helps assemble virions?
vpr	Viral protein R	Positive regulator of transcription. Augments virion production
vpu	Viral protein U	Unique to HIV-1. Down-regulates CD4
nef	So-called negative-regulation factor	Augments viral replication *in vivo* and *in vitro*. Down-regulates CD4

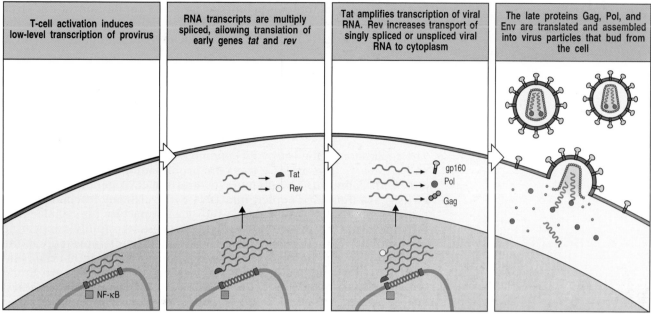

| T-cell activation induces low-level transcription of provirus | RNA transcripts are multiply spliced, allowing translation of early genes *tat* and *rev* | Tat amplifies transcription of viral RNA. Rev increases transport of singly spliced or unspliced viral RNA to cytoplasm | The late proteins Gag, Pol, and Env are translated and assembled into virus particles that bud from the cell |

10-16   **Transcription of the HIV provirus depends on host-cell transcription factors induced upon activation of the infected cell.**

The production of infectious virus particles from the integrated HIV provirus occurs only upon activation of the infected CD4 T cell. Activation of CD4 T cells induces the transcription factor NF-κB, which binds to promoters not only in the cellular DNA but also in the viral LTR, initiating transcription of viral RNA by the cellular RNA polymerase. This transcript is spliced in various ways to produce mRNAs for the viral proteins. At least two of the viral genes, *tat* and *rev*, encode proteins, **Tat** and **Rev** respectively, that promote viral replication in activated T cells. Tat is a potent transcriptional regulator that binds to a sequence in the LTR known as the transcriptional activation region (TAR) and greatly enhances the rate of viral genome transcription.

The *rev* gene has a more complex function. It makes a protein that binds to the RNA transcript of HIV and controls its delivery it to the cytoplasm. To express the Tat and Rev proteins, the viral transcripts must be spliced twice, while for other viral proteins only one splicing event is required. When the provirus is first activated, Rev levels are low, the transcripts are translocated slowly from the nucleus and thus multiple splicing events can occur. Later, when Rev levels have increased, the transcripts are rapidly translocated from the nucleus unspliced or only singly spliced. In the early stages, Tat is required to make multiple transcripts of the proviral genome. At later stages, the structural components of the viral core and envelope are needed, together with the reverse transcriptase, the integrase, and the viral protease, to make new viral particles. Complete, unspliced transcripts must also be exported from the nucleus to be packaged with the proteins as the RNA genomes of the new virus particles (Fig. 10.21).

Recent studies indicate that HIV is probably replicating rapidly at all phases of infection, including the asymptomatic phase, and it is now thought that the immune response to HIV represents a stand-off between the rapidly replicating virus and CD4 T cells, which are almost as rapidly replaced. Eventually, T cell numbers cannot keep up and the

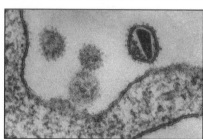

Fig. 10.21   Cells infected with HIV replicate the virus upon activation. Activation of CD4 T cells induces the expression of the transcription factor NF-κB, which binds to the proviral LTR and initiates transcription of the HIV genome into RNA. The viral RNA encodes several regulatory proteins. Tat both enhances transcription from the provirus, and also binds to the RNA transcripts, stabilizing them in a form that can be translated. The protein Rev binds the RNA transcripts and transports them to the cytosol. The viral RNA also encodes the structural proteins of the virus that eventually lead to the production of many new viral particles. Early in the infectious cycle, levels of Rev are low and the transcript is retained in the nucleus and processed extensively: this produces mRNAs encoding the regulatory proteins, such as Tat, that are required for viral replication. Later, as levels of Rev increase, Rev acts to transport less-extensively spliced and unspliced transcripts out of the nucleus. The spliced transcripts encode the structural proteins of the virus and the unspliced transcripts are packaged with these to form new virus particles. Photograph courtesy of H Gelderblom.

patient loses immune competence. The rapid replication of the virus meanwhile contributes to the very high mutation rate that generates the many variants of HIV that arise in a single infected patient in the course of infection.

10-17 | HIV accumulates mutations in the course of infection in a single individual.

The replication of the retroviral genome depends upon two error-prone steps. Reverse transcriptase lacks the proofreading mechanisms associated with cellular DNA polymerases and the RNA genomes of retroviruses are therefore copied into DNA with relatively low fidelity; the transcription of the proviral DNA into RNA copies by the cellular RNA polymerase is a similarly low-fidelity process. A rapidly replicating persistent virus that is going through these two steps repeatedly in the course of an infection can thereby accumulate many mutations, and numerous variants of HIV, sometimes called quasi-species, are found within a single infected individual. This very high mutability was first recognized in HIV and has since proved to be common to the other lentiviruses.

The generation of many mutants of HIV poses a problem for the design of vaccines aimed at eliciting neutralizing antibodies, and may also contribute to the failure of the immune system to overcome the infection in the long term. In some cases, for example, variant peptides produced by the virus have been found to act as antagonists (see Section 4-29) for T cells responsive to the wild-type epitope, thus allowing both mutant and wild-type viruses to survive. Mutant peptides acting as antagonists have also been reported in hepatitis B virus infections, and these may contribute to the persistence of some viral infections, especially where, as sometimes happens, the immune response of an individual is dominated by T cells specific for a particular epitope.

10-18 | An immune response controls but does not eliminate HIV.

Infection with HIV generates an adaptive immune response that controls production of the virus but usually cannot eliminate it. The time course of various elements of the adaptive immune response to HIV is shown, with the levels of infectious virus in plasma, in Fig. 10.22.

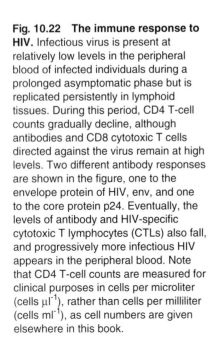

Fig. 10.22 The immune response to HIV. Infectious virus is present at relatively low levels in the peripheral blood of infected individuals during a prolonged asymptomatic phase but is replicated persistently in lymphoid tissues. During this period, CD4 T-cell counts gradually decline, although antibodies and CD8 cytotoxic T cells directed against the virus remain at high levels. Two different antibody responses are shown in the figure, one to the envelope protein of HIV, env, and one to the core protein p24. Eventually, the levels of antibody and HIV-specific cytotoxic T lymphocytes (CTLs) also fall, and progressively more infectious HIV appears in the peripheral blood. Note that CD4 T-cell counts are measured for clinical purposes in cells per microliter (cells μl^{-1}), rather than cells per milliliter (cells ml^{-1}), as cell numbers are given elsewhere in this book.

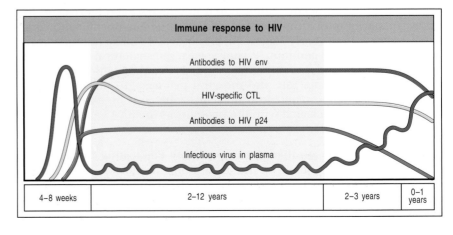

Immune response to HIV

Antibodies to HIV env

HIV-specific CTL

Antibodies to HIV p24

Infectious virus in plasma

| 4–8 weeks | 2–12 years | 2–3 years | 0–1 years |

Seroconversion is the clearest evidence for an adaptive immune response to infection with HIV but the generation of T lymphocytes responding to infected cells is thought by most people to be central in controlling the infection. Both CD8 cytotoxic T cells and inflammatory CD4 T cells specifically responsive to infected cells are associated with the decline in detectable virus after the initial infection. These T-cell responses are, however, also thought to contribute to the pathology of the disease.

Although HIV levels are usually measured in peripheral blood lymphocytes, the highest viral load is in the lymph nodes where most lymphocytes are found. Functional studies on T lymphocytes from AIDS patients suggest that memory CD4 T cells are particularly susceptible to infection. Activation of the infected memory cells in the lymph nodes would then result in viral replication and the destruction of the infected cell. There is, however, evidence from recent studies on infected individuals that the infected cells may be destroyed by cytotoxic lymphocytes rather than by the virus itself.

Strong circumstantial evidence for destruction of infected cells by cytotoxic lymphocytes comes from studies on peripheral blood cells of infected individuals, in which cytotoxic T cells specific for viral peptides can be shown to kill infected cells *in vitro*. In one striking case, rapid progression of the disease was associated with the appearance of mutant viral peptides followed by the appearance of cytotoxic T cells capable of recognizing the mutant peptides, and a rapid loss of CD4 T cells. CD8 T cells specific for HIV-infected cells in a given patient often have a single dominant Vβ-chain gene rearrangement that enables them to be identified. Using such a dominant Vβ rearrangement as a marker for HIV-specific cytotoxic cells, it has been possible to show that these cells are present around the splenic white pulps in infected individuals, suggesting that the splenic white pulps are sites where replication of HIV within infected CD4 T cells and elimination of infected cells by cytotoxic cells occur simultaneously. These studies also showed that different white pulps contain different quasi-species of HIV, suggesting that the original infecting virion is replicating and diversifying within each white pulp. Whatever the mechanism, the result of HIV infection in the lymphoid tissues is the gradual disruption of the lymphoid architecture, leading eventually to the destruction of the lymphoid follicles in the late stages of the disease.

Macrophages, which are also infected by HIV, seem to be able to harbor replicating virus without necessarily being killed by it, and are believed to be an important reservoir of infection, as well as a means of spreading virus to other tissues, such as the brain. Although the function of macrophages as antigen-presenting cells does not seem to be compromised by HIV infection, it is thought that the virus may cause abnormal patterns of cytokine secretion that could account for the wasting that commonly occurs in AIDS patients.

10-19 | **Drugs that block HIV replication lead to a rapid fall in titer of infectious virus and a rise in CD4 T cells, followed by the outgrowth of drug-resistant variant virus.**

Two viral proteins in particular have been the target of drugs aimed at arresting viral replication. These are the viral reverse transcriptase, which is required for synthesis of the provirus, and the viral protease, which cleaves the viral polyproteins to produce the virion proteins and viral enzymes. Inhibitors of these enzymes prevent the establishment of further infection in uninfected cells, although cells that are already infected can continue for a limited time to produce virions. Studies of the effects of two of the protease inhibitors show that almost all the virus present in an individual's circulation is the product of recently infected cells. After as little as two days, these drugs can reduce viral titer in the blood by 100-fold or more. At the same time, there is a surge in CD4 T-cell numbers, which suggests that CD4 T cells are continuously being produced and just as rapidly becoming infected by HIV.

Although most studies to date have focused on the picture observable in the blood, HIV replication is at least as active in lymphoid tissues in the periphery. It is therefore important to look at the lymph nodes and spleen as we seek an answer to two questions raised by these studies. First, what is happening to all the virus that was in the blood originally; how is infectious virus removed so rapidly from the circulation? It seems most likely that infectious HIV particles have been opsonized by specific antibody and removed by phagocytic cells of the reticulo-endothelial system. Opsonized HIV particles may also be trapped on the surface of follicular dendritic cells, which are known to capture antigen:antibody complexes and retain them for prolonged periods (see Chapters 8 and 9).

The second question is: what is the source of the new CD4 T cells that appear once treatment is started? It seems highly unlikely that these are the recent progeny of stem cells that have developed in the thymus, because CD4 T cells are not normally produced in large numbers from the adult thymus. Some investigators believe that these cells are emerging from sites of margination along the blood vessels, and add little to the total numbers of CD4 T cells in the body, while others advocate their origin from mature CD4 T cells that replicate.

As the anti-viral drugs continue to be administered, the virus becomes resistant to their effects, probably because of the expansion of quasi-species in the original viral population that carry mutations conferring resistance. Resistance to the protease inhibitors appears after only a few days. Resistance to the reverse transcriptase inhibitor AZT, the most widely used drug for treating AIDS, takes months to develop. This is because resistance to AZT requires three or four mutations in the viral reverse transcriptase, whereas a single mutation can confer resistance to the protease inhibitors. As a result of the relatively rapid appearance of resistance to all known anti-HIV drugs, successful drug treatment may depend upon the development of a range of anti-viral drugs that can be used in combination, thereby destroying the virus before any one strain has had a chance to accumulate all the necessary mutations to resist the entire cocktail.

10-20   HIV infection leads to low levels of CD4 T cells, increased susceptibility to opportunistic infection, and eventually to death.

The way in which HIV ultimately kills CD4 T cells is still being debated; the only fact on which all parties agree is that it does. Probably the leading hypothesis is that actively infected CD4 T cells are killed by the CD8 cytotoxic lymphocytes that are found in abundance in fragments of spleen from infected individuals.

Alternatively, it may be the binding of CD4 by gp120 that damages CD4 T cells. There is some experimental support for this; CD4 T cells from HIV-infected patients are more susceptible to apoptosis driven by receptor crosslinking, and this effect can be replicated in normal CD4 T cells *in vitro* by crosslinking CD4 either with anti-CD4 or with gp120 complexed with anti-gp120. Moreover, memory CD4 T cells have been shown to be much more susceptible to inhibition through CD4 than naive T cells, perhaps accounting for the early effects of HIV infection on memory T cells.

When CD4 T cell numbers decline below a critical level, cell-mediated immunity is lost, and infections with a variety of opportunistic infectious agents appear. Typically, resistance is lost early to oral *Candida* spp. and to *Mycobacterium tuberculosis*, manifesting as an increased prevalence of thrush and tuberculosis. Later, patients suffer from shingles, caused by the activation of latent herpes zoster, B-cell lymphomas, and Kaposi's sarcoma, an invasive tumor of blood vessels that probably represents a response both to cytokines produced in the infection and to a novel strain of herpes simplex virus that was recently identified in these lesions. At a still later date, *Pneumocystis carinii* pneumonia tends to appear. Finally, Cytomegalovirus or infection with *Mycobacterium avium* complex are more prominent. It is important to note that not all patients with AIDS get all these infections or tumors, and there are other tumors and infections that are less prominent but still significant. Rather, this is a list of opportunistic infections and tumors, most of which are normally controlled by robust CD4 T-cell mediated immunity, which wanes as the CD4 T cell counts drop toward zero (Fig. 10.23).

10-21 | **Vaccination against HIV is an attractive solution to the problem of AIDS but poses many difficulties.**

The development of a safe and effective vaccine for the prevention of HIV infection and AIDS is an attractive goal but its development is fraught with difficulties that have not been faced in vaccination campaigns against other diseases. The first problem is that there is no exact animal model that can be used to test for successful vaccination against HIV, nor can the efficacy of vaccines be studied readily in humans. One model system is based on simian immunodeficiency virus (SIV), which is closely related to HIV and which infects macaques. While these animals have been used to test vaccination strategies, the system is limited somewhat by the fact that SIV does not cause a fatal disease in macaques; the extent to which lessons learned from the study of SIV can be applied to the control of HIV is presently unknown.

The second problem is that it is not clear what would be required to establish immunity to HIV. Whereas most infections elicit an immune response that can provide lasting protection, pathogens such as HIV that persist in spite of a vigorous immune response pose special problems. These are compounded in the case of HIV by the state of immunodeficiency that progressively results from the infection itself. This makes particularly interesting those rare patients who have been exposed often enough to make it virtually certain that they should have become infected, yet have not developed the disease. These individuals are a focus of considerable interest to AIDS researchers but the explanation for their resistance to HIV is not yet clear. Some studies suggest that such people were initially infected by a mutant of HIV that lacks one or more gene products essential for establishing HIV infection, while others suggest a possible durable resistance to HIV infection based on CD8 T cells.

A further important question is the type of immunity one wishes to induce by vaccination. It seems likely that the most desirable type of response would be dominated by CD8 T cells, or perhaps inflammatory CD4 T cells (T_H1). AIDS patients tend to produce cytokines typical of helper CD4 T cells (T_H2), while CD4 T-cell responses to HIV peptides in infected but still healthy individuals tend to be dominated by T_H1 cytokines, although the significance of this observation is still hotly debated by

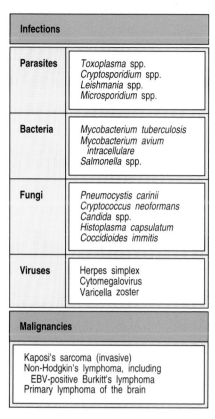

Infections	
Parasites	*Toxoplasma* spp. *Cryptosporidium* spp. *Leishmania* spp. *Microsporidium* spp.
Bacteria	*Mycobacterium tuberculosis* *Mycobacterium avium intracellulare* *Salmonella* spp.
Fungi	*Pneumocystis carinii* *Cryptococcus neoformans* *Candida* spp. *Histoplasma capsulatum* *Coccidioides immitis*
Viruses	Herpes simplex Cytomegalovirus Varicella zoster

Malignancies
Kaposi's sarcoma (invasive) Non-Hodgkin's lymphoma, including EBV-positive Burkitt's lymphoma Primary lymphoma of the brain

Fig. 10.23 A variety of opportunistic pathogens and cancers can kill AIDS patients. Infections are the major cause of death in AIDS, with respiratory infection with *Pneumocystis carinii* being the most prominent. Most of these pathogens require effective macrophage activation by CD4 T cells or effective cytotoxic T cells for host defense. Opportunistic pathogens are present in the normal environment but cause severe disease primarily in immuno-compromised hosts, like AIDS patients and cancer patients. AIDS patients are also susceptible to several rare cancers, such as Kaposi's sarcoma and lymphomas, suggesting that immune surveillance by T cells may normally prevent such tumors (see Chapter 12).

AIDS researchers. In any case, methods have yet to be devised for designing vaccines that reliably elicit a desired type of immune response, as we discuss in Chapter 12.

Attempts have been made to design so-called subunit vaccines, which induce immunity to only some proteins in the virus, and one such has been made from the envelope protein gp120. However, when tested on chimpanzees, this vaccine proved to be specific to the precise strain of virus used to make it, and therefore useless in protection against natural infection.

Finally, there are difficult ethical issues in the development of a vaccine, as seems to be true of all aspects of this deadly disease. When a population is vaccinated, how does one ethically allow them to be exposed to the virus? Does one tell people who have been vaccinated with a placebo that they may not be protected against HIV? This issue is particularly difficult because the consequences of contracting infection with HIV are so serious. These ethical and moral issues are a further impediment to the development of a new vaccine against HIV.

10-22   Prevention and education are one way in which the spread of HIV and AIDS can be controlled.

The one way in which we know we can protect against infection with HIV is by avoiding contact with bodily fluids, such as semen, blood, blood products, or milk, from people who are infected. Indeed, it has been demonstrated repeatedly that this precaution, simple enough in the developed world, is sufficient to prevent infection, as health care workers can take care of AIDS patients for long periods without seroconversion or signs of infection.

For this strategy to work, however, two things are necessary. First, one must be able to test periodically people at risk of infection with HIV, so that they can take the kind of steps necessary to avoid passing the virus to others. For this to work, strict confidentiality is absolutely required. One intelligent suggestion to emerge from President Reagan's AIDS Advisory Group was that before anything could be accomplished in the fight against AIDS, the rights of HIV-infected people would have to be guaranteed in all aspects of life. This step, unfortunately, was never taken. If one cannot test people at risk, then the disease is likely to continue unabated for years.

If, on the other hand, people infected with HIV were guaranteed protection of their rights, then they could begin to act responsibly towards others. Responsibility is at the heart of AIDS prevention, and a law guaranteeing the rights of people infected with HIV might go a long way to encouraging such behavior. The rights of HIV-infected people are protected in the Netherlands and Sweden. The problem in the less developed nations, where elementary health precautions are also virtually impossible to establish, is more profound.

Summary.

Infection with the human immunodeficiency virus (HIV) is the cause of acquired immune deficiency syndrome (AIDS). This worldwide epidemic is now spreading at an alarming rate, especially through heterosexual contact in less developed countries. Infection with HIV causes an acute infectious syndrome that is rapidly controlled but not eliminated by an immune response. HIV establishes a state of persistent infection that responds only very briefly to the anti-viral drugs tested to date.

These anti-viral agents rapidly select viral variants that are resistant to the drug and replicate rapidly even in its continued presence. The use of a combination of drugs may be able to overcome this problem. The main effect of HIV infection is the destruction of CD4 T cells but there is still no agreement about how they are destroyed, whether by a direct cytopathic effect of HIV infection, or indirectly by CD8 cytotoxic T cells, or both. As the CD4 T cell counts wane, the body becomes progressively more susceptible to opportunistic infection with intracellular microbes. Eventually, most HIV-infected individuals develop AIDS and die; some people (3–7%), however, remain healthy for many years, with no apparent ill effects of infection. It is hoped that one can learn from such individuals ways in which infection with HIV is controlled successfully. Analysis of such people appears to be one route to an effective vaccine for HIV.

Summary to Chapter 10.

While most infections elicit protective immunity, some result in serious, persistent disease. This occurs most commonly when the pathogen has developed means to persist despite an adequate immune response. In addition, some individuals have inherited deficiencies in different components of the immune system, making them highly susceptible to certain classes of infectious agents. Persistent infection and immunodeficiency illustrate the importance of effective host defense and present huge challenges for future immunological research. The human immunodeficiency virus (HIV) combines the characteristics of a persistent infectious agent with the ability to create immunodeficiency in its human host, a combination that is lethal to the patient. The key to fighting new pathogens like HIV is to develop more fully our understanding of the basic properties of the immune system and its role in combating infection. When this is achieved, we may be better prepared to combat newly arising pathogens like HIV.

General references.

AIDS 92/93 — A Year in Review. London, Current Science, 1993. Immunodeficiency. London, Current Biology, 1993.

Fauci, A.S.: **Multifactorial nature of human immunodeficiency virus disease: Implications for therapy.** Science 1993, **262**:1011-1018.

Mims, C.A.: The Pathogenesis of Infectious Disease. London, Academic Press, 1987.

Waldmann, T.A.: **Immunodeficiency Diseases: Primary and Acquired.** In Samter, M., Talmage, D.W., Frank, M.M., Austen, K.F., and Claman H.N. (eds): Immunological Diseases, 4th edn. Boston, Little, Brown and Co., 1988, pp. 411-465.

Section references.

10-1 **Antigenic variation can allow pathogens to escape from immunity.**

Borst, P.: **Molecular genetics and antigenic variation.** Immunology Today 1991, **12**:A29-A33.

Murphy, B.R., and Webster, R.G.: **Influenza Viruses.** In Fields, B.N., Knipe, D.M., Chanock, R.M., Hirsch, M.S., Melnick, J.L., Monath, T.P. and Roizman, B. (eds): Virology. New York, Raven Press, 1985, pp. 1179-1239.

10-2 **Some viruses persist in vivo by ceasing to replicate until immunity wanes.**

Garcia-Blanco, M.A., and Cullen, B.R.: **Molecular basis of latency in pathogenic human viruses.** Science 1991, **254**:815-820.

Klein, R.J.: **The pathogenesis of acute, latent and recurrent herpes simplex infections.** Arch. Virol. 1982, **72**:143.

10-3 **Some pathogens resist destruction by host defense mechanisms or exploit them for their own purposes.**

Kaufman, S.H.E.: **Immunity to intracellular bacteria.** Ann. Rev. Immunol. 1993, **11**:129-163.

Steere, A.C.: **Lyme disease.** N. Engl. J. Med. 1989, **321**:586-596.

10-4 **Immunosuppression or inappropriate immune responses can contribute to persistent disease.**

Bloom, B.R., Modlin, R.L., and Salgame, P.: **Stigma variations: Observations on suppressor T cells and leprosy.** Ann. Rev. Immunol. 1992, **10**:453-488.

Salgame, P., Abrams, J.S., Clayberger, C., Goldstein, H., Modlin, R.L., and Bloom, B.R.: **Differing lymphokine profiles of functional subsets of human CD4 and CD8 T-cell clones.** Science 1991, **254**:279.

10-5 Immune responses can contribute directly to pathogenesis.

Golovkina, T.V., Chervonsky, A., Dudley, J.P., and Ross, S.R.: **Transgenic mouse mammary tumor virus superantigen expression prevents viral infection.** *Cell* 1992, **69**:637.

Zinkernagel, R.M., Haenseler, E., Leist, T.P., Cerny, A., Hengartner, H., and Althage, A.: **T-cell mediated hepatitis in mice infected with lymphocytic choriomeningitis virus.** *J. Exper. Med.* 1986, **164**:1075-1092.

10-6 Inherited immunodeficiency diseases are caused by recessive gene defects.

Kinnon, C., and Levinsky, R.J.: **Molecular genetics of inherited immunodeficiency diseases.** *Immunogenet.* 1990, **135**:894-900.

10-7 The main effect of low levels of antibody is an inability to clear extracellular bacteria.

Bruton, O.C.: **Aggamaglobulinemia.** *Pediatrics* 1952, **9**:722-728.

Conley, M.E.: **Molecular approaches to analysis of X-linked immunodeficiencies.** *Ann. Rev. Immunol.* 1992, **10**:215-238.

Preudhomme, J.L., and Hanson, L.A.: **IgG subclass deficiency.** *Immunodef. Rev.* 1990, **2**:129-149.

Vetrie, D., Vorechovsky, I., Sideras, P., Holland, J., Davies, A., Flinter, F., Hammarström, L., Kinnon, C., Levinsky, R., Bobrow, M., Edvard Smith, C.I., and Bentley, D.R.: **The gene involved in X-linked agammaglobulinaemia is a member of the *src* family of protein-tyrosine kinases.** *Nature* 1993, **361**:226-233.

Volanakis, J.E., Zhu, Z.B., Schaffer, F.M., Macon, K.J., Palermos, J., Barger, B.O., Go, R., Campbell, R.D., Schroeder, H.W., and Cooper, M.D.: **Major histocompatibility complex class III genes and susceptibility to immunoglobulin A deficiency and common variable immunodeficiency.** *J. Clin. Invest.* 1992, **89**:1914-1922.

10-8 T-cell defects can result in low antibody levels.

Allen, R.C., Armintage, R.J., Conley, M.E., Rosenblatt, H., Jenkins, N.A., Copeland, N.G., Bedell, M.A., Edelhoff, S., Disteche, C.M., Simoneaux, D.K., Fanslow, W.C., Belmont, J., and Spriggs, M.K.: **CD40-ligand gene defects responsible for X-linked hyper IgM syndrome.** *Science* 1993, **259**:990-993.

Waldmann, T.A., Broder, S., Blaese, R.M., Durm, M., Blackman, M., and Strober, W.: **The role of suppressor T cells in the pathogenesis of common variable hypogammaglobulinemia.** *Lancet* 1974, **2**:609.

10-9 Defects in complement components cause defective humoral immune function and persistence of immune complexes.

Botto, M., Fong, K., So, A.K., Rudge, A., and Walport, M.J.: **Homozygous hereditary C3 deficiency due to a partial gene deletion.** *Proc. Natl. Acad. Sci. USA* 1992, **89**:4957-4961.

Colten, H.R., and Rosen, F.S.: **Complement deficiencies.** *Ann. Rev. Immunol.* 1993, **10**:809-824.

Lachmann, P.J., and Walport, M.J.: **Genetic Deficiency Diseases of the Complement System.** In Ross, G.D. (ed.): *Immunobiology of the complement system*, 1st edn. Orlando, Academic Press, 1986.

10-10 Phagocytic cell defects permit widespread bacterial infections.

Fischer, A., Lisowska-Grospierre, B., Anderson, D.C., and Springer, T.A.: **Leukocyte adhesion deficiency: Molecular basis and functional consequences.** *Immunodef. Rev.* 1988, **1**:39-54.

Rotrosen, D., and Gallin, J.I.: **Disorders of phagocyte function.** *Ann. Rev. Immunol.* 1987, **5**:127-150.

10-11 Defects in T-cell function result in severe combined immunodeficiencies.

Bosma, M.J., and Carroll, A.M.: **The SCID mouse mutant: Definition, characterization, and potential uses.** *Ann. Rev. Immunol.* 1993, **9**:323-350.

Hirschhorn, R.: **Adenosine deaminase deficiency.** *Immunodef. Rev.* 1990, **2**:175-198.

Kara, C.J., and Glimcher, L.H.: **Promoter accessibility within the environment of the MHC is affected in class II-deficient combined immunodeficiency.** *EMBO J.* 1993, **12**:187-193.

Noguchi, M., Yi, H., Rosenblatt, H.M., Filipovich, A.H., Adelstein, S., Modi, W.S., McBride, O.W., and Leonard, W.J.: **Interleukin-2 receptor gamma-chain mutation results in X-linked severe combined immunodeficiency.** *Cell* 1993, **73**:147-157.

Roth, D.B., Menetski, J.P., Nakajima, P.B., Bosma, M.Y., Gellert, M.: **V(D)J recombination: Broken DNA molecules with covalently sealed (hairpin) coding ends in *scid* mouse thymocytes.** *Cell* 1992, **70**:983-991.

Schwartz, K., Hausen-Hagge, T.E., Knobloch, C., Friedrich, W., Kleihauer, E., Bartram, K.: ***Scid* in man: B-cell negative SCID patients exhibit an irregular recombination pattern at the JH locus.** *J. Exper. Med.* 1991, **174**:1039-1048.

10-12 Defective cytokine production or cytokine action can cause immunodeficiency.

Arnaz-Villena, A., Timon, M., Corell, A., Perez-Aciego, P., Martin-Villa, J.M., and Regueiro, J.R.: **Primary immunodeficiency caused by mutations in the gene encoding the C3-γ subunit of the T-lymphocyte receptor.** *N. Engl. J. Med.* 1992, **327**:529-533.

Chatila, T., Wong, R., Young, M., Miller, R., Terhorst, C., and Geha, R.S.: **An immunodeficiency characterized by defective signal transduction in T lymphocytes.** *N. Engl. J. Med.* 1989, **320**:696-702.

Chatila, T., Castigli, E., Pahwa, R., Pahwa, S., Chirmule, S., Oyaizu, N., Godd, R.A., Godd, R.A., Geha, R.S.: **Primary combined immunodeficiency resulting from defective transcription of multiple T-cell lymphokine genes.** *Proc. Natl. Acad. Sci. USA* 1990, **87**:10033-10037.

Disanto, J.P., Keever, C.A., Small, T.N., Nichols, G.L., O'Reilly, R.J., Flombenberg, N.: **Absence of interleukin-2 production in a severe combined immunodeficiency disease syndrome with T cells.** *J. Exper. Med.* 1990, **171**:1697-1704.

Noguchi, M., Nakamura, Y., Russell, S.M., Ziegler, S.F., Tsang, M., Cao, X., and Leonard, W.J.: **Interleukin-2 receptor gamma chain: A functional component of the interleukin-7 receptor.** *Science* 1993, **262**:1877-1880.

Russell, S.M., Keegan, A.D., Harada, N., Nakamura, Y., Noguchi, M., Leland, P., Friedmann, M.C., Miyajima, A., Puri, R.K., Paul, W.E., and Leomard, W.J.: **Interleukin-2 receptor gamma chain: A functional component of the interleukin-4 receptor.** *Science* 1993, **262**:1880-1883.

Soudais, C., de Villartay, J.P., Le Deist, F.: Fischer, A., Lisowska-Grospierre, B.: **Independent mutations of the human CD3ε gene resulting in a T-cell receptor/CD3 complex immunodeficiency.** *Nature Genet.* 1993, **3**:77-81.

Weinberg, K. and Parkman, R.: **Severe combined immunodeficiency due to a specific defect in the production of IL-2**. *N. Engl. J. Med.* 1990, **322**: 1718-1723.

10-13 Transplantation or gene therapy may be useful to correct genetic defects.

Buckley, R.H., Schiff, S.E., Sampson, H.A., Schiff, R.I., Markert, M.L., Knutsen, A.P., Hershfield, M.S., Huang, A.T., Mickey, G.H., and Ward, F.E.: **Development of immunity in severe primary T-cell deficiency following haploidentical bone marrow stem cell transplantation**. *J. Immunol.* 1986, **136**: 2398-2407.

Cournoyer, D. and Caskey, C.T.: **Gene therapy of the immune system**. *Ann. Rev. Immunol.* 1993, **11**:297-332.

10-14 Most individuals infected with HIV progress over time to AIDS.

Pantaleo, G., and Fauci, A.S.: **New concepts in the immunopathogenesis of HIV infection**. *Ann. Rev. Immunol.* 1995, **13**:487-512.

Darby, S.C., Ewart, D.W., Giangrande, P.L.F., Dolin, P.J., Spooner, R.J.D., and Rizza, C.R.: **Mortality before and after HIV infection in the complete UK population of haemophiliacs**. *Nature* 1995, **377**:79-82.

10-15 HIV is a retrovirus that infects CD4 T cells and macrophages.

Subbramanian, R.A., and Cohen, E.A.: **Molecular biology of the human immunodeficiency virus accessory proteins**. *J. Virol.* 1994, **68**:6831-6835.

Trono, D.: **HIV accessory proteins: leading roles for the supporting act**. *Cell* 1995, **82**:189-192.

10-16 Transcription of the HIV provirus depends on host-cell transcription factors induced upon activation of the infected cell.

Jones, K.A., and Peterlin, B.M.: **Control of RNA initiation and elongation at the HIV-1 promotor**. *Ann. Rev. Biochem.* 1994, **63**:717-743.

10-17 HIV accumulates mutations in the course of infection in a single individual.

Chynier, R., Henrichwark, S., Hadida, F., Pelletier, E., Ocksenhendler, E., Autran, B., and Wain-Hobson, S.: **HIV and T cell expansion in splenic white pulps is accompanied by infiltration of HIV-specific cytotoxic T lymphocytes**. *Cell* 1995, **78**:373-387.

Coffin, J.M.: **HIV population dynamics *in vivo*: implications for genetic variation, pathogenesis, and therapy**. *Science* 1995, **267**:483-489.

10-18 An immune response controls but does not eliminate HIV.

Chynier, R., Henrichwark, S., Hadida, F., Pelletier, E., Ocksenhendler, E., Autran, B., and Wain-Hobson, S.: **HIV and T cell expansion in splenic white pulps is accompanied by infiltration of HIV-specific cytotoxic T lymphocytes**. *Cell* 1995, **78**:373-387.

Klein, M.R., van Faalen, C.A., Holwerda, A.M., Garde, S.R.K., Bende, R.J., Keet, I.P.M., Eeftinck-Schattenkerk, J.K.M., Oserhaos, A.D.M.E., Schuitemaker, H., and Miedema, F.: **Kinetics of Gag-specific cytotoxic T lymphocyte responses during the clinical course of HIV-1 infection: A longitudinal analysis of rapid progressors and long-term asymptomatics**. *J. Exp. Med.* 1995, **181**:1365-1372.

Rowland Jones, S., Sutton, J., Ariyoshi, K., Dong, T., Gotch, F., McAdam, S., Whitby, D., Sabally, S., Gallimore, A., Corrah, T., Takiguchi, M., Schultz, T.,

McMichael, A., Whittle, H.: **HIV-specific cytotoxic T-cells in HIV-exposed but uninfected Gambian women**. *Nature Medicine.* 1995, **1**:59-64.

10-19 Drugs that block HIV replication lead to a rapid fall in titer of infectious virus and a rise in CD4 T cells, followed by the outgrowth of drug-resistant variant virus.

Ho, D.D., Neumann, A.U., Perelson, A.S., Chen, W., Leonard, J.M., and Markowitz, M.: **Rapid turnover of plasma virions and CD4 lymphocytes in HIV-1 infection**. *Nature* 1995, **373**:123-126.

Wei, X, Ghosh, S.K., Taylor, M.E., Johnson, V.A., Emini, E.A., Deutsch, P., Lifson, J.D., Bonhoeffer, S., Nowak, M.A., Hahn, B.H., Saag, M.S., and Shaw, G.M.: **Viral dynamics in human immunodeficiency virus type 1 infection**. *Nature* 1995, **373**:117-122.

10-20 HIV infection leads to low levels of CD4 T cells, increased susceptibility to opportunistic infection, and eventually to death.

De Rossi, A., Franchini, G., Aldovini, A., Del Mistro, A., Chieco-Bianchi, L., Gallo, R.C., and Wong-Staal, F.: **Differential response to the cytopathic effects of human T-cell lymphotropic virus type III (HTLV-III) superinfection in T4$^+$ (helper) and T8$^+$ (suppressor) T-cell clones transformed by HTLV-1**. *Proc. Natl. Acad. Sci. USA* 1986, **83**:4297-4301.

Katlama, C., and Dickenson, G.: **Update on opportunistic infections**. *AIDS* 1993, **7**:5158-5194.

Koga, Y., Sasaki, M., Yoshida, H., Wigzell, H., Kimura, G., and Nomoto, K.: **Cytopathic effect determined by the amount of CD4 molecules in human cell lines expressing envelope glycoprotein of HIV**. *J. Immunol.* 1990, **144**:94-102.

Siliken, S., and Boyle, M.J.: **Update on HIV and neoplastic disease**. *AIDS* 1993, **7**:203-209.

Somasundaram, M., and Robinson, H.L.: **A major mechanism of human immunodeficiency virus-induced cell killing does not involve cell fusion**. *J. Virol.* 1987, **61**:3114-3119.

10-21 Vaccination against HIV is an attractive solution to the problem of AIDS but poses many difficulties.

Cease, K.B., and Berzofsky, J.A.: **Toward a vaccine for AIDS: The emergence of immunobiology-based vaccine development**. *Ann. Rev. Immunol.* 1994, **12**:923-989.

Fast, P.E., and Walker, M.C.: **Human trials of experimental AIDS vaccines**. *AIDS* 1993, **7**:147-159.

Girard, M.P., and Shearer, G.M.: **Vaccines and immunology**. *AIDS* 1993, **7**:115-116.

Salk, J., Bretscher, P.A., Salk, P.L., Clerici, M., and Shearer, G.M.: **A strategy for prophylactic vaccination against HIV**. *Science* 1993, **260**:1270-1272.

10-22 Prevention and education are one way in which the spread of HIV and AIDS can be controlled.

Decosas, J., and Finlay, J.: **International AIDS aid: The response of development aid agencies to the HIV/AIDS pandemic**. *AIDS* 1993, **7**:281-286.

Dowsett, G.W.: **Sustaining safe sex: Sexual practices, HIV and social context**. *AIDS* 1993, **7**:257-262.

Kimball, A.M., Berkley, S., Ngugi, E., and Gayle, H.: **International aspects of the AIDS/HIV epidemic**. *Ann. Rev. Public Health.* 1995, **16**:253-282.

MacQueen, K.M.: **The epidemiology of HIV transmission: Trends, structure, and dynamics**. *Ann. Rev. Anthropol.* 1994, **23**:509-526.

Immune Responses in the Absence of Infection

11

We have learned in the preceding chapters that the adaptive immune response is a critical component of host defense against infection and therefore essential for normal health. Adaptive immune responses are also sometimes elicited by antigens not associated with infectious agents, and this may cause serious disease. These responses are essentially identical to adaptive immune responses to infectious agents; only the antigens differ. Responses to three particularly important categories of antigen will be examined in this chapter: inappropriate responses to innocuous foreign substances, called **allergy** or **hypersensitivity**; responses to self tissue antigens, called **autoimmunity**, which can lead to **autoimmune diseases** characterized by tissue damage; and responses to transplanted organs that lead to **graft rejection**.

The deleterious consequences of these adaptive responses are mediated by the very same mechanisms used in protective immunity to destroy pathogens and host cells infected with pathogens. They can be divided into several classes depending on the immune mechanism that causes damage to the host, and whether the antigen is cell-associated or soluble (Fig. 11.1). Responses characterized by IgE antibody production, mast cell sensitization, activation of helper CD4 T cells (T_H2), and recruitment of eosinophils are the most important in allergy, while other classes of **hypersensitivity reactions** are seen in different forms of allergy, autoimmunity, and graft rejection. In this chapter, we will examine these disease processes and the mechanisms that lead to the undesirable adaptive immune responses that are their root cause.

	Type I	Type II		Type III	Type IV	
Immune reactant	IgE antibody, T_H2 cells	IgG antibody		IgG antibody	T cells	
Antigen	Soluble antigen	Cell- or matrix-associated antigen	Cell-surface receptors	Soluble antigen	Soluble antigen	Cell-associated antigen
Effector mechanism	Mast-cell activation	Complement, FcR^+ cells (phagocytes, NK cells)	Antibody alters signaling	Complement Phagocytes	Macrophage activation	Cytotoxicity
Example of hypersensitivity reaction	Allergic rhinitis, asthma, systemic anaphylaxis	Some drug allergies (eg penicillin), transfusion reaction, autoimmune hemolytic anemia	Graves' disease (agonist) Myasthenia gravis (antagonist)	Serum sickness, Systemic lupus erythematosus	Contact dermatitis, graft rejection, rheumatoid arthritis	Contact dermatitis, graft rejection, diabetes mellitus

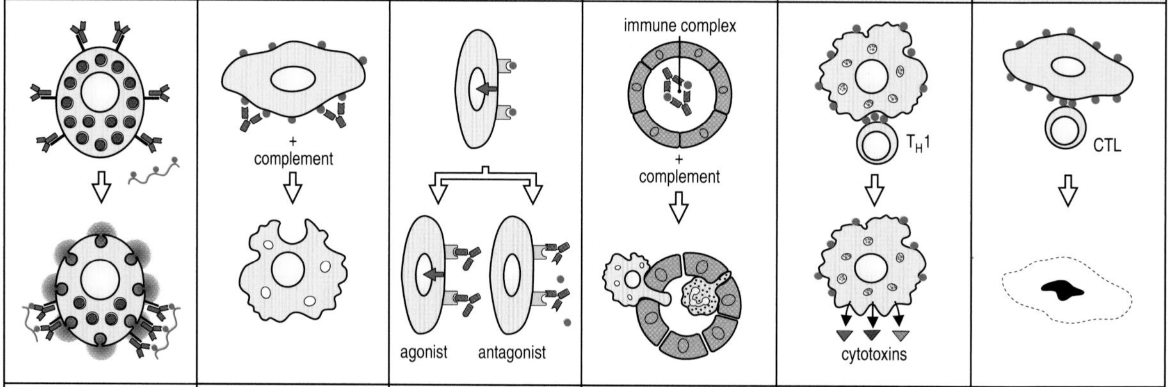

Fig. 11.1   There are four types of immune-mediated tissue damage. Types I–III are antibody-mediated and are distinguished by the different types of antigens recognized and the different classes of antibody involved. Type I responses are mediated by IgE, which induces mast-cell activation, while types II and III are mediated by IgG, which can activate either complement-mediated or phagocytic effector mechanisms. These different effector mechanisms lead to sharply different tissue damage and pathology. Type II responses are directed against cell-surface or matrix-associated antigen, leading to tissue damage, whereas type III responses are directed against soluble antigens, and the tissue damage involved is caused by responses triggered by immune complexes. A special class of type II responses involves IgG antibodies to cell-surface receptors, which disrupt the normal function of the receptor, either by causing uncontrolled activation or by blocking receptor function. Since cell-surface receptors are self proteins, this class of type II reaction is seen only in autoimmune diseases. Type IV is T-cell mediated, and can be subdivided into two classes; in the first class, tissue damage is caused by activation of inflammatory responses by inflammatory T cells (T_H1 cells), mediated mainly by macrophages, and in the second, damage is directly caused by cytotoxic T cells. All of the classes of hypersensitivity responses are seen in both autoimmunity and allergy, with the exception of type I hypersensitivity; IgE responses have not been observed in autoimmunity.

Allergy: responses to innocuous substances.

Allergic reactions occur when an already immune or **sensitized** individual is re-exposed to the same innocuous foreign substance or **allergen**. Allergic responses range from the familiar runny nose and sneezing seen in hay fever to systemic anaphylaxis and death in response to a bee sting or insect bite in highly sensitized individuals. These responses do not occur when a naive individual is first exposed to an allergen; the initial adaptive response takes time, and usually does not cause any symptoms. Once antibody or T cells that react with the allergen have been produced, however, any further exposure will produce symptoms. These responses are identical to the response to a pathogen, but since the foreign substance itself is innocuous the only pathology seen is that caused by the immune response. Allergic responses thus demonstrate further that the immune response itself can cause significant pathology, as it does in some responses to infection (see Section 10-5).

Allergic reactions were initially classified by their clinical effects, since the mechanisms underlying the responses were unknown. Allergic reactions that occur rapidly are called **immediate hypersensitivity reactions** and are dominated by reactions mediated by IgE and helper T cells (T_H2), the latter taking some time to become manifest, and hence being called **late-phase reactions**. Immediate hypersensitivity reactions are also known as **atopic allergy** or **atopy**. **Delayed-type hypersensitivity** reactions are caused by responses involving inflammatory CD4 T cells (T_H1) and cytotoxic CD8 T cells, which may take a day or two to reach their maximum effect. In some cases, allergic responses are complex in their development and cannot be classified readily into a single type. We do not yet understand what causes some individuals to become allergic to a substance while others do not, but MHC genotype clearly plays a role in determining susceptibility to allergy.

11-1   Allergic reactions occur when extrinsic antigens are recognized by a pre-sensitized individual.

Many common allergies are caused by allergens carried by inhaled particles or are directed against substances that make contact with the skin; these are antigens that originate outside the body and are thus termed extrinsic. The first exposure generates antibodies and T cells; re-exposure to the same allergen, usually by the same route, leads to an **allergic reaction**. The response can involve any of the mechanisms shown in Fig. 11.1.

Hay fever is a typical allergic reaction. Initial exposure to proteins in inhaled pollen grains elicits an IgE antibody response presumably by eliciting a predominantly helper T-cell response; IL-4 produced by activated helper T cells will induce B cells to switch the isotype of antibody they produce to IgE. When the same pollen is later inhaled, the proteins diffuse across the respiratory epithelium of the upper airway where they bind to this preformed IgE on submucosal mast cells (see Section 8-20), activating the mast cells lining the airways so that hay fever or asthma develops (Fig. 11.2). Once an individual is sensitized, the allergic reactions often become worse with each exposure, as each re-exposure not only produces allergic symptoms but also increases the level of antibody and helper T cells present.

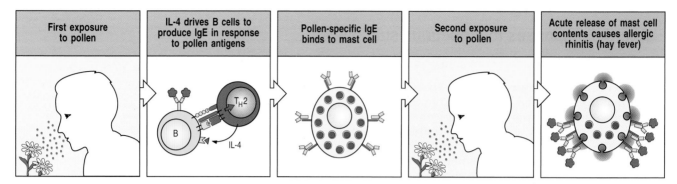

| First exposure to pollen | IL-4 drives B cells to produce IgE in response to pollen antigens | Pollen-specific IgE binds to mast cell | Second exposure to pollen | Acute release of mast cell contents causes allergic rhinitis (hay fever) |

Fig. 11.2 Allergic reactions require prior exposure to the allergen. In this example, the first exposure to pollen induces the production of IgE anti-pollen antibodies, driven by the production of IL-4 by helper T cells (T_H2). The IgE binds to mast cells via FcεRI. Once enough IgE antibody is present on mast cells, exposure to the same pollen induces mast-cell activation and an acute allergic reaction, here allergic rhinitis or hay fever. All allergic reactions require pre-sensitization to the antigen or allergen, and several exposures may be needed before the allergic reaction is initiated.

In the case of IgE-mediated responses, allergists use carefully controlled and repeated exposure to the allergen to **desensitize** the patient, which is believed to gradually divert the response to one dominated by inflammatory T cells and may involve production of IgG and IgA antibodies specific for the allergen. This has been termed **immune deviation**. Although this reduces the impact of inhaled allergens, we shall see in a subsequent section that IgG antibodies and inflammatory T-cell responses can cause tissue damage when they interact with high levels of antigen.

11-2   The nature of the allergic reaction depends on the nature of the immune response.

The antibody-mediated hypersensitivity reactions can be divided into three classes, as shown in Fig. 11.1. Most common allergies result from the production of IgE antibody, which elicits a type I hypersensitivity reaction. This is the classic immediate hypersensitivity reaction occurring within seconds or minutes of antigen contact. The IgE activates mast cells to release vasoactive amines, leukotrienes, and cytokines, exactly as if the mast cell were responding to an infection (see Section 8-21). IgE-mediated allergic reactions are a major cause of symptoms in otherwise healthy individuals. Some of the allergic diseases caused by type I hypersensitivity reactions are summarized in Fig. 11.3.

Some allergic responses involve antibody isotypes other than IgE. If the allergen is cell-bound, the reactions are classified as type II hypersensitivity; the antibody activates complement and Fc-mediated effector reactions, and the cells are attacked much as if they were bacteria (see Sections 8-18 and 8-22–8-30). If the allergen is soluble, immune complexes form in the tissues where antigen is present, and this causes local inflammation, classified as a type III hypersensitivity reaction. While type I responses occur within minutes of allergen contact, type II and type III reactions generally occur within a few hours of exposure.

In type IV hypersensitivity reactions, the allergen may be a foreign protein or a chemical substance that reacts with self proteins. When self proteins are modified chemically, their modified self peptides appear foreign to T cells. Once a person is sensitized to a modified self peptide or a foreign protein, re-exposure leads to a T-cell response that evolves over several days, so these reactions are called delayed-type hypersensitivity.

IgE-mediated allergic reactions			
Syndrome	Common allergens	Route of entry	Response
Systemic anaphylaxis	Drugs Serum Venoms	Intravenous	Edema Vasodilation Tracheal occlusion Circulatory collapse Death
Wheal and flare	Insect bites Allergy testing	Subcutaneous	Local vasodilation Local edema
Allergic rhinitis (hay fever)	Pollens (ragweed, timothy, birch) Dust mite feces	Inhaled	Edema of nasal mucosa Irritation of nasal mucosa
Bronchial asthma	Pollens Dust mite feces	Inhaled	Bronchial constriction Increased mucus production Airway inflammation
Food allergy	Shellfish Milk Eggs Fish Wheat	Oral	Vomiting Diarrhea Pruritis (itching) Urticaria (hives)

Fig. 11.3 IgE-mediated reactions to extrinsic antigens. All IgE-mediated responses involve mast-cell degranulation, but the symptoms experienced by the patient can be very different depending on whether the allergen is injected, inhaled or eaten, and depending on the dose of the allergen (see also Fig. 11.5).

Such responses usually result from direct contact of the skin with the source of the allergen and therefore are also known as **contact hypersensitivity reactions**. The T-cell response can be caused by either CD4 or CD8 T cells, and can damage tissues either by the release of inflammatory cytokines (see Section 7-25) or by direct cytotoxicity, rather as if the host cell presenting the modified peptide is virus-infected (see Section 7-21).

Thus, the class of antibody or T cell produced in response to an allergen determines what type of allergic reaction will follow re-exposure to it. Because IgE responses are driven by helper T cells, which are a prominent feature of allergy, it is important to determine why certain allergens are particularly good at eliciting T$_H$2 cells that help IgE antibody production, and why some people are more susceptible to allergies than others. The current approaches to this problem will be examined in the next few sections.

11-3   Allergens that elicit IgE responses are often delivered transmucosally at low dose.

Much human allergy is caused by a limited number of inhaled protein allergens that reproducibly elicit helper T cells that help the IgE antibody response. Since we inhale many different proteins that do not induce IgE production, this has led researchers to ask what is unusual about the proteins that are common allergens. Although we still do not understand this completely, some general principles have emerged (Fig. 11.4).

Most allergens are relatively small, highly soluble protein molecules that are inhaled in desiccated particles such as pollen grains or mite feces. The allergen elutes from the particle because it is readily soluble and diffuses into the mucosa. Allergens are presented to the immune system at very low doses. It has been estimated that the maximum exposure of a

Features of inhaled allergens that may promote IgE responses	
Protein	Only proteins induce T-cell responses
Low dose	Favors activation of IL-4-producing CD4 T cells
Low molecular weight	Diffuses out of particle into mucus
High solubility	Readily eluted from particle
Stable	Allows survival in desiccated particle
Contains peptides that bind host MHC class II	Required for T-cell priming (see Section 11-14)

Fig. 11.4 Properties of inhaled allergens.

person to common pollen allergens in ragweed cannot exceed 1 µg per year! Yet many people develop irritating and even life-threatening T_H2-driven IgE antibody responses to these minute doses of allergen. It is important to note that only a fraction of people who are exposed to these substances make IgE antibody to them. The host factors that influence which individuals will respond to allergens are considered in the next section.

It seems likely that transmucosal presentation of very low doses of allergen is particularly efficient at inducing IgE responses. As we learned in Chapter 8, IgE antibody production requires IL-4-producing helper T cells and can be inhibited by interferon-γ (IFN-γ)-producing inflammatory T cells (see Fig. 8.7). We have learned (see Section 9-16) that the low doses at which allergens enter the body across mucosal surfaces can favor activation of helper T cells over inflammatory T cells. The dominant antigen-presenting cell type in the respiratory mucosa is a cell with characteristics similar to Langerhans' cells (see Chapters 7 and 9), which are thought to bind allergens and transport them to local lymph nodes where naive CD4 T cells first encounter their peptides. These cells take up protein antigens poorly, but are highly co-stimulatory and, while they may produce small amounts of IL-12, they are unlikely to direct the priming of inflammatory T cells, which is favored by exposure to IL-12 (see Section 9-15).

11-4 Genetic factors contribute to the preferential priming of helper T cells and IgE-mediated allergy.

There are several factors that predispose an individual to develop IgE antibody responses driven by helper T cells. One factor is the individual's MHC class II genotype, which controls responses to specific allergens. IgE production is tightly regulated, as can be seen by the very low serum levels of IgE in most individuals in industrialized countries (see Fig. 3.23). However, very high levels of IgE antibodies are stimulated by infection with parasitic worms, perhaps because IgE is protective against worm infestation (see Fig. 8.28).

Most allergic individuals tend to make IgE antibody to only one or a few allergens. In such patients, there is a clearly discernible relationship between IgE antibody production to a given allergen and genotype at the MHC class II locus HLA-DR. As we saw in Section 11-1, patients with high IgE levels are sometimes given increasing doses of allergen in an attempt to switch the predominant type of T cell to inflammatory T cells and favor an antibody response dominated by IgG. This has indicated that the HLA-DR genotypes that make a patient more likely to produce IgE antibodies to natural allergen exposure also favor the switch to inflammatory T cells and the production of IgG. This strongly suggests that these HLA-DR molecules bind peptides of the allergen particularly well, presenting them to T cells at high levels when the allergen is used to desensitize the patient; effective peptide binding to MHC class II molecules would enhance both the likelihood of the initial IgE response and the likelihood of switching that response to IgG when large amounts of allergen are given, because increasing the amount of specific peptide:MHC complex favors the priming of inflammatory T cells (see Section 9-16).

A second genetic factor has been identified from population studies of IgE levels. Some individuals appear to respond to many antigens by making high levels of IgE, and these persons frequently develop IgE-mediated allergic responses, a condition known as atopy. In family studies, the gene (or genes) responsible for the high IgE levels has been linked to the gene for IL-4; since IL-4 is required to induce B cells to undergo isotype switching to produce IgE, it is possible that the underlying cause of the high IgE levels in atopic individuals is excessive production of IL-4.

Finally, some people appear to be more able to respond to all antigens. This trait is not fully understood but may also be associated with MHC genotype. Two frequent HLA haplotypes are associated with a propensity to develop autoimmune disease and allergic reactions. It is far from clear whether this heightened responsiveness is beneficial to the host, but, if we suppose that these individuals also respond more rapidly and effectively to pathogens, it may have provided an evolutionary advantage. These genetic factors must be understood before we will know why only some people develop allergic reactions.

11-5 | IgE-mediated responses have different consequences depending on the dose of allergen and its route of entry.

Type I hypersensitivity reactions are triggered when the allergen binds to specific IgE antibodies bound to FcεRI on mast cells. When the bound IgE antibodies are crosslinked by allergen, mast cells are activated to release stored preformed mediators that alter the blood vessels and smooth muscle cells in their immediate vicinity. The clinical syndrome produced depends critically on three variables: the amount of IgE antibody present; the route by which the allergen is introduced; and its dose (summarized in Fig. 11.5).

If the allergen is given systemically, the connective tissue mast cells associated with all blood vessels may be activated. This causes a very dangerous syndrome called **systemic anaphylaxis**. Disseminated mast-cell activation causes widespread vasodilation leading to a catastrophic loss of blood pressure, constriction of the airways, and epiglottal swelling that often leads to suffocation, a syndrome called **anaphylactic shock**. This can occur if drugs are administered to allergic people, or after an insect bite in individuals allergic to insect venom. This syndrome is rapidly fatal but can usually be controlled by immediate injection of epinephrine.

The most frequent allergic reaction to drugs occurs with penicillin and its relatives. In people with IgE antibodies to penicillin, intravenous administration can cause anaphylaxis and even death. Great care should therefore be taken to determine whether a person is allergic to penicillin before it is given. Penicillin acts as a hapten (see Section 8-2); it is a small molecule with a highly reactive β-lactam ring, crucial for its antibiotic activity. This ring reacts with amino groups on host proteins forming covalent conjugates. When penicillin is ingested or injected, it forms conjugates with self proteins and alters them sufficiently to induce helper T cells specific for penicillin-modified self peptides. These helper T cells then activate penicillin-binding B cells to produce antibody to the penicillin hapten; for unknown reasons, these are usually IgE antibodies. Thus, penicillin acts both as the B-cell antigen and, by modifying self peptides, as the T-cell antigen. When penicillin is injected intravenously into allergic individuals, the penicillin-modified proteins crosslink IgE molecules on the mast cells to cause anaphylaxis.

Local administration of small amounts of allergen in the skin leads to a much more limited allergic reaction. Local mast-cell activation in the skin causes a local vasodilation and extravasation of fluid called a **wheal and flare reaction**; it is one standard way of testing people for allergy. Another standard test for allergy is to measure IgE antibody levels to a particular allergen in a sandwich ELISA or radioimmuno-assay (see Section 2-7).

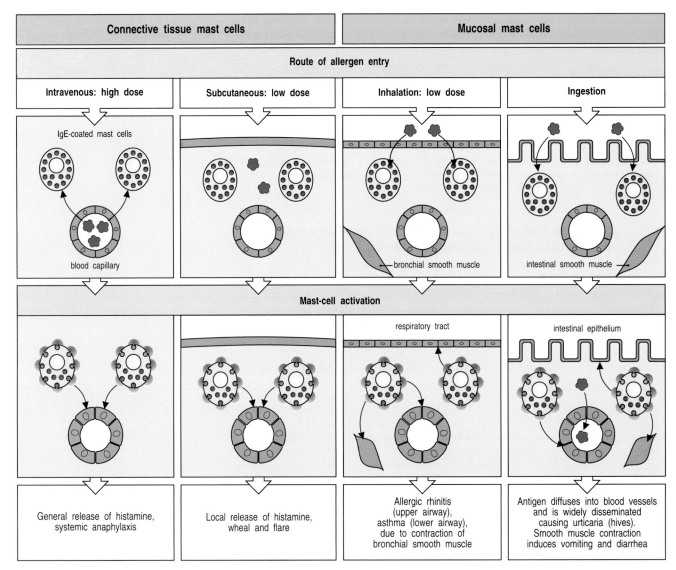

Fig. 11.5   The dose and route of allergen administration determines the type of IgE-mediated allergic reaction that results. There are two main classes of mast cells, those associated with blood vessels, called connective tissue mast cells, and those found in submucosal layers, called mucosal mast cells. In an allergic individual, all of these are loaded with IgE directed against a particular allergen. The overall response to an allergen then depends on which mast cells are activated. Allergen in the bloodstream activates connective tissue mast cells throughout the body, resulting in systemic release of histamine and other mediators. Subcutaneous administration of allergen activates only local connective tissue mast cells, leading to a local inflammatory reaction. Inhaled allergen, penetrating across epithelia, activates mainly mucosal mast cells, increasing the local secretion of mucus and causing irritation. It also causes smooth muscle contraction in the lower airways, leading to bronchoconstriction and difficulty in expelling inhaled air. Similarly, ingested allergen penetrates across gut epithelia, causing vomiting due to smooth muscle contraction; the food allergen is also disseminated in the bloodstream causing urticaria (hives).

Inhalation is the most common route for allergen entry. Many people have mild allergies to inhaled antigens, manifest as sneezing and runny nose. This is called **allergic rhinitis** or hay fever, and results from activation of mucosal mast cells beneath the nasal epithelium by allergens that diffuse across the mucous membrane of the nasal passages. This is annoying but causes little lasting damage. A more serious syndrome is **allergic asthma**, which is caused by activation of submucosal mast cells in the lower airways. This leads to bronchial constriction and increased fluid and mucus secretion, making breathing more difficult by trapping inhaled air in the lungs. Patients with allergic asthma often need treatment, and asthmatic attacks can be life-threatening.

Finally, when the allergen is eaten, two types of allergic response are seen. Activation of mucosal mast cells associated with the gastrointestinal tract can lead to transepithelial fluid loss and smooth muscle contraction, generating vomiting and diarrhea. Connective tissue mast cells in the deeper layers of the skin are also activated, presumably by IgE binding to the ingested and absorbed allergen borne by the blood, producing **urticaria** or hives — large red swellings beneath the skin. This is a common reaction when penicillin is ingested by an allergic patient. Exactly why urticaria results from ingesting allergens is not known.

| 11-6 | **Treatment with anti-histamines affects only the first phase of the IgE-mediated response.** |

The initial response to IgE triggering of mast cells is immediate release of preformed mast-cell granule contents (see Fig. 8.30), particularly the vasoactive amine histamine and various enzymes. Later on, arachidonic acid metabolism in the mast cells generates leukotrienes (see Fig. 8.31), which are also pro-inflammatory, causing a more sustained increase in blood flow and vascular permeability. Cytokines such as IL-3, IL-4, IL-5, and tumor necrosis factor-α (TNF-α) are also produced both by helper T cells and by activated mast cells and these further prolong the allergic reaction. The mediators and cytokines released by mast cells and by helper T cells cause an influx of monocytes, T cells, and eosinophils into the site of allergen entry. Thus, within six to twelve hours a late-phase reaction appears that is dominated by a cellular infiltrate, made up of eosinophils and other inflammatory cells, which make a variety of toxic products. Much of the tissue damage that is associated with chronic allergic reactions is thought to occur in this way. Allergic reactions are often treated with anti-histamine drugs, which affect only the early-phase reaction. The late-phase reaction is best inhibited by corticosteroids.

The changes that occur in many IgE-mediated allergic reactions are transient and resolve when the antigen is removed. However, if these responses recur many times, chronic inflammation can result. In asthma, the repetitive stimulation of antigen-sensitive helper T cells and mast cells bearing bound IgE leads to an abnormal airway that is chronically inflamed and therefore much more susceptible to other types of stimuli, such as changes in temperature or airborne pollutants. The chronically inflamed airway is not significantly affected by anti-histamines or other drugs that may be effective in the immediate-phase response.

| 11-7 | **Some immediate hypersensitivity reactions are mediated by IgG antibodies.** |

The hypersensitivity reactions mediated by helper T cells and IgE are by far the most prevalent allergic reactions. However, there are some medically important hypersensitivity reactions that are due to IgG antibodies. These are called type II and type III hypersensitivity reactions (see Fig. 11.1); they do not involve the activation of mast cells.

Type II hypersensitivity reactions involve binding of IgG (and occasionally IgM) antibodies to cell surfaces or to extracellular matrix molecules. The bound antibodies activate complement and Fc receptor-bearing accessory cells, as they would in host defense against infectious agents. Red blood cells and platelets are particularly vulnerable to this type of response, as they have lower levels of complement regulatory proteins than other cells. Certain drugs such as quinidine, which is used to treat cardiac arrhythmias, can bind to cell membranes; IgG antibodies to these drugs can bind to the modified cell membranes. The most obvious result of such a reaction is the lysis of red blood cells via complement activation. This is an uncommon but important form of allergic reaction.

Type III hypersensitivity reactions arise when the allergen is soluble. The pathology is caused by deposition of antigen:antibody aggregates or **immune complexes** in certain tissue sites. Immune complexes are generated in every antibody response. The pathogenic potential of immune complexes is determined in part by their size. Larger aggregates fix complement and are readily removed by phagocytes, while the small complexes that form at antigen excess (see Fig. 2.13) tend to deposit in blood vessel walls, and it is here that they cause tissue damage. When a sensitized individual has IgG antibodies directed against an antigen, immune complexes can be generated locally by injection of the antigen. If the antigen is injected into the skin, IgG antibody that has diffused into the tissues forms immune complexes locally. The immune complexes activate complement, releasing C5a, which creates a local inflammatory response with increased vascular permeability. The enhanced vascular permeability allows fluid and cells, especially polymorphonuclear leukocytes, to enter the site from the local vessels. This is called an **Arthus reaction** (Fig. 11.6).

A somewhat different reaction occurs when foreign proteins are injected in large amounts into healthy individuals. In the pre-antibiotic era, immune horse serum was often used to treat pneumococcal pneumonia. Specific antibodies in the horse serum would help the patient to clear the infection. In much the same way, anti-venin (serum from horses immunized with snake venoms) is still used today as a source of neutralizing antibodies to treat people suffering from the bites of poisonous snakes. However, such treatments also stimulate the immune system to make IgG antibody to the foreign serum proteins, and after a period of time immune complexes form throughout the body.

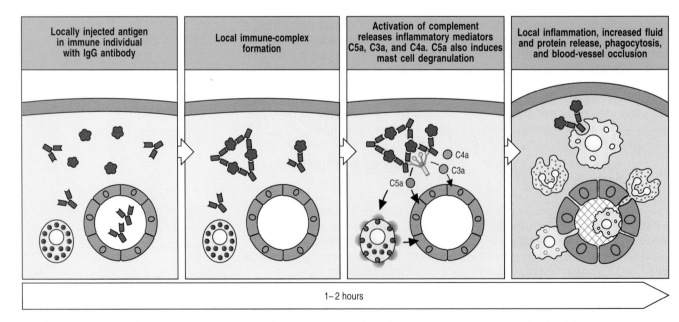

Fig. 11.6   The deposition of immune complexes in local tissues causes a local inflammatory response known as an Arthus reaction (Type III). In individuals who have already made IgG antibody to allergen, allergen injected into the skin forms immune complexes with IgG antibody that has diffused out of the capillaries. Since the dose of antigen is low, the immune complexes are only formed close to the site of injection, where they activate complement, releasing inflammatory mediators such as C5a which in turn can activate mast cells (see Fig. 8.30). As a result, inflammatory cells invade the site and blood-vessel permeability and blood flow are increased. Platelets also accumulate at the site, ultimately leading to vessel occlusion.

Fig. 11.7 Serum sickness is a classical example of a transient immune-complex-mediated syndrome. An injection of a foreign protein or proteins, in this case derived from horse serum, leads to an antibody response. These antibodies form immune complexes with the circulating foreign proteins. These complexes activate complement and phagocytes, inducing fever, and are deposited in small vessels, inducing symptoms of vasculitis, nephritis and arthritis. All these effects are transient and resolve when the foreign protein is cleared.

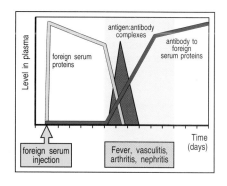

This produces a disease called **serum sickness**, with a clinical picture of fever, joint tenderness, urticaria, and proteinuria. Fortunately, serum sickness resolves completely when the antigen has been eliminated and leaves no obvious pathology behind (Fig. 11.7). This is an unusual type of allergy; because serum proteins (the allergen) are given in large amounts and are long-lived, the sensitization and the allergic reaction both take place after only one dose of allergen. Immune complexes also form in autoimmune diseases such as systemic lupus erythematosus where, because the antigen persists, the deposition of immune complexes continues, and serious disease can result (see Section 11-13).

Several different clinical outcomes are possible for IgG-mediated reactions to a soluble antigen (Fig. 11.8). As for IgE-mediated hypersensitivities, the dose and route of antigen administration is of critical importance. A large dose of antigen delivered systemically leads to a serum-sickness-like syndrome. Provided antigen administration is not sustained or repeated frequently, the immune complexes are solubilized by complement or digested by phagocytic cells, and the patient returns to normal. When antigen is injected locally into the skin, an Arthus reaction results. This can also resolve when the antigen has been cleared, but if the response is very intense it can lead to local clotting and tissue necrosis.

Some inhaled allergens provoke IgG rather than IgE antibody responses, perhaps because they are present at much higher levels in inhaled air. When a person is re-exposed to high doses of such inhaled antigens, immune complexes form in the alveolar wall of the lung. This leads to the accumulation of fluid, protein and cells in the alveolar wall, slowing blood–gas interchange and compromising lung function. This type of reaction occurs in certain occupations such as farming, where exposure to hay dust or mold spores is repetitive. The disease that results is therefore called **farmer's lung**. It can lead to permanent damage to the alveolar membranes if exposure is sustained.

Route	Resulting disease	Site of immune complex deposition
Intravenous (high dose)	Vasculitis	Blood vessel walls
	Nephritis	Renal glomeruli
	Arthritis	Joint spaces
Subcutaneous	Arthus reaction	Perivascular area
Inhaled	Farmer's lung	Alveolar/capillary interface

Fig. 11.8 The dose and route of antigen delivery determines the pathology observed in type III allergic reactions.

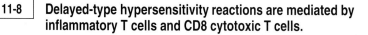

11-8   Delayed-type hypersensitivity reactions are mediated by inflammatory T cells and CD8 cytotoxic T cells.

Unlike the immediate hypersensitivity reactions, which are mediated by antibodies, delayed-type hypersensitivity or type IV hypersensitivity reactions are mediated by specific T cells. Allergic diseases in which type IV hypersensitivity responses predominate are shown in Fig. 11.9. These responses are clearly caused by T cells, since they can be seen in agammaglobulinemic individuals. Such responses can also be transferred between experimental animals using pure T cells or cloned T-cell lines.

The prototypic delayed-type hypersensitivity reaction is an artifact of modern medicine, the tuberculin test (see Section 2-30). This is not an allergic reaction, but a way of determining whether an individual has previously been infected with *Mycobacterium tuberculosis*. When

Fig. 11.9 Type IV responses in allergy. Depending on the source of antigen and its route of introduction, these clinical conditions have different names and consequences.

Type IV hypersensitivity reactions are mediated by specifically immune T cells		
Syndrome	**Antigen**	**Consequence**
Delayed-type hypersensitivity	Proteins: Insect venom Mycobacterial proteins (tuberculin, lepromin)	Local skin swelling: Erythema Induration Cellular infiltrate Dermatitis
Contact hypersensitivity	Haptens: Pentadecacatechol (poison ivy) DNFB Small metal ions: Nickel Chromate	Local epidermal reaction: Erythema Cellular infiltrate Contact dermatitis
Gluten-sensitive enteropathy (Celiac disease)	Gliadin	Villous atrophy in small bowel Malabsorption

small amounts of a protein from *M. tuberculosis* are injected into subcutaneous tissue, a T-cell mediated local inflammatory reaction evolves over 24–72 hours in individuals who have previously responded to this pathogen (Fig. 11.10). The response is mediated by inflammatory T cells that enter the site of antigen injection, recognize complexes of peptide:MHC class II on antigen-presenting cells, and release inflammatory cytokines that increase local blood vessel permeability, bringing fluid and protein into the tissue and recruiting accessory cells to the site (Fig. 11.11). Each of these phases takes several hours and so the mature response appears only 24–48 hours after challenge.

Very similar reactions are observed in several allergic responses. For instance, the rash produced by poison ivy is caused by a T-cell response to a chemical in the poison ivy leaf called **pentadecacatechol**. This compound binds covalently to host proteins. These modified self proteins are then cleaved into modified self peptides, which may bind to self MHC class II molecules where they can be recognized by inflammatory CD4 T cells. When specifically sensitized T cells recognize these complexes they can produce extensive inflammation. Because the chemical is delivered by contact with the skin, this is called a

Fig. 11.10 The time course of a delayed-type hypersensitivity reaction. The first phase involves uptake, processing, and presentation of the antigen by local antigen-presenting cells. In the second phase, T$_H$1 cells that were primed by a previous exposure to the antigen migrate into the site of injection and become activated. Since these specific cells are rare, and since there is no inflammation to attract cells into the site, it may take several hours for a T cell of the correct specificity to arrive. These cells release mediators that activate local endothelial cells, recruiting an inflammatory cell infiltrate dominated by macrophages and causing accumulation of fluid and protein. At this point, the lesion becomes apparent.

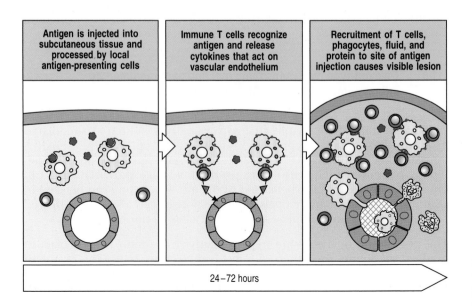

Antigen is injected into subcutaneous tissue and processed by local antigen-presenting cells	Immune T cells recognize antigen and release cytokines that act on vascular endothelium	Recruitment of T cells, phagocytes, fluid, and protein to site of antigen injection causes visible lesion

24–72 hours

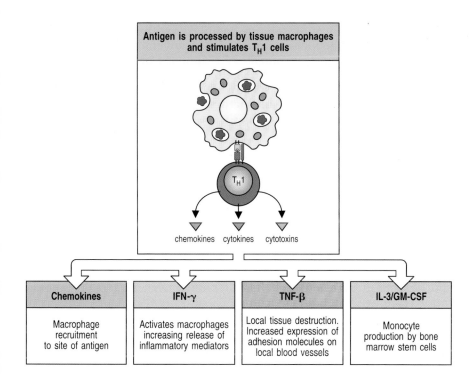

Antigen is processed by tissue macrophages and stimulates T$_H$1 cells

chemokines   cytokines   cytotoxins

Chemokines	IFN-γ	TNF-β	IL-3/GM-CSF
Macrophage recruitment to site of antigen	Activates macrophages increasing release of inflammatory mediators	Local tissue destruction. Increased expression of adhesion molecules on local blood vessels	Monocyte production by bone marrow stem cells

Fig. 11.11 The delayed-type (type IV) hypersensitivity response is directed by cytokines released by T$_H$1 cells stimulated by antigen. Antigen in the local tissues is processed by antigen-presenting cells and presented on MHC class II molecules. Antigen-specific T$_H$1 cells can recognize the antigen locally at the site of injection, and release chemokines and cytokines that recruit macrophages to the site of antigen deposition. Antigen presentation by the newly-recruited macrophages then amplifies the response. T cells may also affect local blood vessels through release of TNF-β and stimulate the production of macrophages through the release of IL-3 and GM-CSF (granulocyte–macrophage colony-stimulating factor). Finally, T$_H$1 cells activate macrophages through release of IFN-γ, and kill macrophages and other sensitive cells through release of TNF-β or by expression of Fas ligand.

contact hypersensitivity reaction. The compounds that cause such reactions must be chemically active so that they can form stable complexes with host proteins.

Some insect proteins also elicit delayed-type hypersensitivity responses. However, the early phases of the host reaction to an insect bite are often IgE-mediated or the result of direct effects of insect venoms. Finally, some unusual delayed-type hypersensitivity responses to divalent cations have been observed, for example to nickel, which may alter the conformation or peptide binding of MHC class II molecules.

Type IV hypersensitivity reactions can also involve CD8 T cells that damage tissues mainly by cell-mediated cytotoxicity. Some chemicals are soluble in lipid and can therefore cross the cell membrane and modify proteins that are inside cells. These modified proteins generate modified peptides within the cytosol, which are translocated into the endoplasmic reticulum and delivered to the cell surface by MHC class I molecules. These CD8 T cells can cause damage either by killing the eliciting cell or by secreting cytokines such as IFN-γ.

Summary.

Allergies or hypersensitivity diseases result from immune responses to non-infectious foreign substances. The allergic reactions occur when preformed antibody or T cells interact with the allergen. Immediate hypersensitivity responses are antibody mediated; the isotype of antibody and the dose and route of allergen entry determine what type of allergic reaction occurs. Most common allergies are immediate hypersensitivity reactions mediated by IgE antibodies, which activate mast cells upon binding allergen. Despite intense study of the nature of allergens, the IgE-antibody response, and mast cells, much remains to be learned about allergy, and its treatment is not yet in any way satisfactory. This may reflect the recent realization that helper CD4 T cells (T$_H$2) play a very important role in allergic reactions. Some immediate hypersensitivity reactions are the result of IgG antibodies binding to allergens on cell surfaces or forming immune complexes with them. Delayed-type hypersensitivity reactions are mediated by inflammatory CD4 T cells (T_H1) that activate local inflammatory responses in the site of antigen deposition or cytotoxic CD8 T cells that can kill tissue cells directly. Allergic reactions are mechanistically identical to protective responses, differing only in the source and nature of the antigen; however, the repeated elicitation of these reactions by repeated exposure to the allergen makes them appear distinctive.

Autoimmunity: responses to self antigens.

Autoimmune disease occurs when a specific adaptive immune response is mounted against self. It is not known what triggers the autoimmune response, but both environmental and genetic factors, especially MHC genotype, are important. Autoimmune responses are common, but it is only when they are sustained and cause lasting tissue damage that they attract medical attention. This presumably reflects the response of T and B cells to self antigens that can only be removed from the system by destroying the cells that produce them. The mechanisms of tissue damage in autoimmune diseases are essentially the same as those that operate in protective immunity and in allergy, with the exception of the IgE-mediated reactions, which dominate allergy but are not known to occur in autoimmunity. It is believed that autoimmunity is initiated by a response involving T cells; cytotoxic T-cell responses and inappropriate activation of macrophages can cause extensive tissue damage, while inappropriate T-cell help can initiate a harmful antibody response to self antigens. Autoimmune responses are a natural consequence of the open repertoires of both B-cell and T-cell receptors that allows them to recognize any pathogen, as such receptors will also include those reactive to self antigens. In this section, we shall examine the nature of autoimmune responses and how autoimmunity leads to tissue damage. In the last section of this chapter, we shall examine the mechanisms by which autoimmune responses are initiated.

11-9   Specific adaptive immune responses to self antigens can cause autoimmune disease.

It was realized early in the study of immunity that the powerful effector mechanisms used in host defense could, if turned against the host, lead to severe tissue damage; Ehrlich termed this *horror autotoxicus*. Normal individuals do not mount sustained adaptive immune responses to their own antigens and, although transient responses to damaged self tissues do occur, these rarely cause additional tissue damage. However, while self tolerance is the general rule, sustained immune responses to self tissues do occur, and these autoimmune responses cause the severe tissue damage that Ehrlich predicted.

In humans, autoimmunity usually arises spontaneously; that is, we do not know what events initiated the immune response to self that leads to the autoimmune disease. However, as we shall learn in the last section of this chapter, there is a strong association between infection and the onset of autoimmunity, suggesting that infectious agents play a critical role in the process. In experimental animals, autoimmune disease can be induced artificially by mixing tissues with strong adjuvants containing bacteria (see Section 2-3) and injecting them into a genetically identical animal. This shows that autoimmunity involves a specific, adaptive immune response to self antigens and forms the basis for our understanding of how autoimmune disease arises.

11-10   Susceptibility to autoimmune diseases is controlled by environmental and genetic factors, especially MHC genes.

Susceptibility to most autoimmune diseases shows a significant genetic component; indeed, familial associations are common. Furthermore, certain inbred mouse strains reliably develop particular spontaneous or experimentally induced autoimmune diseases. These findings have led to an extensive search for human genes that determine disease susceptibility.

To date, the only clear-cut and consistent genetic marker for susceptibility to any autoimmune disease has been the MHC genotype. Many human autoimmune diseases show HLA-linked disease associations (Fig. 11.12), and these associations become stronger as HLA genotyping becomes more accurate (see Section 2-27). For example, there is a strong association with DQβ genotype in insulin-dependent diabetes mellitus; the normal DQβ amino acid sequence has an aspartic acid at position 57, whereas in Caucasoid populations, patients with diabetes most often have valine,

Associations of HLA genotype with susceptibility to autoimmune disease			
Disease	HLA allele	Relative risk	Sex ratio (♀:♂)
Ankylosing spondylitis	B27	87.4	0.3
Acute anterior uveitis	B27	10.04	<0.5
Goodpasture's syndrome	DR2	15.9	?
Multiple sclerosis	DR2	4.8	10
Graves' disease	DR3	3.7	4–5
Myasthenia gravis	DR3	2.5	~1
Systemic lupus erythematosus	DR3	5.8	10–20
Insulin-dependent diabetes mellitus	DR3 and DR4	3.2	~1
Rheumatoid arthritis	DR4	4.2	3
Pemphigus vulgaris	DR4	14.4	?
Hashimoto's thyroiditis	DR5	3.2	4–5

Fig. 11.12 Associations of HLA genotype and of sex with susceptibility to autoimmune disease. The 'relative risk' for an HLA allele in an autoimmune disease is calculated by comparing the observed number of patients carrying the HLA allele with the number that would be expected, given the prevalence of the HLA allele in the general population. HLA-DR3 and DR4 are tightly linked to HLA-DQ, which thus also shows an association with disease susceptibility in insulin-dependent diabetes mellitus (see Section 2-26). Some diseases show a significant bias in the sex ratio; this is taken to imply that sex hormones are involved in pathogenesis. Consistent with this, the difference in the sex ratio in these diseases is greatest just after the onset of puberty when levels of such hormones are highest (~ stands for approximately).

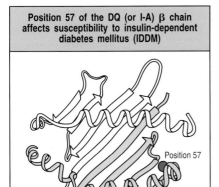

Position 57 of the DQ (or I-A) β chain affects susceptibility to insulin-dependent diabetes mellitus (IDDM)

Position 57

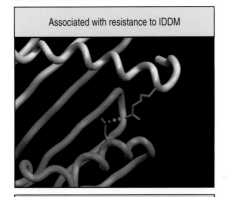

Associated with resistance to IDDM

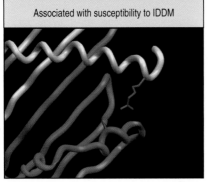

Associated with susceptibility to IDDM

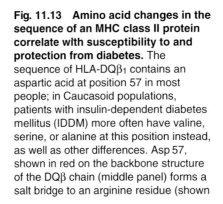

Fig. 11.13 Amino acid changes in the sequence of an MHC class II protein correlate with susceptibility to and protection from diabetes. The sequence of HLA-DQβ₁ contains an aspartic acid at position 57 in most people; in Caucasoid populations, patients with insulin-dependent diabetes mellitus (IDDM) more often have valine, serine, or alanine at this position instead, as well as other differences. Asp 57, shown in red on the backbone structure of the DQβ chain (middle panel) forms a salt bridge to an arginine residue (shown in purple) in the adjacent α chain (gray). The change to an uncharged residue (for example, alanine, shown in red in the bottom panel) disrupts this salt bridge, altering the stability of the DQ molecule. In mice, the non-obese diabetic (NOD) strain, which develops spontaneous diabetes, shows a similar replacement of serine for aspartic acid at position 57 of the homologous I-A β chain, and NOD mice transgenic for β chains with Asp 57 have a marked reduction in diabetes. Photographs courtesy of C Thorpe.

serine, or alanine at that position (Fig. 11.13); mice that develop diabetes also have a serine at this position in the homologous MHC class II molecule. In most autoimmune diseases, susceptibility is linked most closely with MHC class II alleles, but in some cases susceptibility is closely linked to MHC class I alleles.

The association of MHC genotype with autoimmune disease makes good sense, since all autoimmune responses involve T cells, and the ability of T cells to respond to a particular antigen depends on MHC genotype. However, this simple model for the way that MHC genotype determines susceptibility to autoimmune disease has not been proven. Thus, while it is plausible that differences in the ability of different allelic variants of MHC molecules to present autoantigenic peptides to autoreactive T cells determine susceptibility, this remains hypothetical. Identification of autoantigenic peptides and a demonstration that they bind selectively to MHC molecules associated with the disease would help to determine whether the binding of a particular autoantigenic peptide to a particular MHC molecule is an essential factor in susceptibility or simply a trait linked to a true susceptibility locus.

The association of MHC genotype with disease is initially assessed by comparing the frequency of different alleles in patients with their frequency in the normal population (Fig. 11.14). For **insulin-dependent diabetes mellitus (IDDM)**, this approach demonstrated an association between the MHC class II alleles HLA-DR3 and HLA-DR4, which are tightly linked to HLA-DQ and disease susceptibility. In addition, such

Fig. 11.14 Population studies show linkage of susceptibility to insulin-dependent diabetes mellitus (IDDM) to HLA genotype. The prevalence of diabetes in individuals varies enormously with HLA genotype. Prevalence here is relative to prevalence of diabetes in the population as a whole, which is 1 person in 300 in North America. Diabetes is clearly more frequent in people who express HLA-DR3 or DR4, and greatest when both DR3 and DR4 are expressed together; these alleles are tightly linked to HLA-DQ alleles that are associated with susceptibility to IDDM.

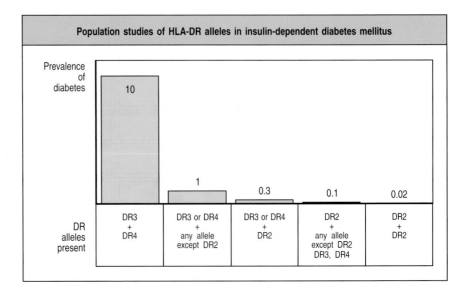

Population studies of HLA-DR alleles in insulin-dependent diabetes mellitus

Prevalence of diabetes

10	1	0.3	0.1	0.02

DR alleles present

DR3 + DR4	DR3 or DR4 + any allele except DR2	DR3 or DR4 + DR2	DR2 + any allele except DR2 DR3, DR4	DR2 + DR2

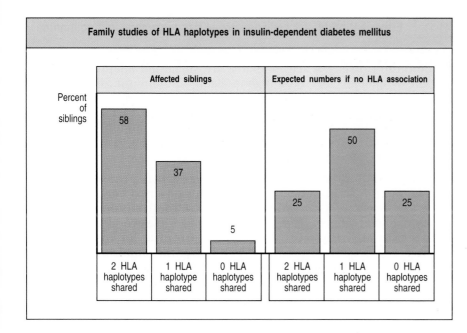

Fig. 11.15 Population and family studies show strong linkage of susceptibility to insulin-dependent diabetes mellitus (IDDM) with HLA genotype. In families in which two or more siblings have IDDM, it is possible to compare the HLA genotypes of affected siblings. Affected siblings share two HLA alleles much more frequently than would be expected if the HLA genotype did not influence disease susceptibility.

studies have shown that the MHC class II allele HLA-DR2 has a dominant protective effect; individuals carrying HLA-DR2, even in association with one of the susceptibility alleles, rarely develop diabetes. Another way to determine whether MHC genes are important in autoimmune disease is to study the families of affected patients. In family studies, it has been shown that two siblings affected with the same autoimmune disease are far more likely than expected to share two MHC haplotypes (Fig. 11.15).

However, MHC genotype alone does not determine whether a person develops disease. Identical twins are far more likely to develop the same autoimmune disease than MHC-identical siblings, demonstrating that genetic factors other than MHC also affect disease susceptibility. Recent studies of the genetics of autoimmune diabetes in humans and mice have shown that there are several independently segregating disease susceptibility loci in addition to MHC. MHC class I alleles also impact on susceptibility to diabetes, which appears to be mediated by both CD4 and CD8 T cells.

Environmental factors also affect susceptibility to autoimmune disease. For instance, if one of a pair of identical twins has diabetes, the other twin does not always develop disease, nor do all members of an inbred strain of diabetes-prone mice. For identical twins, the concordance rate of autoimmune diabetes is around 30%. Therefore, environmental factors such as infection or diet are also likely to play a role in the pathogenesis of autoimmunity.

One very important additional factor in disease susceptibility is the hormonal status of the patient. Many autoimmune diseases show strong sex bias (see Fig. 11.12). In experimental animals where a bias towards disease in one sex is observed, castration normalizes disease incidence between the two sexes. Furthermore, many autoimmune diseases that are more common in females show peak incidence in the years of active child bearing, when maximal production of the female sex hormones estrogen and progesterone occurs. Thorough understanding of how these genetic, environmental, and hormonal factors contribute to disease susceptibility may allow us to prevent the autoimmune response.

11-11 | **Either antibody or T cells can cause tissue damage in autoimmune disease.**

Autoimmune diseases are mediated by sustained adaptive immune responses specific for self antigens. Each autoimmune disease has a characteristic pathogenesis that involves one or more of the four mechanisms of tissue damage summarized in Fig. 11.1. The specific antigen or group of antigens against which the autoimmune response is directed and the mechanism by which the antigen-bearing tissue is damaged together determine the pathology of the disease.

IgE responses to self tissues have been suggested as a cause of intrinsic asthma, but this has not been proven in this or any other autoimmune disease. However, IgG or IgM responses to self antigens on cell surfaces or extracellular matrix lead to tissue damage in several autoimmune diseases. In **autoimmune hemolytic anemia**, for instance, antibodies to self antigens on red blood cells trigger red blood cell destruction (Fig. 11.16). Destruction of nucleated cells is less common, perhaps because such cells are better at resisting the action of complement; when nucleated cells are damaged, it may be by antibody-dependent cellular cytotoxicity mediated by natural killer cells (see Section 8-19). Antibody responses to extracellular matrix molecules are infrequent but can be very damaging when they occur. In **Goodpasture's syndrome**, antibodies are formed to basement membrane collagen and these bind to the basement membranes of renal glomeruli as well as other small vessels, causing a rapidly fatal disease.

In diseases such as systemic lupus erythematosus, chronic IgG antibody production directed at self antigens causes immune complex deposition in the tissues, especially small blood vessels (see Section 11-13). Such diseases are classified as **systemic autoimmune diseases**, as opposed to the **tissue-** or **organ-specific autoimmune diseases** that affect single organs or tissues.

Fig. 11.16 Antibodies specific for cell-surface antigens can destroy cells (type II hypersensitivity). For example, in autoimmune hemolytic anemia, shown here, antibody-coated red cells can be lysed by complement, or cleared by Fc receptor-bearing macrophages in the reticuloendothelial system. Complement deposition on the target cell surface also enhances uptake by macrophages, which bear complement receptors. Red blood cells (RBCs) are relatively poor in proteins that protect against complement activation and are, therefore, particularly vulnerable to this form of tissue damage. Some red cells may also be lysed by the action of complement, but most are lost by uptake in the reticuloendothelial system.

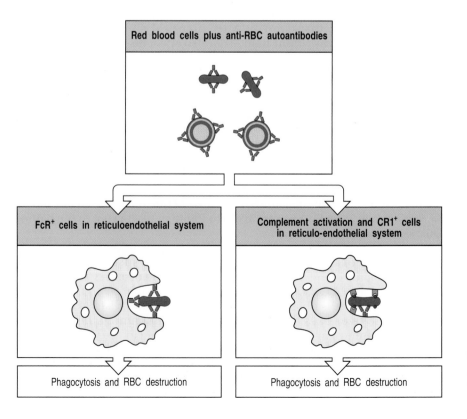

Red blood cells plus anti-RBC autoantibodies

FcR⁺ cells in reticuloendothelial system

Complement activation and CR1⁺ cells in reticulo-endothelial system

Phagocytosis and RBC destruction

Phagocytosis and RBC destruction

Some common autoimmune diseases classified by immunopathogenic mechanism		
Syndrome	**Autoantigen**	**Consequence**
Type II Antibody to surface or matrix antigens		
Autoimmune hemolytic anemia	Rh blood group, I antigen	Destruction of red blood cells by complement and phagocytes, anemia
Autoimmune thrombocytopenia purpura	Platelet integrin gpIIb:IIIa	Abnormal bleeding
Goodpasture's syndrome	Non-collagenous domain of basement membrane collagen type IV	Vasculitis, renal failure Pulmonary hemorrhage
Pemphigus vulgaris	Epidermal cadherin	Blistering of skin
Acute rheumatic fever	Streptococcal cell wall antigens, antibodies cross-react with cardiac muscle	Arthritis, myocarditis, late scarring of heart valves
Type III Immune-complex disease		
Subacute bacterial endocarditis	Bacterial antigen	Glomerulonephritis
Mixed essential cryoglobulinemia	Rheumatoid factor IgG complexes (with or without hepatitis C antigens)	Systemic vasculitis
Systemic lupus erythematosus	DNA, histones, ribosomes, snRNP, scRNP	Glomerulonephritis, vasculitis, arthritis
Type IV T-cell mediated disease		
Insulin-dependent diabetes mellitus	Pancreatic β-cell antigen	β-cell destruction
Rheumatoid arthritis	Unknown synovial joint antigen	Joint inflammation and destruction
Experimental autoimmune encephalomyelitis (EAE), multiple sclerosis	Myelin basic protein, proteolipid protein	Brain invasion by CD4 T cells, paralysis

Fig. 11.17 Autoimmune diseases classified by the mechanism of tissue damage. All the mechanisms outlined in Fig. 11.1 except type I responses also occur in autoimmune diseases.

Finally, immune T cells specific for self peptide:self MHC complexes can cause local inflammation by activating macrophages or can damage tissue cells directly. Thus, autoimmune tissue damage can occur by virtually any of the effector mechanisms utilized in the adaptive immune response (Fig. 11.17).

11-12　Autoantibodies to receptors cause disease by stimulating or blocking receptor function.

A special class of type II hypersensitivity reaction occurs when the autoantibody binds a cell-surface receptor molecule. Antibody binding to a receptor can either stimulate the receptor or block its stimulation by its natural ligand. In **Graves' disease**, autoantibody to the

Fig. 11.18   Feedback regulation of thyroid hormone production is disrupted in Graves' disease. Graves' disease is caused by antibodies specific for the receptor for thyroid-stimulating hormone (TSH). Normally, thyroid hormones are produced in response to TSH and limit their own production by inhibiting the production of TSH by the pituitary (left panels). In Graves' disease, the autoantibodies are agonists for the TSH receptor and therefore stimulate production of thyroid hormones (right panels). The thyroid hormones inhibit TSH production in the normal way, but do not affect production of the autoantibody; the excessive thyroid hormone production induced in this way causes hyperthyroidism.

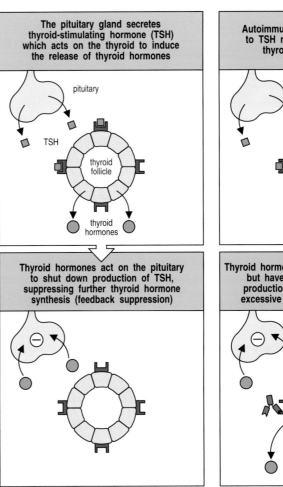

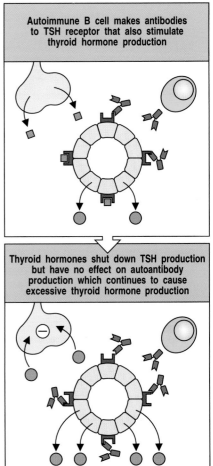

thyroid-stimulating hormone receptor on thyroid cells stimulates the production of excessive thyroid hormone. The production of thyroid hormone is normally controlled by feedback regulation; high levels of thyroid hormone inhibit release of thyroid-stimulating hormone by the pituitary but of course are unable to feedback-inhibit autoantibody production. Thus, in Graves' disease, feedback inhibition fails, and the patients become hyperthyroid (Fig. 11.18).

In **myasthenia gravis**, autoantibodies to the α chain of the acetylcholine receptor found at the neuromuscular junction block neuromuscular transmission. The antibodies are believed to drive internalization and intracellular degradation of acetylcholine receptors (Fig. 11.19). Patients

Fig. 11.19   Autoantibodies inhibit receptor function in myasthenia gravis. Myasthenia gravis is caused by antibodies to the α subunit of the receptor for acetylcholine, which is involved in neuromuscular transmission. These antibodies bind to the receptor without activating it and cause receptor internalization and degradation. As the number of receptors on the muscle is decreased, the muscle becomes less responsive to acetylcholine released by motor neurons.

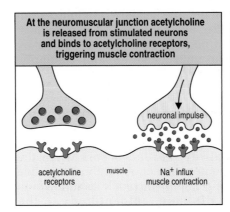

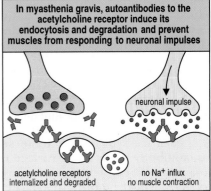

Diseases mediated by antibodies to cellular receptors		
Syndrome	**Antigen**	**Consequence**
Graves' disease	Thyroid-stimulating hormone receptor	Hyperthyroidism
Myasthenia gravis	Acetylcholine receptor	Progressive weakness
Insulin-resistant diabetes	Insulin receptor (antagonist)	Hyperglycemia, ketoacidosis
Hypoglycemia	Insulin receptor (agonist)	Hypoglycemia

Fig. 11.20 Autoimmune diseases caused by autoantibodies to cell-surface receptor molecules. These antibodies produce different effects depending on whether they are agonists, which stimulate, or antagonists, which inhibit, the receptor. Note that different autoantibodies to the insulin receptor can either stimulate or inhibit signaling.

with myasthenia gravis develop progressive weakness and eventually die as a result of their autoimmune disease. Diseases caused by auto-antibodies to cellular receptors acting as agonists or antagonists are listed in Fig. 11.20.

11-13　Chronic generation of immune complexes causes tissue damage in systemic autoimmune diseases.

Immune complexes are produced whenever there is an antibody response to a soluble antigen. Normally, these are cleared efficiently by red blood cells bearing complement receptors and by phagocytes of the reticuloendothelial system that have both complement and Fc receptors, and such complexes cause little tissue damage.

Red blood cells bearing complement receptors gather up the immune complexes and convey them to the liver and spleen where the complex is removed without harming the red blood cell. However, when large amounts of antigen are injected, large amounts of small immune complexes are formed that overwhelm these mechanisms. As we learned in Section 11-7, injection of large amounts of serum proteins causes serum sickness, a transient disease that lasts only until the immune complexes have been cleared.

In certain systemic autoimmune diseases, and also in chronic infections, the production of immune complexes is sustained and the resulting tissue damage can be severe. In the disease **systemic lupus erythematosus (SLE)**, autoantibodies are produced to common cellular constituents such as nucleic acid:protein complexes (see Section 11-15). In this disease, the source of antigen is internal and large quantities of antigen are available, so large numbers of small immune complexes are produced continuously and deposited in the walls of small blood vessels in the renal glomerulus (Fig. 11.21) and in joints, leading to complement fixation and the activation of phagocytic cells. The tissue damage induced releases more nucleopro-tein complexes, which in turn form more immune complexes. Eventually, the inflammation induced in small blood vessel walls, especially in the kidney and brain, can cause sufficient damage to kill the patient. Several diseases are caused by the chronic deposition of immune complexes (see Fig. 11.17).

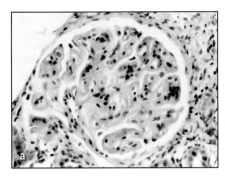
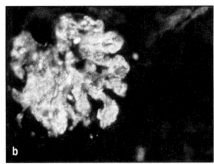
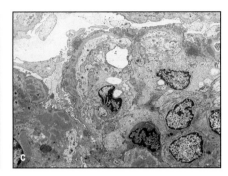

Fig. 11.21   Deposition of immune complexes in the renal glomerulus causes renal failure in systemic lupus erythematosus (SLE). The deposition of immune complexes in SLE causes thickening of the glomerular basement membrane, as shown in panel a. In panel b, such kidney sections have been stained with fluorescent anti-immunoglobulin (see Section 2-13) revealing immunoglobulin in the basement membrane deposits. By electron microscopy, as shown in panel c, dense protein deposits are seen between the glomerular basement membrane and the renal podocytes. Polymorphonuclear neutrophilic leukocytes are also present, attracted by the deposited immune complexes. Photographs courtesy of M Kashgarian.

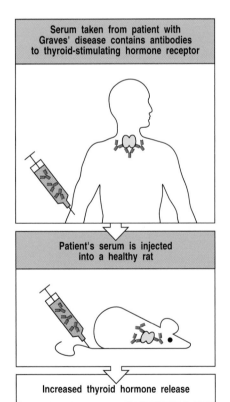

Fig. 11.22   Serum from patients with some autoimmune diseases can transfer the disease to experimental animals. When the autoantigen is well conserved between humans and mice or rats, the transfer of antibody from an affected human can cause the same symptoms in an experimental animal. For example, antibody from patients with Graves' disease produces thyroid activation in rats.

11-14   The mechanism of autoimmune tissue damage can often be determined by adoptive transfer.

To classify a disease as autoimmune one must show that an adaptive immune response to a self antigen causes the observed pathology. Initially, the demonstration that antibodies to the affected tissue could be detected in the serum of patients suffering from various diseases was taken as evidence that the diseases had an autoimmune basis. However, such autoantibodies are also found when tissue damage is caused by trauma or infection. This suggests that autoantibodies can result from, rather than be the cause of, tissue damage. Thus, one must show that the observed autoantibodies are pathogenic before classifying the disease as autoimmune.

Autoantibodies frequently transfer disease to experimental animals, causing pathology similar to that seen in the patient from whom they were obtained (Fig. 11.22). However, this does not always work, presumably because of species differences in autoantigen structure. Another way in which antibody transfer of autoimmune disease can be observed is in newborn babies of diseased mothers (Fig. 11.23). When babies are exposed to IgG autoantibodies transferred across the placenta, they will often manifest pathology similar to the mother's. These symptoms rapidly disappear as the antibody is catabolized. The process can be speeded up by exchange transfusion or plasmapheresis (exchange of plasma) of the infant.

Not all autoimmune diseases are caused by autoantibodies. Many autoimmune diseases are mediated by specifically reactive T cells. Furthermore, it seems likely that autoimmune T cells are required to sustain all autoantibody responses. It is much more difficult to demonstrate the existence of autoimmune T cells than it is to demonstrate the presence of autoantibodies. First, autoimmune human T cells cannot be used to transfer disease to experimental animals because T-cell recognition is MHC restricted and animals have different MHC alleles from humans. Second, it is difficult to identify the antigen recognized by a T cell; for example, autoantibodies can be used to stain self tissues to reveal the distribution of the autoantigen, whereas T cells cannot. Nevertheless, there is strong evidence for involvement of autoreactive T cells in several autoimmune diseases. Insulin-dependent diabetes mellitus is a disease

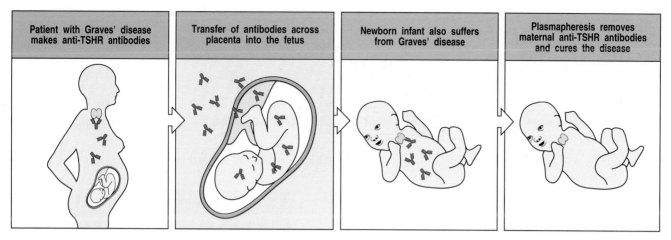

Fig. 11.23   Antibody-mediated autoimmune diseases can appear in the infants of affected mothers as a consequence of transplacental antibody transfer. In pregnant women, IgG antibodies cross the placenta and accumulate in the fetus before birth (see Fig. 8.19). Babies born to mothers with immunoglobulin-mediated autoimmune disease therefore frequently show symptoms similar to the mother in the first few weeks of life. Fortunately, this causes little lasting damage as the symptoms disappear along with the maternal antibody. In Graves' disease, the symptoms are caused by antibodies to the thyroid-stimulating hormone receptor (TSHR). Children of mothers making thyroid-stimulating antibody are born with hyperthyroidism, but this can be corrected by replacing the plasma with normal plasma, removing the maternal antibody.

in which the insulin-producing β cells of the pancreatic islets are selectively destroyed by specific T cells. When such diabetic patients are transplanted with half a pancreas from an identical twin donor, the β cells in the grafted tissue are rapidly and selectively destroyed by CD8 T cells. Recurrence of disease can be prevented by the immunosuppressive drug cyclosporin A (see Chapter 12), which inhibits T-cell activation. Progress towards identifying such autoimmune T cells and proving that they cause disease will be discussed in Section 11-16.

11-15   Autoantibodies can be used to identify the target of the autoimmune process.

When autoantibodies have been shown to be required for pathogenesis, they can be used to purify the autoantigen so that it can be identified. This approach is particularly powerful if the autoantibody causes disease in animals, when large amounts of tissue can be obtained. Autoantibodies can also be used to examine the distribution of the target structure in cells and tissues by immunohistology, often providing clues to the pathogenesis of the disease.

The identification of a critical autoantigen recognized by an antibody may also lead to the identification of the helper T cell responsible for autoantibody production. As we learned in Chapter 8, helper T cells selectively activate B cells that bind epitopes that are physically linked to the peptide recognized by the helper T cell. It follows that autoantibodies can be used to purify proteins or protein complexes that should contain the peptide recognized by the autoreactive helper T cell. For example, in myasthenia gravis the autoantibodies that cause disease bind mainly to the α chain of the acetylcholine receptor. CD4 T cells that recognize peptide fragments of this receptor subunit can also be found in myasthenia patients. Thus, both autoreactive B cells and autoreactive T cells are probably required for this disease (Fig. 11.24).

Another example of the same phenomenon is the antibody-mediated autoimmune disease systemic lupus erythematosus. As we have seen,

Fig. 11.24 Autoantibodies can be used to identify both the B- and T-cell epitopes of some autoantigens.
In myasthenia gravis, autoantibodies immunoprecipitate the α chain of the acetylcholine receptor from lysates of skeletal muscle cells (top panels). This suggests that the same patients should also have helper CD4 T cells that respond to a peptide of the acetylcholine receptor. To investigate this, T cells from myasthenia gravis patients have been isolated and grown in the presence of the acetylcholine receptor plus antigen-presenting cells of the correct MHC type; T cells specific for epitopes of the α chain of the acetylcholine receptor can indeed be identified (center panels). The bottom panels show the probable mechanism for induction of this auto-immune disease; naive autoreactive B cells internalize the α chain of the acetylcholine receptor and present peptides derived from it to the auto-reactive helper T cells. These secrete cytokines such as IL-4, signaling the B cell to produce autoantibodies.

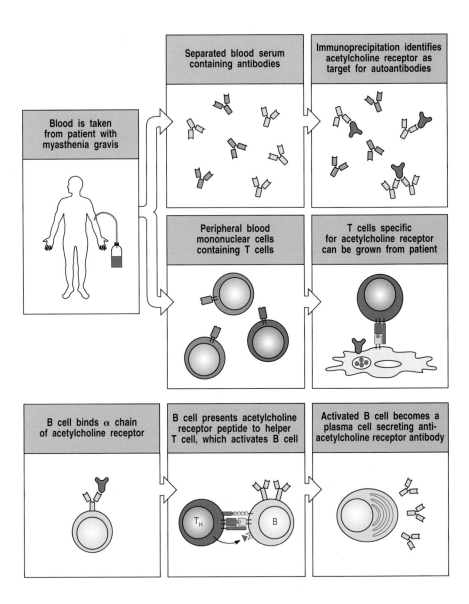

tissue damage in this disease is caused by immune complexes of autoanti-bodies directed against a variety of antigens composed of nucleic acids and proteins, such as nucleosomes, ribosomes, and small ribo-nucleoprotein complexes involved in RNA processing. Interestingly, these antibodies show a high degree of somatic mutation, and the B cells that produce them can be shown to have undergone extensive clonal expansion; these properties are characteristic of antibodies formed in response to chronic stimulation of B cells by antigen and specific helper T cells. This strongly suggests that the autoantibodies in systemic lupus erythematosus must be produced in response to autoantigens that contain peptides recognized by specific autoreactive helper T cells. Further-more, the autoantibodies in any one individual tend to bind all constituents of a particular nucleoprotein particle. This is most readily explained by the presence of helper T cells specific for a peptide constituent of this particle. A B cell whose receptor binds any component of the particle could process and present this peptide to these autoreactive T cells and would then receive help from the T cell (Fig. 11.25). This would account for the observed characteristics of the autoantibody response as well as the clustering of autoantibody specificities in individual patients. To find out whether this is correct, the specific helper T cells involved in this disease need to be isolated.

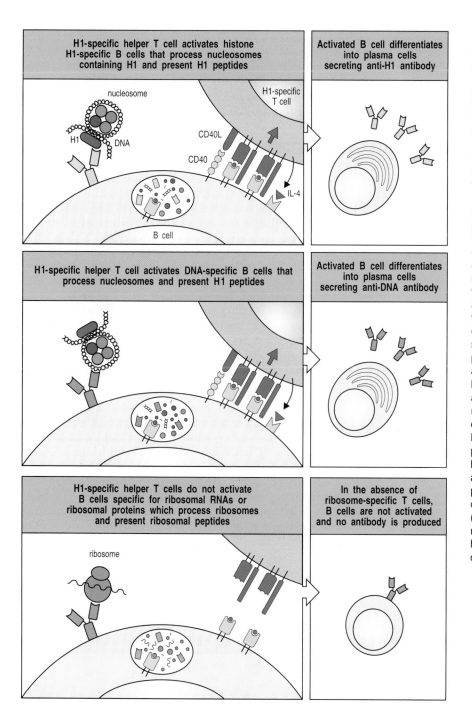

Fig. 11.25 **Autoreactive helper T cells of one specificity can drive the production of autoantibodies with several different specificities.** In systemic lupus erythematosus, patients frequently produce autoantibodies to all of the components of a nucleosome, or all of the components of the ribosome, instead of producing autoantibodies to some components of each of these particles. The most likely explanation is that all the autoreactive B cells are receiving help from a single clone of autoreactive helper T cells specific for a peptide of one of the proteins that make up the particle. Since B cells internalize and process particles that contain the antigen they recognize, any B cell specific for any protein or nucleic acid within the particle can receive help from a T cell that recognizes a peptide derived from a protein found in the particle. For example, if a patient has a helper T cell specific for a peptide of the histone protein H1, any B cell that recognizes any antigen in a nucleosome can present histone peptides to that T cell and be activated by it. Thus, a single auto-reactive helper T cell could give a diverse antibody response. However, B cells able to bind ribosomes cannot present the H1 peptide and so will not be activated to produce anti-ribosomal antibodies (bottom panels). In other patients, responses focusing on ribosomes or small nuclear ribonucleoproteins (snRNP) are observed, presumably reflecting the existence of different helper T cells specific for peptides derived from those particles.

11-16   **The target of T-cell mediated autoimmunity is difficult to identify owing to the nature of T-cell ligands.**

Although there is good evidence for the involvement of T cells in many autoimmune diseases, the specific T cells that cause particular diseases are hard to isolate, and their targets are difficult to identify. In part, this is because one cannot grow the specific T cells needed to identify the autoantigenic peptide without supplying them with their specific antigen. It is also difficult to assay the T cells for their ability to cause disease, since any assay requires target cells of the same MHC genotype as the patient. This problem becomes more tractable in animal models. Since many autoimmune diseases in animals are induced by immunization with self tissue, the nature of the autoantigen can be determined by fractionating an extract of the tissue and testing the fractions for their ability to induce disease. It is also possible to clone T-cell lines that will transfer the disease from an affected animal to another animal with the same MHC genotype.

This has made it possible to identify the autoantigens involved in many experimental autoimmune diseases; they are commonly single peptides that bind to specific MHC molecules. The identified peptide can be used as an immunogen to elicit the entire disease spectrum in animals of the appropriate MHC genotype. For example, cloned T-cell lines can cause a demyelinating disease of the brain called **experimental allergic encephalomyelitis** (**EAE**), which resembles **multiple sclerosis**, when injected into syngeneic mice or rats. Many of these cloned T-cell lines are stimulated by peptides of a protein called myelin basic protein (MBP), which is found in the myelin sheath that surrounds nerve cell axons in the brain and spinal cord. When animals with the appropriate MHC allele are immunized with this peptide, active disease results. Activated T cells specific for myelin basic protein have also been identified in patients with multiple sclerosis (Fig. 11.26). It has not yet been proven that these cells cause the demyelination in multiple sclerosis, but this result suggests that it may be possible to use animal models to gain clues to the identity of autoantigenic proteins in human disease.

In a variety of inflammatory autoimmune diseases, it appears that extracellular self antigens are presented to inflammatory T cells. One example is experimental allergic encephalomyelitis, which is caused by inflammatory, but not helper, T cells specific for myelin basic protein, as shown by the ability of specific inflammatory, but not helper, T cells to cause disease on adoptive transfer. **Rheumatoid arthritis** may also be caused by inflammatory T cells specific for a joint antigen, which triggers them to release lymphokines that initiate local inflammation within the joint, causing swelling, accumulation of polymorphonuclear

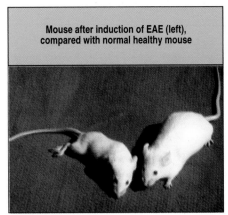

Mouse after induction of EAE (left), compared with normal healthy mouse

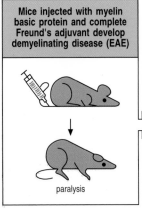

Mice injected with myelin basic protein and complete Freund's adjuvant develop demyelinating disease (EAE)

paralysis

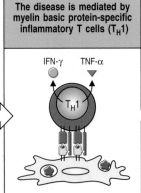

The disease is mediated by myelin basic protein-specific inflammatory T cells (T_H1)

IFN-γ   TNF-α

T_H1

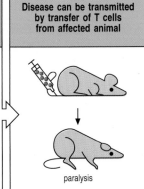

Disease can be transmitted by transfer of T cells from affected animal

paralysis

Fig. 11.26   T cells specific for myelin-specific protein mediate inflammation of the brain in experimental autoimmune encephalomyelitis (EAE). This disease is produced in experimental animals by injecting them with isolated spinal cord homogenized in complete Freunds' adjuvant, causing a progressive paralysis that affects first the tail and hind limbs (as shown in the mouse on the left of the photograph, compared with a healthy mouse on the right) before progressing to forelimb paralysis and eventual death. The disease is caused by T_H1 cells specific for a protein in myelin called myelin basic protein (MBP); immunization with MBP alone can also cause disease, and cloned MBP-specific T_H1 cells can transfer the disease to naive recipients provided that they carry the correct MHC allele. In this system, it has proved possible to identify the peptide:MHC complex recognized by the T_H1 clones that transfer disease.

leukocytes and macrophages, and damage to cartilage, leading to the destruction of the joint. Rheumatoid arthritis is a complex disease and also involves antibodies, often including an IgM anti-IgG autoantibody called **rheumatoid factor**, and some of the tissue damage in this disease is caused by the resultant immune complexes.

Identification of autoantigenic peptides is particularly difficult in the case of diseases mediated by CD8 T cells. Autoantigens recognized by CD4 T cells can come from any extracellular protein or from cells ingested by phagocytes and degraded in cellular vesicles, but autoantigens recognized by CD8 T cells must be made by the target cells themselves (see Chapter 4). Therefore, one can use cellular extracts to identify the autoantigen recognized by autoimmune CD4 T cells, but intact cells from the target tissue of the patient must be used to study autoimmune CD8 T cells that cause tissue damage. Conversely, the pathogenesis of the disease can itself give clues to the identity of the antigen in some CD8 T-cell mediated diseases. For example, since insulin-producing β cells of the pancreatic islets of Langerhans appear to be specifically destroyed by CD8 T cells in insulin-dependent diabetes mellitus it is likely that a protein uniquely expressed by β cells is the source of the peptide that is recognized by pathogenic CD8 T cells in this disease (Fig. 11.27).

There is also evidence for a role of CD4 T cells in insulin-dependent diabetes mellitus, consistent with the linkage of disease susceptibility to particular MHC class II alleles as discussed earlier in this chapter (see Fig. 11.14 and Fig. 11.15). Identifying the autoantigen recognized by T cells in these diseases is an important goal. Not only may it help us to understand disease pathogenesis, but it may also result in several innovative approaches to treatment (see Chapter 12).

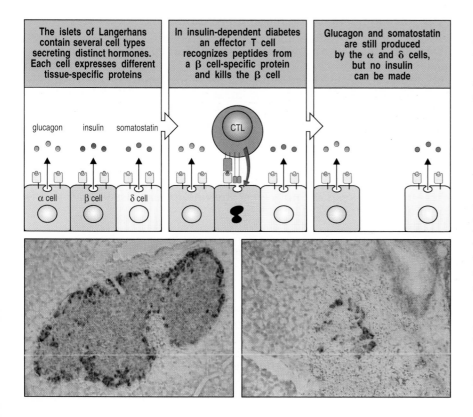

Fig. 11.27 Selective destruction of pancreatic β cells in insulin-dependent diabetes mellitus indicates that the autoantigen is produced in β cells and recognized on their surface. In diabetes there is highly specific destruction of insulin-producing β cells in the pancreatic islets of Langerhans, sparing other islet cell types (α and δ). This is shown schematically in the upper panels. In the lower panels, islets from normal (left) and diabetic (right) mice are stained for insulin (brown), showing the β cells, and glucagon (black), which shows the α cells. Note the lymphocytes infiltrating the islet in the diabetic mouse (right) and the selective loss of the β cells (brown) while the α cells (black) are spared. The characteristic morphology of the islet is also disrupted with the loss of the β cells. It is likely that cytotoxic CD8 T cells are responsible for β-cell destruction; they probably recognize peptides derived from β cell-specific proteins presented by MHC class I molecules. The autoantigen in insulin-dependent diabetes mellitus has not yet been identified, however. Photographs courtesy of I Visintin.

Summary.

To define a disease as autoimmune, the tissue damage must be shown to be caused by an immune response to self antigens. Autoimmune diseases can be caused by autoantibodies or by autoimmune T cells, and tissue damage may result from direct attack on the cells bearing the antigen, from immune complex formation, or from local inflammation. Autoimmune diseases caused by antibodies that bind to cellular receptors, causing either excess activity or inhibition of receptor function, fall into a special class. T cells may be involved directly in inflammation or cellular destruction, and they are also required to sustain autoantibody responses. The most convincing form of proof that the immune response is causal in autoimmunity is transfer of disease by transferring the active component of the immune response to an appropriate recipient. However, this is often not possible. The current challenge is to identify the autoantigens recognized by T cells in autoimmunity, and to use this information to control the activity of these T cells or to prevent their activation in the first place. The deeper, more important question is how the autoimmune response is induced. This issue is most commonly studied by examining the response to non-self tissues in transplantation experiments. We will therefore examine the immune response to grafted tissues in the next section before turning to the problem of how tolerance is maintained normally and why responses occur in autoimmune disease.

Transplant rejection: responses to alloantigens.

The transplantation of tissues to replace diseased organs is now an important medical therapy. Adaptive immune responses to the grafted tissues are the major impediment to successful transplantation in most cases. These responses are very similar to the responses that damage tissues in autoimmunity. In blood transfusion, which is the earliest and still most common transplantation of tissues, blood must be matched for ABO and Rh blood group antigens, to avoid the rapid destruction of mismatched red blood cells by antibodies (see Fig. 2.12). Since there are only four major ABO types and two Rh blood types, this is relatively easy. However, when tissues containing nucleated cells are transplanted, T-cell responses to the highly polymorphic MHC molecules almost always trigger a response against the grafted organ. Matching the MHC type of donor and recipient increases the success rate of grafts, but perfect matching is possible only when donor and recipient are related, and in these cases, genetic differences at other loci still trigger rejection. In this section, we will examine the immune response to tissue grafts, and ask why such responses do not reject the one foreign tissue graft that is routinely tolerated, the mammalian fetus.

11-17 The rejection of grafts is an immunological response mediated primarily by T cells.

The basic rules of tissue grafting were first elucidated using skin transplanted between inbred strains of mice. Skin can be grafted with 100% success between different sites on the same animal or person (an **autograft**), or between genetically identical animals or people (a **syngeneic graft**). However, when skin is grafted between unrelated or **allogeneic** individuals (an **allograft**), the graft is initially accepted and is then rejected about 11–15 days after grafting. This is called a **first set rejection**. This response is quite consistent. It depends on a recipient

T-cell response, since skin grafted onto *nude* mice, which lack T cells, is not rejected. The ability to reject skin can be restored to *nude* mice by the adoptive transfer of normal T cells.

When a recipient that has previously rejected a graft is regrafted with skin from the same donor, the second graft is rejected more rapidly (6–8 days) in a **second set rejection** (Fig. 11.28). Skin from a third-party donor grafted onto the same recipient at the same time does not show this faster response, but follows a first set rejection course. The rapid course of second set rejection can be transferred to normal or irradiated recipients by transferring T cells from the initial recipient, showing that graft rejection is caused by a specific immunological reaction.

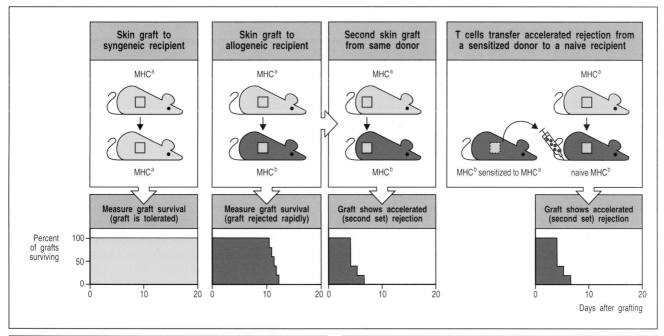

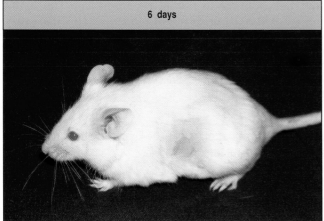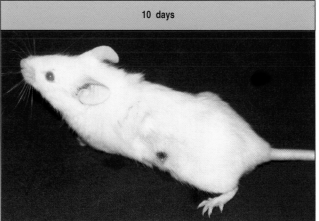

Fig. 11.28   Skin graft rejection is due to a T-cell-mediated anti-graft response. Grafts that are syngeneic are permanently accepted (left panels), but grafts differing at the MHC are rejected around 10–14 days after grafting (first set rejection); when a mouse is grafted for a second time with skin from the same donor, it rejects the second graft faster (center panels). This is called a 'second set rejection' and the accelerated response is MHC-specific; skin from a second donor of the same MHC type is rejected equally fast, while skin from an MHC-different donor is rejected in a first-set pattern (not shown). Naive mice that are given T cells from a sensitized donor behave as if they had already been grafted (right panels). The bottom panels show mice grafted with allogeneic skin six days (left panel) and ten days (right panel) after grafting. Between six and ten days, activated T cells migrate into the graft and proceed to destroy it.

Immune responses are a major barrier to effective tissue transplantation, destroying grafted tissue by an adaptive immune response to its foreign proteins. These responses may be mediated by cytotoxic CD8 T cells, by inflammatory T cells, or by both. Antibodies may also contribute to second set rejection of tissue grafts. Thus, the response to grafted organs bearing non-self antigens is similar to the response to self tissues in autoimmunity.

11-18   Matching donor and recipient at the MHC improves the outcome of transplantation.

When donor and recipient differ at the MHC, the immune response is directed at the non-self MHC molecule or molecules expressed by the graft. Once a recipient has rejected a graft of a particular MHC type, any graft bearing the same non-self MHC molecule will be rejected in a second set response. As we learned in Chapter 4, the frequency of T cells specific for any non-self MHC molecule is high, making differences at MHC the most potent trigger of the rejection of initial grafts; indeed, the major histocompatibility complex was named for this central role in rejection of initial grafts. As we also saw in Chapter 4, the exact nature of T-cell responses to non-self MHC is controversial to this day; T cells may recognize MHC polymorphisms directly, or they may recognize peptides that are presented by non-self MHC proteins but not by self MHC proteins, or both (see Fig. 4.24 and Section 4-18 for a detailed consideration).

Once it became clear that recognition of non-self MHC molecules is a major determinant of graft rejection, a considerable amount of effort was put into MHC matching between recipient and donor. This significantly improves the success rate of clinical organ transplantation. However, HLA matching does not prevent rejection. There are two main reasons for this. First, HLA typing is imprecise, owing to the great polymorphism and complexity of the human MHC. This means that unrelated individuals who type as HLA-identical with the use of antibodies to MHC proteins rarely have identical MHC genotypes (see Section 2-27). However, this should not be a problem with HLA-identical siblings; because siblings inherit their MHC genes as a haplotype, one sibling in four should be truly HLA-identical to a graft recipient (see Fig. 2.47). Nevertheless, grafts between HLA-identical siblings are invariably rejected, albeit more slowly, unless donor and recipient are identical twins. This rejection is due to minor histocompatibility antigens, the nature of which will be discussed in the next section. Therefore, all graft recipients must receive immunosuppressive drugs to prevent rejection unless donor and recipient are identical twins.

11-19   In MHC-identical grafts, rejection is caused by non-self peptides bound to graft MHC molecules.

When donor and recipient are identical at the MHC but differ at other genetic loci, graft rejection is not so rapid (Fig. 11.29). The genetic polymorphisms responsible for rejection of MHC-identical grafts are therefore termed **minor histocompatibility antigens** or **minor H antigens**. Responses to single minor H antigens are much less potent than responses to MHC differences because the frequency of responding T cells is much lower; indeed, minor H antigen-specific T cells need to be primed *in vivo* before they can be detected in a mixed lymphocyte culture. However, most inbred mouse strains that are identical at MHC differ at multiple minor H antigen loci, so grafts between them are still uniformly and relatively rapidly rejected. The cells that respond to minor H antigens

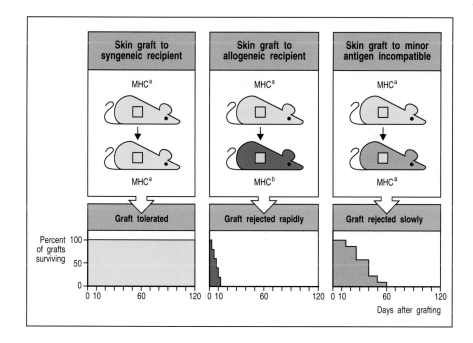

Fig. 11.29 **Even complete matching at the MHC does not ensure graft survival.** Although syngeneic grafts are not rejected (left panels), MHC-identical grafts from donors that differ at other loci are rejected (right panels), albeit more slowly than MHC-disparate grafts (center panels).

are generally CD8 T cells, implying that most minor H antigens are peptides bound to self MHC class I molecules. However, peptides bound to self MHC class II molecules can also participate in the response to MHC-identical grafts.

Minor H antigens are now known to be peptides derived from polymorphic proteins that are presented by MHC molecules on the graft (Fig. 11.30). Virtually any protein made by a cell has the potential to produce peptides that are recognized as minor H antigens. One set of proteins that induce minor H responses are encoded on the male-specific Y chromosome; these are known collectively as H-Y. Because these Y-chromosome specific genes are not expressed in females, female anti-male minor H responses occur; male anti-female responses are not seen, since both males and females express X chromosome genes. The response to minor H antigens is in every way analogous to the response to viral infection. As all cells in the graft express the minor H antigen, the entire graft is destroyed in such responses, just as the analogous responses to tissue-specific peptides can destroy an entire tissue in autoimmunity. Thus, even though MHC genotype may be exactly matched, polymorphism in any protein may elicit potent T-cell responses that will destroy the entire graft. It is no wonder that successful transplantation requires the use of potent immunosuppressive drugs.

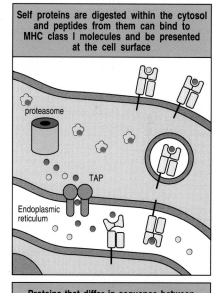

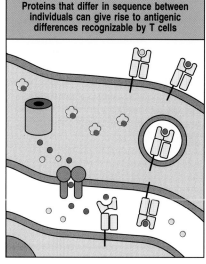

Fig. 11.30 **Minor H antigens are peptides derived from polymorphic cellular proteins bound to MHC class I molecules.** Self proteins are routinely digested by proteasomes within the cell's cytosol, and peptides derived from them are delivered to the rough endoplasmic reticulum where they can bind to MHC class I molecules and be delivered to the cell surface (top panel; see also Section 4-8). If any polymorphic protein differs between the graft donor and the recipient, it may give rise to a peptide that can be recognized by T cells as non-self and elicit an immune response (lower panel).

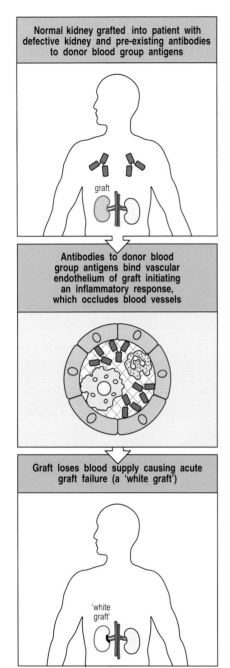

Normal kidney grafted into patient with defective kidney and pre-existing antibodies to donor blood group antigens

graft

Antibodies to donor blood group antigens bind vascular endothelium of graft initiating an inflammatory response, which occludes blood vessels

Graft loses blood supply causing acute graft failure (a 'white graft')

'white graft'

Fig. 11.31 Antibody to donor graft antigens can cause acute graft rejection. In some cases, recipients have antibodies to donor antigens. When the donor organ is grafted into such recipients, these antibodies bind to vascular endothelium, initiating the complement and clotting cascades. This blocks blood flow to the graft, leading to necrosis of the graft because of lack of perfusion. The absence of blood causes the graft to look white, so such grafts are called 'white grafts'.

11-20 **Antibodies reacting with endothelium cause hyperacute graft rejection.**

Most grafts that are routinely transplanted in clinical medicine are vascularized organ grafts linked directly to the recipient's circulation. In some cases, the recipient may already have antibodies to donor graft antigens that were produced in response to a previous transplant or a blood transfusion. Such antibodies can cause very rapid rejection of vascularized grafts, since they react with antigens on the vascular endothelial cells of the graft and initiate the complement and clotting cascades, blocking the vessels of the graft and causing its immediate death (Fig. 11.31). Because such grafts are not perfused with blood, they have a white appearance and are called white grafts. This problem can be avoided by **cross-matching** donor and recipient. Cross-matching, as in blood transfusion, involves determining whether the recipient has antibodies that react with the white blood cells of the donor. If antibodies of this type are found, they are a serious contraindication to transplantation, as they lead to near-certain hyperacute rejection.

A very similar problem prevents the routine use of xenogeneic transplantation of animal organs into humans. Most humans have antibodies that react with endothelial cell antigens of common domestic animals, such as pigs. When pig xenografts are placed in humans, these antibodies trigger hyperacute rejection by reacting with endothelial cell antigens and initiating the complement and clotting cascades. The problem is more difficult in the case of xenografts because complement regulatory proteins such as CD59, DAF, and MCP (CD46) (see Section 8-31) show strict species specificity, so that the complement regulatory proteins of xenogeneic endothelial cells cannot protect them from attack by human complement. If xenogeneic grafts could be used, it would avoid a major barrier to organ replacement therapy, namely, a stable supply of donor organs.

11-21 **A variety of organs are routinely transplanted in clinical medicine.**

Although the immune response makes organ transplantation difficult, there are few alternative therapies for organ failure diseases. Three major advances have made it possible to use organ transplantation routinely in the clinic. First, the technical skill to carry out organ replacement surgery has been mastered by many people. Second, networks of transplantation centers have been organized to ensure that the few healthy organs that are available are HLA-typed and so matched with the most suitable recipient. Third, use of potent immunosuppressive drugs, especially cyclosporin A and FK-506 to inhibit T-cell activation (see Chapter 12) has increased graft survival rates dramatically. A list of the different organs that are transplanted in the clinic is given in Fig. 11.32. Some of these operations are performed routinely with a very high success rate. By far the most frequently transplanted organ is the kidney, the organ first successfully transplanted between identical twins in the 1950s. Transplantation of the cornea gives the highest success rate; this tissue is a special case, as it is not vascularized, and corneal grafts between unrelated people are usually successful even without immunosuppression (see Section 11-27).

As well as graft rejection, there are many other problems associated with organ transplantation. First, donor organs are difficult to obtain; this is especially a problem when the organ involved is a vital one, such as the heart or liver. Because there is no supportive therapy that would allow survival, the time available to find a suitable donor organ is limited. Second, the disease that destroyed the patient's organ may also destroy the graft. Third, the immunosuppression required to prevent graft rejection increases the risk of cancer and infection. Finally, the procedure is very costly. All of these problems need to be addressed before clinical transplantation can become commonplace. The problem most amenable to scientific solution is the development of more effective means of immunosuppression or the induction of graft-specific tolerance.

11-22   The fetus is an allograft that is tolerated repetitively.

All of the transplants discussed in this section are artifacts of modern medical technology. However, one tissue that is repeatedly grafted and repeatedly tolerated is the mammalian fetus. The fetus carries paternal MHC and minor H antigens that differ from those of the mother (Fig. 11.33), and yet a mother can bear many children expressing the same non-self MHC proteins derived from the father. The mysterious lack of rejection of the fetus has puzzled generations of reproductive immunologists, and no comprehensive explanation has yet emerged. One problem is that acceptance of the fetal allograft is so much the norm that it is difficult to study the mechanism that prevents rejection; if the mechanism for rejecting the fetus is rarely activated, how can one analyze the mechanisms that control it?

Various hypotheses have been advanced to account for the tolerance normally shown to the fetus. It has been proposed that, for some reason, the fetus is simply not recognized as foreign in the first place. This seems unlikely, since women who have borne several children usually have antibodies directed at the father's MHC proteins; indeed, this is the best source of antibodies for human MHC typing. However, the placenta, which is a fetus-derived tissue, appears to sequester the fetus away from the mother's T cells. The trophoblast cells that form the outer layer of the placenta in contact with maternal tissues do not express classical MHC proteins, perhaps due to a transcriptional inhibitor whose cDNA was recently isolated from placental cells. This gene can suppress expression of MHC molecules in many cell types, and such transfectants are not rejected. This holds real promise for xenotransplantation.

A second possible factor in fetal tolerance is the presence of high levels of α-fetoprotein in fetal blood. This is the fetal form of albumin; it is also a naturally occurring immunosuppressive molecule. If maternal lymphocytes enter the fetal circulation, α-fetoprotein may prevent them from responding to fetal antigens and damaging the fetus.

The fetus is thus tolerated for two main reasons: it occupies a site protected by a non-immunogenic tissue barrier, and its environment is immunosuppressive. We shall see in Section 11-27 that several sites in the body have these characteristics and allow prolonged acceptance of foreign tissue grafts. They are usually called immunologically privileged sites.

Summary.

Clinical transplantation is now an everyday reality, its success built on MHC matching, immunosuppressive drugs, and technical skill. However, even accurate MHC matching does not prevent graft rejection; any genetic difference between host and donor may encode a protein whose peptides are presented as minor H antigens by MHC molecules on the grafted tissue, and responses to these can lead to rejection. Because we lack the ability to suppress the response to the graft specifically without compromising host defense, most transplants require generalized

Tissue transplanted	5 year graft survival*	No. of grafts in USA (1992)
Kidney	80–90%	9736
Liver	40–50%	3064
Heart	70%	2172
Lung	Low	535
Skin	Transient	N/A
Cornea	>90%	N/A
Bone marrow	80%	N/A

Fig. 11.32   Tissues commonly transplanted in clinical medicine. All grafts except corneal and some bone marrow grafts require long-term immunosuppression. The number of organ grafts performed in the USA in 1992 is shown (N/A = not available). *The five year survival values are an average; closer matching between donor and recipient generally gives better survival.

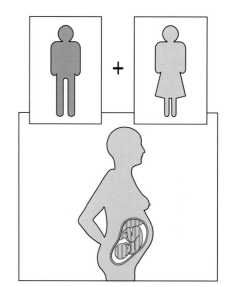

Fig. 11.33   The fetus is an allograft that is not rejected. Although the fetus carries MHC molecules derived from the father, and other foreign antigens, it is not rejected. Even when the mother bears several children to the same father, no sign of immunological rejection is seen.

immunosuppression of the recipient that may cause significant toxicity and increases the risk of cancer and infection. The fetus is a natural allograft that must be accepted or the species will not survive; it almost always is. Tolerance to the fetus may hold the key to specific graft tolerance, or it may be a special case not applicable to organ replacement therapy.

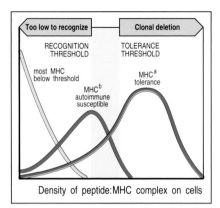

Fig. 11.34 An autoantigenic peptide will be presented at different levels on different MHC molecules. Peptides bind to different MHC molecules with varying affinities; in this example, the peptide binds to MHC^a well, MHC^b less well, and poorly to all other MHC types. The graph shows the number of cells expressing a given density of antigen: MHC complex. For MHC^a, most cells express high levels of the complex, and reactive T-cell clones are therefore deleted in the thymus or anergized in the periphery. For MHC^b, and for all other MHC types, few thymic cells express levels of antigen:MHC complex above the tolerance threshold, and therefore T cells whose receptors could recognize this self peptide mature. However, on all MHC haplotypes other than MHC^b, the peptide is presented so poorly on tissue cells that even T cells with receptors that can recognize the peptide do not respond. Only MHC^b presents the peptide at an intermediate level so that significant levels of the peptide:MHC^b complex are present in the periphery. Normally this would not cause problems, since the peptide would not normally be presented on cells that carry co-stimulatory molecules. However, if the autoreactive T-cell clones are activated inappropriately, they may be able to attack self cells bearing the peptide:MHC^b complex. It is probably rare for a peptide to be presented at this intermediate level by any of the MHC molecules in the population. This situation probably arises most frequently when the antigen is expressed selectively in a tissue rather than ubiquitously, since tissue-specific antigens are less likely to induce clonal deletion in the thymus.

Tolerance and response to self and non-self tissues.

Tolerance to self is acquired by clonal deletion or inactivation of developing lymphocytes, and its loss leads to autoimmune disease, a rare occurrence. Tolerance to antigens expressed by grafted tissues can be induced artificially, but it is very difficult to establish once a full repertoire of functional lymphocytes has been produced, which occurs in fetal life in humans and around the time of birth in mice. We have already learned about the two important mechanisms of self tolerance, clonal deletion by ubiquitous self antigens, and clonal inactivation by tissue-specific antigens presented in the absence of co-stimulatory signals (see Chapters 5–7). These processes were first discovered by studying tolerance to non-self, where the absence of tolerance can be studied in the form of graft rejection. In this section, we shall consider tolerance to self and tolerance to non-self as two aspects of the same basic mechanism. We also examine the instances where tolerance to self or non-self is lost in an attempt to understand the related phenomena of autoimmunity and graft rejection.

11-23   **Autoantigens are not so abundant that they induce clonal deletion or anergy, but are not so rare as to escape recognition entirely.**

We have learned in Chapter 6 that clonal deletion removes T cells that recognize ubiquitous self antigens, and in Chapter 7 that antigens expressed abundantly in the periphery induce anergy or clonal deletion in lymphocytes that encounter them on tissue cells. Most self proteins are expressed at levels that are too low to serve as targets for T-cell recognition on any cell type and thus cannot serve as autoantigens. It is likely that only rare proteins contain peptides that are presented by a given MHC molecule at a level that is sufficient for effector T-cell recognition but too low to induce tolerance (Fig. 11.34). The nature of such peptides will vary depending on the MHC genotype of the individual, since MHC polymorphism profoundly affects peptide binding (see Section 4-16). T cells able to recognize such antigens will be present in the individual but will not normally be activated; they are said to be in a state of **immunological ignorance**. Most autoimmunity is likely to reflect the activation of such immunologically ignorant cells.

Autoimmunity is unlikely to reflect the failure of the main mechanisms of tolerance, clonal deletion and clonal inactivation, because these are such efficient processes. For example, clonal deletion of developing lymphocytes mediates tolerance to self MHC molecules. If such tolerance were not induced, the reaction to self tissues would be similar to those seen in graft-versus-host disease (see Section 10-13). To estimate the impact of clonal deletion on the developing T-cell repertoire, we should remember that the frequency of T cells able to respond to any set of non-self MHC molecules can be as high as 5% (see Section 4-18), yet responses to self MHC antigens are not detected in naturally self-tolerant individuals. Moreover, mice given bone marrow cells from a foreign donor at birth, before any T cells have achieved functional maturity, can be rendered fully and permanently tolerant to the bone marrow donor's tissues, provided the bone marrow donor's cells continue to be produced so as to induce tolerance of each new cohort of developing T cells (Fig. 11.35). This experiment, performed by Medawar, validated Burnet's prediction that developing lymphocytes with an open repertoire of receptors must be purged of self-reactive cells before they achieve functional maturity; it won them a Nobel Prize.

As clonal deletion reliably removes all of the T cells that can mount aggressive responses against self MHC molecules, autoimmune diseases, which involve rare T-cell responses to a particular self peptide bound to a self MHC molecule, are unlikely to reflect a general failure in clonal deletion. Rather, the lymphocytes that mediate autoimmune responses appear not to be subject to clonal deletion and such autoreactive cells are present in all of us. They do not normally cause autoimmunity because they are only activated under special circumstances. Similar arguments apply to the idea that autoimmunity is caused by a random failure in the mechanisms responsible for anergy. Therefore it seems unlikely that naturally occurring autoimmune diseases arise because of a failure in these mechanisms responsible for self-tolerance.

A striking demonstration that autoreactive T cells can be present in healthy individuals comes from a strain of mice carrying transgenes encoding an autoreactive T-cell receptor specific for a peptide of myelin basic protein (MBP) bound to self MHC class II molecules. The autoreactive receptor is present on every T cell, and yet the mice are healthy unless their T cells are activated deliberately. We will discuss these mice further in Section 11-27. Because the level of the specific peptide:MHC class II complex is low outside the central nervous system, a site not visited by naive T cells, the autoreactive T cells remain in a state of immunological ignorance. When these T cells are activated, for example by deliberate immunization, they migrate into all the tissues, including the central nervous system, where they can recognize their MBP:MHC ligand. This triggers cytokine production by the activated T cells, causing inflammation in the brain and the destruction of myelin and neurons that ultimately causes the symptoms of paralysis in this disease.

It is likely that only a small fraction of proteins will be able to serve as autoantigens, since if a self protein is abundant, naive T cells specific for its peptides will be deleted or rendered anergic, while many proteins will be expressed at levels too low to be detected by T cells (see Fig. 11.34). It has been estimated that we can make approximately 10^5

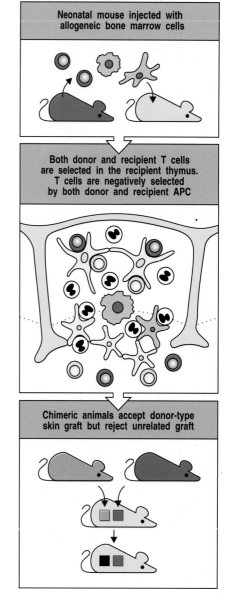

Chimeric animals accept donor-type skin graft but reject unrelated graft

Fig. 11.35 Tolerance to allogeneic skin can be established in bone marrow chimeric mice. In normal mice, T cells that would respond to peptides borne by self antigen-presenting cells (APCs) are negatively selected in the thymus, while T cells reactive to non-self MHC molecules mature, allowing the mouse to reject allogeneic skin grafts (not illustrated). If mice are injected with allogeneic bone marrow at birth (top panel) before they achieve immune competence, they become chimeric, with T cells and APCs deriving from both host and donor bone marrow stem cells. T cells developing in these mice are negatively selected on APCs of both host and donor, so that mature T cells are tolerant to the MHC molecules of the bone marrow donor (center panel). This allows the chimeric mouse to accept skin derived from the bone marrow donor. Such acquired tolerance is specific, since skin from an unrelated or 'third party' donor is rejected normally (bottom panel). This tolerance lasts only while the recipient is chimeric; if donor bone marrow ceases to produce APCs, then tolerance is lost as new T cells develop, and the mice acquire the ability to reject donor skin.

proteins of average length 300 amino acids, capable of generating about 3×10^7 distinct self peptides. Since MHC molecules are rarely expressed at levels above 10^5 molecules per cell, and since the MHC molecules on a cell must bind 10–100 identical peptides for T-cell recognition to occur, fewer than 10 000 self peptides can be presented by a given MHC molecule at levels detectable by T cells. Many of these will be presented at a high enough level to induce tolerance. Therefore, most self peptides will be presented at levels that are too low to induce tolerance in naive T cells by any mechanism, and will also be displayed on tissue cells at levels insufficient for recognition by armed effector T cells and thus cannot serve as autoantigens. However, as shown in Fig. 11.34, a few peptides may fail to induce tolerance yet are present at high enough levels for recognition by T cells. This argument leaves aside the crucial issue of how such effector T cells are activated, which we shall consider in a later section (see Section 11-28).

If the idea that only a few peptides can act as autoantigens is correct, then it is not surprising that there are relatively few distinct autoimmune syndromes, and that all individuals with a particular autoimmune disease tend to recognize the same antigen. If all antigens could give rise to autoimmunity, one would expect that different individuals with the same disease might recognize different antigens on the target tissue, which does not appear to be the case. Finally, since the level of auto-antigenic peptide presented is determined by polymorphic residues in MHC molecules that govern the affinity of peptide binding, this idea could also explain the association of autoimmune diseases with particular MHC genotypes (see Fig. 11.12).

| 11-24 | ## The induction of a tissue-specific response requires expression of co-stimulator activity on antigen-presenting cells. |

As we learned in Chapter 7, only professional antigen-presenting cells that express co-stimulator activity can initiate clonal expansion of T cells — an essential step in all specific immune responses, including graft rejection and presumably autoimmunity. In tissue grafts, it is the donor antigen-presenting cells in the graft that stimulate the host T cells, initiating the response that leads to graft rejection. If the grafted tissue is depleted of antigen-presenting cells by treatment with antibodies or by prolonged incubation, rejection occurs only after a much longer time. The normal route for sensitization to a graft appears to involve the antigen-presenting cells leaving the graft and migrating to regional lymph nodes (Fig. 11.36); when the site of grafting lacks lymphatic drainage, no response against the graft results. Thus, to induce an efficient immune response, antigen-presenting cells bearing both graft antigens and co-stimulatory activity must travel to regional lymph nodes. Here, they are examined by large numbers of host T cells and can activate those that have specific receptors. This clearly reflects the way that responses to infection are normally induced (see Section 9-14).

Although grafts depleted of antigen-presenting cells are tolerated for long periods of time, such grafts are eventually rejected. This process appears to involve host antigen-presenting cells. Interestingly, when grafts that are MHC-identical to the host but mismatched at minor H antigens are depleted of antigen-presenting cells, they are rejected more rapidly than similarly depleted grafts that are MHC-different from the host but identical at minor H antigens. This suggests that host antigen-presenting cells pick up proteins from the graft and present their peptides, including those that contain minor H antigens, to MHC-restricted host T cells. As MHC-different grafts present different peptides and lack self MHC molecules, they may evade this type of response. These grafts are

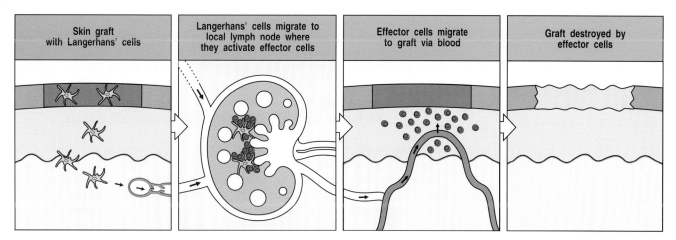

| Skin graft with Langerhans' cells | Langerhans' cells migrate to local lymph node where they activate effector cells | Effector cells migrate to graft via blood | Graft destroyed by effector cells |

Fig. 11.36 The initiation of graft rejection normally involves migration of donor antigen-presenting cells from the graft to local lymph nodes. Here they encounter recirculating T cells, some of which are specific for graft antigens, stimulating these T cells to divide. The resulting activated effector T cells migrate via the thoracic duct to the blood and home to the grafted tissue, which they rapidly destroy. Destruction is highly specific for donor-derived cells, suggesting that it is mediated by direct cytotoxicity and not by non-specific inflammatory processes.

rejected by inflammation, probably triggered when host T cells recognize graft peptides presented by host antigen-presenting macrophages, rather than by the direct attack of cytotoxic T cells on cells of the graft. These experiments also show that the co-stimulation needed to induce a response to the non-self MHC molecules on the graft cannot be delivered separately by host antigen-presenting cells. The ability of professional antigen-presenting cells to pick up antigens in tissues and initiate graft rejection is important, as it may play a role in the initiation of autoimmune tissue damage as well. However, the mechanism by which graft antigens are presented is not currently understood.

11-25   In the absence of co-stimulation, tolerance is induced.

As we learned in Section 7-4, T-cell activation requires that one cell express both peptide:MHC and co-stimulatory molecules; in the absence of co-stimulation, specific antigen recognition leads to anergy or deletion of mature T cells (see Section 7-10). For instance, expression of foreign antigens in peripheral tissues is not sufficient to induce autoimmunity, but co-expression of antigen and B7 in the same target tissue will do so. As B7 expression on peripheral tissue cells is not by itself a sufficient stimulus for autoimmunity, it is clear that the loss of tolerance to self tissues requires both a suitable target antigen (see Section 11-23) and co-stimulation expressed by one cell. As tissue cells are not known to express B7 or other co-stimulatory molecules, tolerance to self tissues is the norm.

From these experiments, it seems likely that autoimmunity results when an antigen-presenting cell that has co-stimulatory activity picks up a tissue-specific antigen. Once an autoantigen is expressed on a cell with co-stimulatory potential, T cells specific for the autoantigen may become activated and can home to the tissues where they produce tissue damage.

A second level at which autoimmune responses to tissue cells may be controlled is that armed effector T cells kill only a limited number of antigen-expressing tissue cells if these lack co-stimulatory activity; after killing a few targets, the effector cell dies. Thus, not only can responses not be initiated in the absence of co-stimulatory activity, they also cannot be sustained in its absence. Thus, in addition to the question of how autoimmunity is avoided, we must ask why does it ever occur? How are responses to self initiated, and how are they sustained? It is thought that one trigger for autoimmunity is infection (see Section 11-28).

| 11-26 | **Dominant immune suppression can be demonstrated in models of tolerance and can affect the course of autoimmune disease.** |

In some models of tolerance, it can be demonstrated that specific T cells play an active role in suppressing the activity of other T cells that are capable of causing tissue damage. Tolerance in these cases is dominant in that it can be transferred by T cells, which are usually called **suppressor T cells**. Furthermore, depletion of the suppressor T cells leads to aggravated responses to self or graft antigens. Although it is clear that these phenomena of immune suppression exist, the mechanisms responsible have been the subject of much controversy. The current thinking on this issue is discussed in greater detail in Chapter 12. Here, we will examine the phenomenon in three animal models.

In a skin graft rejection model, neonatal rats can be rendered tolerant to allogeneic grafts by injection of allogeneic bone marrow. The tolerance induced is highly specific and can be transferred to normal adult recipient rats. This shows that tolerance in this model is dominant and active, as the lymphocytes of the recipient are prevented from mediating graft rejection by the transferred cells. Transfer requires cells of both the allogeneic donor and the original tolerized host. Depletion of either cell type abolishes the transfer of tolerance. This finding is reminiscent of the studies of Medawar on tolerance in neonatal bone marrow chimeric mice discussed in Section 11-23. In both cases, even injection of massive numbers of normal syngeneic lymphocytes, which would react vigorously against the foreign cells in the normal environment of the cell donor, did not break tolerance. Tolerance could only be broken with cells that had been immunized before transfer; such cells probably break tolerance by killing the allogeneic donor cells. Thus, an active host response prevents graft rejection in this model. Since the tolerance is specific for cells of the original donor, the suppression must also be specific.

In mouse diabetes, an autoimmune disorder, transfer of certain islet-specific T-cell clones can prevent the destruction of pancreatic β cells by cytotoxic T cells. This suggests that these cells can suppress the activity of autoaggressive T cells in an antigen-dependent manner. There are interesting hints that such cells naturally affect the course of the auto-immune response that causes diabetes; β-cell destruction in humans occurs over a period of several years before diabetes is manifest, yet when new islets are transplanted from an identical twin into his or her diabetic sibling, they are destroyed within a few weeks. This suggests that in the normal course of the disease, specific cells protect the β cells from attack by effector T cells and the disease therefore progresses slowly. It may be that after the host islets have been destroyed these protective mechanisms decline in activity, but the effector cells responsible for rejection do not.

If specific suppression of autoimmune responses could be elicited at will, autoimmunity would not be a problem. While this has not yet been documented in human autoimmunity, experimental studies in which tissue antigens are fed to mice have shown some protective effects, and early studies of this procedure in humans have also shown benefits. Feeding of specific antigen is known to elicit a local immune response in the intestinal mucosa, while responses to the same antigen given sub-sequently by a systemic route are suppressed (see Section 2-4). This has been exploited in experimental autoimmune diseases by feeding proteins from target tissues to mice; mice fed insulin are protected from diabetes, while mice fed myelin basic protein are resistant to experimental allergic encephalomyelitis (Fig. 11.37). This disease is normally caused by inflammatory T cells that produce IFN-γ in response to myelin basic protein; in mice fed with this protein, CD4 T cells that produce cytokines such as transforming growth factor-β (TGF-β) and IL-4 are found in the brain instead. In both of these cases, the protection appears to be tissue rather than antigen-specific. Thus, feeding insulin protects against diabetes, yet insulin is not thought to be the target of autoimmune attack on the β cells. Likewise, feeding myelin basic protein protects against experimental allergic encephalomyelitis elicited by other brain antigens. Feeding with antigen induces the production of T cells producing TGF-β and IL-5, because these cytokines are also required for IgA production to antigens ingested in food. If feeding with antigen works as a clinical therapy, it would have the advantage over treatments with immunosuppressive drugs that it does not alter the general immune competence of the host. This intriguing potential therapeutic approach will be discussed further in Chapter 12.

Like human diabetes, multiple sclerosis is a chronic, relapsing disease with acute episodes followed by periods of quiescence. This again suggests a balance between autoimmune and protective T cells that may alter at different stages of the disease. However, it remains to be proven whether the specific suppressive cells discussed in this section exist

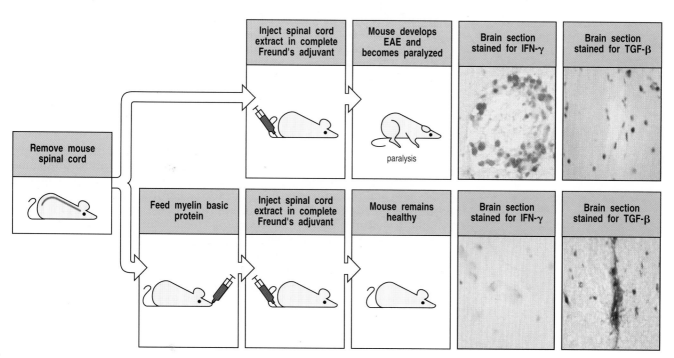

Fig. 11.37   Antigen given orally can lead to protection against autoimmune disease. The autoimmune disease experimental allergic encephalomyelitis (EAE) is induced in mice or rats by immunizing them with spinal cord in complete Freund's adjuvant (top panels); the disease is caused by T_H1 cells specific for myelin basic protein (MBP). When mice or rats are first fed with MBP, later immunization with spinal cord or MBP fails to induce the disease. T_H1 cells that produce IFN-γ are found in the brains of diseased rats (upper left photograph, where the brown staining reveals the presence of IFN-γ). These T cells are presumably responsible for the damage that results in paralysis. Note that cells expressing TGF-β are not seen in diseased rats (upper right photograph). In orally tolerized rats, IFN-γ-producing cells are absent (lower left photograph) while TGF-β-producing T cells are found in the brain in place of the autoaggressive T_H1 cells (lower right photograph, the brown stain in this case reveals the presence of TGF-β), and presumably protect the brain from autoimmune attack. Photographs courtesy of S Khoury, W Hancock, and H Weiner.

naturally and contribute to self tolerance, or whether they only arise upon artificial stimulation or in response to autoimmune attack. Nevertheless, as they can play an active, dominant role in self tolerance, they are particularly attractive targets for immunotherapy of autoimmune disease.

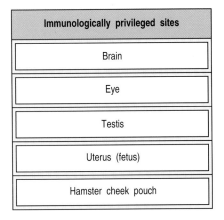

Fig. 11.38 **Some body sites are immunologically privileged.** Tissue grafts placed in these sites often last indefinitely, and antigens placed in these sites do not elicit destructive immune responses.

11-27 | **Antigens in immunologically privileged sites do not induce immune attack but can serve as targets.**

Tissue grafts placed in some sites in the body do not elicit immune responses. For instance, the brain and the anterior chamber of the eye are sites in which tissues can be grafted without inducing graft rejection. Such locations in the body are termed **immunologically privileged sites** (Fig. 11.38). It was originally believed that immunological privilege arose from the failure of antigens to leave privileged sites and induce responses. However, subsequent studies have shown that antigens do leave immunologically privileged sites, and that these antigens do interact with T cells; instead of eliciting a destructive immune response, they induce tolerance or a response that is not destructive to the tissue. Immunologically privileged sites appear to be unusual in two ways. First, the communication between the privileged site and the body is atypical in that extracellular fluid in these sites does not pass through conventional lymphatics, although proteins placed in these sites do leave them and can have immunological effects. Second, humoral factors, presumably cytokines, which affect the behavior of the immune response are produced in privileged sites and leave them together with antigens. The cytokine TGF-β appears to be particularly important in this regard, and antigens mixed with TGF-β appear to induce T-cell responses that do not damage tissues, such as helper rather than inflammatory CD4 T-cell responses.

Paradoxically, it is often the antigens sequestered in immunologically privileged sites that are the targets of autoimmune attack; for example, multiple sclerosis is directed at brain autoantigens such as myelin basic protein and is one of the most prevalent autoimmune diseases. As we have seen, experimental allergic encephalomyelitis is induced in some strains of rats and mice upon immunization with spinal cord or myelin basic protein in adjuvant. It is therefore clear that this antigen does not induce deletional tolerance and anergy. As we saw in Section 11-23, mice transgenic for a T-cell receptor specific for myelin basic protein carry this autoreactive receptor on most of their T cells, yet develop normally. These T cells are readily activated by the appropriate peptide of the protein. Nevertheless, the mice do not become diseased unless they are immunized with myelin basic protein, in which case they become acutely sick, show severe infiltration of the brain with specific inflammatory T cells, and often die. The non-transgenic littermates have a milder, transient illness. Thus, at least some antigens expressed in immunologically privileged sites induce neither tolerance nor activation, but if activation is induced elsewhere they may become targets for autoimmune attack. It seems plausible that T cells specific for antigens that are sequestered in immunologically privileged sites are more likely to remain in the state of immunological ignorance described in Section 11-23. This is further shown in the eye disease **sympathetic ophthalmia** (Fig. 11.39). If one eye is ruptured by a blow or other trauma, an autoimmune response to eye proteins can occur. Once the response is induced, it often attacks both eyes. Immunosuppression and removal of the damaged eye, the source of antigen, is frequently required to preserve vision in the undamaged eye.

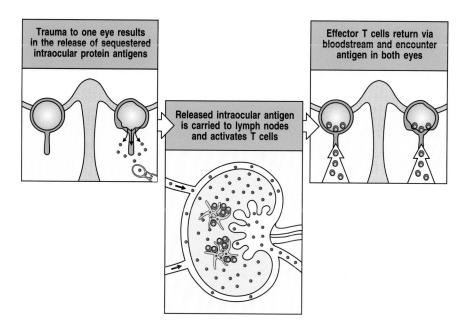

Fig. 11.39 Damage to an immunologically privileged site can induce an autoimmune response. In the disease sympathetic ophthalmia, trauma to one eye releases the sequestered eye antigens into the surrounding tissues, making them accessible to T cells. The effector cells elicited attack the traumatized eye, and also infiltrate and attack the healthy eye. Thus, although the sequestered antigens do not induce a response by themselves, if a response is induced elsewhere they can serve as targets for attack.

It is not surprising that effector T cells can enter immunologically privileged sites: such sites can become infected, and effector cells must be able to enter these sites during infection. As we learned in Chapter 9, effector T cells enter most or all tissues after activation, but accumulations of cells are only seen when antigen is recognized in the site, triggering the production of cytokines that alter tissue barriers.

11-28   Autoimmunity could be triggered by infection in a variety of ways.

Human autoimmune diseases often appear gradually, making it difficult to find out how the process is initiated. Nevertheless, there is a strong suspicion that infections can trigger autoimmune disease in genetically susceptible individuals. Indeed, many experimental autoimmune diseases are induced by mixing tissue cells with adjuvants that contain bacteria. For example, to induce experimental allergic encephalomyelitis (see Fig. 11.37), it is necessary to emulsify the spinal cord or myelin basic protein used for immunization in complete Freund's adjuvant, which includes killed *Mycobacterium tuberculosis* (see Section 2-3); when the mycobacteria are omitted from the adjuvant, not only is no disease elicited, but the animals become refractory to disease induction with antigen in complete Freund's adjuvant, and T cells can transfer this resistance to syngeneic recipients (Fig. 11.40). There are several other systems in which infection is important in the induction of disease; for example, the transgenic mice that express a T-cell receptor specific for myelin basic protein (see Sections 11-23 and 11-27) often develop spontaneous autoimmunity if they become infected. One possible mechanism for this loss of tolerance is that the infectious agents induce co-stimulatory activity on cells expressing low levels of peptides from myelin basic protein, thus activating the autoreactive T cells.

It has also been suggested that autoimmunity may be initiated by a mechanism known as **molecular mimicry**, in which antibodies or T cells generated in the response to an infectious agent cross-react with self antigens. To show that infectious agents can trigger responses that have the capacity to destroy tissues, mice were made transgenic for a viral nuclear protein driven by the insulin promoter, so that the protein was expressed only in pancreatic β cells. Because the amount of protein expressed was low, the T cells that recognized the viral protein remained

Fig. 11.40 Bacterial adjuvants are required to induce experimental autoimmune disease. Mice immunized with spinal cord homogenate in complete Freund's adjuvant, which contains large numbers of killed *Mycobacterium tuberculosis* organisms, get experimental allergic encephalomyelitis (EAE). Mice immunized with the same antigen in incomplete Freund's adjuvant, which lacks the *M. tuberculosis*, not only do not become diseased, but are actually protected from subsequent disease induction. Moreover, T cells from these mice can transfer protection from disease to naive, syngeneic recipients.

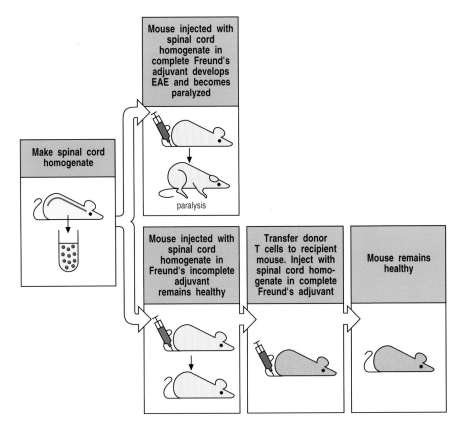

ignorant, that is, they were neither tolerant to the viral protein nor activated by it, and the animals showed no sign of disease. However, if they were infected with the live virus, they responded by making cytotoxic CD8 T cells specific for the viral protein and these could destroy the β cells, causing diabetes (Fig. 11.41). Recent data also suggest that the immune response to natural infection occasionally elicits T cells that cause autoimmune disease by recognizing cross-reacting self peptides.

In antibody-mediated autoimmunity, it is clear that molecular mimicry can operate; microbial antigens can elicit antibody responses that react not only with the pathogen but also with host antigens that are similar in structure. This type of response occurs after infection with some

Fig. 11.41 Virus infection can break tolerance to a transgenic viral protein expressed in pancreatic β cells. Mice that express a protein from the lymphocytic choriomeningitis virus (LCMV) in pancreatic β cells do not respond to the protein and therefore do not get diabetes. However, if the transgenic mice are infected with LCMV, a potent anti-viral cytotoxic T-cell response is elicited, and this kills the β cells, leading to diabetes. It is thought that infectious agents may sometimes elicit T-cell responses that cross-react with self peptides, a process known as molecular mimicry, and that this could cause autoimmune disease in a similar way.

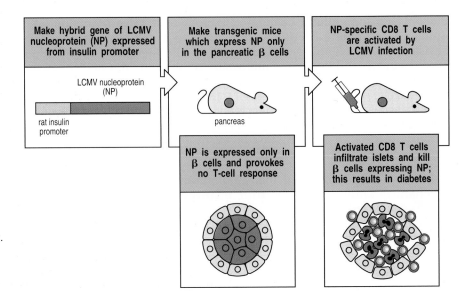

Streptococcus species that elicit antibodies that cross-react with kidney, joint, and heart antigens to produce pathology. However, such responses are usually transient and do not lead to sustained autoantibody production since the helper T cells are specific for the microbe and not for self proteins. Host proteins that complex with bacteria can induce a similar transient response; in this case, the antibody response is not cross-reactive, but the bacterium is acting as a carrier, allowing B cells that express an autoreactive receptor to receive inappropriate T-cell help. These and some other mechanisms that could allow an infectious agent to break tolerance are summarized in Fig. 11.42. All of these mechanisms can be shown to act in experimental systems, and some evidence supports their importance in human autoimmune disease.

The argument that autoimmunity may be initiated by infection is strengthened by the fact that there are several human autoimmune diseases in which a prior infection with a specific agent or class of agents leads to a particular disease (Fig. 11.43). Again, disease susceptibility in these cases is determined largely by MHC genotype. However, in most autoimmune diseases there is still no firm evidence that a particular infectious agent is associated with onset of the disease; this may be partly because it often takes many years for a patient with an autoimmune disease to show noticeable symptoms.

The persistence of autoimmune phenomena is also puzzling. Even if an infection initiates disease by, for example, inducing co-stimulatory activity on cells in a tissue, the co-stimulation would have to be sustained once the infection has been cleared. One way in which this has been accomplished in mice is through antigen-specific B cells, which are rendered immunogenic by induction of B7.2 by T cells expressing CD40 ligand. If these B cells also bind and present an autoantigen, then the high efficiency of antigen presentation by these cells could explain

Mechanism	Disruption of cell or tissue barrier	Infection of antigen-presenting cell	Binding of pathogen to self protein	Molecular mimicry	Superantigen
Effect	Release of sequestered self antigen; activation of non-tolerized cells	Induction of co-stimulator activity	Pathogen acts as carrier to allow anti-self response	Production of cross-reactive antibodies or T cells	Polyclonal activation of autoreactive T cells
Example	Sympathetic ophthalmia	Effect of adjuvants: induction of EAE	? Interstitial nephritis	Rheumatic fever ? Diabetes ? Multiple sclerosis	? Rheumatoid arthritis

Fig. 11.42 There are several ways in which infectious agents could break self tolerance. Since some antigens are sequestered from the circulation, either behind a tissue barrier or within the cell, it is possible that an infection that breaks cell and tissue barriers may expose hidden antigens (first panel). A second possibility is that the local inflammation in response to an infectious agent may trigger expression of MHC molecules and co-stimulators on tissue cells, inducing an autoimmune response (second panel). In some cases, infectious agents may bind to self proteins. Since the infectious agent induces a helper T-cell response, any B cell that recognizes the self protein will also receive help. Such responses should be self-limiting once the infectious agent is eliminated, since at this point the T-cell help will no longer be provided (third panel). Infectious agents may induce either T- or B-cell responses that can cross-react with self antigens. This is termed molecular mimicry (fourth panel). T-cell polyclonal activation by a bacterial superantigen could overcome clonal anergy, allowing an autoimmune process to begin (fifth panel). There is little evidence for most of these mechanisms in human autoimmune disease (see text).

Fig. 11.43 Association of infection with autoimmune diseases. Several autoimmune diseases occur after specific infections and are presumably triggered by the infection. The case of post-streptococcal disease is best known but is now rare since effective antibiotic therapy of Group A streptococcal infection usually prevents post-infection complications. Most of these post-infection autoimmune diseases also show susceptibility linked to MHC.

Associations of infection with immune-mediated tissue damage		
Infection	HLA association	Consequence
Group A streptococcus	?	Rheumatic fever (carditis, polyarthritis)
Chlamydia trachomatis	HLA-B27	Reiter's syndrome (arthritis)
Shigella flexneri, Salmonella typhimurium, S. enteritidis, Yersinia enterocolitica, Campylobacter jejuni	HLA-B27	Reactive arthritis
Borrelia burgdorferi	HLA-DR2, DR4	Chronic arthritis in Lyme disease

epitope spreading, the finding that responses to autoantigens tend to become more diverse as the response persists. It is possible that analysis of the expression of co-stimulatory activity on cells in tissues that are damaged in active autoimmune disease may improve our understanding of autoimmunity. If we could learn to modulate the expression of co-stimulatory activity, perhaps these sustained and damaging responses could be prevented.

Summary.

Tolerance to self is a normal state that is maintained chiefly by clonal deletion of developing cells and clonal or deletion inactivation of mature, peripheral cells. In addition, some antigens are ignored by the immune system, many by being present in immunologically privileged sites. When the state of self tolerance is disrupted, perhaps by infection, then autoimmunity can result. The process of clonal deletion sets limits on the kinds of autoimmune diseases that can occur; only antigens that do not trigger clonal deletion in the thymus, either because they are not abundant enough or because they are tissue-specific and not expressed in the thymus, are candidate autoantigens. Tolerance to non-self can be acquired by mimicking the mechanisms responsible for tolerance to self. A third mechanism for self tolerance, dominant suppression, has been noted in several experimental systems of autoimmunity and graft rejection; if this mechanism could be understood, it is possible that it could be used to prevent both graft rejection and autoimmunity, which are closely related problems.

Summary to Chapter 11.

The response to non-infectious antigens causes three types of medical problem, allergy, autoimmunity, and graft rejection. These responses have many features in common because all use the normal mechanisms of the adaptive immune response to produce symptoms and pathology (Fig. 11.44). What is unique to these syndromes is their initiation and the nature of the antigens recognized, not the underlying nature of the response itself. For each of these undesirable categories of response, the question is how to control them without adversely affecting protective immunity to infection. The answer may lie in a more complete understanding of the regulation of the immune response, especially the suppressive mechanisms that appear to be important in tolerance. The control of the immune response is examined further in the next chapter.

Classification	Effector mechanism	Examples		
		Allergy	Graft rejection	Autoimmune disease
Type I	IgE activation of mast cells ($T_H2 >> T_H1$)	Allergic rhinitis Allergic asthma Wheal and flare Systemic anaphylaxis	None	None
Type II	Antibody:FcR interaction Complement fixation at cell surface ($T_H1 >> T_H2$)	Some drug allergies where drug binds to cell surface eg penicillin	Transfusion reaction (antibody to donor erythrocytes) White graft (antibody to blood vessel wall)	Autoimmune hemolytic anemia Goodpasture's syndrome
	Antibody to surface receptor	None	None	Myasthenia gravis (antagonist) Graves' disease (agonist)
Type III	Immune complexes Activation of complement and FcR+ cells	Serum sickness Arthus reaction Farmer's lung	None	Systemic lupus erythematosus
Type IV	Macrophage activation by T cells ($T_H1 > T_H2$)	Contact dermatitis Tuberculin reaction	MHC class II disparate graft rejection (?)	Rheumatoid arthritis Multiple sclerosis (?)
	Cytotoxic T cells	Contact dermatitis (?)	Tissue-graft rejection	Diabetes mellitus

Fig. 11.44   Allergy, autoimmunity and graft rejection all share the same effector mechanisms as the adaptive immune response to pathogens. Most effector mechanisms are active in all three types of response, with the exception of type I responses, which play the major role in allergy. The symptoms generated by the different responses are distinct, owing to the fact that antigens differ in localization and route of delivery. In some cases the mechanism of tissue damage is uncertain; these cases are marked with (?).

General references.

Coombs, R.R.A. and Gell, P.G.H.: **Classification of allergic reactions for clinical hypersensitivity and disease.** In: Gell, P.G.H., Coombs, R.R.A., and Lachmann, P.J. (eds): *Clinical Aspects of Immunology.* Oxford, Blackwell Scientific, 1975, 761-781.

Holgate, S.T. and Church, M.K.: *Allergy,* 1st edn. London, Gower Medical Publishing, 1993.

Moller, G. (ed.): **Chronic graft rejection.** *Immunol. Rev.* 1993, **134**:1116.

Moller, G. (ed.): **Models of autoimmunity.** *Immunol. Rev.* 1993, **118**:1-310.

Moller, G. (ed.): **Transgenic mice and immunological tolerance.** *Immunol. Rev.* 1992, **122**:1-204.

Moller, G. (ed.): **Peripheral T-cell immunological tolerance.** *Immunol. Rev.* 1993, **133**:1-240.

Rose, N.R. and MacKay, I.R. (eds): *The Autoimmune Diseases II,* 2nd edn. Orlando, Academic Press, 1992.

Samter, M., Talmage, D.W., Frank, M.M., Austen, K.F., and Claman, H.N. (eds.): *Immunological Diseases, Volumes 1 and 2,* 4th edn. Boston, Little, Brown and Co., 1988.

Sutton, B.J. and Gould, H.J.: **The human IgE network.** *Nature* 1993, **366**:421-428.

Section references.

11-1   Allergic reactions occur when extrinsic antigens are recognized by a pre-sensitized individual.

Kitamura, Y.: **Heterogeneity of mast cells and phenotypic change between subpopulations.** *Ann. Rev. Immunol.* 1989, **7**:59-76.

Lictenstein, L.M.: **Allergy and the immune system.** *Sci. Amer.* 1993, **269**:117-124.

Norman, P.S.: **Modern concepts of immunotherapy.** *Curr. Opin. Immunol.* 1993, **5**:968-973.

11-2   The nature of the allergic reaction depends on the nature of the immune response.

Dombrowicz, D., Flamand, V., Brigman, K.K., Koller, B.H., and Kinet, J.P.: **Abolition of anaphylaxis by targeted disruption of the high-affinity immunoglobulin E receptor α chain gene.** *Cell* 1993, **75**:969-976.

11-3   Allergens that elicit IgE responses are often delivered transmucosally at low dose.

Marsh, D.G. and Norman, P.S.: **Antigens that cause atopic disease.** In: Samter, M., Talmage, D.W., Frank, M.M., Austen, K.F., Claman, H.N. (eds): *Immunological Diseases.* Little, Brown, and Co., 1988, 982-1008.

Parronchi, P., Macchia, D., Biswas, M.P., Simonelli, C., Maggi, E., Ricci, M., Ansari, A.A., and Romagnani, S.: **Allergen- and bacterial-antigen-specific T-cell clones established from atopic donors show a different profile of cytokine production**. *Proc. Natl Acad. Sci. USA* 1991, **88**:4538.

Ricci, M., Rossi, O., Bertoni, M., and Matucci, A.: **The importance of T$_H$2-like cells in the pathogenesis of airway allergic inflammation**. *Clin. Exper. Allergy* 1993, **23**:360-369.

Romagnani, S.: **Regulation of the development of type 2 T-helper cells in allergy**. *Curr. Opin. Immunol.* 1994, **6**:838-846

Varney, V., Hamid, Q.A., Gag, M., Ying, S., Jacobson, M., Frew, A.J., Kay, A.B., and Durham, S.R.: **Influence of grass pollen immunotherapy on cellular infiltration and cytokine mRNA expression during allergen-induced late- phase cutaneous responses**. *J. Clin. Invest.* 1993, **92**:644-651.

Wierenga, E.A., Snoek, M., De Grast, C., Chretein, I., Bos, J.D., Jansen, H.M., and Kapsenberg, M.L.: **Evidence of compartmentalization of functional subsets of CD4$^+$ T lymphocytes in atopic patients**. *J. Immunol.* 1990, **144**:4651.

11-4   Genetic factors contribute to the preferential priming of helper T cells and IgE-mediated allergy.

Huang, S.K., and Marsh, D.G.: **Genetics of allergy**. *Ann. Allergy* 1993, **70**:347-358.

Marsh, D.G. and Bias, W.B.: **The genetics of atopic allergy**. In: Samter, M., Talmage, D.W., Frank, M.M., and Claman, H.N. (eds): *Immunologic Diseases.* Boston, Little, Brown and Co., 1988, 981-1008.

Meyers, D.A., Bias, W.B., and Marsh, D.G.: **A genetic study of total IgE levels in the Amish**. *Hum. Hered.* 1982, **32**:15.

11-5   IgE-mediated responses have different consequences depending on the dose of allergen and its route of entry.

Anderson, J.A.: **Allergic reactions to drugs and biological agents**. *JAMA* 1992, **268**:2845-2857.

11-6   Treatment with anti-histamines affects only the first phase of the IgE-mediated response.

Davies, P., Bailey, P.J., Goldenberg, M.M., and Ford-Hutchinson, A.W.: **The role of arachidonic acid oxygenation products in pain and inflammation**. *Ann. Rev. Immunol.* 1993, **2**:335-357.

Galli, S.J., Gordon, J.R., and Wershii, B.K.: **Cytokine production by mast cells and basophils**. *Curr. Opin. Immunol.* 1991, **3**:865-873.

Ishizaka, T., Mitsui, H., Yanagida, M., Miura, T., and Dvorak, A.: **Development of human mast cells from their progenitors**. *Curr. Opin. Immunol.* 1993, **5**:937-943.

Parker, C.W.: **Lipid mediators produced through the lipoxygenase pathway**. *Annu. Rev. Immunol.* 1993, **5**:65-84.

Zweiman, B.: **The late-phase reaction: role of IgE, its receptor and cytokines**. *Curr. Opin. Immunol.* 1993, **5**:950-955.

11-7   Some immediate hypersensitivity reactions are mediated by IgG antibodies.

Dixon, F.J., Cochrane, C.C., and Theofilopoulos, A.N.: **Immune complex injury**. In: Samter, M., Talmage, D.W., Frank, M.M., Austen, K.F., and Claman, H.N.: *Immunologic Diseases.* Little, Brown and Co., 1988, 233-259.

Stankus, R.P., and Salvaggio, J.E.: **Infiltrative lung disease: Hypersensitivity pneumonitis, allergic bronchopulmonary aspergillosis, and the inorganic dust pneumoconioses**. In: Samter, M., Talmage, D.W., Frank, M.M., Austen, K.F., and Claman, H.N. (eds): *Immunologic Diseases.* Little Brown and Co., 1988, 1561-1585.

11-8   Delayed-type hypersensitivity reactions are mediated by inflammatory T cells and CD8 cytotoxic T cells.

Cher, D., and Mosmann, T.: **Two types of murine helper T-cell clone. II. Delayed type hypersensitivity is mediated by Th1 clones**. *J. Immunol.* 1987, **138**:3688.

Kirkpatrick, C.H.: **Delayed hypersensitivity**. In: Samter, M., Talmage, D.W., Frank, M.M., Austen, K.F., and Claman, H.N. (eds): *Immunologic Diseases.* Little, Brown and Co., 1988, 261-277.

Stout, R., and Bottomly, K.: **Antigen-specific activation of effector macrophages by interferon-gamma producing (T$_H$1) T-cell clones. Failure of IL-4 producing (T$_H$2) T-cell clones to activate effector functions in macrophages**. *J. Immunol.* 1989, **142**:760.

11-9   Specific adaptive immune responses to self antigens can cause autoimmune disease.

Acha-Orbea, H., Steinman, L., and McDevitt, H.O.: **T-cell receptors in murine autoimmune diseases**. *Ann. Rev. Immunol.* 1993, **7**:371-405.

Naparstek, Y., and Plotz, P.H.: **The role of autoantibodies in autoimmune disease**. *Ann. Rev. Immunol.* 1993, **11**:79-104.

Rose, N.R., and MacKay, I.R.: **The immune response in autoimmunity and autoimmune disease**. In: Rose, N.R. and MacKay, I.R. (eds): *The Autoimmune Diseases II.* Academic Press, 1992, 1-26.

11-10   Susceptibility to autoimmune diseases is controlled by environmental and genetic factors, especially MHC genes.

Campbell, R.D., and Milner, C.M.: **MHC genes in autoimmunity**. *Curr. Opin. Immunol.* 1993, **5**:887-893.

Moller, E., Bohme, J., Valugerdi, M.A., Ridderstad, A., and Olerup, O.: **Speculations on mechanisms of HLA associations with autoimmune diseases and the specificity of autoreactive T lymphocytes**. *Immunol. Rev.* 1993, **118**:5-19.

Nepom, G.T., and Erlich, H.: **MHC class II molecules and autoimmunity**. *Annu. Rev. Immunol.* 1991, **9**:493-525.

Nepom, G.T., and Concannon, P.: **Molecular genetics of autoimmunity**. In: Rose, N.R. and MacKay, I.R. (eds): *The Autoimmune Diseases II.* Academic Press, 1992, 127-152.

11-11   Either antibody or T cells can cause tissue damage in autoimmune disease.

Wieslander, J., Barr, J.F., Butkowski, R.J., Edwards, S.J., Bygren, P., Heinegard, D., and Hudson, B.G.: **Goodpasture antigen of the glomerular basement membrane: Localization to noncollagenous regions of type IV collagen**. *Proc. Natl Acad. Sci. USA* 1984, **81**:3838-3842.

11-12   Autoantibodies to receptors cause disease by stimulating or blocking receptor function.

Adams, D.D., and Purves, H.D.: **Abnormal responses in the assay of thyrotropin**. *Proc. Univ. Otago Med. School* 1956, **34**:11.

Lindstrom, J., Shelton, D., and Fuji, Y.: **Myasthenia gravis**. *Adv. Immunol.* 1988, **42**:233-284.

Weetman, A.P., Yateman, M.E., Ealey, P.A., Black, C.M., Reimer, C.B., Williams, R.C. Jr, Shine, B., and Marshall, N.J.: **Thyroid stimulating antibody activity between different immunoglobulin G subclasses**. *J. Clin. Invest.* 1990, **86**:723-727.

Willcox, N.: **Myasthenia gravis**. *Curr. Opin. Immunol.* 1993, **5**:910-917.

11-13 Chronic generation of immune complexes causes tissue damage in systemic autoimmune diseases.

Ferrell, P.B., and Tan, E.M.: **Systemic lupus erythematosus**. In: Rose, N.R. and MacKay, I.R. (eds): *The Autoimmune Diseases.* Academic Press, 1985, 29-57.

Reichlin, M.: **Disease-specific autoantibodies in the systemic rheumatic diseases**. In: Rose, N.R. and MacKay, I.R. (eds): *The Autoimmune Diseases II.* Academic Press, 1992, 195-212.

Tan, E.M.: **Antinuclear antibodies: diagnostic markers for autoimmune diseases and probes for cell biology**. *Adv. Immunol.* 1989, **44**:93.

11-14 The mechanism of autoimmune tissue damage can often be determined by adoptive transfer.

Lindstom, J.M., Seybold, M.E., Lennon, V.A., Whittingham, S., and Duane, D.: **Antibody to acetylcholine receptor in myasthenia gravis**. *Neurology* 1976, **26**:1054.

Zamvil, S., Nelson, P., Trotter, J., Mitchell, D., Knobler, R., Fritz, R., and Steinman, L.: **T-cell clones specific for myelin basic protein induce chronic relapsing paralysis and demyelination**. *Nature* 1985, **317**:355.

11-15 Autoantibodies can be used to identify the target of the autoimmune process.

Craft, J., Mamula, M.J., Ohosone, H., Boire, G., Gold, H., and Hardin, J.A.: **snRNPs and scRNPs as autoantigens: clues to etiology of connective tissue diseases**. *Clin. Rheumatol.* 1990, **9**:1.

11-16 The target of T-cell mediated autoimmunity is difficult to identify owing to the nature of T-cell ligands.

Baekkeskov, S., Aanstoot, H.J., Christgau, S., Reetz, A., Solimena, M., Cascalho, M., Folli, F., Richter-Olesen, H., and De Camilli, P.: **Identification of the 64kD autoantigen in insulin-dependent diabetes as the GABA-synthesizing enzyme glutamic acid decarboxylase**. *Nature* 1990, **347**:151-156.

Lanchbury, J.S., and Pitzalis, C.: **Cellular immune mechanisms in rheumatoid arthritis and other inflammatory arthritides**. *Curr. Opin. Immunol.* 1993, **5**:918-924.

MacLaren, N., and Lafferty, K.: **Perspectives in diabetes. The 12th international immunology and diabetes workshop**. *Diabetes* 1993, **42**:1099-1104.

Martin, R., McFarland, H.F., and McFarlin, D.E.: **Immunological aspects of demyelinating diseases**. *Annu. Rev. Immunol.* 1992, **10**:153-187.

Protti, M.P., Manfredi, A.A., Horton, R.M., Bellone, M., and Conti-Tronconi, B.M.: **Myasthenia gravis: recognition of a human autoantigen at the molecular level**. *Immunol. Today* 1993, **14**:363-368.

Willcox, N., Baggi, F., Batocchi, A.-P., Beeson, D., Harcourt, G., Hawke, S., Jacobson, L., Matsuo, H. and Moody, A.-M.: **Approaches for studying the pathogenic T cells in autoimmune patients**. *Ann. NY Acad. Sci.* 1993, **681**:219-237.

11-17 The rejection of grafts is an immunological response mediated primarily by T cells.

Manning, D.D., Reed, N.D., and Schaffer, C.F.: **Maintenance of skin xenografts of widely divergent phylogenetic origin on congenitally athymic (*nude*) mice**. *J. Exper. Med.* 1973, **138**:488.

Medawar, P.B.: **The immunology of transplantation**. *Harvey Lect.* 1958, **1956**:144.

Morris, P.S.: *Tissue transplantation*, 1st edn. Edinburgh, Churchill Livingstone, 1982.

Sprent, J., Schaefer, M., Lo, D., and Korngold, R.: **Properties of purified T-cell subsets**. *J. Exper. Med.* 1986, **163**:998-1011.

11-18 Matching donor and recipient at the MHC improves the outcome of transplantation.

Ayoub, G. and Terasaki, P.: **HLA-DR matching in multicenter, single-typing laboratory data**. *Transplantation* 1982, **33**:515.

Opelz, G., Mytilineos, J., Scherer, S., Dunckley, H., Trejaut, J., Chapman, J., Middleton, D., Savage, D., Fischer, O., Bignon, J.-D., Bensa, J.-C., Albert, E., and Noreen, H.: **Survival of DNA HLA-DR typed and matched cadaver kidney transplants**. *Lancet* 1991, **338**:461-463.

11-19 In MHC-identical grafts, rejection is caused by non-self peptides bound to graft MHC molecules.

Roopenian, D.C.: **What are minor histocompatibility loci? A new look at an old question**. *Immunol. Today* 1992, **13**:7-10.

Scott, D.M., Ehrmann, I.E., Ellis., P.S., Bishop, C.E., Agulnik, A.I., Simpson, E., and Mitchell, M.J.: **Identification of a mouse male-specific transplantation antigen, H-Y**. *Nature* 1995, **376**:695-698.

Walny, H.-J. and Rammensee, H.-G.: **Identification of classical minor histocompatibility antigen as cell-derived peptide**. *Nature* 1990, **343**:275-278.

11-20 Antibodies reacting with endothelium cause hyperacute graft rejection.

Kissmeyer-Nielsen, F., Olsen, S., Petersen, V.P., and Fjeldborg. O.: **Hyperacute rejection of kidney allografts, associated with pre-existing humoral antibodies against donor cells**. *Lancet* 1966, **2**:662.

Williams, G.M., Hume, D., Hudson, R., Morris, P., Kano, K., and Milgrom, F.: **Hyperacute renal homograft rejection in man**. *N. Engl. J. Med.* 1968, **279**:611-618.

11-22 The fetus is an allograft that is tolerated repetitively.

Hunt, J.S.: **Immunobiology of pregnancy**. *Curr. Opin. Immunol.* 1992, **4**:591-596.

Kovats, S., Main, E.L., Librach, C., Stubblebine, M., Fischer, S.J., and DeMars, R.: **A class I antigen, HLA-G, expressed in human trophoblasts**. *Science* 1990, **248**:220-223.

11-23 Autoantigens are not so abundant that they induce clonal deletion or anergy, but are not so rare as to escape recognition entirely.

Billingham, R.E., Brent, L., and Medawar, P.B.: **Actively acquired tolerance of foreign cells**. *Nature* 1953, **172**:603-606.

Brent, L.: **Tolerance: Past, present, and future**. *Transplant. Proc.* 1991, **23**:2056-2060.

Goverman, J., Woods, A., Larson, L., Weiner, L.P., Hood, L., and Zaller, D.M.: **Transgenic mice that express a myelin basic protein-specific T-cell receptor develop spontaneous autoimmunity**. *Cell* 1993, **72**:551-560.

Katz, J., Wang, B., Haskins, K., Benoist, C., and Mathis, D.: **Following a diabetogenic T cell from genesis through pathogenesis**. *Cell* 1993, **74**:1089-1100.

Ohashi, P.S., Oehen, S., Burki, K., Pircher, H.P., Ohashi, C., Odermatt, C.T., Odermatt, B., Malissen, B., Zinkernagel, R., and Hengertner, H.: **Ablation of tolerance and induction of diabetes by virus infection in viral antigen transgenic mice**. *Cell* 1991, **65**:305-317.

11-24 **The induction of a tissue-specific response requires expression of co-stimulator activity on antigen-presenting cells.**

Benichou, G., Takizawa, P.A., Olson, C.A., McMillan, and M., Sercarz, E.E.: **Donor major histocompatibility complex (MHC) peptides are presented by recipient MHC molecules during graft rejection**. *J. Exper. Med.* 1992, **175**:918-924.

Lafferty, K., Prowse, S., Simeonovic, C., and Warren, H.S.: **Immunobiology of tissue transplantation: a return to the passenger leucocyte concept**. *Ann. Rev. Immunol.* 1983, **1**:143-173.

11-25 **In the absence of co-stimulation, tolerance is induced.**

Guerder, S., Picarella, D.E., Linsley, P.S., and Flavell, R.A.: **Co-stimulator B7 confers APC function to parenchymal tissue and in conjunction with TNF-α leads to autoimmunity in transgenic mice**. *Proc. Natl Acad. Sci. USA* (in press).

Liu, Y. and Janeway, C.A. Jr.: **Interferon γ plays a critical role in induced cell death of effector T cell: A possible third mechanism of self-tolerance**. *J. Exper. Med.* 1990, **172**:1735-1739.

11-26 **Dominant immune suppression can be demonstrated in models of tolerance and can affect the course of autoimmune disease.**

Qin, S., Cobbold, S.P., Pope, H., Elliott, J., Kioussis, D., Davies, J., and Waldmann, H.: **Infectious transplantation tolerance**. *Science* 1993, **259**: 974-977.

Reich, E.-P., Scaringe, D., Yagi, J., Sherwin, R.S., and Janeway, C.A. Jr.: **Prevention of diabetes in NOD mice by injection of autoreactive T lymphocytes**. *Diabetes* 1989, **38**:1647-1651.

11-27 **Antigens in immunologically privileged sites do not induce immune attack but can serve as targets.**

Streilein, J.W.: **Immune privilege as the result of local tissue barriers and immunosuppressive microenvironments**. *Curr. Opin. Immunol.* 1993, **5**:428-432.

Williams, G.A., Mammolenti, M.M., and Streilein, J.W.: **Studies on the induction of anterior chamber-associated immune deviation (ACAID). III. Induction of ACAID depends upon intraocular transforming growth factor-β**. *Eur. J. Immunol.* 1992, **22**:165-173.

11-28 **Autoimmunity could be triggered by infection in a variety of ways.**

Fujinami, R.S.: **Molecular mimicry**. In: Rose, N.R. and McaKay, I.R. (eds): *The autoimmune diseases II*. Academic Press, 1992, 153-171.

Nossal, G.J.V.: **Autoimmunity and self-tolerance**. In: Rose, N.R. and MacKay, I.R. (eds): *The autoimmune diseases II*. Academic Press, 1992, 27-46.

Rook, G.A.W., Ludyard, P.M., and Stanford, J.L.: **A reappraisal of the evidence that rheumatoid arthritis and several other idiopathic diseases are slow bacterial infections**. *Ann. Rheum. Dis.* 1993, **52**:S30-S38.

Wucherpfennig, K.W., and Strominger, J.L.: **Molecular mimicry in T cell mediated autoimmunity: Viral peptides activate human T cell clones specific for myelin basic protein**. *Cell* 1995, **80**:695-705.

Control and Manipulation of the Immune Response

In this book, we have learned how adaptive immune responses are induced in resting lymphocytes, and how both innate immunity and adaptive immune responses protect us from infectious diseases. We have also learned about failures to contain certain infections and about deleterious adaptive immune responses, such as inappropriate responses to allergens and to autoantigens, and the rejection of grafted tissues. Immunologists seek to understand how the immune system works so that they can devise effective treatments for these problems. In this chapter, we shall consider the current methods used to treat immunological diseases, as well as new approaches to controlling and manipulating the immune response. To introduce these concepts, we first look at what we know about endogenous or intrinsic regulation of immune responses.

How can we hope to inhibit only the harmful responses and enhance only the desirable ones? Probably the best approach is to stimulate the mechanisms the body itself uses to regulate its own responses. The nature of the effector mechanisms engaged in all immune responses is essentially the same: what determines whether a response is desirable or undesirable is the nature of the antigen. Therefore, some diseases are caused by a normal response to an inappropriate antigen, as we saw in Chapter 11: those directed at allergens, at autoantigens, and at grafts are harmful to the host and one would like to be able to inhibit them. By contrast, some diseases result from a failure to make an appropriate response, and one would like to stimulate protective responses directed at pathogens such as malaria and HIV, or at the transformed cells that cause cancer. In the last two sections of this chapter, we will examine immunity to tumors and current approaches to vaccination against tumors or pathogens. Vaccination, by far the most successful application of immunology to date, takes advantage of the specificity of immunological responses. These approaches are based increasingly on the improved understanding of basic immunological processes that has been achieved in this century.

Intrinsic regulation of immunity.

All biological systems are to some extent self-regulating, and thus it has long been the belief of immunologists that endogenous or intrinsic regulation of immune responses occurs. Indeed, there is a vast literature on this subject. However, unlike most biological systems, the immune system must also make specific responses to extrinsic substances whose nature cannot be anticipated, and these responses must be prompt enough and sufficiently strong to control a rapidly growing pathogen. Thus, the system must allow large deviations from homeostasis when called upon to do so.

Basically, one can break endogenous regulation down into three effects. The first is the consequence of producing antibodies and T cells, which we shall call feedback inhibition. This mechanism controls the responses of lymphocytes by removing its stimulus — the antigen. It also allows later responses to the same pathogen to engage those cells that participated in the initial response. Second, we can imagine a regulatory mechanism based on receptor:receptor interactions, which Niels Jerne called the idiotypic network. Third, the type of immune response, which we think of mainly as cell-mediated or humoral, is controlled by the cytokines produced by T cells; such responses can be protective or harmful depending on the target antigen. It is the hope of the people who study these problems to learn how to control immune responses of all types, so that harmful immune responses can be inhibited, and helpful ones encouraged.

12-1 **In immune individuals, secondary and subsequent responses are mediated solely by memory lymphocytes.**

In the normal course of an infection, a pathogen first proliferates to a level sufficient to elicit an adaptive immune response and then stimulates the production of antibodies and effector T cells that eliminate the pathogen from the body. As we learned in Chapter 9, most of the effector T cells die and antibody levels gradually decline after the pathogen is eliminated because the antigens that elicited the response are no longer present at a level needed to sustain it; we can think of this as feedback inhibition of the response. However, memory T and B cells remain and maintain a heightened ability to mount a response to a recurrence of the infection (see Sections 9-21–25).

The antibody and effector T cells remaining in an immunized individual also prevent the activation of naive B and T cells by the same antigen. This can be shown by passively transferring antibody or effector T cells to naive recipients; when the recipient is then immunized, naive lymphocytes do not respond to the original antigen, whereas responses to other antigens are unaffected. This has been put to practical use to prevent the response of Rh$^-$ mothers to their Rh$^+$ children (see Section 2-9): if anti-Rh antibody is given to the mother before she reacts to her child's red blood cells, her response will be inhibited. While the precise mechanism of suppression is unclear, it is known that crosslinking of the antigen receptor on B cells to FcγRII on the B-cell surface inhibits the activation of naive B cells (Fig. 12.1), which may explain this kind of suppression. For some reason, memory B-cell responses are not inhibited by antibody to the Rh$^+$ antigen, so for this treatment to be useful the Rh$^-$ mothers at risk must be identified before a response has occurred. This also shows that memory B cells can be activated to produce antibody even when they are exposed to pre-existing antibody, which allows secondary antibody responses to occur in immune individuals.

Adoptive transfer of immune T cells to naive syngeneic mice also prevents the activation of naive T cells by antigen. This has been shown most clearly for cytotoxic T cells. It is possible that the memory CD8 T cells that are transferred are activated to regain cytotoxic activity sufficiently rapidly that they kill the antigen-presenting cells that are required to activate naive CD8 T cells, thereby inhibiting their activation.

These mechanisms may also explain the phenomenon known as **original antigenic sin**. This term describes the tendency of people to make antibodies only to epitopes expressed on the first influenza virus variant to which they were exposed, even in subsequent infections with variants that bear additional, highly immunogenic epitopes (Fig. 12.2). Antibodies to the original virus will tend to suppress responses of naive B cells specific for the new epitopes by crosslinking their antigen receptors to FcγRII. This may benefit the host by using only those B cells that can respond most rapidly and effectively to the virus. This pattern is broken only if the person is exposed to an influenza virus that lacks all epitopes seen in the original infection, since now no pre-existing antibodies bind the virus and naive B cells are able to respond.

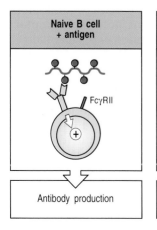
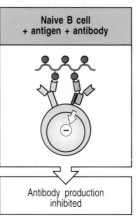
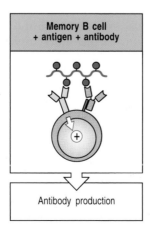

Naive B cell + antigen	Naive B cell + antigen + antibody	Memory B cell + antigen + antibody
FcγRII		
Antibody production	Antibody production inhibited	Antibody production

Fig. 12.1 Antibody can suppress naive B-cell activation by crosslinking the specific antigen receptor on B cells to the Fcγ receptor II (FcγRII). Antigen binding to the B-cell antigen receptor delivers an activating signal (left panel), while simultaneous signaling via the antigen receptor and FcγRII delivers a negative signal to naive B cells (center panel). Such crosslinking does not appear to affect memory B cells (right panel). This mechanism may play a role in suppressing naive B-cell responses in already primed individuals.

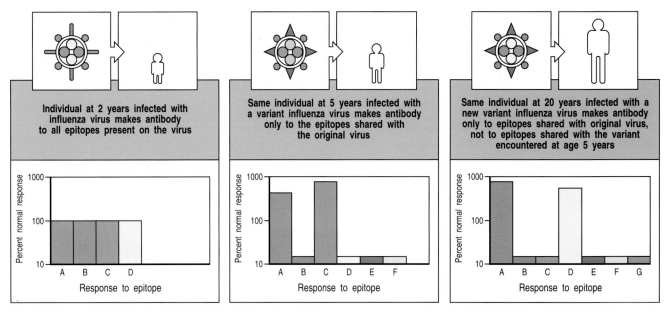

Fig. 12.2 Individuals who have already been infected with one variant of influenza virus make antibodies only to epitopes that were present on the initial virus variant when infected with other variants. A child infected for the first time with an influenza virus makes a response to all epitopes (left panel). At five years of age, the same child exposed to a variant virus responds preferentially to those epitopes shared with the original virus, and makes a less than normal response to new epitopes on the virus (middle panel). Even at 20 years of age, this commitment to respond to epitopes shared with the original virus, and the subnormal response to new epitopes, is retained (right panel). This phenomenon is called 'original antigenic sin'.

<hr>

12-2 | Interactions between lymphocyte receptors may regulate the repertoire.

A second type of regulatory interaction between lymphocytes can occur when the receptors on one lymphocyte recognize the receptors on a second lymphocyte. Such interactions were proposed by Niels Jerne to regulate antibody production through what he termed an **idiotypic network**. We learned in Chapter 3 (see Fig. 3.32) that antibodies directed at the variable region of another antibody molecule define the unique features or **idiotype** of the antibody, and such antibodies are called anti-idiotype antibodies. When it was shown that anti-idiotype antibodies would suppress the responses of B cells bearing that idiotype, Jerne proposed that such interactions would link the B cells of the immune system into a regulatory network. We now tend to think more generally of immune networks, since interactions between receptors on all classes of lymphocytes have been demonstrated experimentally.

The conceptual basis of Jerne's idiotypic network hypothesis is simple. Since antibodies can bind to a very large number of antigen epitopes, each with its own characteristic shape, the shapes of the antibody variable regions themselves must also be very diverse. Jerne termed the shapes on antibody variable domains **idiotopes**, since they are epitopes on the antigen-binding region of a given receptor; the idiotype is the sum of idiotopes on that receptor. There is no reason to think that the shapes of the set of epitopes presented by foreign antigens are distinct from the shapes of the set of idiotopes found on antibodies (Fig. 12.3), and therefore it is not surprising that one can raise anti-idiotope antibodies specific for virtually any antibody molecule.

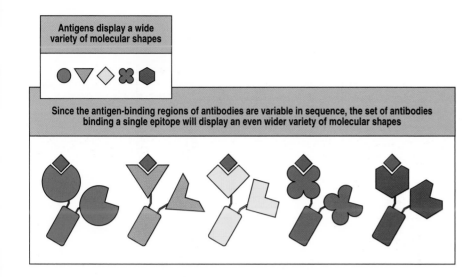

Fig. 12.3   The Jerne idiotypic network hypothesis is based on the idea that the set of shapes of antigen epitopes will largely overlap with the set of shapes of receptor idiotopes. The immune system can respond specifically to an almost infinite array of epitopes. In responding to a single epitope, many different antibodies are made, each of which carries many different epitopes on the variable region of the antibody, called idiotopes. The range of idiotopes available is essentially as great as the range of external antigenic epitopes. This internal array of idiotopes should therefore include many, and perhaps all, of the epitopes of the external antigenic universe. These internal antigenic images cannot render the immune system tolerant, or there would be no responsive cells left. It is therefore possible to make antibodies that recognize the idiotype of an antibody (the idiotopes collectively), called anti-idiotype antibodies, in the same way that one would raise antibodies to an epitope on a foreign antigen.

Anti-idiotope antibodies can be of two types. One type, called **internal images**, mimic epitopes of the original antigen, and can be used as surrogate antigens for immunization. The internal image antibodies must have an idiotope with the same shape as an epitope on the original antigen, and must bind to the antibody used to raise them in the same way as antigen. In other words, they are virtually immunologically indistinguishable from external antigen. However, most anti-idiotope antibodies do not resemble antigen but can, nevertheless, regulate the behavior of the initial responding cells. They are known as the anti-idiotypic regulatory set. This second type of anti-idiotope antibodies also regulate the behavior of cells bearing related idiotopes, known as the non-specific parallel set (Fig. 12.4). This set of cells are regulated in parallel with the antigen-specific antibodies, although they themselves are not specific for the same antigen.

It has also been reported that T cells can recognize peptides derived from the variable regions of T-cell receptors bound to self MHC molecules on other T cells; again, it would be surprising if the set of peptides available from T-cell receptor variable regions did not overlap with the set of peptides derived from antigen. Thus, the immune system can recognize its own receptors, and there is no apparent distinction between the scope of receptor recognition and the scope of recognition of antigen.

Since it is possible to raise anti-idiotope antibodies to most antibodies, it is clear that the lymphocyte repertoire is not tolerant to most antibody idiotopes, presumably because most idiotopes are present at low levels. Indeed, since antibodies bear internal images of antigen, tolerance to all idiotopes would potentially destroy the ability to respond to most antigens. In consequence, many receptors will be able to recognize and respond to one or more other receptors within the system.

Experimental studies have shown that early B-cell differentiation produces cells whose receptors are multi-specific and highly interconnected; that is, they bind to many different antigens including important bacterial pathogens, and they also bind the receptors of other B cells that arise slightly later in ontogeny. The second wave of B cells, whose development is stimulated by interaction with the first wave, also make anti-bacterial antibodies. Thus, the very first B cells to develop produce receptors that are immediately useful for host defense and also promote

Fig. 12.4 Two types of anti-idiotype antibody can be made in the course of a response to antigen. When antigen activates the proliferation of a set of responding cells (the 'induced set'; shown here as B cells, although the same applies to T cells), the receptors on this set of cells can activate two further sets of cells via receptor:receptor interactions. The first is the internal image set, whose receptors carry epitopes that resemble the antigen (left panels); the second is a set of cells called the anti-idiotypic regulatory set (right panels), which recognize epitopes on the receptors of the induced set but whose receptors do not resemble the original antigen. Cells from the internal image set can themselves induce a second set of cells with receptors specific for the antigen (bottom left). The receptors on cells from this set may or may not also carry the idiotype of the initial, induced set of antibodies. The regulatory set can also induce a second set of cells; these usually carry one or more of the idiotopes of the induced set but do not bind antigen. This is called the non-specific parallel set (bottom right). All these interactions can operate in either direction, as the network has no inherent directionality, direction being determined by the abundance of each set of cells. Since each receptor carries several distinct idiotopes, the network is much more complex than shown here, and can in theory ramify indefinitely. This diagram simply depicts the minimum elements in the network as conceived by Jerne.

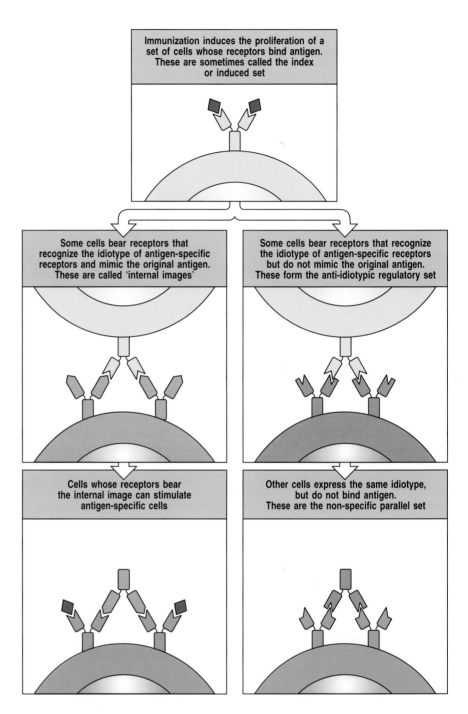

the expansion of further B cells that express other potentially useful receptors. Network interactions thus appear to direct the early expansion of the most useful components of the repertoire. These highly interactive B cells are probably all CD5 B cells, whose function in broad anti-bacterial responses we discussed in Section 9-13, and it is not clear whether similar network interactions affect the development of conventional B cells.

It is interesting to note that anti-idiotype antibodies injected into fetal or neonatal mice often enhance production of the corresponding idiotype, whereas injection of anti-idiotypic antibodies in adult mice almost always inhibits idiotype production. Thus, network interactions in adult mice are likely to be suppressive.

Fig. 12.5 Idiotypic interactions may be important for maintaining the diversity of the lymphocyte receptor repertoire. The adaptive immune response must be able to recognize all possible non-self molecules. To do so, a broadly distributed repertoire of receptors, each present at low frequency, is ideal, as depicted in the top panel. An antigenic challenge causes a major perturbation in the repertoire (center panel), with expansion in some sets of receptors (D and H) and presumed decreases in other parts of the repertoire, especially those that interact with the expanded set and are thereby suppressed. Over time, this could generate a repertoire with significant 'holes' if there were not some way to modulate the distribution of receptors. Network interactions could provide this modulatory effect (bottom panel), serving to maintain the distribution of receptors as relatively even, while allowing some increase in the frequency of receptors of proven utility. These effects would be difficult to detect and have not yet been identified.

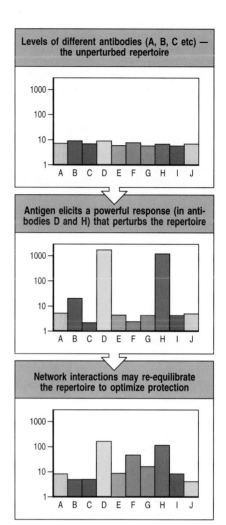

Such suppressive network interactions could serve the important function of maintaining the distribution of the repertoire of receptor specificities in a fully developed immune system. To respond as swiftly as possible to any challenge, the repertoire of receptors on naive lymphocytes needs to be diverse enough to contain receptors specific for virtually any molecular shape. In theory, if the generation of receptors is completely random, the repertoire should always be broadly distributed. In the real world, however, the distribution of receptors is continually being distorted by responses to antigen. Network interactions may be the only way for the immune system itself to monitor repertoire distribution (Fig. 12.5).

12-3 | **CD4 T-cell subsets can regulate one another's growth.**

As we learned in Chapter 7, the two subsets of CD4 T cells, T$_H$1 or inflammatory CD4 T cells, and T$_H$2, or helper CD4 T cells, have very different functions: helper T cells are the most effective activators of B cells, especially in primary responses, while inflammatory T cells are crucial for activating macrophages. Two major factors that determine which effector cell type develops are the cytokines present in the early phases of the CD4 T-cell response, and the nature, route, and dose of antigen used for priming (see Sections 9-16 and 9-17). It is also clear that the two CD4 T-cell subsets regulate each other; once one subset becomes dominant, it is often hard to shift the response to the other type. One reason for this is that cytokines from one type of CD4 T cell inhibit the activation of the other. Thus, IL-10, a product of helper T cells, can inhibit the development of inflammatory T cells by acting on the antigen-presenting cell, while interferon-γ (IFN-γ), a product of inflammatory T cells, can prevent the activation of helper T cells (Fig. 12.6). If a particular CD4 T-cell subset is activated first or preferentially in a response, it can suppress the development of the other subset. The overall effect is that certain responses are dominated by either humoral or cell-mediated immunity.

This interplay of cytokines plays an important role in human disease but, to date, it has been explored mainly in mouse models, where such polarized responses are easier to study. For example, when CD4 T cells in BALB/c mice are stimulated with *Leishmania* spp., their macrophages fail to make IL-12 and thus fail to induce differentiation of their CD4 T cells into inflammatory T cells; instead, they preferentially make helper T cells in response to these antigens. Helper T cells are unable to activate macrophages to inhibit leishmanial growth, resulting in susceptibility to disease. By contrast, macrophages in C57BL/6 mice make IL-12 when infected with *Leishmania* spp., and the mice respond by producing inflammatory T cells that protect the host by activating macrophages infected with the parasite to kill the *Leishmania* spp.

Fig. 12.6 The two subsets of CD4 T cells each produce cytokines that can negatively regulate the other subset. Helper T cells (T$_H$2) cells make IL-10, which acts on macrophages to inhibit inflammatory T cell (T$_H$1) activation, perhaps by blocking macrophage IL-12 synthesis, and TGF-β, which is directly inhibitory to T$_H$1 cells (left panel). T$_H$1 cells make IFN-γ, which blocks the growth of T$_H$2 cells (right panels). These effects allow either subset to dominate a response by suppressing outgrowth of cells of the other subset.

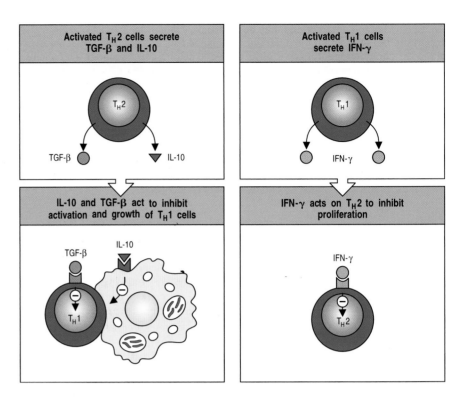

| Activated T$_H$2 cells secrete TGF-β and IL-10 | Activated T$_H$1 cells secrete IFN-γ |

| IL-10 and TGF-β act to inhibit activation and growth of T$_H$1 cells | IFN-γ acts on T$_H$2 to inhibit proliferation |

12-4   CD4 T-cell subsets can regulate one another's effector functions.

A second aspect of this balancing is that one type of effector CD4 T cell can directly inhibit the effector functions of the other type. Thus, armed inflammatory T cells can block B-cell activation by armed helper T cells, at least in some systems. This occurs mainly through killing of activated B cells by armed inflammatory T cells, which express the Fas ligand (see Section 7-20), which binds Fas on activated B cells (Fig. 12.7). Likewise, there is evidence that armed helper T cells may prevent expression of armed inflammatory T-cell function by secreting the cytokine IL-10. As we discussed in Chapter 10, a shift to a predominance of helper T cells has been suggested to be important in the pathogenesis of AIDS (see Section 10-21). Studies of CD4 T cells activated by oral presentation of antigen has suggested that yet another functional subset, which some have called **T$_H$3**, makes predominantly the cytokine transforming growth factor-β (TGF-β). Cells secreting TGF-β are very potent inhibitors of inflammatory

Fig. 12.7 Inflammatory T cells (T$_H$1) can suppress the activation of B cells by helper T cells (T$_H$2). T$_H$2 cells activate B cells to produce antibody. When both T$_H$2 cells and T$_H$1 cells that are recognizing peptides from the same antigen are added to antigen-specific B cells, suppression can dominate so that no antibody production is seen. Most T$_H$1 cells can kill B cells by expressing Fas ligand, which binds Fas that is expressed on activated B cells and kills them, perhaps explaining their suppressive effects.

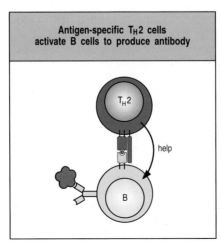

Antigen-specific T$_H$2 cells activate B cells to produce antibody

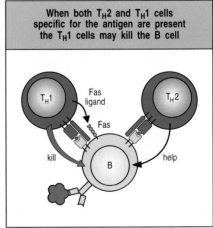

When both T$_H$2 and T$_H$1 cells specific for the antigen are present the T$_H$1 cells may kill the B cell

An antigen has peptides presented by both I-A and I-E molecules	In mice expressing only I-A molecules, T cells respond to peptides bound to I-A	In mice that also express I-E, I-A-restricted T-cell responses are not observed	Anti-I-E antibodies block responses of I-E-restricted T cells, restoring response
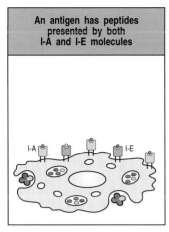	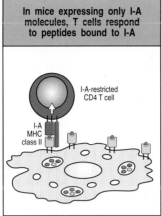	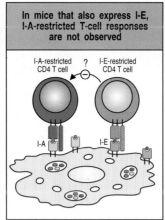	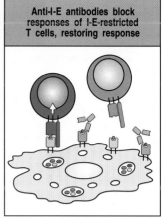

Fig. 12.8　CD4 T cells responding to peptides from the same antigen bound to different MHC class II molecules may have opposing effects. Some antigens elicit T-cell proliferative responses when used to immunize mice that carry I-A but not I-E molecules (second panel). When the same antigen is used to prime mice that have both I-A and I-E molecules, no response is observed (third panel). However, CD4 T cells recognizing peptide bound to I-A have been primed, as anti-I-E antibody added to the cultures of primed T cells reveals a T-cell proliferative response (far right panel). This may occur because I-A molecules elicit T_H1 responses while I-E molecules elicit T_H2 responses that inhibit the response of T_H1 cells, or it may occur by some other mechanism.

T-cell action in local inflammation, for instance in the brain in the mouse model for multiple sclerosis, called experimental autoimmune encephalo-myelitis.

One peculiar phenomenon that may be accounted for in this way is the finding that, for some antigens, presentation by one MHC class II molecule can suppress the T-cell response to the same antigen presented by a different MHC class II molecule (Fig. 12.8); this has been described in both mice and humans. The two different MHC class II molecules presumably bind different peptides of the same antigen or bind the same peptide with different affinities. It may be that the resulting density of specific peptide:MHC complexes is very different for the two MHC class II molecules, so that one of these MHC class II molecules elicits a helper T-cell response and the other an inflammatory T-cell response (see Section 9-16). Since only one of these responses can dominate, such effects will appear as suppression if only one type of response is measured, such as disease induction, proliferation, or help to B cells.

Since cytokines appear to regulate the balance between T_H1, T_H2, and T_H3 cells, one might expect that it would be possible to shift this balance by administering appropriate cytokines. IL-2 and IFN-γ have been used to stimulate cell-mediated immunity in diseases such as lepromatous leprosy and can cause both a local resolution of the lesion and a systemic change in T-cell responses. IL-12, which is a potent inducer of inflammatory T cells, may be an even more attractive potential therapy. If a failure to generate inflammatory T cells is really important in the initial phases of infection with HIV, as discussed in Chapter 10, then early intervention with cytokines such as IL-12 or other such therapies could be crucially important.

12-5　Cytokines released by CD8 T cells can affect CD4 T cells, B cells and macrophages.

CD8 T cells have long been a focus of attention for those who want to control the immune response by manipulating the natural regulatory processes, as it was believed early on that CD8 T cells were especially potent in this function. Initially, it was proposed that a subset of

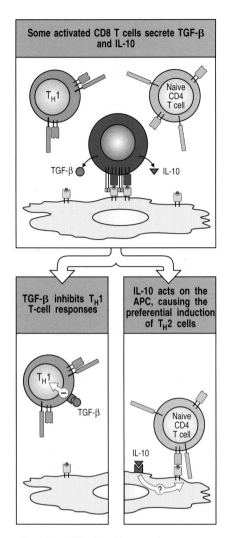

Some activated CD8 T cells secrete TGF-β and IL-10

T$_H$1   Naive CD4 T cell

TGF-β   IL-10

TGF-β inhibits T$_H$1 T-cell responses

T$_H$1

TGF-β

IL-10 acts on the APC, causing the preferential induction of T$_H$2 cells

Naive CD4 T cell

IL-10

?

Fig. 12.9   CD8 T cells can also regulate responses by secreting cytokines that suppress T-cell subsets. When stimulated, some CD8 T cells respond by secreting IL-10 and TGF-β. These cytokines are able to suppress other T-cell responses; TGF-β acts directly on T$_H$1 T cells to inhibit their responses, while IL-10 acts on antigen-presenting cells (APC), causing them to inhibit the differentiation of CD4 T cells into T$_H$1 effector cells and thus increase the production of T$_H$2 cells. How this effect is mediated is unknown.

CD8 T cells could secrete a factor able to suppress the response of other T cells in an antigen-specific manner. Although it was often possible to obtain soluble factors from hybrids of these cells, it was never proven that they had a definable molecular structure. These factors were variously described as consisting of secreted α chains of the T-cell receptor, or of whole T-cell receptors, which also possessed the ability to directly bind the same protein antigen whose peptide fragment was recognized by the T cell. These factors also carried information for MHC or immunoglobulin V gene segment restriction in recognition and effector functions, typically for inhibiting the response. These claims have been met with skepticism by most investigators. Rather, while the phenomena of immune regulation have been repeatedly confirmed, the reality of the secreted factors has remained a source of mystery. Regulation is now considered in the light of the new paradigms of immunology: most T cells recognize antigen in the form of peptide fragments bound to MHC molecules, and T cells in general carry out their effector functions by secreting non-specific cytokines.

Indeed, it has recently become clear that CD8 T cells can, in addition to their common cytolytic function, also respond to antigen by secreting cytokines typical of either inflammatory or helper T cells. Furthermore, some CD8 cells appear to resemble T$_H$3 cells, and can be induced by much the same procedures of feeding antigen. Such cells appear to be responsible for the polar forms of leprosy, which are discussed in detail in Chapter 10 (see Fig. 10.5). Patients with lepromatous leprosy had CD8 cells that suppressed the inflammatory T-cell response seen in tuberculoid leprosy by making IL-10 and TGF-β; patients with tuberculoid leprosy only made inflammatory T cells and these could activate macrophages to rid the body of leprosy bacilli. Thus, suppression by CD8 T cells may again be explained by the production of a particular set of cytokines (Fig. 12.9).

Summary.

The major regulatory influence on the adaptive immune response is the presence of antigen. Introduction of antigen elicits a response, and its clearance causes the response to cease. However, there is strong evidence that the immune system also regulates itself. The most important regulatory mechanism is the selective activation of inflammatory (T$_H$1) or helper T cells (T$_H$2), which can inhibit each other's growth and effector functions, leading to dominance of one or the other subset in a response. There is also evidence for a network of idiotypic interactions between lymphocyte receptors. The network may help to establish and maintain a distributed repertoire of receptors at all times. Finally, there is evidence that CD8 T cells have antigen-specific suppressor activity, perhaps by also secreting cytokines that differentially inhibit CD4 T-cell subsets. A better understanding of these regulatory mechanisms may make it possible to exploit them to control unwanted responses such as graft rejection, allergy, or autoimmunity, and to provoke adaptive immunity to tumors or to pathogens.

Extrinsic regulation of unwanted immune responses.

Current treatments for immunological disorders are nearly all empirical in origin; many drugs that suppress immune responses were identified by screening large numbers of natural and synthetic compounds. Studying how these drugs act has revealed some interesting features of the immune system, and we will therefore first examine the drugs and biological agents currently used to treat immunological diseases. The drugs currently available are very broad in their actions and usually affect all responses, the protective as well as the harmful. These drugs thus fail to take advantage of the most important feature of the adaptive immune response, which is its clonal specificity, and fall far short of the ideal, a treatment that affects only the clones mediating the pathogenic response. However, it may be that the use of antibodies themselves in therapy will be able to exploit the specificity of the immune response, leading to more effective treatments.

12-6 Cytotoxic drugs and steroids cause immunosuppression by killing dividing cells and have serious side effects.

For the first 30 years of organ transplantation, the most commonly used immunosuppressive agents were cytotoxic drugs such as **azathioprine**, **cyclophosphamide** and corticosteroids such as **prednisone** (Fig. 12.10). Cytotoxic drugs kill rapidly dividing cells, and it is believed that they suppress graft rejection by killing the host lymphocytes that proliferate in response to graft antigens on donor antigen-presenting cells. With time, donor antigen-presenting cells die and are replaced with host cells. As these provide less potent stimulation of the response to the graft, the dose of drug can be reduced. However, the graft will be rejected if the drug is discontinued at any time.

As might be expected, cytotoxic drugs have several unwanted side effects. First, like all broad-spectrum immunosuppressive agents, they inhibit both beneficial and harmful immune responses. Second, they also kill other rapidly proliferating cell types, such as the cells in the bone marrow that produce all the cellular elements of blood. Third, and most disturbing, prolonged treatment with these drugs is associated with a marked increase in the incidence of lymphomas. It is not known why this happens but it provides a strong motivation to find other, less dangerous immunosuppressive agents.

The **corticosteroids** are potent inhibitors of inflammatory responses, well known for their beneficial effects when used in salves or local injections. When given systemically they are toxic to lymphocytes, especially the immature cortical thymocytes. They also inhibit the inflammatory activity of macrophages and other phagocytic cells, further hampering the immune response to pathogens. The combination of a cytotoxic drug with a powerful corticosteroid like prednisone is a useful treatment for acute episodes of graft rejection. However, prolonged treatment with steroids causes weakening of bone and connective tissues and atrophy of the adrenal glands due to inhibition of the release of adrenocorticotropic hormone (ACTH) from the pituitary gland. This reduces the ability of the body to make important adrenal responses to stress. Like the cytotoxic drugs, corticosteroids also increase the risk of infection. Thus, these drugs are not favored for long-term treatment, although they are still used in short courses when other drugs are ineffective.

12-7 Cyclosporin A, FK506, and rapamycin are powerful immunosuppressive agents that interfere with T-cell signaling.

Cyclosporin A, a cyclic decapeptide derived from the soil fungus *Tolypocladium inflatum* (see Fig. 12.13), is widely used in clinical transplantation because it is both effective and relatively non-toxic. An unrelated compound with similar activity is **FK506**. Interestingly, the study of these drugs has led to the identification of a previously unsuspected step in T-cell activation; cyclosporin A and FK506 prevent the synthesis of IL-2 by blocking a late stage of the signaling pathways initiated by the T-cell receptor. Their mode of action is now fairly well understood.

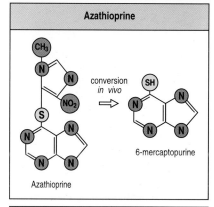

Immunosuppressive drugs kill dividing cells or inhibit inflammation

Azathioprine

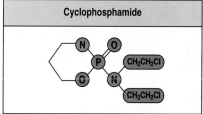

Cyclophosphamide

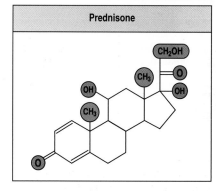

Prednisone

Fig. 12.10 Structures of the cytotoxic immunosuppressive drugs azathioprine and cyclophosphamide and the potent anti-inflammatory corticosteroid prednisone. Azathioprine is converted into an active toxic substance *in vivo*, as shown in the upper panel.

Cyclosporin A and FK506 bind to molecules inside cells called immuno-philins, the cyclophilins and FK-binding proteins (FKBP) respectively. These immunophilins are peptidyl-prolyl *cis-trans* isomerases. However, the isomerase activity of the binding proteins seems to be unrelated to the immunosuppressive activity of these drugs. Rather, the immunophilin:drug complex binds to the Ca^{2+}-activated serine/threonine phosphatase **calcineurin** and inhibits its activity. Calcineurin is activated when intracellular calcium ion levels rise following T-cell receptor binding to appropriate antigen:MHC complexes. When calcineurin is active, it leads to the dephosphorylation of the cytosolic component of the transcription factor NF-AT, NF-ATc, which migrates to the nucleus where it pairs with a second, nuclear component, NF-ATn and induces transcription of the IL-2 gene (see Sections 4-27 and 7-9) (Fig. 12.11). It

Fig. 12.11 Cyclosporin A and FK506 inhibit T-cell activation by interfering with the serine/threonine-specific phosphatase calcineurin. Signaling via T-cell receptor-associated tyrosine kinases (see Section 4-28) leads to increased synthesis of the nuclear component of the nuclear factor of activated T cells (NF-ATn), as well as increasing the concentration of calcium in the cytoplasm (left panels). This increase in calcium concentration activates calcineurin to dephosphorylate the cytoplasmic component of NF-AT, namely NF-ATc (or to activate a phosphatase, which then dephosphorylates NF-ATc). Once dephosphorylated, the active NF-ATc migrates to the nucleus to form a complex with NF-ATn; the NF-AT complex can then induce transcription of genes required for T-cell activation, including the IL-2 gene. When cyclosporin A (CsA) or FK506 are present, they form complexes with their immunophilin targets, cyclophilin (CyP) and FK-binding protein (FKBP), respectively (right panels). The complex of cyclophilin with cyclosporin A can bind to calcineurin, blocking its ability to activate NF-ATc. Similarly, the complex of FK506 with FKBP binds to calcineurin at the same site, also blocking its activity.

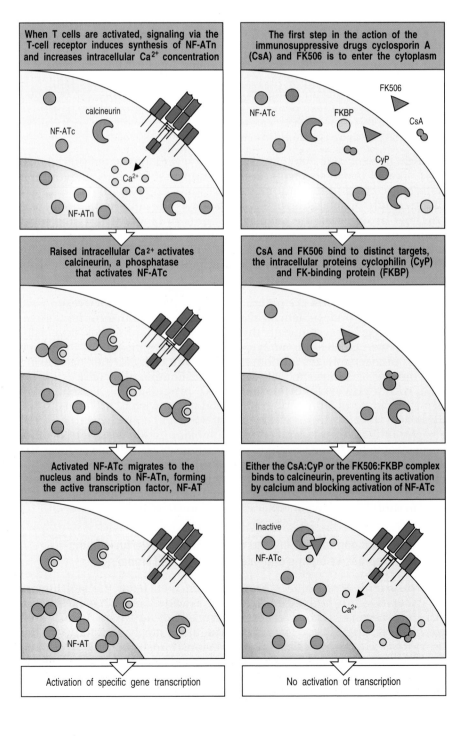

is so far unclear why calcineurin binds to these two complexes of drug and immunophilin. It is tempting to speculate that there are endogenous equivalents for cyclosporin A and FK506 that perform similar regulatory functions but, to date, none has been discovered. Physiological roles for each of the members of the immunophilin families also remain to be uncovered.

Cyclosporin A and FK506 inhibit clonal expansion of T cells by blocking IL-2 synthesis. A second type of immunosuppressive agent, **rapamycin**, instead inhibits the signaling pathway used by the IL-2 receptor by interfering with protein kinases (Fig. 12.12). Rapamycin and FK506 are related compounds (Fig. 12.13) produced by different species of *Streptomyces*, and they compete for binding to the same cellular receptor, FKBP. Rapamycin does not inhibit production of IL-2, however, because the complex of FKBP with rapamycin does not bind to calcineurin. Thus, paradoxically, rapamycin can prevent the inhibition of IL-2 synthesis by FK506, yet inhibits the response to the IL-2 once it is produced. However, rapamycin does not bind to cyclophilin and therefore does not prevent cyclosporin A from inhibiting IL-2 synthesis. Cyclosporin A and rapamycin therefore make a very effective combination, one inhibiting IL-2 production and the other the response to any IL-2 that is produced.

Although these compounds are relatively non-toxic, they are not free from problems. First, as with the cytotoxic agents, they are indiscriminate in their effects on immune responses. The only control available over their immunosuppressive action is the dose; at the time of grafting, high doses are required, but once the graft is established, the dose can be reduced in an attempt to allow useful protective immune responses while maintaining adequate suppression of the residual response to the grafted tissue. This is a difficult balance that is not always achieved successfully. Furthermore, as the immunophilins are found in many cells, it is to be expected that these drugs will have effects on other tissues. Cyclosporin A and FK506 are both toxic to kidneys and other organs. Finally, treatment with cyclosporin A is expensive, since it is a complex natural product that must be taken indefinitely. Thus, there is considerable room for improvement on these drugs, and better and less expensive analogs are being sought. Nevertheless, at present, these are the drugs of choice in clinical transplantation, and are also being tested in a variety of autoimmune diseases, especially those that are mediated by T cells and so resemble graft rejection.

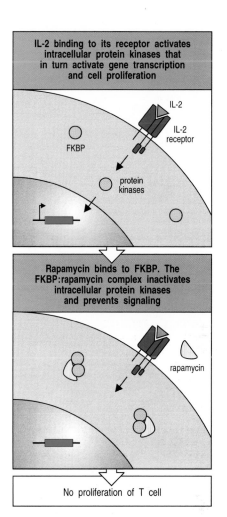

Fig. 12.12 Rapamycin binds to FK-binding protein (FKBP) but does not block calcineurin activation. Unlike cyclosporin A and FK506, rapamycin therefore does not inhibit the activation of NF-AT-responsive genes. Instead, it blocks the signaling pathway initiated by the IL-2 receptor. Thus, rapamycin can antagonize the activity of FK506 but is synergistic with cyclosporin A.

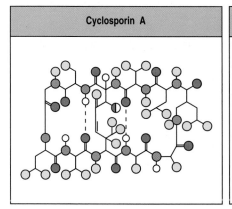
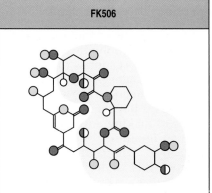
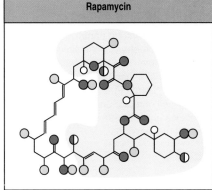

Fig. 12.13 Structures of the powerful immunosuppressive drugs cyclosporin A, FK506, and rapamycin. Red = oxygen; green = nitrogen; white = hydrogen; and yellow = methyl group.

Note that rapamycin and FK506 share a large part of their structure (shaded) and bind to the same cellular receptor.

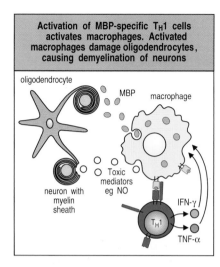

Activation of MBP-specific T$_H$1 cells activates macrophages. Activated macrophages damage oligodendrocytes, causing demyelination of neurons

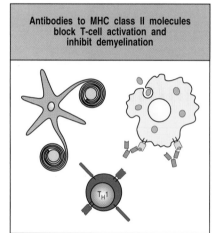

Antibodies to MHC class II molecules block T-cell activation and inhibit demyelination

Fig. 12.14 Anti-MHC class II antibody can inhibit the development of experimental autoimmune encephalomyelitis (EAE). Oligodendrocytes make the myelin sheath of neurons. In mice immunized with myelin basic protein (MBP), CD4 T cells activate macrophages (top panel), which damage oligodendrocytes, leading to inflammation of the brain and spinal cord. Anti-MHC class II antibodies prevent the CD4 T cell from recognizing MBP peptides bound to MHC class II molecules on the macrophages (bottom panel). This prevents macrophage activation and inhibits disease. This treatment also blocks normal antigen recognition (see Section 2-25 and Fig. 2.46). Antibodies to the T-cell receptor and to accessory molecules have similar effects but by a different mechanism.

12-8 **Antibodies to cell-surface molecules have been used to remove specific lymphocyte subsets or to inhibit cell function.**

Cytotoxic drugs kill all proliferating cells and therefore affect indiscriminately all types of activated lymphocytes and any other cell that is proliferating. Cyclosporin A, FK506, and rapamycin are more selective but still inhibit most adaptive responses. It would be better to be able to remove only the lymphocytes responsible for the unwanted response. One approach to this, anti-lymphocyte globulin (a preparation of immunoglobulin from horses immunized with human lymphocytes), has been used for many years and has shown benefit in treating acute graft-rejection episodes. However, anti-lymphocyte globulin does not discriminate between useful lymphocytes and those responsible for unwanted responses. With the advent of monoclonal antibodies, it has become possible to increase the accuracy of these therapeutic tools. Some monoclonal antibodies are referred to as depleting, killing lymphocytes *in vivo*, while others are non-depleting and show beneficial effects by blocking the function of their target protein without killing the cell that bears it.

Antibodies to the T-cell receptor, to the CD4 and CD8 co-receptors, to MHC class II molecules, to the integrins involved in T-cell binding to antigen-presenting cells and to vascular endothelium, and to the B7.1 and B7.2 co-stimulator molecules, have all been tested for benefit in experimental models of autoimmune disease. For instance, antibodies to T-cell receptor V$_\beta$ domains, to CD4, to α_4 integrins, and to MHC class II molecules (Fig. 12.14) have all been successful in preventing or treating the autoimmune disease in mice known as experimental allergic encephalomyelitis. None of these treatments requires depletion of the relevant cells in order to be effective.

In animal studies of graft rejection, a fusion protein made from CTLA-4 and the Fc portion of human immunoglobulin has allowed long-term survival of certain grafted tissues. Presumably this fusion protein, which binds to both B7.1 and B7.2, blocks co-stimulation of the T cells that recognize donor antigen, and thus allows the cells to induce anergy in the alloreactive cells in the recipient.

Perhaps even more interesting, certain non-depleting anti-CD4 antibodies, when given for a short time during primary exposure to grafted tissue, lead to a state of tolerance in the recipient (Fig. 12.15). This tolerant state is long-lived and can be transferred to naive recipients with CD4 T cells producing cytokines typical of helper T cells (T$_H$2). The presence of anti-CD4 at the time of transplantation may involve selective activation of either inflammatory or helper T cells, as discussed in the previous part of this chapter.

The major impediment to this type of therapy in humans is that most monoclonal antibodies are made in mice, and humans rapidly develop an antibody response to mouse antibodies, inhibiting their activity and producing allergic reactions such as anaphylaxis on continued treatment (see Section 11-7). Once this has happened, all mouse monoclonal antibodies become useless in that patient. To avoid this problem, three ways of making antibodies that are not recognized as foreign by the human immune system are being explored. One approach is to clone human V regions into a phage display library and select for binding to human cells, as described in Section 2-11. In this way, monoclonal antibodies that are entirely human in origin can be obtained. Second, mice that lack endogenous immunoglobulin genes can be made transgenic (see Section 2-38) for human heavy and light immunoglobulin chain loci using yeast artificial chromosomes. B cells in these mice should have receptors encoded by human immunoglobulin genes but would not be

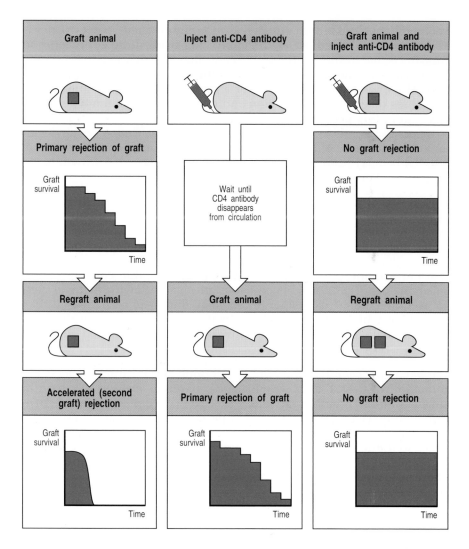

Fig. 12.15 A tissue graft given together with anti-CD4 antibody can induce specific tolerance. Mice grafted with tissue from a genetically different mouse reject that graft. Having been primed to respond to the antigens in the graft, they then reject a subsequent graft of identical tissue more rapidly (left panels). Mice injected with anti-CD4 antibody alone can recover immune competence when the antibody disappears from the circulation, as shown by a normal primary rejection of graft tissue (center panels). However, when tissue is grafted and anti-CD4 antibody is administered at the same time, the primary rejection response is markedly inhibited (right panels). An identical graft made later in the absence of anti-CD4 antibody is not rejected, showing that the animal has become tolerant to the graft antigen. This tolerance can be transferred to naive recipients with T cells.

tolerant to most human proteins. It is therefore possible to produce monoclonal antibodies that are indistinguishable from human antibodies by immunizing such mice with human cells or proteins. Finally, one may graft the antigen-binding loops or CDRs of a mouse monoclonal antibody onto the framework of a human immunoglobulin molecule, a process known as **humanization**. Since antigen-binding specificity is determined by the structure of the CDRs, and because the overall framework of mouse and human antibodies is so similar, this approach produces a monoclonal antibody that is identical to human immunoglobulin but binds the same antigen as the mouse monoclonal antibody from which the CDR sequences were derived. These recombinant antibodies are far less immunogenic in humans than the parent mouse monoclonal antibodies, and thus they can be used for treatments of humans with far less risk of anaphylaxis.

12-9 | CD4 subset activation can be manipulated with cytokines, anti-cytokine antibodies, the route and dose of antigen administration, or the structure of the antigen.

As we saw in Chapter 9, both the cytokine environment and the nature and density of the ligand for CD4 T-cell receptors is important in determining which subset of CD4 T cells is activated in response to immunization. Impressive results have been obtained by injection of recombinant cytokines or anti-cytokine antibodies, although the latter is generally more effective. The difficulty with using these approaches in humans is that in animal studies, it seems that the anti-cytokine antibody or the cytokine needs to be present at the first encounter with the antigen. Thus, while one can clear certain leprosy lesions by injection of cytokines directly into the lesion and cause reversal of the type of leprosy seen, this does not appear to be the case in experimental leishmaniasis in the mouse. Here, the susceptible BALB/c mice injected with anti-IL4 at the time of infection clear their infection. If administration of anti-IL4 is delayed by just one week, there is progressive growth of the parasite and dominant helper T-cell responses (Fig. 12.16).

High doses of peptide that engage the T-cell receptor strongly result in the activation of inflammatory T cells, while low doses of peptide that bind the T-cell receptor weakly preferentially induce helper T cells. Thus, manipulating the effective dose of antigen by using a peptide with known affinity for a particular MHC class II molecule is one way to control the priming of CD4 T cells. At very high peptide concentrations, inflammatory T cells may become tolerant, again allowing helper T cells to predominate. Thus, helper T cells may dominate responses at very low or very high antigen doses. Injecting different doses or different antigen analogs may therefore allow one to control which subset of effector CD4 T cells is induced in a response.

We have also seen that the route of peptide administration affects the induction of CD4 T cells. For instance, peptides given orally tend to prime helper T cells that make IL-4 or T_H3 cells that make predominantly TGF-β. When a soluble peptide is given intravenously, it binds preferentially to MHC class II molecules on resting B cells and tends to induce anergy in inflammatory T cells. Thus, careful choice of the dose or structure of antigen, or its route of administration, may allow us to control the type of response that results.

The formulation of antigen for injection is a third factor. A peptide in incomplete Freund's adjuvant (see Fig. 2.4), which is an oil-in-water emulsion, tends either to induce tolerance or to activate only helper T cells. The same peptide in complete Freund's adjuvant, which contains mycobacteria as well, activates inflammatory T cells that often dominate the response. The addition of the bacterial component may provoke different early cytokine responses, such as the production of IL-12 by tissue macrophages, which favors the generation of inflammatory T cells.

Thus, in a naive immune system, which type of effector CD4 T cell is activated can be affected by: injection of antigen at different doses; subtle changes in the structure of the immunizing peptide that affect its interaction with the T-cell receptor; different routes of delivery; and antigen in different formulations (see Fig. 2.17). It is not yet clear, however, whether these manipulations can affect an ongoing immune response. One drawback of this approach, even if it can be effective

Fig. 12.16 Treatment with anti-IL-4 antibody clears *Leishmania* infection. The left panel shows a hematoxylin-eosin stained section through the footpad of a Balb/c mouse infected with *Leishmania major*. Large numbers of parasites are present in tissue macrophages. The right panel shows a similar preparation from a mouse infected in the same experiment but simultaneously treated with a single injection of anti-IL-4 monoclonal antibody. Very few parasites are present. Photographs courtesy of R Locksley.

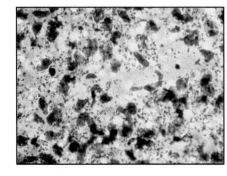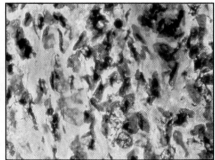

in manipulating established immune responses, is that one must first identify the specific antigen against which the response is directed. In most cases of autoimmune disease, as we learned in Section 11-16, the autoantigens recognized by T cells are unknown. It will therefore be necessary to carry out extensive testing to identify the correct antigen before one can think of actually treating disease in this way. This could make such treatments very expensive and difficult to establish. A more generic approach to manipulating CD4 T-cell subset balance in ongoing immune responses, such as novel drugs that selectively inhibit responses by T_H1, T_H2, or T_H3 cells, would undoubtedly be much more useful.

Summary.

Attempts to inhibit deleterious immune responses, such as those that drive allergic reactions, autoimmune disease, or graft rejection, have to date been carried out largely with broad-spectrum immunosuppressive drugs. However, as we understand the endogenous regulation of immune responses better, we can begin to look to these mechanisms to control unwanted immune responses or to elicit desirable ones. The manipulation of CD4 T-cell subsets by antigen or by cytokines seems feasible, and has been shown to work in model systems. So far, such treatments have not been shown to be effective in diseases in which the CD4 T-cell pattern has already been established; drugs that affect the balance between inflammatory T cells (T_H1) and helper T cells (T_H2), or T_H3 cells, in ongoing responses would be enormously useful. Knowledge of normal regulatory mechanisms, and agents that allow their manipulation, are vitally important if we are to control responses to the benefit of the patient.

Using the immune response to attack tumors.

Cancer is one of the three leading causes of death in industrialized nations. As treatments for infectious diseases and the prevention of cardio-vascular disease continues to improve, and the average life expectancy increases, cancer is likely to become the most common fatal disease in these countries. Cancers are caused by the progressive growth of the progeny of a single transformed cell. Therefore, curing cancer requires that all the malignant cells be removed or destroyed without killing the patient. An attractive way to achieve this would be to induce an immune response against the tumor that would discriminate between the cells of the tumor and their normal cellular counterparts. Immunological approaches to the treatment of cancer have been attempted for over a century with tantalizing but not sustainable results. It is now clear that T cells are a critical mediator of tumor immunity and recent advances in our understanding of antigen presentation and the molecules involved in T-cell activation have provided for new immunotherapy strategies based on a better molecular understanding of the immune response. These are beginning to show increased success in animal models and are now being tested in human patients.

12-10 | Some tumors can be recognized and rejected by the immune system.

We saw in Chapter 2 (Section 2-23) that rejection of allogeneic tumors was used to develop the first MHC-congenic strains of mice. This shows that foreign MHC molecules on transplantable tumors can be recognized by the immune system, leading to complete destruction of the tumor. Specific immunity to tumors must therefore be studied in inbred strains, so that host and tumor can be matched for MHC type. Several of these studies have been performed with murine tumors that have been induced experimentally by either carcinogenic chemicals or ultraviolet irradiation. These experimental tumors exhibit quite a variable pattern of growth when injected into syngeneic recipients. Most tumors, termed 'progressor tumors', grow progressively and eventually kill the host but some tumors, called 'regressor tumors', grow for a period of time and then regress (Fig. 12.17). When animals that have rejected regressor tumors are rechallenged with cells from that same tumor, no tumor growth is observed. Among progressor tumors, there is a spectrum of immunogenicity as defined by the ability of injected irradiated cells to induce protective immunity against a challenge injection of viable tumor cells at a distant site. Experiments carried out in T-cell deficient mice show the need for T cells to mediate all these effects, as does the observation that adoptive transfer of T cells from immune mice confers tumor-specific immunity on T-cell deficient recipients.

The absolute requirement for T cells in either the elimination of regressor tumors or the generation of immunity against challenge with progressor tumors indicates that these tumors express specific antigenic peptides

Fig. 12.17 The different growth patterns of transplantable tumors are governed by immune responses. Many tumors will grow progressively in T-cell deficient *nude* or irradiated mice (left panels). These tumors show two patterns of growth in normal syngeneic recipient mice, progressor or regressor (center panels). The regressor pattern is due to an adaptive immune response to the tumor, and therefore regrafting the same tumor leads to accelerated rejection. These tumors are rejected in allogeneic mice by T cells specific for MHC molecules on the tumor (right panels). † indicates death of the animal.

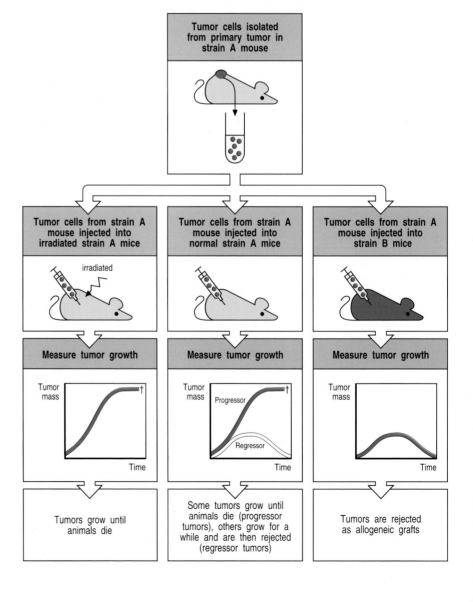

capable of being recognized by T cells. Thus, immunization with irradiated tumor cells from tumor A would protect a syngeneic mouse from challenge with live cells from tumor A but not from challenge with a syngeneic tumor B, and vice versa. The antigens expressed by experimentally induced murine tumors, often termed **tumor-specific transplantation antigens (TSTA),** are usually found to be tumor specific, although some appear to be shared by tumors of a similar cellular origin (Fig. 12.18).

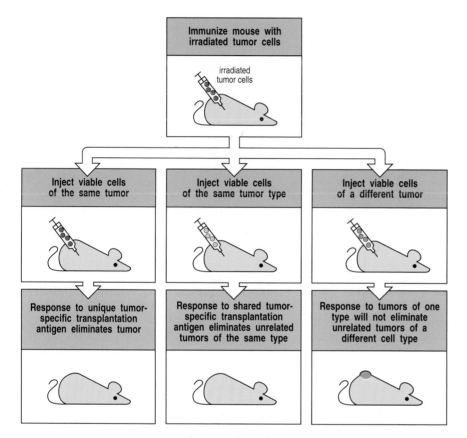

Fig. 12.18   Tumor-specific transplantation antigens are defined by growth patterns in immunized mice. Mice immunized with an irradiated tumor and challenged with viable cells of the same tumor can reject a lethal dose of that tumor in some cases (left panels). This is due to an immune response to tumor-specific transplantation antigens (TSTAs). Some TSTAs are unique to a given tumor, while others are shared by closely related tumors (middle panels) but not by unrelated tumors (right panels).

Molecular identification of the TSTA has shown that they can represent either mutations in cytoplasmic proteins that yield novel peptides capable of being presented on MHC class I to CD8 T cells, changes in the level of expression of normal cellular proteins or reactivation of embryonic genes that are expressed in the tumor but not in the tissue from which the tumor arose (Fig. 12.19). Currently, human tumor antigens recognized by autologous T cells have only been identified in melanoma (Fig. 12.20). This may be because melanoma appears to be somewhat unique among human tumors in that functional melanoma-specific T cells can be propagated from either peripheral blood lymphocytes, tumor-infiltrating lymphocytes, or draining lymph nodes of patients in whom the melanoma is growing. Interestingly, none of the melanoma-specific tumor antigens arise from mutated proto-oncogenes or tumor suppressor genes; these molecules are likely to be responsible for the initial transformation of the cell into a cancer cell. Rather, they fall into three categories. Antigens of the MAGE family are not expressed in any normal adult tissues with the exception of the testes, which we have learned in Chapter 11 is an immunologically privileged site. They probably represent early developmental antigens re-expressed in the process of tumorigenesis. Most melanoma patients do not possess T cells reactive

Fig. 12.19 Tumor-specific transplant-ation antigens are peptides of cellular proteins presented by self MHC class I molecules. Tumor-specific transplant-ation antigens (TSTAs) are peptides of cellular proteins presented by self MHC class I molecules. TSTAs arise mainly in two ways. In some cases, proteins that are normally expressed only in embryonic tissues are re-expressed by the tumor cells (lower left panel). As these proteins are normally expressed at a time when the immune system is not fully developed, T cells are not tolerant of these self antigens and can respond to them as if they were foreign proteins. In other tumors, overexpression of a self protein increases the density of presentation of a normal self peptide on tumor cells (lower right panel). Such peptides are then presented at high enough levels to be recognized by T cells. It is often the case that the same embryonic or self proteins are over-expressed in many tumors of a given type, giving rise to shared TSTAs.

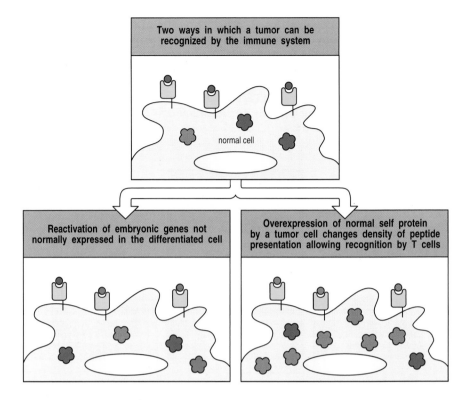

Origin of tumor antigen	Tumor antigen	Normal tissue of expression
Reactivated embryonic gene products	MAGE-1	Testes
	MAGE-3	Testes
Over-expressed normal gene products	MART 1	Melanocytes
	gp100	Melanocytes
	tyrosinase	Melanocytes

Fig. 12.20 Human melanoma-defined tumor-specific transplantation antigens.

with the MAGE family of antigens, indicating that they represent a tumor antigen that is not expressed or is not immunogenic in the majority of cases. The most common melanoma antigens are peptides from the enzyme tyrosinase or from three proteins — gp100, Mart 1, or gp75. These are differentiation antigens specific to the melanocyte lineage from which melanomas arise. In this case, it is likely that overexpression of these proteins in the tumor cells now renders them immunogenic. Tyrosinase has also been shown to stimulate CD4 T-cell responses in some melanoma patients by being ingested by cells expressing MHC class II and presented to CD4 T cells. Finally, a few melanoma antigens seem to represent the products of mutations.

TSTAs shared between most examples of a tumor, and against which tolerance can be broken, represent candidates for successful immunotherapy of these cancers. The MAGE family of antigens certainly represents excellent candidates because of their limited tissue distribution and their shared expression by many melanomas. It might seem risky to use tumor vaccines based on antigens that are not truly tumor specific because of the risk of inducing autoimmunity. Often, however, the tissues from which tumors arise are dispensable; the prostate is perhaps the best example of this. In the case of melanoma, however, some melanocyte-specific TSTAs are also expressed in certain retinal cells, in the inner ear, in the brain and in the skin. Despite this, melanoma patients receiving immunotherapy, while occasionally developing vitiligo, a destruction of pigmented cells in the skin that correlates well with a good response to the tumor, do not develop abnormalities in the visual, vestibular, and central nervous systems, perhaps because of the low expression of MHC class I molecules in these sites (see Section 4-5).

12-11   Tumors can escape immune surveillance in many ways.

Burnet called the ability of the immune system to detect tumor cells and destroy them **immune surveillance**. However, it is difficult to show that tumors are subject to surveillance by the immune system; after all, cancer is a common disease, and most tumors show little evidence for immunological control. Mice that lack lymphocytes show an incidence of the common tumors that is little different from the incidence of the same tumors in control mice with normal immune systems; the same is true for humans deficient in T cells. The major tumor type that occurs with increased frequency in immunodeficient mice or humans are virus-associated tumors; it can thus be said that immune surveillance is critical for control of virus-associated tumors, while the immune system does not normally respond to the neoantigens derived from the multiple genetic alterations in spontaneously arising tumors.

Why do T cells from animals or patients with spontaneously arising tumors fail to recognize tumor-specific antigens? The reason may be that when a new antigen arises in a tumor cell, it is tolerated by the T cells of the immune system in the same way as tissue-specific antigens. The goal in the development of cancer vaccines is thus to break the tolerance that exists within the immune system for antigens expressed by the tumor. Tumors can use other mechanisms to avoid or evade immune attack (Fig. 12.21). Some may lack distinctive antigenic peptides, while others may lack the adhesion or co-stimulatory molecules necessary to elicit T-cell responses. Even when an immune response does arise, tumor cells can lose their antigens by mutation, since they tend to be genetically unstable. This would generate escape variants that then cause cancer. Some tumors, such as colon cancers, lose expression of a particular MHC class I molecule, perhaps through immunoselection by T cells specific for that MHC class I molecule. In experimental studies, when a tumor loses expression of all MHC class I molecules, it can no longer be recognized by cytotoxic T cells, although it may become susceptible to NK cells. However, tumors that lose only one MHC class I molecule may be able to avoid recognition by specific CD8 cytotoxic T cells while remaining resistant to NK cells, giving them a selective advantage *in vivo* (Fig. 12.22).

Furthermore, many tumors make immunosuppressive cytokines, although little is known of their precise nature; transforming growth factor-β (TGF-β) was first identified in the culture supernatant of a tumor (hence its name), and, as we have seen, tends to suppress inflammatory T-cell responses and the cell-mediated immunity needed to control tumor growth. Thus, there are many ways in which tumors avoid recognition and destruction by the immune system.

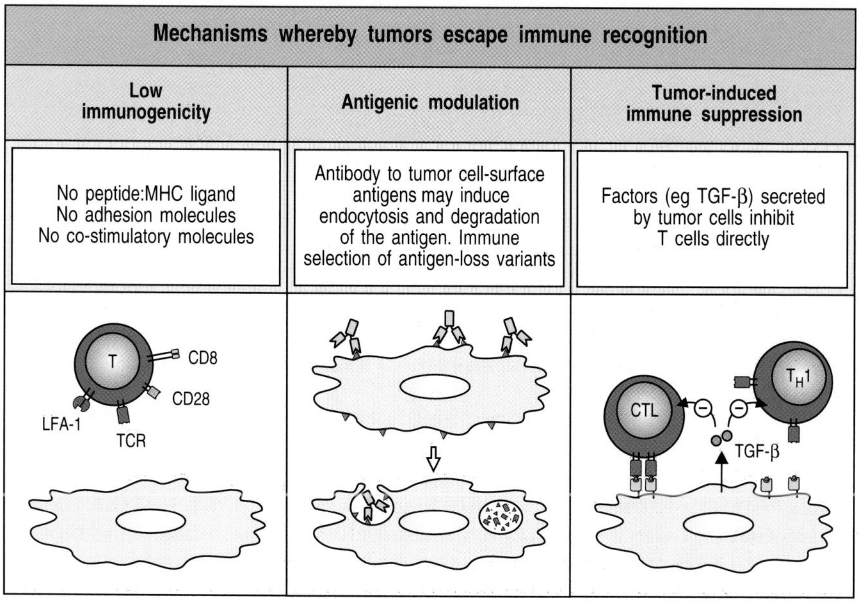

Mechanisms whereby tumors escape immune recognition		
Low immunogenicity	Antigenic modulation	Tumor-induced immune suppression
No peptide:MHC ligand No adhesion molecules No co-stimulatory molecules	Antibody to tumor cell-surface antigens may induce endocytosis and degradation of the antigen. Immune selection of antigen-loss variants	Factors (eg TGF-β) secreted by tumor cells inhibit T cells directly

Fig. 12.21 **Tumors may escape immune surveillance in a variety of ways**. First, tumors may have low immunogenicity (left panel). Some tumors do not have peptides of novel proteins that can be presented by MHC molecules, and therefore appear normal to the immune system. Others have lost one or more MHC molecules, or fail to express co-stimulatory proteins. Second, tumors may initially express antigens that the immune system can recognize but lose them due to antibody-induced internalization or antigenic variation. When tumors are attacked by cells responding to a particular antigen, any tumor that does not express that antigen will have a selective advantage (center panel). Third, tumors often produce substances, such as TGF-β, that suppress immune responses directly (right panel).

Fig. 12.22 Tumors that lose expression of all MHC class I molecules as a mechanism of escape from immune surveillance are more susceptible to natural killer (NK) cell killing. Normally, tumor growth is largely controlled by cytotoxic T cells (CTL) (left panels). NK cells have inhibitory receptors that bind MHC class I molecules (see Fig. 9.18), so variants of the tumor that have low MHC class I levels, although they are less sensitive to CD8 cytotoxic T cells, become susceptible to NK cells (center panels). Although *nude* mice lack T cells, they have higher than normal levels of NK cells, and so tumors that are sensitive to NK cells grow less well in *nude* mice than in normal mice. Transfection with MHC class I genes can restore both resistance to NK cells and susceptibility to CD8 cytotoxic T cells. Tumors that lose only one MHC class I molecule may escape a specific cytotoxic CD8 T-cell response while remaining NK resistant, however. The bottom panels show scanning electron micrographs of NK cells attacking leukemia cells. Left panel: shortly after binding to the target cell the NK cell has put out numerous microvillous extensions and established a broad zone of contact with the leukemia cell. The NK cell is the smaller cell on the left in both photographs. Right panel: 60 min after mixing, long microvillous processes can be seen extending from the NK cell (bottom left) to the leukemia cell and there is extensive damage to the leukemia cell membrane; the plasma membrane of the leukemia cell has rolled up and fragmented under the NK cell attack. Photographs courtesy of J Hiserodt.

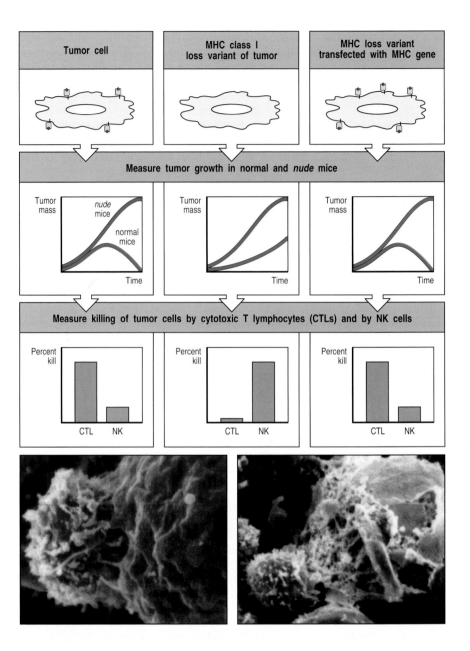

12-12   **Monoclonal antibodies to tumor antigens, alone or linked to toxins, can control tumor growth.**

The advent of monoclonal antibodies suggested that tumors might be targeted and destroyed by making antibodies against tumor-specific antigens (Fig. 12.23). In contrast to tumor antigens recognized by T cells, only cell-surface molecules make suitable targets for monoclonal antibodies. To date, there has been limited success using this approach, although as an adjunct to other therapies, it holds promise.

The first report of successful treatment of a tumor with monoclonal antibodies utilized anti-idiotypic antibodies to target B-cell lymphomas, whose surface immunoglobulin expressed the specific idiotype. The initial course of treatment usually leads to a remission, but the tumor always reappears in a somatically mutated form that no longer binds to the antibody used for the initial treatment. This case represents a clear example of a tumor using its inherent genetic instability to evade treatment.

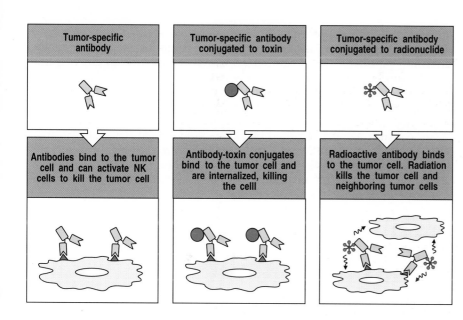

Fig. 12.23   A monoclonal antibody coupled to a toxin chain or a radio-isotope can eliminate or reduce the size of a tumor. Antibodies that recognize tumor-specific antigens can be used in a variety of ways to help eliminate tumors. If they are of the correct isotypes, the antibodies themselves may be able to direct the lysis of the tumor cells by NK cells, activating the NK cells via their Fcγ receptor (left panels). A more useful strategy may be to couple the antibody to a powerful toxin (center panels). When the antibody binds to the tumor cell and is endocytosed, the toxin is released from the antibody and can kill the tumor cell. If the antibody is coupled to a radionuclide, binding of the antibody to a tumor cell will deliver a dose of radiation sufficient to kill the tumor cell. In addition, nearby tumor cells may also receive a lethal radiation dose, even though they may not bind the antibody.

Other problems with tumor-specific or tumor-selective monoclonal antibodies as therapeutic agents include inefficient killing of cells after binding of the monoclonal antibody and inefficient penetration of the antibody into the tumor mass. The first problem can often be circumvented by linking the antibody to a toxin, producing a reagent called an **immunotoxin**; two favored toxins are ricin A chain and *Pseudomonas* toxin. Both approaches require the antibody to be internalized to allow the cleavage of the toxin from the antibody in the endocytic compartment (Fig. 12.23), allowing the toxin chain to penetrate and kill the cell.

Two other approaches using monoclonal antibody conjugates involve linking the antibody molecule to chemotherapeutic drugs such as adriamycin, or to radioisotopes. In the first case, the specificity of the monoclonal antibody for a cell surface antigen on the tumor concentrates the drug to the site of the tumor. After internalization, the drug is released in the endosomes and exerts its cytostatic or cytotoxic effect. Monoclonal antibodies linked to radionuclides (see Fig. 12.23) concentrate the radioactive source in the tumor site. Both these approaches have the advantage of producing bystander killing since the released drug or radioactive emissions can affect cells adjacent to those that actually bind the antibody. Ultimately, combinations of toxin-, drug-, or radionuclide-linked monoclonal antibodies together with T-cell vaccination approaches may provide the most effective cancer immunotherapy.

12-13   Enhancing the immunogenicity of tumors holds promise for cancer therapy.

While antigen-specific vaccines utilizing dominant shared tumor antigens are conceptually the ideal approach to T-cell mediated cancer immunotherapy, it will probably be many decades before the dominant tumor antigens for common cancers are identified. Even when these are identified, it will be uncertain how widely the relevant epitopes are shared.

Thus, the use of the individual patient's tumor removed at surgery as a source of vaccine antigens remains an important therapeutic strategy. Until recently, most cell-based cancer vaccines have involved mixing either irradiated tumor cells or tumor extracts with bacterial adjuvants such as BCG or *Corynebacterium parvum* (see Section 2-3). These adjuvants have generated modest therapeutic results in melanoma, but have been disappointing in general.

More recently, new molecular approaches to modifying tumor cells have been introduced with an enhanced ability to generate tumor-specific immune responses. These approaches involve introducing genes that encode co-stimulatory molecules or cytokines into tumors. Introducing co-stimulatory molecules is intended to make the tumor itself more immunogenic. The basic scheme of such experiments is shown in Fig. 12.24. A tumor cell transfected with the gene encoding the co-stimulator molecule B7 (see Section 7-4) is implanted in a syngeneic animal. These B7-positive cells are able to activate naive T cells that recognize TSTAs and reject the tumor cells. These effector T cells can recognize the tumor cells whether they express B7 or not; this can be shown by re-implanting non-transfected tumor cells, which are also rejected.

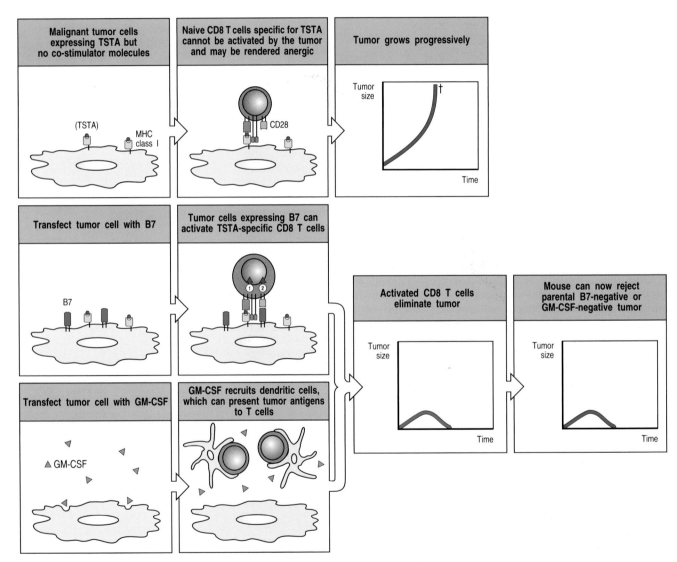

Fig. 12.24 Transfection of tumors with the gene for B7 or GM-CSF enhances tumor immunogenicity. A tumor that does not express co-stimulator molecules will not induce an immune response, even though it may express tumor-specific transplantation antigens (TSTAs), because naive CD8 T cells specific for the TSTA cannot be activated by the tumor. The tumor therefore grows progressively in normal mice (top panels). If such tumor cells are transfected with a co-stimulator molecule, such as B7, TSTA-specific CD8 T cells now receive both signal 1 and signal 2 from the same cell (see Section 7-4) and can therefore be activated (center panels). The same effect can be obtained by transfecting the tumor with the gene encoding GM-CSF, which attracts and induces the differentiation of the precursors of dendritic cells (bottom panels). Both of these strategies have been tested in mice and shown to elicit memory T cells, although results with GM-CSF are more impressive. Since TSTA-specific CD8 cells have now been activated, even the original B7-negative or GM-CSF negative tumor cells can be rejected. †indicates death of animal.

The second strategy, transducing cytokine genes into tumors so that they secrete the product of that gene, is aimed at attracting antigen-presenting cells to the tumor and takes advantage of the paracrine nature of cytokines. It has now been shown that the most effective tumor vaccines are tumor cells that secrete granulocyte-macrophage colony-stimulating factor (GM-CSF), which attracts hematopoietic precursors to the site and induces their differentiation into dendritic cells. It is believed that these cells process the tumor antigens and migrate to the local lymph nodes where they induce potent anti-tumor responses. Indeed, these GM-CSF-transfected tumor cells seem to be more potent inducers of anti-tumor T-cell responses than B7-transfected cells, perhaps because the bone marrow derived dendritic cells express more of the molecules required for naive T-cell activation than do B7-transfected tumor cells, which express both antigen and co-stimulator molecules but which lack various other molecules required for activating naive T cells (see Fig. 12.24).

What is not certain is whether people with established cancers can generate sufficient T-cell responses to eliminate all their tumor cells under circumstances where any tumor-specific naive T cells may have been rendered tolerant to the tumor. Moreover, there is always the risk that such transfectants will elicit an autoimmune response against the normal tissue from which the tumor derived. Clinical trials are in progress to determine the safety and efficacy of such approaches.

Summary.

Tumors represent outgrowths of a single abnormal cell, and in some instances it is clear that the immune system can distinguish tumor cells from normal cells. Nevertheless, the immune system seems to have been rendered tolerant to these tumor antigens, probably by the same processes that generate tolerance to normal peripheral tissue antigens (see for example, Sections 5-9 and 7-10). By utilizing current knowledge about antigen presentation to T cells, including the co-stimulatory signals that distinguish T-cell activation from inactivation, together with knowledge of the molecular nature of tumor-specific antigens, it may be possible to generate effective immune responses to tumors that can control their growth or even eliminate them entirely.

Manipulating the immune response to fight infection.

Modern immunology grew from Jenner's and Pasteur's original successes with vaccination. Many vaccines have been developed following these initial triumphs over smallpox and rabies (see Fig. 1.30). However, while these vaccines have virtually eliminated a number of diseases, their rare harmful side effects have led to a search for better ways to vaccinate against such illnesses. Moreover, great challenges remain in vaccine development against the many diseases for which no vaccine exists, including malaria and AIDS. The recent explosion in knowledge about the immune system and its interaction with pathogens has made vaccine development a highly attractive approach to disease control. Recombinant DNA technology has opened new avenues for manipulating microbial genomes and has the potential to improve vaccines tremendously. This, coupled with a growing awareness of the need for vaccines to prevent diseases prevalent in developing countries, those newly described diseases such as AIDS, and animal diseases important in agriculture, has created a resurgence of interest in this area. In this section, some current approaches to vaccine development will be outlined.

Features of effective vaccines	
Safe	Vaccine must not itself cause illness or death
Protective	Vaccine must protect against illness resulting from exposure to live pathogen
Gives sustained protection	Protection against exposure must last for several years
Induces neutralizing antibody	Some pathogens (like poliovirus) infect cells that cannot be replaced (eg neurons). Neutralizing antibody is essential to prevent infection of such cells
Induces protective T cells	Some pathogens, particularly intracellular, are more effectively dealt with by cell-mediated responses
Practical considerations	Low cost-per-dose Biological stability Ease of administration Few side effects

Fig. 12.25   There are several criteria for an effective vaccine.

12-14   There are several requirements for an effective vaccine.

For a vaccine to be useful, it must first and foremost be safe. Vaccines must be given to huge numbers of people, relatively few of whom are likely to die of the disease that the vaccine is designed to prevent, and this means that even a low level of toxicity is unacceptable (Fig. 12.25). Second, the vaccine must be able to produce protective immunity in a very high proportion of the people to whom it is given. Since it is impractical to give large or dispersed, rural populations regular 'booster' vaccinations, a successful vaccine must generate long-lived immunological memory. This means that both B and T lymphocytes must be primed by the vaccine. Third, vaccines must be very cheap if they are to be administered to large populations. Vaccines are one of the most cost-effective measures in health care but this benefit is eroded as the cost-per-dose rises.

Finally, for some infectious agents, protective immunity requires preexisting serum antibody. This is particularly necessary in the case of intracellular pathogens, such as the poliomyelitis virus, which infect critical host cells within a short period after entering the body. Some infectious agents have a prolonged incubation period before they invade critical host cells, and for these, pre-existing antibody is not necessary for protection, since there is time to elicit a secondary antibody response before the disease becomes established. Immune responses to infectious agents usually involve antibodies directed at multiple epitopes; only some of these antibodies confer protection. Thus, an effective vaccine must lead to the generation of antibodies and T cells directed at the correct epitopes of the infectious agent. For some of the modern vaccine techniques, in which only one or a few epitopes are used, this consideration is particularly important.

While existing vaccines may be improved by the modern approaches to vaccine development described in the following sections, it is worth noting that the existing vaccines largely mimic a natural infection that generates lasting protective immunity in patients who survive the disease. By contrast, many of the diseases for which vaccines are now being developed do not elicit protective immunity in their post-infectious phase; indeed, in many of these cases, the primary infection is not cleared. Thus, vaccines for these diseases cannot simply mimic natural immune responses but must improve upon them. This is a formidable challenge.

12-15   Recombinant DNA technology can be used to reduce the virulence of viruses or to insert genes for protective antigens into established vaccine strains.

Most anti-viral vaccines currently in use consist of dead or live attenuated viruses. Live attenuated virus vaccines are generally far more potent, perhaps because they elicit all relevant effector mechanisms, including cytotoxic CD8 T cells; dead viruses cannot produce proteins in the cytosol, so peptides from the viral antigens cannot be presented by MHC class I molecules and thus cytotoxic CD8 T cells are not generated by these vaccines.

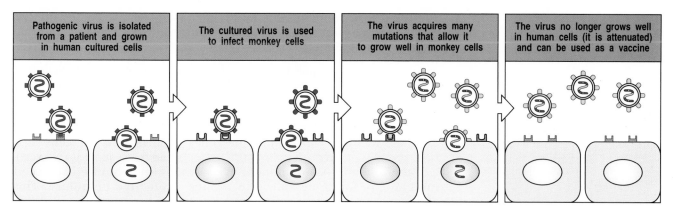

Fig. 12.26 Traditionally, viruses are attenuated by selecting for growth in non-human cells. To produce an attenuated virus, the virus must first be isolated by growing it in cultured human cells. This stock is then adapted to growth in cells of a different species, until it grows only poorly in human cells. The adaptation is a result of mutation, usually a combination of several point mutations. It is usually hard to tell which of the mutations in the genome of an attenuated viral stock are critical to attenuation. An attenuated virus will grow poorly in the human host, and will therefore produce immunity but not disease.

Traditionally, attenuation is achieved by growing the virus in non-human host cells. Viruses are selected for preferential growth in non-human cells and in the course of selection become less able to grow in human cells (Fig.12.26). Since these attenuated strains replicate poorly in human hosts, they induce immunity but not disease when given to people. Although attenuated virus strains contain multiple mutations in genes encoding several of their proteins, it may be possible for a pathogenic virus strain to re-emerge by a further series of mutations. This empirical approach to attenuation is still in use but may be superseded by two new approaches that use recombinant DNA technology. One is the isolation and *in vitro* mutagenesis of specific viral genes. The mutated genes are used to replace the wild-type gene in a reconstituted virus genome, and this deliberately attenuated virus can now be used as a vaccine (Fig. 12.27). The advantage of this approach is that mutations can be engineered so that reversion to wild type is virtually impossible. The second approach is to identify genes involved in virulence and to delete the entire gene from the virus. In some cases, this approach can give rise to replicating avirulent viruses that nevertheless induce protective immune responses against the wild-type virus. Again, the deletion of the gene virtually eliminates the possibility of genetic reversion to virulence. Similar approaches can be used for bacterial vaccine development.

These approaches might be particularly useful in developing influenza vaccines. As we learned in Chapter 10, the influenza virus can re-infect the same host several times, because it undergoes antigenic shift and thus escapes the original immune response. If the new virus strain can be isolated early in an epidemic and attenuated using the relatively rapid techniques described above, it might be possible to contain the epidemic. Recombinant DNA technology can alter virulence without

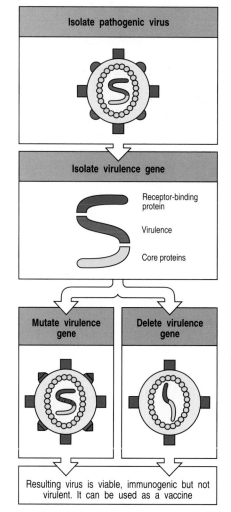

Fig. 12.27 Attenuation may be achieved more rapidly and reliably using recombinant DNA techniques. If a gene in the virus can be identified that is required for virulence but not for growth or immunogenicity, this gene may either be crippled by multiple mutations (left lower panel) or deleted from the genome (right lower panel) using recombinant DNA techniques. This procedure creates an avirulent (non-pathogenic) virus that can be used as a vaccine. The mutations in the virulence gene are usually large, so that it is very difficult for the virus to revert to the wild type.

altering the antigenicity or immunogenicity of viruses, allowing the rapid generation of effective vaccine strains, even in highly variable viruses such as influenza.

An alternative approach to vaccine generation involves the isolation of genes encoding antigens that elicit protective immunity, known as protective antigens, and their transfer to established avirulent vaccine strains such as the vaccinia virus. This approach requires an understanding of the nature of protective immunity against the infectious agent, so that one can identify the genes for protective antigens. It is now possible, using recombinant DNA technology, to separate a microbial genome into its component parts so that they can be examined individually for their ability to induce protective immunity. This approach has already succeeded in identifying both T- and B-cell epitopes from several different microorganisms (Fig. 12.28).

Once the critical epitopes have been identified, the genes that encode them can be introduced into a host organism and used to generate

Fig. 12.28   T- and B-cell epitope genes can be identified in pathogen DNA by cloning in vaccinia virus. Individual genes from a virulent virus can be cloned and inserted into the genome of the vaccinia virus, producing several recombinant viruses, each of which expresses only one gene of the pathogen. These recombinant viruses can then be tested for expression of antigens recognized by human antibodies or T cells from immune individuals. Thus, if antibodies found in the serum of an immune individual bind to the variant virus, the gene cloned into that variant must contain a B-cell epitope (left and center panels). The same variants can also be used to infect human cells, to determine their ability to render these cells targets for cytotoxic T cells from immune individuals (bottom panels). If killing of the target is detected (center and right panels) the gene contains a T-cell epitope. Vaccinia virus carrying genes for both B- and T-cell antigens may have potential use as a vaccine. Vaccinia is an attractive vaccine vector because it is known to be safe for immunization in most people and because it is highly immunogenic.

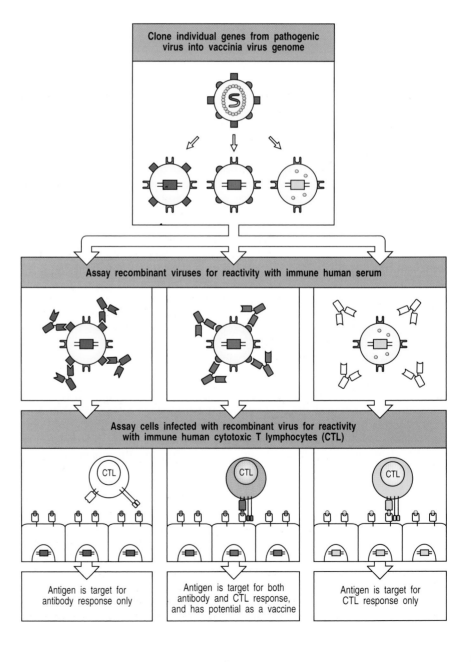

vaccines in a variety of ways. The gene can be incorporated in an expression system, so that the antigenic protein is produced in large quantities that can be used as a non-living vaccine. The first genetically engineered vaccine for human use, the hepatitis B vaccine, is of this type. Alternatively, the gene can be inserted into an existing attenuated viral vaccine strain of known immunogenicity, such as the vaccinia virus used in Jenner's original vaccine, so that it is expressed in an immunogenic form by the vaccinia virus. The attenuated mycobacterial vaccine strain, Bacille Calmette-Guérin (BCG), is also a candidate carrier for vaccine development. In this way, antigens can be used to elicit protective immunity using a vaccine strain that is known to be acceptably safe and effective at inducing long-term immunity to itself. This approach can be used for both viral and bacterial antigens. It has been proposed to place genes encoding protective antigens from several different organisms in a single vaccine strain. This approach makes it possible to immunize individuals against several different pathogens at once. This kind of approach combines the analytical power of recombinant DNA methods with their ability to manipulate the structure of genes.

12-16 | Synthetic peptides of protective antigens can elicit protective immunity.

The identification and isolation of protective antigens by recombinant DNA technology allows the complete characterization of their amino acid sequence by DNA sequencing of their genes. This, in turn, allows peptides representing different parts of the molecule to be chemically synthesized and tested for their ability to elicit protective immunity. In principle, this could allow the production of an entirely synthetic vaccine, avoiding the safety hazards involved in using live vaccine strains. However, there are also problems associated with peptide vaccines that may ultimately limit their use in humans.

Peptide synthesis is expensive, and it becomes progressively more difficult technically as the peptides become longer. Thus, most synthetic peptides used for immunization are 20 amino acids in length or less. Immunization of animals with such small synthetic peptides usually does not elicit an antibody response, probably because the peptide lacks any sequences that bind to MHC class II molecules. To overcome this, the peptide is treated as a hapten and is coupled to a protein carrier that does contain peptides that bind to human MHC class II molecules. Animals immunized with these peptide:protein conjugates make antibody to the peptide, and some of these antibodies also bind to the native protein; indeed, animals can be immunized in this way to make neutralizing antibodies that confer protective immunity against infection. However, the duration of this immunity has not been tested and, as the helper T cells in this case are directed at the artificial carrier and not at peptides from the pathogen, re-infection may not elicit a secondary antibody response since there will be no pathogen-specific memory T cells available.

To overcome this difficulty, complex peptide vaccines containing both peptides recognized by antibodies and peptides recognized by T cells can be prepared. Here, the choice of a peptide for recognition by T cells becomes critical. As we have learned, different MHC class II molecules bind different peptides, so a single peptide able to bind to MHC class II molecules in all individuals may be difficult to identify. Moreover, to be effective, this peptide must also be presented by MHC class II molecules during natural infection. Such peptides can be identified in three ways. First, one can synthesize a whole set of peptides from the sequence of the gene and test each one for its ability to stimulate T cells from infected individuals. Second, one can use known peptide motifs to identify candidate peptides and synthesize only this subset of peptides in similar tests. Third, one can purify MHC molecules from infected cells and examine their bound peptides for those derived from the pathogen. The virtue of this last approach is that it only detects peptides that are actually processed and presented by infected cells. This approach has been used with MHC class II to predict successfully the sequence of a gene for a protective antigen in *Leishmania* spp. that is abundantly expressed in the correct site for processing and presentation by MHC class II molecules, allowing this gene to be cloned for use in vaccines. Similar approaches to MHC class I associated peptides could also be attempted.

A final problem with synthetic peptide vaccines is that, even as conjugates, they are poorly immunogenic. Thus, they need to be delivered together with adjuvants. As we shall see in the next section, the development of adjuvants that can elicit potent protective immune responses to peptides is a separate area of investigation that needs to be developed.

12-17 | New adjuvants and new delivery systems are needed for peptide, protein, and carbohydrate vaccines.

Protective B-cell epitopes to an infectious agent may be protein or carbohydrate in nature. Peptides, proteins, and carbohydrate antigens are usually poorly immunogenic, or not immunogenic at all, when administered on their own. We learned in Section 8-2 that carbohydrate antigens can be linked chemically to immunogenic proteins to overcome this deficiency and this is also applicable to peptide antigens. Even this approach leads to vaccines that are only weakly immunogenic. Better delivery systems and adjuvants are needed to improve the ease of delivery and immunogenicity of such carbohydrates and peptides. Better adjuvants are also needed for some protein vaccines; the most widely used protein vaccines, diphtheria and tetanus toxoids, are initially given mixed with killed *Bordetella pertussis*, which serves as an adjuvant as well as an antigen, so that useful immunity to three pathogens is elicited by one immunization. However, untoward reactions to *B. pertussis* have sometimes occurred, and better adjuvants are needed here as well.

In addition to their weak immunogenicity, another problem associated with peptide and protein vaccines is their inability to enter certain cellular compartments. In particular, the generation of MHC class I-specific responses by *in vivo* immunization with peptides and proteins has proved difficult. One possible technique to solve these two problems is the use of **ISCOMs** (see Section 2-3). ISCOMs (immune stimulatory complexes) are lipid carriers that act as adjuvants but have minimal toxicity. They also appear to load peptides and proteins into the cell cytoplasm, allowing MHC class I-restricted T-cell responses to peptides (Fig. 12.29). These carriers are being developed for use in human immunization.

Several small molecules, for example muramyl dipeptide extracted from the mycobacterial cell wall, also act as adjuvants, although their mechanism of action is not known. They may act by stimulating the expression of co-stimulatory activity in antigen-presenting cells or by mimicking co-stimulatory signals in T cells. Alternatively, they may enhance uptake of the antigen by dendritic cells that already express co-stimulatory molecules. To date, adjuvant development has been largely an empirical exercise; as we learn what makes a good adjuvant, we should be able to approach this problem in a more direct fashion.

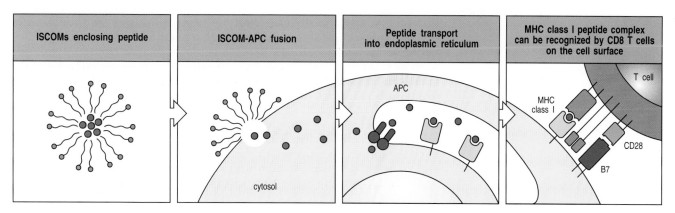

Fig. 12.29 ISCOMs can be used to deliver peptides to the MHC class I processing pathway. ISCOMs (immune stimulatory complexes) are lipid micelles that will fuse with cell membranes. Peptides trapped in ISCOMs can be delivered to the cytosol of an antigen-presenting cell (APC), allowing the peptide to be transported into the endoplasmic reticulum where it may be bound by nascent MHC class I molecules and hence transported to the cell surface as peptide:MHC class I complexes. This is a possible means for using peptides to activate CD8 cytotoxic T-cell responses. ISCOMs can also be used to deliver proteins to the cytosol of other types of cell, where they can be processed and presented as though they were a protein produced by the cell.

| 12-18 | **Protective immunity can be induced by injecting DNA encoding microbial antigens and human cytokines into muscle.** |

The latest development in vaccination has come as a surprise even to the scientists who initially developed the method. The story begins with attempts to use modified adenoviruses for gene therapy. To avoid responses to the viral proteins, it was decided to inject the modified adenoviral DNA in the form of plasmids containing the gene of interest into muscle cells. When DNA encoding a viral immunogen is injected, it leads to the development of antibody responses and cytotoxic T cells that allow the mice to reject a later challenge with whole virus (Fig. 12.30). This response does not appear to damage the muscle tissue, is safe and effective, and, since it uses only a single microbial gene, it does not carry the risk of active infection. This procedure has been termed genetic immunization. Techniques for mass immunization using DNA coated onto minute metal projectiles that can be administered by an air gun, so

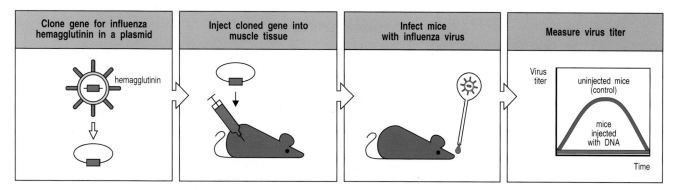

Fig. 12.30 Genetic immunization with DNA encoding a protective antigen and cytokines injected into muscle. Influenza hemagglutinin contains both B- and T-cell epitopes. When a naked DNA plasmid containing the gene for this protein is injected directly into muscle, a flu-specific immune response consisting of both antibody and cytotoxic CD8 T cells results. The response can be enhanced by including a plasmid encoding GM-CSF. Presumably, the plasmid DNAs are expressed by some of the cells in the muscle tissue into which it was injected, allowing an immune response that involves both antibody and cytotoxic T cells. The details of this process are not yet understood.

that several metal particles penetrate through the skin into the muscle beneath, have been shown to be effective in animals. This approach has yet to be tested in humans. Mixing in plasmids that encode cytokines such as GM-CSF allows these immunizations with genes encoding protective antigens to become much more effective, as has been seen earlier in attempts to induce tumor immunity.

It is not yet clear how genetic immunization actually works. Why is plasmid DNA effectively expressed in muscle tissue? Do the muscle cells elicit the immune response, or do tissue dendritic cells take up the DNA and express it? How do lymphocytes encounter the antigen if it is expressed in muscle cells? How safe is the approach, and how generally applicable will it be?

This intriguing new development may change the face of vaccines more than any other advance. Or it may be superseded by some other unexpected approach. Few were impressed with Jenner's vaccine when it was introduced nearly 200 years ago, yet attempts to understand how that vaccine works lie at the root of much of the progress in immunology that has been made since then. We clearly have many surprises ahead, and some will surely come from the development of new vaccines.

Summary.

The greatest triumphs of modern immunology have come from vaccination, which has eradicated or virtually eliminated several human diseases. It is the single most successful manipulation of the immune system to date because it takes advantage of its natural specificity and inducibility. Nevertheless, there remains much work to do. There are no vaccines against a variety of important infectious diseases, existing vaccines need to be safer and more effective, and the speed of the process of generating vaccines for newly emerging pathogens must be increased. The growing understanding of microbiology and immunology, together with the power of molecular biology, have already made it possible to develop new approaches to vaccine development. The ultimate aim must be to achieve the improvement in world health that is the required precursor to population control and economic development.

Summary to Chapter 12.

One of the great future challenges of immunology is the control of the immune response, so that unwanted immune responses can be suppressed and desirable responses elicited. Current approaches to the control of unwanted responses involve drugs that suppress adaptive immunity indiscriminately and are thus inherently flawed. The immune system can suppress its own responses in an antigen-specific manner, and by studying these endogenous regulatory events it may be possible to devise strategies to manipulate specific responses, while sparing general immune competence. This should allow the suppression of the responses that lead to allergy, autoimmunity, or the rejection of grafted organs. Similarly, as we learn more about tumors and infectious agents, better strategies to mobilize the immune system against cancer and infection should become possible. To do this, we need to learn more about the induction of immunity and the biology of the immune system, and to apply what we have learned to human disease.

General references.

Ada, G.: **Vaccination in Third World countries.** *Curr. Opin. Immunol.* 1993, **5**:683-686.

Brines, R. (ed.): **Immunopharmacology.** *Immunol. Today* 1993, **14**:241-332.

Klein, G. and Boon, T.: **Cancer, Editorial Overview.** *Curr. Opin. Immunol.* 1993, **5**:687-692.

Lanzavecchia, A.: **Identifying strategies for immune intervention.** *Science* 1993, **260**:937-944.

Moller, G. (ed.): **New immunosuppressive drugs.** *Immunol. Rev.* 1993, **136**: 1-109.

Moller, G. (ed.): **Engineered antibody molecules.** *Immunol. Rev.* 1992, **130**: 1-212.

Moller, G. (ed.): **Antibodies in disease therapy.** *Immunol. Rev.* 1992, **129**: 1-201.

Plotkin, S.A. and Mortimer, E.A.: *Vaccines*, 1st edn. Philadelphia, W.B. Saunders Co., 1988.

Section references.

12-1 | In immune individuals, secondary and subsequent responses are mediated solely by memory lymphocytes.

Amigorena, S., Bonnerot, C., Drake, J., Choquet, D., Hunziker, W., Guillet, J.G., Webster, P., Sautes, C., Mellman, I., and Fridman, W.H.: **Cytoplasmic domain heterogenicity and functions of IgG Fc receptors in B lymphocytes.** *Science* 1992, **256**:1808-1812.

Fazekas de St Groth, B., and Webster, R.G.: **Disquisitions on original antigenic sin. I. Evidence in man.** *J. Exper. Med.* 1966, **140**:2893-2898.

Fridman, W.H.: **Regulation of B cell activation and antigen presentation by Fc receptors.** *Curr. Opin. Immunol.* 1993, **5**:355-360.

Pollack, W. *et al.*: **Results of clinical trials of RhoGAm in women.** *Transfusion* 1968, **8**:151.

Uhr, J.W. and Moller, G.: **Regulatory effect of antibody on the immune response.** *Adv. Immunol.* 1968, **8**:81-127.

12-2 | Interactions between lymphocyte receptors may regulate the repertoire.

Jerne, N.K.: **Toward a network theory of the immune system.** *Ann. Immunol.* 1974, **125C**:373-389.

Holmberg, D., Andersson, A., Carlsson, L., and Forsgren, S.: **Establishment and functional implications of B cell connectivity.** *Immunol. Rev.* 1989, **110**:89-103.

Perelson, A.S.: **Immune network theory.** *Immunol. Rev.* 1989, **110**:5-36.

Pollok, B.A., and Kearney, J.F.: **Identification and characterization of an apparent germline set of auto-anti-idiotypic regulatory B lymphocytes.** *J. Immunol.* 1984, **132**:114-121.

Rajewsky, K., and Takemori, T.: **Genetics, expression and function of idiotypes.** *Ann. Rev. Immunol.* 1983, **1**:569-607.

12-3 | CD4 T cell subsets can regulate one another's growth.

Baxevanis, C.N., Nagy, Z.A., and Klein, J.: **A novel type of T-T interaction removes the requirement for I-B region in the H-2 complex.** *Proc. Natl. Acad. Sci. USA* 1981, **78**:3809-3813.

de Waal Malefyt, R., Haanen, J., Spits, H., Roncarolo, M.-G., te Velde, A., Figdor, C., Johnson, K., Kastelein, R., Yssel, H., and de Vries, J.E.: **IL-10 and viral IL-10 strongly reduce antigen-specific human T cell proliferation by** diminishing the antigen-presenting capacity of monocytes via downregulation of class II major histocompatibility complex expression. *J. Exper. Med.* 1991, **174**:915.

Gajewski, T.F., and Fitch, F.W.: **Anti-proliferative effect of IFN-γ in immune regulation. I. IFN-gamma inhibits the proliferation of Th2 but not Th1 murine helper T lymphocyte clones.** *J. Immunol.* 1988, **140**:4245.

Ruegemer, J.J., Ho, S.N., Augustine, J.A., Schlager, J.W., Bell, M.P., McKean, D.J., and Abraham, R.T.: **Regulatory effects of transforming growth factor β on IL-2 and IL-4 dependent T cell cycle progression.** *J. Immunol.* 1990, **144**:1767-1776.

12-4 | CD4 T-cell subsets can regulate one another's effector functions.

DelPrete, G.F., De Carli, M., Ricci, M., and Romagnani, S.: **Helper activity for immunoglobulin synthesis of T helper type 1 (Th1) and Th2 human T cell clones: the help of Th1 clones is limited by their cytolytic capacity.** *J. Exper. Med.* 1991, **174**:908-913.

Sher, A., Gazzinelli, R.T., Oswald, I.P., Clerici, M., Kullberg, M., Pearce, E.J., Berzofsky, J.A., Mosmann, T.R., James, S.L., Morse, H.C. III, and Shearer, G.M.: **Role of T cell derived cytokines in the downregulation of immune responses in parasitic and retroviral infection.** *Immunol. Rev.* 1992, **127**:183-204.

12-5 | Cytokines released by CD8 T cells can affect CD4 T cells, B cells and macrophages.

Powrie, F., and Coffman, R.L.: **Cytokine regulation of T cell function: Potential for therapeutic intervention.** *Immunol. Today* 1993, **14**:270-274.

Salgamme, P., Yamamura, M., Bloom, B.R., and Modlin, R.L.: **Evidence for functional subsets of CD4⁺ and CD8⁺ T cells in human disease – lymphokine patterns in leprosy.** *Chem. Immunol.* 1992, **54**:44-59.

12-6 | Cytotoxic drugs and steroids cause immunosuppression by killing dividing cells and have serious side effects.

Chan, G.L.C., Canafax, D.M., and Johnson, C.A.: **The therapeutic use of azathioprine in renal transplantation.** *Pharmacotherapy* 1987, **7**:165-177.

Cupps, T.R., and Fauci, A.S.: **Corticosteroid-mediated immunoregulation in man.** *Immunol. Rev.* 1982, **65**:133-155.

12-7 | Cyclosporin A, FK506, and rapamycin are powerful immuno- suppressive agents that interfere with T-cell signaling.

Bierer, B.E., Hollander, G., Fruman, D., and Burakoff, S.J.: **Cyclosporin A and FK506: molecular mechanisms of immunosuppression and probes for transplantation biology.** *Curr. Opin. Immunol.* 1993, **5**:763-773.

Clipstone, N.E., and Crabtree, G.R.: **Identification of calcineurin as a key signaling enzyme in T lymphocyte activation.** *Nature* 1992, **357**:695.

Flanagan, W.M., Firpo, E., Roberts, J.M., and Crabtree, G.R.: **The target of rapamycin defines a restriction point in late G1.** *Mol. Cell Biol.* 1993.

Schreiber, S.L.: **Chemistry and biology of the immunophilins and their immunosuppressive ligands.** *Science* 1991, **251**:283.

Schreiber, S.L., and Crabtree, G.R.: **The mechanism of action of cyclosporin A and FK506.** *Immunol. Today* 1992, **13**:136.

12-8 | Antibodies to cell-surface molecules have been used to remove specific lymphocyte subsets or to inhibit cell function.

Cobbold, S.P., Qin, S., Leong, L.Y.W., Martin, G., and Waldmann, H.: **Reprogramming the immune system for peripheral tolerance with CD4 and CD8 monoclonal antibodies.** *Immunol. Rev.* 1992, **129**:165-201.

Lenschow, D.J., Zeng, Y., Thistlewaite, J.R., Montag, A., Brady, W., Gibson, M.G., Linsley, P.S., and Bluestone, J.A.: **Long-term survival of xenogeneic pancreatic islet cell grafts induced by CTLA4Ig.** *Science* 1992, **257**:789-792.

Lenschow, D.J. and Bluestone, J.A.: **T cell costimulation and** *in vivo* **tolerance.** *Curr. Opin. Immunol.* 1993, **5**:747-752.

Waldmann, H., and Cobbold, S.: **The use of monoclonal antibodies to achieve immunological tolerance.** *Immunol. Today* 1993, **14**:247-251.

Winter, G., and Harris, W.J.: **Humanized antibodies.** *Immunol. Today* 1993, **14**:243-246.

12-9   CD4 subset activation can be manipulated with cytokines, anti-cytokine antibodies, the route and dose of antigen administration, or the structure of the antigen.

Constant, S., Pfeiffer, C., Pasqualini, T., and Bottomly, K.: **Extent of T cell ligation determines the functional differentiation of naive CD4 T cells.** *J. Exper. Med.* 1995.

De Magistris, M.T., Alexander, J., Coggeshall, M., Altman, A., Gaeta, F.C.A, Grey, H.M., and Sette, A.: **Antigen analog-major histocompatibility complex acts as antagonists of the T cell receptor.** *Cell* 1992, **68**:625-634.

Gammon, G., and Sercarz, E.E.: **How some T cells escape tolerance induction.** *Nature* 1989, **342**:183-185.

Pfeiffer, C., Murray, J., Madri, J., and Bottomly, K.: **Selective activation of Th1- and Th2-like cells** *in vivo* **- response to human collagen IV.** *Immunol. Rev.* 1991, **123**:65-84.

12-10   Some tumors can be recognized and rejected by the immune system.

Boel, P., Wildmann, C., Sensi, M.L., Brasseur, R., Renauld, J.C., Coulie, P., Boon, T., and Van, D.B.P.: **BAGE: A new gene encoding an antigen recognized on human melanomas by cytolytic T lymphocytes.** *Immunity* 1995, **2**:167-175.

Brichard, V., Van, P.A., Wolfel, T., Wolfel, C., Lethe, B., Coulie, P., and Boon, T.: **The tyrosinase gene codes for an antigen recognized by autologous cytolytic T lymphocytes on HLA-A2 melanomas.** *J. Exper. Med.* 1993, **178**:489-495.

Coulie, P.G., Brichard, V., Van, P.A., Wolfel, T., Schneider, J., Traversari, C., Mattei, S., De, P.E., Lurquin, C., Szikora, J.P., Renauld, J.C., and Boon, T.: **A new gene coding for a differentiation antigen recognized by autologous cytolytic T lymphocytes on HLA-A2 melanomas.** *J. Exper. Med.* 1994, **180**:35-42.

Cox, A.L., Skipper, J., Chen, Y., Henderson, R.A., Darrow, T.L., Shabanowitz, J., Engelhard, V.H., Hunt, D.F., and Slingluff, C.J.: **Identification of a peptide recognized by five melanoma-specific human cytotoxic T cell lines.** *Science* 1994, **264**:716-719.

De, P.E., Arden, K., Traversari, C., Gaforio, J.J., Szikora, J.P., De, S.C., Brasseur, F., Van, D.B.P., Lethe, B., Lurquin, C., Brasseur, R., Chomez, P., De, B.O., Cavenee, W., and Boon,T.: **Structure, chromosomal localization, and expression of 12 genes of the MAGE family.** *Immunogenetics* 1994, **40**:360-369.

Kawakami, Y., Eliyahu, S., Delgado, C.H., Robbins, P.F., Sakaguchi, K., Appella, E., Yannelli, J.R., Adema, G.J., Miki, T., and Rosenberg, S.A. **Identification of a human melanoma antigen recognizes by tumor-infiltrating lymphocytes associated with** *in vivo* **tumor rejection.** *Proc. Natl. Acad. Sci. USA* 1994, **901**:6458-6462.

Topalian, S.L., Rivoltini, L., Mancini, M., Markus, N.R., Robbins, P.F., Kawakami, Y., and Rosenberg, S.A.: **Human CD4+ T cells specifically recognize a shared melanoma-associated antigen encoded by the tyrosine gene.** *Proc. Natl. Acad. Sci. USA.* 1994, **91**:9461-9465.

12-11   Tumors can escape immune surveillance in many ways.

Moller, P., and Hammerling, G.J.: **The role of surface HLA-A,B,C molecules in tumor immunity.** *Cancer Surv.* 1992, **13**:101-127.

Storkus, W.J., Howell, D.N., Slater, R.D., Dawson, I.R., and Cresswell, P.: **NK susceptibility varies inversely with target cell class I HLA antigen expression.** *J. Immunol.* 1987, **138**:1657-1659.

Travers, P.J., Arklie, J.L., Trowsdale, J., Patillo, R.A., and Bodner, W.F.: **Lack of expression of HLA-ABC antigens in choriocarcinoma and other human tumor cell lines.** In: Greenwald, P. (ed.): *Research Frontiers in Aging and Cancer.* Natl. Cancer Inst. Monogr. 1982, **60**:175-180.

Uyttenhove, C., Maryanski, J., and Boon, T.: **Escape of mouse mastocytoma P815 after nearly complete rejection is due to antigen loss variants rather than immunosuppression.** *J. Exper. Med.* 1983, **157**:1040-1052.

12-12   Monoclonal antibodies to tumor antigens, alone or linked to toxins, can control tumor growth.

Miller, R.A., Maloney, D.G., Warnke, R., and Levy, R.: **Treatment of B cell lymphoma with monoclonal anti-idiotype antibody.** *N. Engl. J. Med.* 1982, **306**:517-522.

Riethmuller, G., Schneider-Gadicke, E., and Johnson, J.P.: **Monoclonal antibodies in cancer therapy.** *Curr. Opin. Immunol.* 1993, **5**:732-739.

Vitetta, E., Thorpe, P.E., and Uhr, J.W.: **Immunotoxins: magic bullets or misguided missiles?** *Immunol. Today* 1993, **14**:252-259.

12-13   Enhancing the immunogenicity of tumors holds promise for cancer therapy.

Baskar, S., Ostrand-Rosenberg, S., Nabavi, N., Nadler, L.M., Freeman, G.J., and Glimcher, L.H.: **Constitutive expression of B7 restores immunogenicity of tumor cells expressing truncated MHC class II molecules.** *Proc. Natl. Acad. Sci. USA* 1993, **90**:5687-5690.

Brunda, M.J., Luistro, L., Warrier, R.R., Wright, R.B., Hubbard, B.R., Murphy, M., Wolf, S.F., and Gately, M.K.: **Antitumor and antimetastatic activity of interleukin 12 against murine tumors.** *J. Exper. Med.* 1993, **178**:1223-1230.

Dranoff, G., Jaffee, E., Lazenby, A., Golumbek, P., Levitsky, H., Brose, K., Jackson, V., Hamada, H., Pardoll, D., and Mulligan, R.C.; **Vaccination with irradiated tumor cells engineered to secrete murine granulocyte-macrophage colony-stimulating factor stimulates potent, specific, and long-lasting anti-tumor immunity.** *Proc. Natl. Acad. Sci. USA* 1993, **90**:3539-3543.

Laning, J., Kawasaki, H., Tanaka, E., Luo, Y., and Dorf, M.E.: **Inhibition of** *in vivo* **tumor growth by the beta chemokine TCA3.** 1994, *J. Immunol.* **153**:4625-4635.

Pardoll, D.M.: **New strategies for enhancing the immunogenicity of tumors.** *Curr. Opin. Immunol.* 1993, **5**:719-725.

Pardoll, D.M.: **Cancer vaccines.** *Curr. Opin. Immunol.* 1993, **14**:310-316.

Townsend, S.E. and Allison, J.P.: **Tumor rejection after direct costimulation of CD8+ T cells by B7-transfected melanoma cells.** *Science* 1993, **259**:368- 370.

12-14   There are several requirements for an effective vaccine.

Cryz, S.J. Jr (ed.): *Vaccines and Immunotherapy*, 1st edn. New York, Pergamon Press, 1991 .

Institute of Medicine: *New Vaccine Development: Establishing Priorities. Diseases of Importance in the United States, Vol. 1,* 1st edn. Washington, DC, National Academy Press, 1985.

12-15   Recombinant DNA technology can be used to reduce the virulence of viruses or to insert genes for protective antigens into established vaccine strains.

Aldovani, A. and Young, R.A.: **Humoral and cell-mediated responses to live recombinant BCG-HIV vaccines.** *Nature* 1991, **351**:479-482.

Cox, W.I., Tartaglia, J., and Paoletti, E.: **Poxvirus recombinants as live vaccines.** In: Binns, M. and Smith, G.L. (eds.): *Recombinant Poxviruses*, 1st edn. Boca Raton, FL, CRC Press, 1992.

Kit, S., Kit, M., and Pirtle, E.C.: **Attenuated properties of thymidine kinase - negative deletion mutants of pseudorabies virus.** *Am. J. Vet. Res.* 1985, **46**:1359-1367.

Omata, T., Kohara, M., Kuge, S., Komatsu, T., *et al*: **Genetic analysis of the attenuation phenotype poliovirus type I.** *J. Virol.* 1986, **58**:348-358.

Stover, C.K., de la Cruz, V.F., Fuerst, T.R., Burlein, J.E., Benson, L.A., Bennett, L.T., Bansal, G.P., Young, J.F., Lee, M.H., Hatfull, G.F., Snapper, S.B., Barletta, R.G., Jacobs Jr, W.R., and Bloom, B.R..: **New use of BCG for recombinant vaccines.** *Nature* 1991, **351**:456-460.

12-16 Synthetic peptides of protective antigens can elicit protective immunity.

Brown, F.: **The potential of peptides as vaccines.** *Semin. Virol.* 1990, **1**:67- 74.

12-17 New adjuvants and new delivery systems are needed for peptide, protein, and carbohydrate vaccines.

Audibert, F.M. and Lise, L.D.: **Adjuvants: current status, clinical perspectives and future prospects.** *Immunol. Today* 1993, **14**:281-284.

Rhodes. J., Chen. H., Hall, S.R., Beesley, J.E., Jenkins, D.C., Collins, P., and Zheng, B.: **Therapeutic potentiation of the immune system by costimulatory Schiff-base-forming drugs.** *Nature* 1995, **377**:71-75.

Takahasshi, H., Takeshita, T., Morein, B., Putney, S., Germain, R.N., and Berzofsky, J.A.: **Induction of CD8$^+$ cytotoxic T cells by immunization with purified HIV-1 envelope protein in ISCOMs.** *Nature* 1990, **344**:873-875.

12-18 Protective immunity can be induced by injecting DNA encoding microbial antigens and human cytokines into muscle.

Ulmer, J.B., Donnelly, J.J., Parker, S.E., Gromkowski, S.H., Deck, R.R., DeWitt, C.M., Friedman, A., Hawe, L.A., Leander, K.R., Martinez, D., Perry, H.C., Shiver, J.W., Montgomery, D.L., and Liu, M.A.: **Heterologous protection against influenza by injection of DNA encoding a viral protein.** *Science* 1993, **259**:1745-1749.

APPENDICES

Appendix I. The CD antigens. (Gray indicates the CD antigens that are mentioned in the text.)					
CD antigen	**Cellular expression**	**Molecular weight (kDa)**	**Functions**	**Other names**	**Family relationships**
CD1a,b,c,d	Cortical thymocytes, Langerhans' cells, dendritic cells, B cells (CD1c), intestinal epithelium (CD1d)	43–49	MHC class I-like molecule, associated with β_2-microglobulin. May have specialized role in antigen presentation		Immunoglobulin superfamily (IgSF)
CD2	T cells, thymocytes, natural killer cells	45–58	Adhesion molecule, binding CD58 (LFA-3). Can activate T cells	T11, LFA-2	Immunoglobulin superfamily
CD2R	Activated T cells	45–58	Activation-dependent conformational form of CD2	T11-3	Immunoglobulin superfamily
CD3	Thymocytes, T cells	γ: 25–28 δ: 20 ϵ: 20 ζ: 16 η: 22	Associated with the T-cell antigen receptor. Required for cell-surface expression of and signal transduction by T-cell receptor	T3	Immunoglobulin superfamily ($\gamma\delta\epsilon$) ζ/η related to FcRγ chain
CD4	Thymocyte subsets, helper and inflammatory T cells (about two thirds of peripheral T cells), monocytes, macrophages	55	Co-receptor for MHC class II molecules. Binds lck on cytoplasmic face of membrane. Receptor for HIV-1 and HIV-2 gp120	T4, L3T4	Immunoglobulin superfamily
CD5	Thymocytes, T cells, subset of B cells	67	Unknown, may bind to CD72	T1, Ly1	Scavenger receptor
CD6	Thymocytes, T cells, B-cell chronic lymphatic leukemia	100–130	Binds ligand (ALCAM) on thymic epithelium	T12	Scavenger receptor
CD7	Pluripotential hematopoietic cells, thymocytes, T cells	40	Unknown. Marker for T-cell acute lymphatic leukemia and pluripotential stem cell leukemias		Immunoglobulin superfamily
CD8	Thymocyte subsets, cytotoxic T cells (about one third of peripheral T cells)	α: 32–34 β: 32–34	Co-receptor for MHC class I molecules. Binds lck on cytoplasmic face of membrane	T8, Lyt2,3	Immunoglobulin superfamily
CD9	Pre-B cells, eosinophils, basophils, platelets	22–27	Possible role in platelet aggregation and activation		Tetraspanning membrane protein also called serpentine or Transmembrane 4 superfamily
CD10	B- and T-cell precursors, bone marrow stromal cells	100	Zinc metalloproteinase, marker for pre-B acute lymphatic leukemia	Neutral endopeptidase, common acute lymphocytic leukemia antigen (CALLA)	
CD11a	Lymphocytes, granulocytes, monocytes and macrophages	180	α^L subunit of integrin LFA-1 (associated with CD18); binds to CD54 (ICAM-1), ICAM-2, and ICAM-3	LFA-1	

CD antigen	Cellular expression	Molecular weight (kDa)	Functions	Other names	Family relationships
CD11b	Myeloid and natural killer cells	170	α^M subunit of integrin CR3 (associated with CD18); binds CD54, complement component iC3b, and extracellular matrix proteins	Mac-1	
CD11c	Myeloid cells	150	α^X subunit of integrin CR4 (associated with CD18); binds fibrinogen	gp150,95	
CDw12	Monocytes, granulocytes, platelets	90–120	Unknown		
CD13	Myelomonocytic cells	150–170	Zinc metalloproteinase	Aminopeptidase N	
CD14	Myelomonocytic cells	53–55	Receptor for complex of lipopolysaccharide and lipopolysaccharide binding protein (LBP)		
CD15	Neutrophils, eosinophils, monocytes		Branched pentasaccharide, expressed on glycolipids and many cell-surface glycoproteins; the sialylated form CD15S is a ligand for CD62E (ELAM)	Lewis x (Le^x)	
CD16	Neutrophils, natural killer cells, macrophages	50–80	Component of low affinity Fc receptor, FcγRIII, mediates phagocytosis and antibody-dependent cell-mediated cytotoxicity	FcγRIII	Immunoglobulin superfamily
CDw17	Neutrophils, monocytes, platelets		Lactosyl ceramide, a cell-surface glycosphingolipid		
CD18	Leukocytes	95	Integrin β_2 subunit, associates with CD11a, b, and c		
CD19	B cells	95	Forms complex with CD21 (CR2) and CD81 (TAPA-1); co-receptor for B cells		Immunoglobulin superfamily
CD20	B cells	33–37	Possible role in regulating B-cell activation		
CD21	Mature B cells, follicular dendritic cells	145	Receptor for complement component C3d, Epstein-Barr virus. With CD19 and CD81, CD21 forms co-receptor for B cells	CR2	Complement control protein (CCP) superfamily
CD22	Mature B cells	140	Adhesion of B cells to monocytes, T cells	BL-CAM	Immunoglobulin superfamily
CD23	Mature B cells, activated macrophages, eosinophils, follicular dendritic cells, platelets	45	Low affinity receptor for IgE, ligand for CD19:CD21:CD81 co-receptor	FcεRII	C-type lectin
CD24	B cells, granulocytes	35–45	Unknown	Possible human homolog of mouse heat stable antigen (HSA) or J11d	
CD25	Activated T cells, B cells, and monocytes	55	IL-2 receptor α chain associates with CD122 and IL-2Rγ chain	Tac	Complement control protein superfamily
CD26	Activated B and T cells, macrophages	110	Protease. Recently implicated in HIV entry into cells	Dipeptidyl peptidase IV	
CD27	Medullary thymocytes, T cells	50–55 homodimer	Binds TNF-like ligand, CD70		NGF receptor superfamily

CD antigen	Cellular expression	Molecular weight (kDa)	Functions	Other names	Family relationships
CD28	T-cell subsets, activated B cells	44	Activation of naive T cells, receptor for co-stimulatory signal (signal 2) binds CD80 (B7.1) and B7.2	Tp44	Immunoglobulin superfamily
CD29	Leukocytes	130	Integrin β_1 subunit, associates with CD49a in VLA-1 integrin		
CD30	Activated B and T cells	105–120	Binds TNF-like membrane protein, CD30-L	Ki-1	NGF receptor superfamily
CD31	Monocytes, platelets, granulocytes, B cells, endothelial cells	130–140	Possibly an adhesion molecule	PECAM-1	Immunoglobulin superfamily
CD32	Monocytes, granulocytes, B cells, eosinophils	40	Low affinity Fc receptor for aggregated immunoglobulin/immune complexes	FcγRII	Immunoglobulin superfamily
CD33	Myeloid progenitor cells, monocytes	67	Unknown		Immunoglobulin superfamily
CD34	Hematopoietic precursors, capillary endothelium	105–120	Ligand for CD62L (L-selectin)		
CD35	Erythrocytes, B cells, monocytes, neutrophils, eosinophils, follicular dendritic cells	250	Complement receptor 1, binds C3b and C4b, mediates phagocytosis	CR1	Complement control protein superfamily
CD36	Platelets, monocytes	88	Unknown	Platelet GPIV	
CD37	Mature B cells, mature T cells, myeloid cells	40–52	Unknown	gp52–40	Tetraspanning membrane protein
CD38	Early B and T cells, activated T cells, germinal center B cells, plasma cells	45	Unknown	T10	
CD39	Activated B cells, activated natural killer cells, macrophages, dendritic cells	78	Unknown, may mediate adhesion of B cells	gp80	
CD40	B cells, monocytes, dendritic cells	50	Receptor for co-stimulatory signal for B cells, binds CD40 ligand (CD40-L)	gp50	NGF receptor superfamily
CD40-L	Activated CD4 T cells	39	Ligand for CD40	T-BAM, gp39	TNF-like
CD41	Platelets, megakaryocytes	125/122 dimer	α^{IIb} integrin, associates with CD61 to form GPIIb, binds fibrinogen, fibronectin, von Willebrand factor, and thrombospondin	GPIIb	
CD42a,b,c,d	Platelets, megakaryocytes	a: 23 b: 135,23 c: 22 d: 85	Binds von Willebrand factor, thrombin; essential for platelet adhesion at sites of injury	a: GPIX b: GPIbα c: GPIbβ d: GPV	
CD43	Leukocytes, except resting B cells	115–135 (neutrophils) 95–115 (T cells)	Mucin-like glycoprotein	Leukosialin, sialophorin	
CD44	Leukocytes, erythrocytes	80–95	Binds hyaluronic acid, mediates adhesion of leukocytes	Hermes antigen Pgp-1	Link
CD45	Leukocytes	180–240	Phosphotyrosine phosphatase, augments signaling through antigen receptor of B and T cells, multiple isoforms result from alternative splicing (see below)	Leukocyte common antigen (LCA), T200, B220	
CD45RO	T-cell subsets, B-cell subsets, monocytes, macrophages	180	Isoform of CD45 containing none of the A, B, and C exons		

CD antigen	Cellular expression	Molecular weight (kDa)	Functions	Other names	Family relationships
CD45RA	B cells, T-cell subsets (naive T cells), monocytes	205–220	Isoforms of CD45 containing the A exon		
CD45RB	T-cell subsets, B cells, monocytes, macrophages, granulocytes	190–220	Isoforms of CD45 containing the B exon	T200	
CD46	Hematopoietic and non-hematopoietic nucleated cells	56/66 (splice variants)	Membrane co-factor protein, binds to C3b and C4b to permit their degradation by Factor I	MCP	Complement control protein superfamily
CD47	All cells	47–52	Integrin-associated glycoprotein, associated with Rh blood group		Immunoglobulin superfamily
CD48	Leukocytes	40–47	Unknown	Blast-1	Immunoglobulin superfamily
CD49a	Activated T cells, monocytes	210	α^1 integrin, associates with CD29, binds collagen, laminin	VLA-1	
CD49b	B cells, monocytes, platelets	165	α^2 integrin, associates with CD29, binds collagen, laminin	VLA-2	
CD49c	B cells	125	α^3 integrin, associates with CD29, binds laminin, fibronectin	VLA-3	
CD49d	B cells, thymocytes	150	α^4 integrin, associates with CD29, binds fibronectin, Peyer's patch HEV, VCAM-1	VLA-4	
CD49e	Memory T cells, monocytes, platelets	135,25 dimer	α^5 integrin, associates with CD29, binds fibronectin	VLA-5	
CD49f	Memory T cells, thymocytes, monocytes	120,25 dimer	α^6 integrin, associates with CD29, binds laminin	VLA-6	
CD50	Thymocytes, T cells, B cells, monocytes, granulocytes	130	Binds integrin CD11a/CD18	ICAM-3	Immunoglobulin superfamily
CD51	Platelets, megakaryocytes	125,24 dimer	α^v integrin, associates with CD61, binds vitronectin, von Willebrand factor, fibrinogen and thrombospondin	Vitronectin receptor	
CD52	Thymocytes, T cells, B cells (not plasma cells), monocytes, granulocytes	21–28	Unknown, target for antibodies used therapeutically to deplete T cells from bone marrow	CAMPATH-1	
CD53	Leukocytes	35–42	Unknown	MRC OX44	Tetraspanning membrane protein
CD54	Hematopoietic and non-hematopoietic cells	85–110	Intercellular adhesion molecule (ICAM)-1, binds CD11a/CD18 integrin (LFA-1) and CD11b/CD18 integrin (Mac-1), receptor for rhinovirus	ICAM-1	Immunoglobulin superfamily
CD55	Hematopoietic and non-hematopoietic cells	60–70	Decay accelerating factor (DAF), binds C3b, disassembles C3/C5 convertase	DAF	Complement control protein superfamily
CD56	Natural killer cells	175–185	Isoform of neural cell adhesion molecule (NCAM), adhesion molecule	NKH-I	Immunoglobulin superfamily
CD57	Natural killer cells, subsets of T cells, B cells, and monocytes		Oligosaccharide, found on many cell-surface glycoproteins	HNK-1, Leu-7	
CD58	Hematopoietic and non-hematopoietic cells	55–70	Leukocyte function-associated antigen-3 (LFA-3), binds CD2, adhesion molecule	LFA-3	Immunoglobulin superfamily
CD59	Hematopoietic and non-hematopoietic cells	19	Binds complement components C8 and C9, blocks assembly of membrane-attack complex	Protectin, Mac inhibitor	Ly-6 superfamily
CD60	T-cell subsets, platelets, monocytes		Oligosaccharide present on gangliosides		

CD antigen	Cellular expression	Molecular weight (kDa)	Functions	Other names	Family relationships
CD61	Platelets, megakaryocytes, macrophages	105	Integrin β_3 subunit, associates with CD41 (GPIIb/IIIa) or CD51 (vitronectin receptor)		
CD62E	Endothelium	140	Endothelium leukocyte adhesion molecule (ELAM), binds sialyl-Lewis x, mediates rolling interaction of neutrophils on endothelium	ELAM-1, E-selectin	C-type lectin EGF and CCP superfamily
CD62L	B cells, T cells, monocytes, natural killer cells	150	Leukocyte adhesion molecule (LAM), binds CD34, GlyCAM, mediates rolling interactions with endothelium	LAM-1, L-selectin, LECAM-1	C-type lectin EGF and CCP superfamily
CD62P	Platelets, megakaryocytes, endothelium	140	Adhesion molecule, binds sialyl-Lewis x, mediates interaction of platelets with neutrophils, monocytes, and rolling interaction of neutrophils on endothelium	P-selectin, PADGEM	C-type lectin EGF and CCP superfamily
CD63	Activated platelets, monocytes, macrophages	53	Unknown, is lysosomal membrane protein translocated to cell surface after activation	Platelet activation antigen	Tetraspanning membrane protein
CD64	Monocytes, macrophages	72	High affinity receptor for IgG	FCγRI	Immunoglobulin superfamily
CDw65	Myeloid cells		Oligosaccharide component of a ceramide dodecasaccharide		
CD66a	Neutrophils	160–180	Unknown, member of carcinoembryonic antigen (CEA) family (see below)	Biliary glycoprotein-1 (BGP-1)	Immunoglobulin superfamily
CD66b	Granulocytes	95–100	Unknown, member of carcinoembryonic antigen (CEA) family	Previously CD67	Immunoglobulin superfamily
CD66c	Neutrophils, colon carcinoma	90	Unknown, member of carcinoembryonic antigen (CEA) family	Non-specific cross-reacting antigen (NCA)	Immunoglobulin superfamily
CD66d	Neutrophils	30	Unknown, member of carcinoembryonic antigen (CEA) family		Immunoglobulin superfamily
CD66e	Adult colon epithelium, colon carcinoma	180–200	Unknown, member of carcinoembryonic antigen (CEA) family	Carcinoembryonic antigen (CEA)	Immunoglobulin superfamily
CD68	Monocytes, macrophages, neutrophils, basophils, large lymphocytes	110	Unknown	Macrosialin	
CD69	Activated T and B cells, activated macrophages, natural killer cells	28,32 homodimer	Unknown, early activation antigen	Activation inducer molecule (AIM)	C-type lectin
CD70	Activated B cells, activated T cells, macrophages	75,95,170	Ligand for CD27	Ki-24	TNF-like
CD71	Activated leukocytes	90–95 homodimer	Transferrin receptor	T9	
CD72	B cells	42 homodimer	Unknown, may be ligand for CD5	Lyb-2	C-type lectin
CD73	B-cell subsets, T-cell subsets	69	Ecto-5′-nucleotidase, dephosphorylates nucleotides to allow nucleoside uptake		

CD antigen	Cellular expression	Molecular weight (kDa)	Functions	Other names	Family relationships
CD74	B cells, macrophages, monocytes, MHC class II positive cells	33, 35, 41, 43 (alternative initiation and splicing)	MHC class II-associated invariant chain	Ii, Iγ	
CDw75	Mature B cells, T-cell subsets		Unknown, possibly oligosaccharide, dependent on sialylation		
CD76	Mature B cells, T-cell subsets		Unknown, possibly oligosaccharide, dependent on sialylation		
CD77	Germinal center B cells		Unknown	Globotriaocylcer-amide (Gb₃), Pᵏ blood group	
CDw78	B cells		Unknown	Ba	
CD79α,β	B cells	a: 32–33 β: 37–39	Components of B-cell antigen receptor analogous to CD3, required for cell-surface expression and signal transduction	Igα, Igβ	Immunoglobulin superfamily
CD80	B-cell subset	60	Co-stimulator, ligand for CD28 and CTLA-4	B7 (now B7.1), BB1	Immunoglobulin superfamily
CD81	Lymphocytes	26	Associates with CD19, CD21 to form B cell co-receptor	Target of antiproliferative antibody (TAPA-1)	Tetraspanning membrane protein
CD82	Leukocytes	50–53	Unknown	R2	Tetraspanning membrane protein
CD83	Activated B cells, activated T cells, circulating dendritic cells (veil cells)	43	Unknown	HB15	
CDw84	Monocytes, platelets, circulating B cells	73	Unknown	GR6	
CD85	Monocytes, circulating B cells	120,83	Unknown	GR4	
CD86	Monocytes, activated B cells	80	Unknown	FUN-1, GR65	
CD87	Granulocytes, monocytes, macrophages, activated T cells	50–65	Urokinase plasminogen activator receptor	UPA-R	Ly-6 superfamily
CD88	Polymorphonuclear leukocytes, macrophages, mast cells	40	Receptor for complement component C5a	C5aR	Rhodopsin superfamily
CD89	Monocytes, macrophages, granulocytes, neutrophils, B-cell subsets, T-cell subsets	50–70	IgA receptor	FcαR	Immunoglobulin superfamily
CDw90	CD34⁺ prothymocytes (human) thymocytes, T cells (mouse)	18	Unknown	Thy-1	Immunoglobulin superfamily
CD91	Monocytes	600	α₂-macroglobulin receptor		
CDw92	Neutrophils, monocytes, platelets, endothelium	70	Unknown	GR9	
CD93	Neutrophils, monocytes, endothelium	120	Unknown	GR11	
CD94	T-cell subsets, natural killer cells	43	Unknown	KP43	
CD95	Wide variety of cell lines, in vivo distribution uncertain	43	Binds TNF-like Fas ligand, induces apoptosis	Apo-1, Fas	NGF receptor superfamily

CD antigen	Cellular expression	Molecular weight (kDa)	Functions	Other names	Family relationships
CD96	Activated T cells	160	Unknown	T-cell activation increased late expression (TACTILE)	
CD97	Activated cells	74,80,90	Unknown	GR1	
CD98	T cells, B cells, natural killer cells, granulocytes, all human cell lines	80,40 heterodimer	Unknown	4F2	
CD99	Peripheral blood lymphocytes, thymocytes	32	Unknown	MIC2, E2	
CD100	Broad expression on hematopoietic cells	150	Unknown	GR3	
CDw101	Granulocytes, macrophages	140	Unknown	BPC#4	
CD102	Resting lymphocytes, monocytes, vascular endothelial cells (strongest)	55–65	Binds CD11a/CD18 (LFA-1) but not CD11b/CD18 (Mac-1)	ICAM-2	Immunoglobulin superfamily
CD103	Intraepithelial lymphocytes, 2–6%, peripheral blood lymphocytes	150,25	α_E integrin	HML-1, α_6, α_E integrin	
CD104	Epithelia, Schwann cells, some tumor cells	220	β_4 integrin	β_4 integrin chain	
CD105	Endothelial cells, bone marrow cell subset, in vitro activated macrophages	95 homodimer	Binds TGF-β	Endoglin	
CD106	Endothelial cells	100,110	Adhesion molecule, ligand for VLA-4	VCAM-1	Immunoglobulin superfamily
CD107a	Activated platelets	110	Unknown, is lysosomal membrane protein translocated to the cell surface after activation	Lysosomal associated membrane protein-1 (LAMP-1)	
CD107b	Activated platelets	120	Unknown, is lysosomal membrane protein translocated to the cell surface after activation	LAMP-2	
CDw108	Activated T cells in spleen, some stromal cells	80	Unknown	GR2	
CDw109	Activated T cells, platelets, endothelial cells	170/50	Unknown	Platelet activation factor, GR56	
CD110–CD114	Not yet assigned				
CD115	Monocytes, macrophages	150	Macrophage colony stimulating factor (M-CSF) receptor	M-CSFR, c-fms	Immunoglobulin superfamily
CDw116	Monocytes, neutrophils, eosinophils, endothelium	70–85	Granulocyte macrophage colony stimulating factor (GM-CSF) receptor α chain	GM-CSFRα	Cytokine receptor superfamily, fibronectin type III superfamily
CD117	Hematopoietic progenitors	145	Stem cell factor (SCF) receptor	c-kit	Immunoglobulin superfamily, tyrosine kinase
CD118	Broad cellular expression		Interferon-α,β receptor	IFN-α,βR	
CD119	Macrophages, monocytes, B cells, endothelium	90–100	Interferon-γ receptor	IFN-γR	
CD120a	Hematopoietic and non-hematopoietic cells, highest on epithelial cells	50–60	TNF receptor, binds both TNF-α and TNF-β	TNFR-I	NFG receptor superfamily

CD antigen	Cellular expression	Molecular weight (kDa)	Functions	Other names	Family relationships
CD120b	Hematopoietic and non-hematopoietic cells, highest on myeloid cells	75–85	TNF receptor, binds both TNF-α and TNF-β	TNFR-II	NGF receptor superfamily
CDw121a	Thymocytes, T cells	80	Type I interleukin-1 receptor, binds IL-1α and IL-1β	IL-1R type I	Immunoglobulin superfamily
CDw121b	B cells, macrophages, monocytes	60–70	Type II interleukin-1 receptor, binds IL-1α and IL-1β	IL-1R type II	Immunoglobulin superfamily
CD122	Natural killer cells, resting T-cell subpopulation, some B-cell lines	75	IL-2 receptor β chain	IL-2Rβ	
CD123	Bone marrow stem cells, granulocytes, monocytes, megakaryocytes	70	IL-3 receptor α chain	IL-3Rα	Cytokine receptor superfamily, fibronectin type III superfamily
CD124	Mature B and T cells, hematopoietic precursor cells	130–150	IL-4 receptor	IL-4R	Cytokine receptor superfamily, fibronectin type III superfamily
CD125	Eosinophils, basophils	55–60	IL-5 receptor α chain	IL-5Rα	Cytokine receptor superfamily, fibronectin type III superfamily
CD126	Activated B cells and plasma cells (strong), most leukocytes (weak)	80	IL-6 receptor α subunit	IL-6Rα	Immunoglobulin superfamily, cytokine receptor superfamily, fibronectin type III superfamily
CDw127	Bone marrow lymphoid precursors, pro-B cells, mature T cells, monocytes	68–79, possibly forms homodimers	IL-7 receptor	IL-7R	Fibronectin type III superfamily
CDw128	Neutrophils, basophils, T-cell subset	58–67	IL-8 receptor	IL-8R	Rhodopsin superfamily
CD129	Not yet assigned				
CDw130	Activated B cells and plasma cells (strong), most leukocytes (weak), endothelial cells	130	Common subunit of IL-6, IL-11, oncostatin M (OSM) and leukemia inhibitory factor (LIF) receptors	IL-6Rβ, IL-11Rβ, OSMRβ, LIFRβ	Immunoglobulin superfamily, cytokine receptor superfamily, fibronectin type III superfamily

	Appendix II. Cytokines and their receptors.					
Family	Cytokine (alternative names)	Size (no. of amino acids) and form*	Receptors (c denotes common subunit)	Producer cells	Actions	Effect of cytokine or receptor knock-out (where known)
Hematopoietins* (four-helix bundles)	Epo (erythropoietin)	165, monomer*	EpoR	Kidney	Stimulates erythroid progenitors	
	IL-2 (T-cell growth factor)	133, monomer	CD25 (α), CD122 (β),γ_c	T cells	T-cell proliferation	IL-2: decreased T-cell proliferation; Receptor γ chain: incomplete T-cell development
	IL-3 (multicolony CSF)	133, monomer	CD123, β_c	T cells, thymic epithelial cells	Synergistic action in early hematopoiesis	
	IL-4 (BCGF-1, BSF-1)	129, monomer	CD124, γ_c	T cells, mast cells	B-cell activation, IgE switch	Decreased IgE synthesis
	IL-5 (BCGF-2)	115, homodimer	CD125, β_c	T cells, mast cells	Eosinophil growth, differentiation	
	IL-6 (IFN-β_2, BSF-2, BCDF)	184, monomer	CD126,CD$_W$130	T cells, macrophages	T- and B-cell growth and differentiation, acute phase protein production	Decreased acute phase reaction
	IL-7	152, monomer*	CD$_W$127, γ_c	Bone marrow stroma	Growth of pre-B cells and pre-T cells	
	IL-9	125, monomer	IL-9R, γ_c	T cells	Mast cell enhancing activity	
	IL-11	178, monomer	IL-11R, CD$_W$130	Stromal fibroblasts	Synergistic action with IL-3 and IL-4 in hematopoiesis	
	IL-13 (P600)	132, monomer	IL-13R, γ_c	T cells	B-cell growth and differentiation, inhibits macrophage inflammatory cytokine production	
	G-CSF	? monomer*	G-CSFR	Fibroblasts	Stimulates neutrophil development	
	IL-15 (T-cell growth factor)	114, monomer	IL-15R, γ_c	T cells	IL-2-like, stimulates growth of intestinal epithelium	
	GM-CSF (granulocyte macrophage colony stimulating factor)	127, monomer*	CD$_W$116, β_c	Macrophages, T cells	Stimulates growth and differentiation of myelomonocytic lineage	
	OSM (OM, oncostatin M)	196, monomer	OMR, CD$_W$130	T cells, macrophages	Stimulates Kaposi sarcoma cells, inhibits melanoma growth	
	LIF (leukemia inhibitory factor)	179, monomer	LIFR, CD$_W$130	Bone marrow stroma, fibroblasts	Maintains embryonic stem cells, like IL-6, IL-11, OSM	
Interferons	IFN-γ	143, monomer	CD119	T cells, natural killer cells	Macrophage activation, increased MHC expression	Susceptibility to intracellular infection
	IFN-α	166, monomers	CD118	Leukocytes	Anti-viral, increased MHC class I expression	
	IFN-β	166, monomer	CD118	Fibroblasts	Anti-viral, increased MHC class I expression	
Immunoglobulin superfamily	B7.1 (CD80)	262 dimer	CD28, CTLA-4	Antigen-presenting cells	Co-stimulation of T-cell responses	
	B7.2 (B70)		CD28, CTLA-4	Antigen-presenting cells	Co-stimulation of T-cell responses	

* May function as dimers

Family	Cytokine (alternative names)	Size (no. of amino acids) and form	Receptors (c denotes common subunit)	Producer cells	Actions	Effect of cytokine or receptor knock-out (where known)
TNF family	TNF-α (cachectin)	157, trimers	p55, p75 CD120a, CD120b	Macrophages, natural killer cells	Local inflammation, endothelial activation	Receptor: resistance to septic shock, susceptibility to *Listeria*
	TNF-β (lymphotoxin, LT, LT-α)	171, trimers	p55, p75 CD120a, CD120b	T cells, B cells	Killing, endothelial activation	Absent lymph nodes, increased antibody
	LT-β	Transmembrane, trimerizes with TNF-β		T cells, B cells	Unknown	
	CD40 ligand (CD40-L)	Trimers	CD40	T cells, mast cells	B-cell activation, class switching	Poor antibody response, no class switch
	Fas ligand	Trimers	CD95 (Fas)	T cells, stroma?	Apoptosis, Ca^{2+}-independent cytotoxicity	Lymphoproliferation
	CD27 ligand	Trimers (?)	CD27	T cells	Stimulates T-cell proliferation	
	CD30 ligand	Trimers (?)	CD30	T cells	Stimulates T- and B- cell proliferation	
	4-1BBL	Trimers (?)	4-1BB	T cells	Co-stimulates T- and B- cells	
Chemokines	IL-8 (NAP-1)	69–79, dimers	CDw128	Macrophages, others	Chemotactic for neutrophils, T cells	
	MCP-1 (MCAF)	76, monomer(?)		Macrophages, others	Chemotactic for monocytes	
	MIP-1α	66, monomer (?)		Macrophages, others	Chemoattractant for monocytes, T cells, eosinophils	
	MIP-1β	66, monomer (?)		T cells, B cells, monocytes	Chemoattractant for monocytes, T cells	
	RANTES	66, monomer (?)		T cells, platelets	Chemoattractant for monocytes, T cells, eosinophils	
Unassigned	TGF-β	112, homo- and heterotrimers		Chondrocytes, monocytes, T cells	Inhibits cell growth, anti-inflammatory	
	IL-1α	159, monomer	CDw121a	Macrophages, epithelial cells	Fever, T-cell activation, macrophage activation	
	IL-1β	153, monomer	CDw121a	Macrophages, epithelial cells	Fever, T-cell activation, macrophage activation	
	IL-1 RA	? monomer		Macrophages	Binds to but doesn't trigger IL-1 receptor, acts as a natural antagonist of IL-1 function	
	IL-10 (cytokine synthesis inhibitor F)	160, homodimer		T cells, macrophages, Epstein-Barr virus	Potent suppressant of macrophage functions	
	IL-12 (natural killer cell stimulatory factor)	197 and 306, heterodimer		B cells, macrophages	Activates natural killer cells, induces CD4 T cell differentiation to T_H1-like cells	
	MIF	115, monomer		T cells, others	Inhibits macrophage migration	

BIOGRAPHIES

Emil von Behring (1854–1917) discovered antitoxin antibodies with Shibasaburo Kitasato.

Baruj Benacerraf (1920–) discovered immune response genes and collaborated in the first demonstration of MHC restriction.

Jules Bordet (1870–1961) discovered complement as a heat-labile component in normal serum that would enhance the antimicrobial potency of specific antibodies.

Frank Macfarlane Burnet (1899–1985) proposed the first generally accepted clonal selection hypothesis of adaptive immunity.

Jean Dausset (1916–) was an early pioneer in the study of the human major histocompatibility complex or HLA.

Gerald Edelman (1929–) made crucial discoveries about the structure of immunoglobulins, including the first complete sequence of an antibody molecule.

Paul Ehrlich (1854–1915) was an early champion of humoral theories of immunity, and proposed a famous side-chain theory of antibody formation that bears a striking resemblance to current thinking about surface receptors.

James Gowans (1924–) discovered that adaptive immunity is mediated by lymphocytes, focusing the attention of immunologists on these small cells.

Michael Heidelberger (1888–1991) developed the quantitative precipitin assay, ushering in the era of quantitative immunochemistry.

Edward Jenner (1749–1823) described the successful protection of humans against smallpox infection by vaccination with cowpox or vaccinia virus. This founded the field of immunology.

Niels Jerne (1911–1994) developed the hemolytic plaque assay and several important immunological theories, including an early version of clonal selection, a prediction that lymphocyte receptors would be inherently biased to MHC recognition, and the idiotype network.

Shibasaburo Kitasato (1892–1931) discovered antibodies in collaboration with Emil von Behring.

Robert Koch (1843–1910) defined the criteria needed to characterize an infectious disease, known as Koch's postulates.

Georges Köhler (1946–1995) pioneered monoclonal antibody production from hybrid antibody-forming cells with Cesar Milstein.

Karl Landsteiner (1868–1943) discovered the ABO blood group antigens. He also carried out detailed studies of the specificity of antibody binding using haptens as model antigens.

Peter Medawar (1915–1987) used skin grafts to show that tolerance is an acquired characteristic of lymphoid cells, a key feature of clonal selection theory.

Elie Metchnikoff (1845–1916) was the first champion of cellular immunology, focusing his studies on the central role of phagocytes in host defense.

Cesar Milstein (1927–) pioneered monoclonal antibody production with Georges Köhler.

Louis Pasteur (1822–1895) was a French microbiologist and immunologist who validated the concept of immunization first studied by Jenner. He prepared vaccines against chicken cholera and rabies.

Rodney Porter (1920–1985) worked out the polypeptide structure of the antibody molecule, laying the groundwork for its analysis by protein sequencing.

George Snell (1903–) worked out the genetics of the murine major histocompatibility complex and generated the congenic strains needed for its biological analysis, laying the groundwork for our current understanding of the role of the MHC in T cell biology.

Susumu Tonegawa (1939–) discovered the somatic recombination of immunological receptor genes that underlies the generation of diversity in human and murine antibodies and T-cell receptors.

GLOSSARY

The **ABO blood group system** antigens are expressed on red blood cells. They are used for typing human blood for transfusion. People naturally form antibodies to the A or B blood group antigens if they do not express them on their red blood cells.

The removal of antibodies specific for one antigen from an antiserum to render it specific for another antigen or antigens is called **absorption**.

Accessory cells in adaptive immunity are cells that aid in the response but do not directly mediate specific antigen recognition. They include phagocytes, mast cells, and natural killer cells, and are also known as **accessory effector cells**.

The **acquired immune deficiency syndrome (AIDS)** is a disease caused by infection with the human immunodeficiency virus. AIDS occurs when an infected patient has lost most of his or her CD4 T cells, so that infections with opportunistic pathogens occur.

Acquired immune response: see **adaptive immune response**.

Immunization with antigen is called **active immunization** to distinguish it from the transfer of antibody to a naive individual, which is called passive immunization.

Acute phase proteins are a series of proteins found in the blood shortly after the onset of an infection. These proteins participate in early phases of host defense against infection. An example is the mannose-binding protein.

The **acute phase response** is a change in the blood that occurs during early phases of an infection. It includes the production of acute phase proteins and also of cellular elements.

The **adaptive immune response** or **adaptive immunity** is the response of antigen-specific lymphocytes to antigen, including the development of immunological memory. Adaptive immune responses are generated by clonal selection of lymphocytes. Adaptive immune responses are distinct from innate and non-adaptive phases of immunity, which are not mediated by clonal selection of antigen-specific lymphocytes. Adaptive immune responses are also known as **acquired immune responses**.

The **adenoids** are **mucosal-associated lymphoid tissues** located in the nasal cavity.

The enzyme defect **adenosine deaminase deficiency** leads to the accumulation of toxic purine nucleosides and nucleotides, resulting in the death of most developing lymphocytes within the thymus. It is a common cause of severe combined immunodeficiency.

Adhesion molecules mediate the binding of one cell to other cells or to extracellular matrix proteins. Integrins, selectins, members of the immunoglobulin gene superfamily, and CD44 and related proteins are all adhesion molecules important in the operation of the immune system.

An **adjuvant** is any substance that enhances the immune response to an antigen with which it is mixed.

Adoptive immunity is immunity conferred on a naive or irradiated recipient by transfer of lymphoid cells from an actively immunized donor. This is called **adoptive transfer** or **adoptive immunization**.

Afferent lymphatic vessels drain fluid from the tissues and carry antigens from sites of infection in most parts of the body to the lymph nodes.

Affinity is the strength of binding of one molecule to another at a single site, such as the binding of a monovalent Fab fragment of antibody to a monovalent antigen (also see **avidity**).

Affinity chromatography is the purification of a substance by means of its affinity for another substance immobilized on a solid support; an antigen can be purified by affinity chromatography on a column of specific antibody molecules covalently linked to beads.

Affinity maturation refers to the increase in the affinity of the antibodies produced during the course of a humoral immune response. It is particularly prominent in secondary and subsequent immunizations.

Agammaglobulinemia: see **X-linked agammaglobulinemia**.

Agglutination is the clumping together of particles, usually by antibody molecules binding to antigens on the surfaces of adjacent particles. When the particles are red blood cells, the phenomenon is called hemagglutination.

Alleles are variants of a single genetic locus.

Allelic exclusion refers to the expression of immunoglobulin encoded by a single heavy-chain and a single light-chain immunoglobulin constant-region allele on the surface of B cells in heterozygous animals or people. It has come to be used more generally to describe the expression of a single receptor specificity in cells with the potential to express two or more receptors.

Allergens are antigens that elicit hypersensitivity or allergic reactions.

Allergic asthma is constriction of the bronchial tree due to an allergic reaction to inhaled antigen.

An **allergic reaction** is a response to innocuous environmental antigens or allergens due to pre-existing antibody or T cells There are various immune mechanisms of allergic reactions, but the most common is the binding of allergen to IgE antibody on mast cells that causes asthma, hay fever, and other common allergic reactions.

Allergic rhinitis is an allergic reaction in the nasal mucosa, also known as hay fever, that causes runny nose, sneezing and tears.

Allergy is the symptomatic reaction to a normally innocuous environmental antigen. It results from the interaction between the antigen and antibody or T cells produced by earlier exposure to the same antigen.

Two individuals or two mouse strains that differ at the MHC are said to be **allogeneic**. The term can also be used for allelic differences at other loci (see also **syngeneic**, **xenogeneic**).

Rejection of grafted tissues from unrelated donors usually results from T-cell responses to **allogeneic MHC molecules** expressed by the grafted tissues.

An **allograft** is a graft of tissue from an allogeneic or non-self donor of the same species; such grafts are invariably rejected unless the recipient is immunosuppressed.

Alloreactivity describes the stimulation of T cells by MHC molecules other than self; it marks the recognition of **allogeneic** MHC.

Allotypes are allelic polymorphisms detected by antibodies; in immunology, allotypic differences in immunoglobulin molecules were important in deciphering the genetics of antibodies.

The **altered ligand hypothesis** states that the ligand selecting the T cell receptor is unable to trigger a mature T cell with the same T cell receptor. It stands in contrast to the avidity hypothesis, which says that the same exact peptide at different levels can select a T cell either positively or induce deletional tolerance.

The **alternative pathway** of complement activation is not triggered by antibody, as is the classical pathway of complement activation, but by the binding of complement protein C3b to the surface of a pathogen; it is therefore a feature of innate immunity. The alternative pathway also amplifies the classical pathway of complement activation.

Anaphylactic shock is an allergic reaction to systemically administered antigen that causes circulatory collapse and suffocation due to tracheal swelling. It results from binding of antigen to IgE antibody on connective tissue mast cells throughout the body, leading to the disseminated release of inflammatory mediators .

Anaphylatoxins are small fragments of complement proteins released by cleavage during complement activation. The fragments C5a, C3a, and C4a are all anaphylatoxins, listed in order of decreasing potency *in vivo*. They serve to recruit fluid and inflammatory cells to sites of antigen deposition.

Peptide fragments of antigens are bound to specific MHC class I molecules by **anchor residues** which are amino acid side chains of the peptide that bind into pockets lining the peptide-binding groove of the MHC class I molecule. Each MHC class I molecule binds different patterns of anchor residues called a motif, giving some specificity to peptide binding. Anchor residues are less obvious for peptides that bind to MHC class II molecules.

Anergy is a state of non-responsiveness to antigen. People are said to be **anergic** when they cannot mount delayed-type hypersensitivity reactions to challenge antigens, while T and B cells are said to be anergic when they cannot respond to their specific antigen under optimal conditions of stimulation.

Antagonist peptides are able to inhibit the response of a cloned T-cell line to agonist peptides that are usually closely related in amino acid sequence.

Antibody molecules are plasma proteins that bind specifically to particular molecules known as antigens. Antibody molecules are produced in response to immunization with antigen. They are the specific molecules of the humoral immune response that bind to and neutralize pathogens or prepare them for uptake and destruction by phagocytes. Each antibody molecule has a unique structure that allows it to bind its specific antigen, but all antibodies have the same overall structure and are known collectively as **immunoglobulins**.

Antibody-dependent cell-mediated cytotoxicity (ADCC) is the killing of antibody-coated target cells by cells with Fc receptors that recognize the Fc region of the bound antibody. Most ADCC is mediated by natural killer (NK) cells that have the Fc receptor FcγRIII or CD16 on their surface.

The **antibody repertoire** describes the total variety of antibodies that an individual can make.

Antigens are molecules that react with antibodies. Their name arises from their ability to **gen**erate **anti**bodies. However, some antigens do not, by themselves, elicit antibody production; only those antigens that can induce antibody production are called **immunogens**.

Antigen:antibody complexes are non-covalently associated groups of antigen and antibody molecules which may vary in size from small, soluble complexes to large, insoluble complexes that precipitate out of solution; they are also known as **immune complexes**.

The **antigen-binding site** or **antigen-combining site** of an antibody is the surface of the antibody molecule that makes physical contact with the antigen. Antigen-binding sites are made up of six hypervariable loops, three from the light-chain variable region and three from the heavy-chain variable region.

Both T and B lymphocytes bear on their surface highly diverse **antigen receptors** capable of recognizing a wide diversity of antigens. Each lymphocyte bears receptors of a single antigen specificity.

An **antigenic determinant** is the portion of an antigenic molecule bound by a given antibody; it is also known as an **epitope**.

Influenza virus varies from year to year by a process of **antigenic drift** in which point mutations of viral genes cause small differences in the structure of viral surface antigens. Periodically, influenza viruses undergo an **antigenic shift** through reassortment of their segmented genome with another influenza virus, changing their surface antigens radically. Such antigenic shift variants are not recognized by individuals immune to influenza, so when antigenic shift variants arise, there is widespread and serious disease.

Many pathogens evade the adaptive immune response by **antigenic variation** in which new antigens are displayed that are not recognized by antibodies or T cells elicited in earlier infections.

Antigen presentation describes the display of antigen as peptide fragments bound to MHC molecules on the surface of a cell; all T cells recognize antigen only when it is presented in this way.

Antigen-presenting cells are highly specialized cells that can process antigens and display their peptide fragments on the cell surface together with molecules required for lymphocyte activation. The main antigen-presenting cells for T cells are dendritic cells, macrophages, and B cells, while the main antigen-presenting cells for B cells are follicular dendritic cells.

Antigen processing is the degradation of proteins into peptides that can bind to MHC molecules for presentation to T cells. All antigens except peptides must be processed into peptides before they can be presented by MHC molecules.

Anti-immunoglobulin antibodies are antibodies to immunoglobulin constant domains, useful for detecting bound antibody molecules in immunoassays and other applications.

An **antiserum** (plural: **antisera**) is the fluid component of clotted blood from an immune individual that contains antibodies against the molecule used for immunization. Antisera contain heterogeneous collections of antibodies, which bind the antigen used for immunization, but each has its own structure, its own epitope on the antigen, and its own set of cross-reactions. This heterogeneity makes each antiserum unique.

Aplastic anemia is a failure of bone marrow stem cells so that formation of all cellular elements of the blood ceases; it can be treated by bone marrow transplantation.

Apoptosis, or **programmed cell death**, is a form of cell death in which the cell activates an internal death program. It is characterized by nuclear DNA degradation, nuclear degeneration and condensation, and the phagocytosis of cell residua. Proliferating cells frequently undergo apoptosis, which is a natural process in development, and proliferating lymphocytes undergo high rates of apoptosis in development and during immune responses. It contrasts with necrosis, death from without, which occurs in situations such as poisoning and anoxia.

The **appendix** is a **gut-associated lymphoid tissue** located at the beginning of the colon.

In this book, we have termed activated effector T cells **armed effector T cells**, because these cells are triggered to perform their effector functions immediately upon contact with cells bearing the peptide:MHC complex for which they are specific. They contrast with memory T cells which need to be activated by antigen-presenting cells before they can mediate effector responses.

The **Arthus reaction** is a skin reaction in which antigen is injected into the dermis and reacts with IgG antibodies in the extracellular spaces, activating complement and phagocytic cells to produce a local inflammatory response.

Atopic allergy, or **atopy**, is a condition of increased susceptibility to immediate hypersensitivity usually mediated by IgE antibodies.

Pathogens are said to be **attenuated** when they will grow in their host and induce immunity without producing serious clinical disease.

Antibodies specific for self antigens are called **autoantibodies**.

A graft of tissue from one site to another on the same individual is called an **autograft**.

Diseases in which the pathology is caused by immune responses to self antigens are called **autoimmune diseases**.

Autoimmune hemolytic anemia is a pathological condition with low levels of red blood cells (anemia), due to autoantibodies that bind red blood cell surface antigens and target the red blood cell for destruction.

An adaptive immune response directed at self antigens is called an **autoimmune response**, and likewise, adaptive immunity specific for self antigens is called **autoimmunity**.

Autoreactivity describes immune responses directed at self antigens.

Avidity is the sum total of the strength of binding of two molecules or cells to one another at multiple sites. It is distinct from affinity, which is the strength of binding of one site on a molecule to its ligand.

The **avidity hypothesis** (formerly called affinity hypothesis) of T-cell selection in the thymus states that T cells must have a measurable affinity for self MHC molecules in order to mature, but not so great an affinity as to cause activation of the cell when it matures, as this would require that the cell be deleted to maintain self tolerance.

Azathioprine is a potent immunosuppressive drug that is converted to its active form *in vivo* and then kills rapidly proliferating cells, including lymphocytes responding to grafted tissues.

A **β sheet** is one of the fundamental structural building blocks of proteins, consisting of adjacent, extended strands of amino acids which are bonded together by interactions between backbone amide and carbonyl groups. Along a single strand, amino acid side chains alternate between the two sides of the sheet. β sheets may be parallel, in which case the adjacent strands run in the same direction, or antiparallel, where adjacent strands run in opposite directions. All immunoglobulin domains are made up of antiparallel β sheet structures. A **β strand** is one strand of amino acids in a β sheet.

The major T cell co-stimulatory molecules are closely related members of the immunoglobulin gene superfamily, called **B7.1** and **B7.2**. They are expressed differently in various antigen presenting cell types, and they may have different consequences for the responding T cells.

Many infectious diseases are caused by **bacteria**, which are prokaryotic microorganisms that exist as many different species and strains. Bacteria can live on body surfaces, in extracellular spaces, in cellular vesicles, or in the cytosol, and different bacterial species cause distinctive infectious diseases.

The **bare lymphocyte syndrome** is an immunodeficiency in which MHC class II molecules are not expressed on cells as a result of one of several different regulatory gene defects. Patients with bare lymphocyte syndrome are severely immunodeficient and have few CD4 T cells.

Basophils are white blood cells containing granules that stain with basic dyes, and which are thought to have a function similar to **mast cells**.

B cells, or **B lymphocytes**, are one of the two major classes of lymphocyte. The antigen receptor on B lymphocytes, sometimes called the **B-cell receptor**, is a cell-surface immunoglobulin molecule. Upon activation by antigen, B cells differentiate into cells producing antibody of the same specificity as their initial receptor.

A complex of CD19, TAPA-1 and CR2 makes up the **B-cell co-receptor**; co-ligation of this complex with the B cell antigen receptor increases responsiveness to antigen by about 100-fold.

B1 cells, B1a cells and **B2 cells**: see CD5 B cells.

The **B-cell corona** in the **spleen** is the zone of the **white pulp** primarily made up of B cells.

B-cell mitogens are substances that cause B cells to proliferate.

Blood group antigens are surface molecules on red blood cells that are detectable with antibodies from other individuals. The major blood group antigens are called ABO and Rh (Rhesus), and are used in routine blood banking to type blood. There are many other blood group antigens that can be detected in cross-matching.

In transfusion medicine, **blood typing** is used to determine if donor and recipient have the same ABO and Rh blood group antigens. A cross-match, in which serum from the donor is tested on the cells of the recipient, and vice versa, is used to rule out other incompatibilities. Transfusion of incompatible blood causes a transfusion reaction, in which red blood cells are destroyed and the released hemoglobin causes toxicity.

B lymphocytes: see B cells.

The **bone marrow** is the site of hematopoiesis, the generation of the cellular elements of blood, including red blood cells, monocytes, polymorphonuclear leukocytes, and platelets. The bone marrow is also the site of B-cell development in mammals and the source of stem cells that give rise to T cells upon migration to the thymus. Thus, bone marrow transplantation can restore all the cellular elements of the blood including the cells required for adaptive immunity.

A **bone marrow chimera** is formed by transferring bone marrow from one mouse to an irradiated recipient mouse, so that all of the lymphocytes and blood cells are of donor genetic origin. Bone marrow chimeras have been crucial in elucidating the development of lymphocytes and other blood cells.

The lymphoid cells and organized lymphoid tissues in the respiratory tract have been termed the **bronchial-associated lymphoid tissues** or **BALT**. These tissues are very important in the induction of immune responses to inhaled antigens and respiratory infection.

The **bursa of Fabricius** is an outpouching of the cloaca found in birds. It is an aggregate of epithelial tissue and lymphoid cells and the site of intense early B-cell proliferation. The bursa of Fabricius is required for B-cell development in birds as its removal (bursectomy) early in life causes absence of B cells in adult birds. An equivalent structure has not been detected in humans, where B-cell development follows a different pathway.

C1 inhibitor (C1INH) is a protein that inhibits the activity of activated complement component C1 by binding to and inactivating its C1r:C1s enzymatic activity. Deficiency in C1INH is the cause of the disease **hereditary angioneurotic edema**, in which spontaneous complement activation causes episodes of epiglottal swelling and suffocation.

The generation of the enzyme **C3/C5 convertase** on the surface of a pathogen or cell is a crucial step in complement activation. The C3/C5 convertase then catalyzes the deposition of large numbers of C3 molecules on the pathogen surface, leading to opsonization and the activation of the effector cascade that causes membrane lesions.

The cytosolic serine/threonine phosphatase **calcineurin** plays a crucial but undefined role in signaling via the T-cell receptor. The immunosuppressive drugs cyclosporin A and FK506 form complexes with cellular proteins called immunophilins that bind and inactivate calcineurin, suppressing T-cell responses.

The protein **calnexin** is an 88 kDa protein found in the endoplasmic reticulum. It binds to partially folded members of the immunoglobulin superfamily of proteins and retains them in the endoplasmic reticulum until folding is completed.

Carriers are foreign proteins to which small, non-immunogenic antigens, or haptens, can be coupled to render the hapten immunogenic. *In vivo*, self proteins can also serve as carriers if they are correctly modified by the hapten; this is important in drug allergy.

Caseation necrosis is a form of necrosis seen in the center of large granulomas, such as the granulomas in tuberculosis. The term comes from the white cheesy appearance of the central necrotic area.

CD: see **clusters of differentiation** and Appendix I.

The **CD3 complex** describes a complex of $\alpha\beta$ or $\gamma\delta$ T cell receptor chains with the invariant subunits, cd3γ,δ, and ε, and the dimeric ζ chains.

CD5 B cells are a class of atypical, self-renewing B cells found mainly in the peritoneal and pleural cavities in adults and which have a far less diverse receptor repertoire than conventional B cells.

B-cell growth is triggered in part by the binding of **CD40 ligand** expressed on activated helper T cells to **CD40** on the B-cell surface.

CD45 or the leukocyte common antigen is a transmembrane tyrosine phosphatase that is expressed in various isoforms on different T cells. These **isoforms** are commonly denoted by the designation of CD45R followed by the exon whose presence gives rise to distinctive antibody binding patterns.

CDRs: see **complementarity determining regions**.

The three complementarity-determining regions, **CDR1**, **CDR2**, and **CDR3** are loops at the end of a V domain in antibodies or T cell receptors that make direct contact with antigen or peptide: MHC respectively.

Cell adhesion molecules (CAMs) are cell-surface proteins that are involved in binding cells together in tissues, and also in less permanent cell–cell interactions.

Cell-mediated immunity, or **cell-mediated immune responses**, describes any adaptive immune response in which antigen specific T cells play the main role. It encompasses all adaptive immunity that cannot be transferred to a naive recipient with serum antibody, the definition of humoral immunity.

Cell-surface immunoglobulin is the B-cell receptor for antigen: see **B cell**.

Cellular immunology is the study of the cellular basis of immunity.

Central lymphoid organs are sites of lymphocyte development. In humans, B lymphocytes develop in bone marrow whereas T lymphocytes develop within the thymus from bone marrow derived progenitors.

Central tolerance is tolerance that is established in lymphocytes developing in central lymphoid organs (cf. **peripheral tolerance**).

Centroblasts are large, rapidly dividing cells found in germinal centers, and are the cells in which somatic hypermutation is believed to occur. Antibody-secreting and memory B cells derive from these cells.

Centrocytes are the small, non-proliferating B cells in germinal centers that derive from centroblasts. They may mature into antibody-secreting plasma cells or memory B cells, or may undergo apoptosis, depending on their receptor's interaction with antigen.

Chediak-Higashi syndrome is a defect in phagocytic cell function, due to unknown causes, in which lysosomes fail to fuse properly with phagosomes and which there is impaired killing of ingested bacteria.

Chemokines are small cytokines that are involved in the migration and activation of cells, especially phagocytic cells and lymphocytes. They play a central part in inflammatory responses.

Chronic granulomatous disease is an immunodeficiency disease in which multiple granulomas form as a result of defective elimination of bacteria by phagocytic cells. It is caused by a defect in the NADPH oxidase system of enzymes that generate the superoxide radical involved in bacterial killing.

Class switching: see **isotype switching**.

Classes: see **isotypes**.

The **classical pathway** of complement activation is the pathway activated by antibody bound to antigen, and involves complement components C1, C4, and C2 in the generation of the C3/C5 convertase (see also **alternative pathway**).

According to clonal selection theory, tolerance to self is due to **clonal deletion**, the elimination of immature lymphocytes upon binding to self antigens. Clonal deletion is the main mechanism of central tolerance and can also occur in peripheral tolerance.

Clonal expansion is the proliferation of antigen-specific lymphocytes in response to antigenic stimulation and precedes their differentiation into effector cells. It is an essential step in adaptive immunity, allowing rare antigen-specific cells to increase in number so that they can effectively combat the pathogen that elicited the response.

The **clonal selection theory** is a central paradigm of adaptive immunity. It states that adaptive immune responses derive from individual antigen-specific lymphocytes that are self-tolerant. These specific lymphocytes proliferate in response to antigen and differentiate into antigen-specific effector cells to eliminate the eliciting pathogen, and memory cells to sustain immunity. The theory was formulated by Sir Macfarlane Burnet and in earlier forms by Niels Jerne and David Talmage.

A **clone** is a population of cells all derived from a common progenitor.

A **cloned T cell line** is a continuously growing line of T cells derived from a single progenitor. Cloned T cell lines must be stimulated with antigen periodically to maintain growth. They are useful for studying T-cell specificity, growth, and effector functions.

A feature unique to individual cells or members of a clone is said to be **clonotypic**. Thus, a monoclonal antibody that reacts with the receptor on a cloned T cell line is said to be a clonotypic antibody and to recognize its clonotype or the clonotypic receptor of that cell. See **idiotype** and **idiotypic**.

Clusters of differentiation (CD) are groups of monoclonal antibodies that identify the same cell-surface molecule. The cell surface molecule is designated CD (cluster of differentiation) followed by a number (eg. CD1, CD2, etc.). For a current listing of CD see Appendix I.

The expression of a gene is said to be **co-dominant** when both alleles at one locus are expressed in roughly equal amounts in heterozygotes. Most genes show this property, including the highly polymorphic MHC genes.

A **coding joint** is formed by the imprecise joining of a V gene segment to a (D)J gene segment in immunoglobulin or T cell receptor genes.

co-isogenic: see **congenic**.

Collectins are a structurally related family of calcium-dependent sugar-binding proteins or lectins containing collagen-like sequences, to which **mannose-binding protein** belongs.

Immunological receptors manifest two distinct types of **combinatorial diversity** generated by combination of separate units of genetic information. Receptor gene segments are joined in many different combinations to generate diverse receptor chains, and then two different receptor chains (heavy and light in immunoglobulins, α and β or γ and δ in T-cell receptors) are combined to make the antigen recognition site.

Common lymphoid progenitors are stem cells which give rise to all lymphocytes. They are derived from pluripotent **hemato-poietic stem cells**.

Common variable immunodeficiency is a relatively common deficiency in antibody production whose pathogenesis is not yet understood. There is a strong association with genes mapping within the MHC.

Competitive binding assays are serological assays in which unknowns are detected and quantitated by their ability to inhibit the binding of a labeled known ligand to its specific antibody.

The **complement** system is a set of plasma proteins that act together to attack extracellular forms of pathogens. Complement can be activated spontaneously on certain pathogens or by antibody binding to the pathogen. The pathogen becomes coated with complement proteins that facilitate pathogen removal by phagocytes and may also kill the pathogen.

Complement receptors (CR) are cell-surface proteins on various cells which recognize and bind complement proteins that have bound a pathogen. Complement receptors on phagocytes allow them to identify pathogens coated with complement proteins for uptake and destruction.

The **complementarity determining regions (CDRs)** of immunological receptors are the parts of the receptor that make contact with specific ligand and determine its specificity. The CDRs are the most variable part of the receptor protein, giving receptors their diversity, and are carried on six loops at the distal end of the receptor's variable domains, three loops coming from each of the two variable domains of the receptor.

Some epitopes on a protein antigen are called **conformational** or **discontinuous epitopes** because they are formed from several separate regions in the primary sequence of a protein by protein folding. Antibodies that bind conformational epitopes only bind native, folded proteins.

Congenic strains of mice are genetically identical at all loci except one. Each strain is generated by the repetitive backcrossing of mice carrying the desired trait onto a strain that provides the genetic background for the set of congenic strains. The most important congenic strains in immunology are the **congenic resistant strains**, developed by George Snell, that differ from each other at the MHC.

Constant regions: see **C regions**.

Contact hypersensitivity is a form of delayed-type hypersensitivity in which T cells respond to antigens that are introduced by contact with the skin. Poison ivy is a contact sensitivity reaction due to T-cell responses to the chemical antigen pentadeca-catechol in poison ivy leaves.

Continuous or **linear epitopes** are antigenic determinants on proteins that are contiguous in the protein sequence and therefore do not require protein folding for antibody to bind. See also **conformational** or **discontinuous epitopes**.

A **convertase** is an enzymatic activity that converts a complement protein into its reactive form by cleaving it. Generation of the C3/C5 convertase is the pivotal event in complement activation.

The **Coombs test** is a test for antibody binding to red blood cells. Red blood cells that are coated with antibody are agglutinated if they are exposed to an anti-immunoglobulin antibody. The Coombs test is important in detecting the non-agglutinating antibodies to red blood cells produced in Rh incompatibility.

A **co-receptor** is a cell-surface protein that increases the sensitivity of the antigen receptor to antigen by binding to associated ligands and participating in signaling for activation. CD4 and CD8 are MHC-binding co-receptors on T cells, while CD19 is part of a complex that makes up a co-receptor on B cells.

Corticosteroids are steroids related to those produced in the adrenal cortex, such as cortisone. Corticosteroids can kill lymphocytes, especially developing thymocytes, inducing apoptotic cell death. They are useful anti-inflammatory and immunosuppressive agents.

The proliferation of lymphocytes requires both antigen binding and the receipt of a **co-stimulatory signal**, usually delivered by a cell-surface molecule on the cell presenting antigen. For T cells, the co-stimulatory signals are B7 and B7.2, related molecules that act on the T-cell surface molecules CD28 and CTLA-4. For B cells, CD40 ligand acting on CD40 serves an analogous role.

Cowpox is the common name of the disease produced by vaccinia virus, used by Edward Jenner in the successful vaccination against smallpox, which is caused by the related variola virus.

C-reactive protein is an acute phase protein that binds to phosphatidylcholine which is a constituent of the C-polysaccharide of the bacterium *Streptococcus pneumoniae*, hence its name. Many other bacteria also have surface phosphatidylcholine that is accessible to C-reactive protein, so C-reactive protein can bind many different bacteria and opsonize them for ready uptake by phagocytes.

C regions or **constant regions** of antibody molecules and T-cell receptors are made up of one or more **C domains**, each encoded in a single exon. As only a single gene encodes each C region, it has the same structure in all antibodies or T-cell receptors in which it is expressed.

Cross-matching is used in blood typing and histocompatibility testing to determine whether donor and recipient have antibodies against each other's cells that might interfere with successful transfusion or grafting.

A **cross-reaction** is the binding of antibody to an antigen not used to elicit that antibody. Thus, if antibody raised against antigen A also binds antigen B, it is said to cross-react with antigen B. The term is used generically to describe the reactivity of antibodies or T cells with more than the eliciting antigen.

CTLA-4: High-affinity receptor for B7 molecules on T cells.

Cutaneous T-cell lymphoma is a malignant growth of T cells that home to the skin.

Cyclophosphamide is an alkylating agent that is used as an immunosuppressive drug. It acts by killing rapidly dividing cells including lymphocytes proliferating in response to antigen.

Cyclosporin A is a potent immunosuppressive drug that inhibits signaling from the T-cell receptor, preventing T-cell activation and effector function. It binds to cyclophilin, and this complex binds to and inactivates the serine/threonine phosphatase **calcineurin**.

Cytokines are proteins made by cells that affect the behavior of other cells. Cytokines made by lymphocytes are often called **lymphokines** or **interleukins** (abbreviated IL), but the generic term cytokine is used in this book and most of the literature. Cytokines act on specific cytokine receptors on the cells they affect. Cytokines and their receptors are listed in Appendix II.

Cytokine receptors are cellular receptors for cytokines. Binding of the cytokine to the cytokine receptor induces new activities in the cell, such as growth, differentiation, or death. Cytokine receptors are listed in Appendix II.

Cytotoxic T cells are T cells that can kill other cells. Most cytotoxic T cells are MHC class I-restricted CD8 T cells, but CD4 T cells can also kill in some cases. Cytotoxic T cells are important in host defense against cytosolic pathogens.

Cytotoxins are proteins made by cytotoxic T cells that participate in the destruction of target cells. **Perforins** and **granzymes** or **fragmentins** are the major defined cytotoxins.

Defective endogenous retroviruses are partial retroviral genomes integrated into host cell DNA and carried as host genes. There are a great many defective endogenous retroviruses in the mouse genome.

Delayed-type hypersensitivity is a form of cell-mediated immunity elicited by antigen in the skin. It is mediated by inflammatory CD4 T cells. It is called delayed-type hypersensitivity because the reaction appears hours to days after antigen is injected, as distinct from immediate hypersensitivity in which skin reactions are seen minutes after antigen injection.

Dendritic cells, also known as **interdigitating reticular cells**, are found in T-cell areas of lymphoid tissues. They have a branched or dendritic morphology and are the most potent stimulators of T-cell responses. Non-lymphoid tissues also contain dendritic cells, but these do not appear to stimulate T-cell responses until they are activated and migrate to lymphoid tissues. The dendritic cell derives from bone marrow precursors. It is distinct from the follicular dendritic cell that presents antigen to B cells.

Dendritic epidermal cells (dEC) are a specialized class of γ:δ T cells found in the skin of mice and some other species, but not humans. All dEC have the same γ:δ T-cell receptor; their function is unknown.

Desensitization is a procedure in which an allergic individual is exposed to increasing doses of allergen in hopes of inhibiting their allergic reactions. It probably involves shifting CD4 T-cell types and thus changing antibody from IgE to IgG.

D gene segments, or **diversity gene segments** are short DNA sequences that join the V and J gene segments in immunoglobulin heavy-chain genes and T-cell receptor β and δ chain genes during the somatic generation of a variable-region exon. See **gene segments**.

Diacylglycerol (DAG) is a product of lipid breakdown, most commonly released from inositol phospholipids by the action of phospholipase C-γ, which produces inositol trisphosphate as well as diacylglycerol. Diacylglycerol production is stimulated by ligation of many receptors. It activates cytosolic protein kinase C which further propagates the signal.

Diapedesis is the movement of blood cells, particularly leukocytes, from the blood across blood vessel walls into tissues.

The **differential signaling hypothesis** is one way to explain the distinction between the processes of positive and negative selection in the thymus during T cell maturation.

Differentiation antigens are proteins detected on some cells by means of specific antibodies. Many differentiation antigens play important functional roles characteristic of the differentiated phenotypes of the cell on which they are expressed, such as cell-surface immunoglobulin on B cells.

DiGeorge syndrome is a recessive genetic immunodeficiency disease in which there is a failure to develop thymic epithelium associated with absent parathyroid glands and large vessel anomalies. It appears to be due to a developmental defect in neural crest cells.

The **direct Coombs test** uses anti-immunoglobulin to agglutinate red blood cells as a way of detecting whether they are coated with antibody *in vivo* due to autoimmunity or maternal anti-fetal immune responses (see **Coombs test, indirect Coombs test**).

Discontinuous epitopes: see **conformational epitopes**.

Diversity gene segments: see **D gene segments**.

A truncated heavy chain known as a **Dμ protein** can be produced during B-cell development as a result of heavy-chain transcription from a previously inactive promoter 5' to the D gene segments.

In tissue grafting experiments, the grafted tissues come from a **donor** and are placed in a **recipient** or **host**.

Double-negative thymocytes are immature T cells within the thymus that lack expression of the two co-receptors, CD4 and CD8, whose selective expression parallels T-cell development. The four main intrathymic T-cell populations are double-negative, double-positive, and CD4 and CD8 single-positive thymocytes.

Double-positive thymocytes are an intermediate stage in T-cell development within the thymus characterized by expression of both the CD4 and the CD8 co-receptor proteins.

The genetic defect in scid mice, which cannot rearrange their T or B cell receptor genes, is in the enzyme **DNA dependent kinase**. This enzyme is part of a complex of proteins that bind to the hairpin ends of double stranded breaks in DNA, that includes the DNA-binding Ku proteins.

The **early induced responses** or **early non-adaptive responses** are a series of host defense responses that are triggered by infectious agents early in infection. They are distinct from innate immunity because there is an inductive phase, and from adaptive immunity in that they do not operate by clonal selection of rare, antigen-specific lymphocytes.

Early pro-B cell: see **pro-B cell**.

Effector cells are lymphocytes that can mediate the removal of pathogens from the body without the need for further differentiation, as distinct from naive lymphocytes, which must proliferate and differentiate before they can mediate effector functions, and memory cells which must differentiate and often proliferate before they become effector cells. They are also called **armed effector cells** in this book, to indicate that they can be triggered to effector function by antigen binding alone.

The innate and adaptive immune responses use most of the same **effector mechanisms** to eliminate pathogens.

Lymphocytes leave a lymph node through the **efferent lymphatic vessel**.

Electrophoresis is the movement of molecules in a charged field. In immunology, many forms of electrophoresis are used to separate molecules, especially protein molecules, to determine their charge, size, and subunit composition.

ELISA: see **enzyme-linked immunosorbent assay**.

ELISPOT assay is an adaptation of ELISA in which cells are placed over antibodies or antigens attached to a plastic surface which trap the cells' secreted products. The trapped products are then detected with an enzyme-coupled antibody that cleaves a colorless substrate to make a localized colored spot.

Embryonic stem (ES) cells are continuously growing cells that retain the ability to contribute to all lineages of cells in developing mouse embryos. ES cells can be genetically manipulated in tissue culture and then inserted into mouse blastocysts to generate mutant lines of mice; most often, genes are deleted in ES cells by homologous recombination and the mutant ES cells then used to generate **gene knock-out** mice.

Some bacteria have thick carbohydrate coats that protect them from phagocytosis; these **encapsulated bacteria** can cause extracellular infections and are effectively engulfed and destroyed by phagocytes only if they are first coated with antibody and complement produced in an adaptive immune response.

Some anti-carbohydrate antibodies are called **end-binders** because they bind the ends of oligosaccharide antigens, while others bind the sides of these molecules.

Cytokines that can induce a rise in body temperature are called **endogenous pyrogens**, as distinct from exogenous substances like endotoxin from Gram-negative bacteria that induce fever by triggering endogenous pyrogen synthesis and release.

Endotoxins are bacterial toxins that are only released when the bacterial cell is damaged, as opposed to exotoxins which are secreted bacterial toxins. The most important endotoxin is lipopolysaccharide, a potent inducer of cytokine synthesis found in Gram-negative bacteria.

The **enzyme-linked immunosorbent assay (ELISA)** is a serological assay in which bound antigen or antibody is detected by a linked enzyme that converts a colorless substrate into a colored product. The ELISA assay is widely used in biology and medicine as well as immunology.

Eosinophils are white blood cells thought to be important chiefly in defense against parasitic infections; they are activated by the lymphocytes of the adaptive immune response.

An **epitope** is a site on an antigen recognized by an antibody; epitopes are also called **antigenic determinants**. A T-cell epitope is a short peptide derived from a protein antigen. It binds to an MHC molecule and is recognized by a particular T cell.

Epitope spreading is shorthand used to describe the phenomenon that responses to autoantigens tend to become more diverse as the response persists.

The **Epstein-Barr virus (EBV)** is a herpes virus that selectively infects human B cells by binding to complement receptor 2 (CR2, also known as CD21). It causes infectious mononucleosis and establishes a life-long latent infection in B cells that is controlled by T cells. Some B cells latently infected with EBV will proliferate *in vitro* to form lymphoblastoid cell lines.

The affinity of an antibody can be determined by **equilibrium dialysis**, a technique in which antibody in a dialysis bag is exposed to varying amounts of a small antigen able to diffuse across the dialysis membrane. The amount of antigen inside and outside the bag at the equilibrium diffusion state is determined by the amount and affinity of the antibody in the bag.

E-rosettes are human T cells which will bind to treated sheep red blood cells; the many red blood cells bound to each T cell give it the appearance of a rosette and increase its buoyant density so that the T cells can be isolated by gradient centrifugation. E-rosetting is often used for isolating human T cells.

Erythroblastosis fetalis is a severe form of Rh hemolytic disease in which maternal anti-Rh antibody enters the fetus and produces a hemolytic anemia so severe that the fetus has mainly immature erythroblasts in the peripheral blood.

E-selectin: see **selectins**.

Experimental allergic encephalomyelitis (EAE) is an inflammatory disease of the central nervous system which develops after mice are immunized with neural antigens in a strong adjuvant.

The movement of cells or fluid from within blood vessels to the surrounding tissues is called **extravasation**.

IgG antibody molecules can be cleaved into three fragments by the enzyme papain. Two of these are called the **Fab fragments** because they are the **F**ragment with specific **a**ntigen **b**inding. The Fab fragment consists of the light chain and the amino-terminal half of the heavy chain held together by an interchain disulfide bond. See also **Fc fragment**.

FACS[R]: see **fluorescence-activated cell sorter**.

Factor P: see **properdin**

Farmer's lung is a hypersensitivity disease caused by the reaction of IgG antibodies with large amounts of an inhaled allergen in the alveolar wall of the lung, causing alveolar wall inflammation and compromising gas exchange.

Fas is another member of the TNF receptor gene family; it is expressed on certain target cells that are susceptible to killing by cells expressing the **Fas ligand**, a member of the TNF family of cytokines and cell surface molecules.

When IgG antibodies are cleaved with the enzyme papain, three fragments are generated. Two are the identical **Fab** fragments and one fragment is called the **Fc fragment** for **F**ragment **c**rystallizable. The Fc fragment comprises the carboxy-terminal halves of the two heavy chains disulfide-bonded to each other by the residual hinge region.

Fc receptors are receptors for the Fc piece of various immunoglobulin isotypes. They include the **Fcγ** and **Fcε receptors**.

The high affinity **Fcε receptor (FcεRI)** found on mast cells and basophils binds free IgE. When antigen binds this IgE, it can crosslink the FcεRI and cause mast cell activation.

Fcγ receptors, including **FcγRI, RII,** and **RIII** are cell-surface receptors that bind the Fc domain of IgG molecules. Most Fcγ receptors only bind aggregated IgG, allowing them to discriminate bound antibody from free IgG. They are expressed on phagocytes, B lymphocytes, natural killer cells, and follicular dendritic cells. They play a key role in humoral immunity, linking antibody binding to effector cell functions.

When tissue or organ grafts are placed in naive recipients, they are eventually rejected by an immune response. This is called a **first set rejection**, to distinguish it from subsequent responses to grafts from the same or related donors, which are much more intense and are called **second set rejections**.

FK506 is an immunosuppressive polypeptide drug that inactivates T cells by inhibiting signal transduction from the T-cell receptor. FK506 and cyclosporin A are the most commonly used immunosuppressive drugs in organ transplantation.

Individual cells can be characterized and separated in a machine called a **fluorescence-activated cell sorter (FACS^R)** that measures cell size, granularity, and fluorescence due to bound fluorescent antibodies as single cells pass in a stream past photodetectors. The analysis of single cells in this way is called **flow cytometry** and the instruments that carry out the measurements are called **flow cytometers**.

Lymphoid **follicles** consist of clusters of B cells organized around a dense network of **follicular dendritic cells**, cells of uncertain origin with long, branching processes that make intimate contact with many different B cells. Follicular dendritic cells have non-phagocytic Fc receptors that allow them to hold antigen:antibody complexes on their surface for long periods of time; these play a crucial role in selecting antigen-binding B cells during antibody responses.

Fragmentins or **granzymes** are serine esterases found in the granules of cytotoxic lymphocytes including T cells and natural killer cells. When fragmentins enter the cytosol of other cells they induce apoptosis, inducing nuclear DNA fragmentation into 200 base pair multimers, hence their name.

The variable regions of immunological receptors can be divided into two types of sequence: **framework regions** and **hypervariable regions**. The framework regions are relatively invariant sequences in variable regions that provide a protein scaffold for the hypervariable regions that make contact with antigen.

Fungi are single-cell eukaryotic organisms, yeasts, and molds, that can cause a variety of diseases. Immunity to fungi is complex and involves both humoral and cell-mediated responses.

Most T lymphocytes have α:β heterodimeric T-cell receptors, but the receptor on γ:δ T cells has distinct antigen recognition chains assembled in a **γ:δ heterodimer**. The specificity and function of these cells is uncertain.

Plasma proteins can be separated into albumin and the α, β, and γ globulins on the basis of their electrophoretic mobility. Most antibodies migrate as **γ globulins** (or **gamma globulins**), and patients who lack antibodies are said to have agammaglobulinemia based on the absence of gamma globulins on serum protein electrophoresis.

In birds and rabbits, immunoglobulin receptor diversity is generated mainly by **gene conversion**, in which homologous inactive V gene segments exchange short sequences with an active, rearranged variable-region gene.

Gene knock-out is slang for gene disruption by homologous recombination.

The variable domains of immunological receptors are encoded in **gene segments** that must first undergo somatic recombination to form a complete exon encoding the **variable region**. There are three types of gene segment, **V gene segments** that encode the first 95 amino acids, **D gene segments** that encode about 5 amino acids, and **J gene segments** that form the last 10–15 amino acids of the variable region. There are multiple copies of each type of gene segment in the germline DNA, but only one is expressed in a receptor-bearing lymphocyte.

Gene therapy is the correction of a genetic defect by the introduction of a normal gene into bone marrow or other cell types.

Genetic immunization is a novel technique for inducing adaptive immune responses. Plasmid DNA encoding a protein of interest is injected into muscle, and for unknown reasons is expressed and elicits antibody and T-cell responses to the protein encoded by the DNA.

Germinal centers are sites in secondary lymphoid tissues of intense B-cell proliferation, selection, maturation, and death during antibody responses. Germinal centers form around follicular dendritic cell networks when activated B cells migrate into lymphoid follicles.

Immunological receptor genes are said to be in the **germline configuration** in the DNA of germ cells and in all somatic cells in which somatic recombination has not yet occurred.

Immunological receptors have specificity for antigen because of their diversity of structure. Some of this diversity is due to the inheritance of multiple gene segments that encode variable regions; such diversity is called **germline diversity** and can be distinguished from diversity arising during gene rearrangement or after receptor gene expression, which is somatically generated.

One theory of antibody diversity, the **germline theory**, proposed that each antibody was encoded in a separate germline gene.

GlyCAM-1 is a mucin-like molecule found on the high endothelial venules of lymphoid tissues. It is an important ligand for the **L-selectin** molecule expressed on naive lymphocytes, directing these cells to leave the blood and enter the lymphoid tissues.

Goodpasture's syndrome is an autoimmune disease in which autoantibodies to basement membrane or type IV collagen are produced and cause extensive vasculitis. It is rapidly fatal.

G proteins are proteins that bind GTP and convert it to GDP in the process of cell signal transduction. There are two kinds of G protein, the trimeric (α,β,γ) receptor-associated G proteins, and the small G proteins, like Ras, that act downstream of many transmembrane signaling events.

Tissue and organ grafts between genetically distinct individuals almost always elicit an immune response that causes **graft rejection**, the destruction of the grafted tissue by attacking lymphocytes.

When mature T lymphocytes are injected into a non-identical immuno-incompetent recipient, they can attack the recipient causing a **graft-versus-host (GVH) reaction**; in human patients, mature T cells in allogeneic bone marrow grafts can cause **graft-versus-host disease**.

Granulocyte: another name for **polymorphonuclear leukocyte**.

Granulocyte–macrophage colony-stimulating factor (GM-CSF): is a cytokine involved in the growth and differentiation of myeloid and monocytic lineage cells, including dendritic cells, monocytes and tissue macrophages, and cells of the granulocyte lineage.

granuloma is a site of chronic inflammation usually triggered by persistent infectious agents such as mycobacteria or by a non-degradable foreign body. Granulomas have a central area of macrophages, often fused into multinucleate giant cells, surrounded by T lymphocytes.

Granzymes: another name for **fragmentins**.

Graves' disease is an autoimmune disease in which antibodies to the thyroid-stimulating hormone receptor cause overproduction of thyroid hormone and thus hyperthyroidism.

The **gut-associated lymphoid tissues** or **GALT** are lymphoid tissues closely associated with the gastrointestinal tract, including the palatine tonsils, Peyer's patches, and intraepithelial lymphocytes. The GALT has a distinctive biology related to its exposure to antigens from food and normal intestinal microbial flora.

The major histocompatibility complex of the mouse is called histocompatibility-2 or more commonly **H-2**. Haplotypes are designated by a lower case superscript, as in H-2^b.

A **haplotype** is a linked set of genes associated with one haploid genome. The term is used mainly in connection with the linked genes of the major histocompatibility complex, which are usually inherited as one haplotype from each parent. Some MHC haplotypes are over-represented in the population, a phenomenon known as **linkage disequilibrium**.

Haptens are molecules that can bind antibody but cannot by themselves elicit an adaptive immune response. Haptens must be chemically linked to protein **carriers** to elicit antibody and T-cell responses.

All immunoglobulin molecules have two types of chain, a **heavy (H) chain** of 50–70 kDa and a light chain of 25 kDa. The basic unit of immunoglobulin consists of two identical heavy and two identical light chains. Heavy chains come in a variety of **heavy-chain classes** or **isotypes**, each of which specifies a distinctive functional activity in the antibody molecule.

Helper CD4 T cells are CD4 T cells that can help B cells make antibody in response to antigenic challenge. The most efficient helper T cells are also known as T$_H$2, cells that make the cytokines IL-4 and IL-5. Some experts refer to all CD4 T cells, regardless of function, as **helper T cells;** we do not accept this usage as function can only be determined in cellular assays, and some CD4 T cells kill the cells they interact with.

A **hemagglutinin** is any substance that causes red blood cells to agglutinate, a process known as **hemagglutination**. The hemagglutinins in human blood are antibodies that recognize the ABO blood group antigens. Influenza and some other viruses have hemagglutinin molecules that must bind to glycoproteins on host cells to initiate the infectious process.

A **hematopoiesis** is the generation of the cellular elements of blood, including the red blood cells, leukocytes and platelets. These cells all originate from pluripotent **hematopoietic stem cells** whose differentiated progeny divide under the influence of **hematopoietic growth factors.**

A **hematopoietic lineage** is any developmental series of cells that derives from **hematopoietic stem cells** and results in the production of mature blood cells.

Hemolytic disease of the newborn or **erythroblastosis fetalis** is caused by a maternal IgG antibody response to paternal antigens expressed on fetal red blood cells. The usual target of this response is the **Rh blood group antigen**. The maternal IgG antibodies cross the placenta to attack the fetal red blood cells.

The **hemolytic plaque assay** detects antibody-forming cells by the ability of their secreted antibodies to produce a **hemolytic plaque**, an area of localized destruction of a thin layer of red blood cells around each antibody-producing cell. The antibodies secreted by the B cell are trapped by antigens on the red blood cells immediately surrounding it, and then complement is added that is triggered by the bound antibody to lyse the red blood cells.

The gene segments that recombine to form variable domains of immunological receptors are flanked on one or both sides by recombination signal sequences consisting of a seven-nucleotide **heptamer** followed by a spacer of 23 base pairs followed by a nine-nucleotide nonamer. The sequences of heptamer and nonamer are highly conserved for all receptor gene segments. These recombination signal sequences direct somatic recombination of receptor gene segments and are removed during gene segment joining.

Hereditary angioneurotic edema is the clinical name for a genetic deficiency of the C1 inhibitor of the complement system. In the absence of C1 inhibitor, spontaneous activation of the complement system can cause diffuse fluid leakage from blood vessels, the most serious consequence of which is epiglottal swelling leading to suffocation.

Individuals **heterozygous** for a particular gene have two different alleles of that gene.

High endothelial venules (HEV) are specialized venules found in lymphoid tissues. Lymphocytes migrate from blood into lymphoid tissues by attaching to and migrating across the **high endothelial cells** of these vessels.

Tolerance to injected protein antigens occurs at low or high doses of antigen. Tolerance induced by injection of high doses of antigen is called **high-zone tolerance**, while tolerance produced with low doses of antigen is called **low-zone tolerance**.

The **hinge region** of antibody molecules is a flexible domain that joins the Fab arms to the Fc piece. The flexibility of the hinge region in IgG and IgA molecules allows the Fab arms to adopt a wide range of angles, permitting binding to epitopes spaced variable distances apart.

Histamine is a vasoactive amine stored in mast cell granules. Histamine released by antigen binding to IgE molecules on mast cells causes dilation of local blood vessels and smooth muscle contraction, producing some of the symptoms of immediate hypersensitivity reactions. **Anti-histamines** are drugs that counter histamine action.

Histocompatibility is literally the ability of tissues (Greek: *histo*) to get along. It is used in immunology to describe the genetic systems that determine the rejection of tissue and organ grafts that results from immunological recognition of **histocompatibility (H) antigens.**

HIV: see **human immunodeficiency virus.**

HLA, the acronym for **H**uman **L**eukocyte **A**ntigen, is the genetic designation for the human **major histocompatibility complex**. Individual loci are designated by upper case letters, as in HLA-A, and alleles are designated by numbers, as in HLA-A*0201.

The MHC of humans contains an MHC class II like set of genes that encode **HLA-DM** that is involved in the loading of peptides onto MHC class II molecules. An homologous gene in mice is called **H-2M**.

Hodgkin's disease is a malignant disease in which antigen presenting cells that resemble dendritic cells appear to be the transformed cell type. **Hodgkin's lymphoma** is a form of Hodgkin's disease in which lymphocytes predominate, and it has a much better prognosis than the **nodular sclerosis** form of this disease in which the predominant cell type is non-lymphoid.

Cellular genes can be disrupted by **homologous recombination** with copies of the gene into which erroneous sequences have been inserted. When these exogenous DNA fragments are introduced into cells, they recombine selectively with the cellular gene, replacing the functional gene with a non-functional copy.

The **human immunodeficiency virus (HIV)** is the causative agent of the acquired immune deficiency syndrome (AIDS). HIV is a retrovirus of the lentivirus family that selectively infects CD4 T cells, leading to their slow depletion and eventually resulting in immunodeficiency.

Humanization is a term used to describe the production of antibodies with mainly human sequences. The DNA encoding hypervariable loops of mouse monoclonal antibodies or V regions selected in phage display libraries is inserted into the framework regions of human immunoglobulin genes. This allows production of antibodies of a desired specificity that do not cause an immune response in humans treated with them.

Protective immunity can be divided into cell-mediated immunity and **humoral immunity**, specific immunity mediated by antibodies made in a **humoral immune response**. Humoral immunity can be transferred to naive recipients with immune serum containing specific antibody, whereas cell-mediated immunity can only be transferred by specifically immune cells.

Monoclonal antibodies are produced most commonly by hybrid cell lines or **hybridomas**. These are formed by fusing a specific antibody-producing B lymphocyte with a myeloma cell that is selected for its ability to grow in tissue culture and the absence of immunoglobulin chain synthesis.

Repetitive immunization to achieve a heightened state of immunity is called **hyperimmunization**.

Immune responses to innocuous antigens that lead to symptomatic reactions upon re-exposure are called **hypersensitivity reactions**. These can cause **hypersensitivity diseases** if they occur repetitively. This state of heightened reactivity to antigen is called **hypersensitivity**.

The variable regions of immunological receptor chains can be divided into two types of sequence: **hypervariable (HV) regions**, which occur at sites that make contact with antigen and differ extensively from one receptor to the next, and **framework regions** of much less variable sequence that provide the molecular scaffold for V region structure.

ICAM: see **intercellular adhesion molecule**.

Iccosomes are small fragments of membrane coated with immune complexes that fragment off the processes of follicular dendritic cells in lymphoid follicles early in a secondary or subsequent antibody response.

Each immunoglobulin molecule has the potential of binding to a variety of antibodies directed at its unique features or **idiotype**. An idiotype is made up of a series of **idiotopes**, which can stimulate regulatory responses through an **idiotypic network.**

Lymphocyte receptors can recognize one another through idiotope: anti-idiotope interactions, forming an **idiotypic network** of receptors that may be important for the generation and main-tenance of the repertoire of receptors. The various components of idiotype networks exist, but their functional significance is uncertain.

Ig: standard abbreviation for **immunoglobulin**. Different immunoglobulin isotypes are called **IgM, IgD, IgG, IgA, and IgE**.

Ig α: The **heavy chain of Immunoglobulin A.**

Ig δ: The **heavy chain of Immunoglobulin D.**

Ig ε: The **heavy chain of Immunoglobulin E.**

Ig γ: The **heavy chain of Immunoglobulin G.**

Ig μ: The **heavy chain of Immunoglobulin M.**

Immature B cells are B cells that have rearranged heavy and light chain V-region genes and express a surface IgM receptor, but have not yet matured sufficiently to express a surface IgD receptor as well.

Hypersensitivity reactions that occur within minutes of exposure to antigen are called **immediate hypersensitivity reactions**; such reactions are antibody mediated, whereas **delayed-type hypersensitivity reactions**, which occur hours to days after antigen exposure, are T-cell mediated.

When large amounts of antigen are injected into the blood, they are initially removed slowly by normal catabolic processes that also degrade plasma proteins. However, if the antigen elicits an antibody response, then antigen is removed at an accelerated rate as antigen:antibody complexes, a process known as **immune clearance**.

When antibody reacts with soluble antigen, the binding of antigen by antibody forms **immune complexes**. Larger immune complexes form when sufficient antibody is available; these are readily cleared by the reticuloendothelial system of cells bearing Fc and complement receptors, but small, soluble immune complexes forming when antigen is in excess can deposit in and damage small blood vessels.

Immune deviation is a term used to describe polarization of an immune response to T_H1-dominated or T_H2-dominated by injection of antigen.

The **immune response** is the response made by the host to defend itself against a pathogen.

Immune response (Ir) genes are genetic polymorphisms that control the intensity of the immune response to a particular antigen. Virtually all Ir phenotypes are due to differential binding of peptide fragments of antigen to MHC molecules, especially MHC class II molecules. The term is little used now.

It has been proposed that most tumors that arise are detected and eliminated by **immune surveillance** mediated by lymphocytes specific for tumor antigens. There is little evidence for the efficacy of this proposed process, but it remains an important concept in tumor immunology.

The **immune system** is the name used to describe the tissues, cells, and molecules involved in adaptive immunity, or sometimes the totality of host defense mechanisms.

Immunity is the ability to resist infection.

Immunization is the deliberate provocation of an adaptive immune response by introducing antigen (see also **active immunization** and **passive immunization**).

Immunobiology is the study of the biological basis for host defense against infection.

Immunodeficiency diseases are a group of inherited or acquired disorders in which some aspect or aspects of host defense are absent or functionally defective.

Immunodiffusion is the detection of antigen or antibody by the formation of an antigen:antibody precipitate in a clear agar gel.

Immunoelectrophoresis is a technique in which antigens are identified by first separating them by electrophoretic mobility and then detecting them by **immunodiffusion**.

Immunofluorescence is a technique for detecting molecules using antibodies labeled with fluorescent dyes. The bound fluorescent antibody can be detected by microscopy, by flow cytometry, or by fluorimetry, depending on the application being used. **Indirect immunofluorescence** uses anti-immunoglobulin antibodies labeled with fluorescent dyes to detect binding of a specific, unlabeled antibody.

Any molecule that can elicit an adaptive immune response upon injection into a person or animal is called an **immunogen**. In practice, only proteins are fully **immunogenic** because only proteins can be recognized by T lymphocytes.

Immunogenetics was originally the analysis of genetic traits by means of antibodies to genetically polymorphic molecules such as blood group antigens or MHC proteins. Immunogenetics now includes the genetic analysis of molecules important in immunology by any technique.

All antibody molecules belong to a family of plasma proteins called **immunoglobulins** and abbreviated **Ig**. Surface immunoglobulin serves as the specific antigen receptor of B lymphocytes.

Many molecules are made up in part or in their entirety of blocks of protein known as **immunoglobulin domains** or **Ig domains** because they were first described in the structure of antibody molecules. Immunoglobulin domains are the characteristic feature of proteins of the immunoglobulin superfamily of proteins that includes antibodies, T-cell receptors, MHC molecules, and many other molecules described in this book. The immunoglobulin domain comprises two β-pleated sheets held together by a disulfide bond, called the **immunoglobulin fold**. There are two main types of immunoglobulin domain, C domains with a three-strand and a four-strand sheet, and V domains with an extra strand in each sheet. Domains less closely related to the canonical Ig domains are sometimes also called **Ig-like domains**.

Immunoglobulin fold: see **immunoglobulin domains**.

Many proteins involved in antigen recognition and cell–cell interaction in the immune and other biological systems are members of a family of genes and proteins called the **immunoglobulin superfamily**, or **Ig superfamily**, because their shared structural and genetic features were first defined in immunoglobulin molecules. All members of the immunoglobulin superfamily have at least one **immunoglobulin domain**.

The detection of antigens in tissues by means of visible products produced by the degradation of a colorless substrate by enzymes linked to antibodies is called **immunohistochemistry**. This technique has the advantage that it can be combined with other special stains viewed in the light microscope, whereas immunofluorescent microscopy requires a special dark-field microscope.

Immunological ignorance describes a form of self tolerance in which reactive lymphocytes and their target antigen are both detectable within an individual yet no autoimmune attack occurs. Most autoimmune diseases probably occur when immunological ignorance is broken.

When an antigen is encountered more than once, the adaptive immune response to each subsequent encounter is speedier and more effective, a crucial feature of protective immunity known as **immunological memory**. Immunological memory is specific and long-lived.

Allogeneic tissue placed in certain sites in the body, such as the brain, does not elicit graft rejection. Such sites are called **immunologically privileged sites**. Immunological privilege results from the effects of both physical barriers to cell and antigen migration and soluble immunosuppressive mediators such as certain cytokines.

Immunology is the study of all aspects of host defense against infection and of adverse consequences of immune responses.

Immunophilins are proteins with peptidyl-prolyl *cis-trans* isomerase activity that bind the immunosuppressive drugs cyclosporin A, FK506, and rapamycin.

Soluble proteins, or membrane proteins solubilized in detergents, can be labeled and then detected by **immunoprecipitation analysis** using specific antibodies. The immunoprecipitated labeled protein is usually detected by SDS-PAGE followed by autoradiography.

The T and B cell antigen receptors are associated with transmembrane molecules with **immunoreceptor tyrosine-based activation motifs (ITAMs)** in their cytoplasmic domains. Each ITAM consists of a pair of YXXL motifs spaced by about 10 amino acids. They are sites of tyrosine phosphorylation and association with tyrosine kinases and other phosphotyrosine binding moieties involved in receptor signaling.

The ability of the immune system to sense and regulate its own responses is called **immunoregulation**.

Compounds that inhibit adaptive immune responses are called **immunosuppressive drugs**. They are used mainly in the treatment of graft rejection and severe autoimmune disease.

Antibodies that are chemically coupled to toxic molecules usually derived from plant or microbial toxins are called **immunotoxins**. The antibody targets the toxin moiety to specific cells. Immunotoxins are being tested as anti-cancer agents and as immunosuppressive drugs.

The **indirect Coombs test** is a variation of the **direct Coombs test** in which an unknown serum is tested for antibodies to normal red blood cells by first mixing the two and then washing the red blood cells and reacting them with anti-immunoglobulin antibody. If antibody in the unknown serum binds to the red blood cells, agglutination by anti-immunoglobulin occurs.

Indirect immunofluorescence: see **immunofluorescence**.

Infectious mononucleosis, or glandular fever, is the term used to describe the common form of infection with the Epstein-Barr virus. It consists of fever, malaise, and swollen lymph nodes.

Inflammation is a general term for the local accumulation of fluid, plasma proteins, and white blood cells that is initiated by physical injury, infection, or a local immune response. This is also known as an **inflammatory response**. Acute inflammation is the term used to describe early and often transient episodes, while chronic inflammation occurs when the infection persists or during autoimmune responses. Many different forms of inflammation are seen in different diseases. The cells that invade tissues undergoing inflammatory responses are often called **inflammatory cells** or an **inflammatory infiltrate**.

Inflammatory CD4 T cells, also known as T_H1, are armed effector T cells that make the cytokines interferon-γ and tumor necrosis factor upon recognition of antigen. Their major function is the activation of macrophages. Some T_H1 also have cytotoxic activity.

Influenza hemagglutinin: see **hemagglutinin**.

The early phases of the host response to infection depend on **innate immunity** in which a variety of **innate resistance mechanisms** recognize and respond to the presence of a pathogen. Innate immunity is present in all individuals at all times, does not increase with repeated exposure to a given pathogen, and does not discriminate between pathogens. It is followed by adaptive immunity mediated by clonal selection of specific lymphocytes and leading to long-term protection from disease.

When inositol phospholipid is cleaved by phospholipase C-γ, it yields **inositol trisphosphate** and diacylglycerol. Inositol trisphosphate releases calcium ions from intracellular stores in the endoplasmic reticulum.

In **insulin-dependent diabetes mellitus**, the β cells of the pancreatic islets of Langerhans are destroyed so that no insulin is produced.

The disease is believed to result from an autoimmune attack on the β cells.

The **integrins** are heterodimeric cell-surface proteins involved in cell–cell and cell–matrix interactions. They are important in adhesive interactions between lymphocytes and antigen-presenting cells and in lymphocyte and leukocyte migration into tissues.

The **β₁-integrins** are a family of integrins with shared β₁ chains and distinct α chains that mediate adhesion to other cells and to extracellular matrix proteins. They are also known as the very late antigens (VLA).

The **intercellular adhesion molecules (ICAMs) ICAM-1, ICAM-2,** and **ICAM-3** are cell-surface molecules that are ligands for the leukocyte integrins and play a crucial role in the binding of lymphocytes and other leukocytes to certain cells, including antigen-presenting cells and endothelial cells. They are members of the immunoglobulin superfamily of proteins.

The **intercrines** are a family of small cytokines, also known as chemokines, that are produced by many cell types and play an important role in leukocyte migration into sites of inflammation. They are listed in Appendix II.

Interdigitating reticular cells: see **dendritic cells**.

Interferons are cytokines that can induce cells to resist viral replication. **Interferon-α** (**IFN-α**) and **interferon-β** (**IFN-β**) are produced by leukocytes and fibroblasts respectively, as well as by other cells, while **interferon-γ** (**IFN-γ**) is a product of inflammatory CD4 T cells, CD8 T cells, and natural killer cells. Interferon-g has as its primary action the activation of macrophages.

Interleukin, abbreviated **IL**, is a generic term for cytokines produced by leukocytes. We use the more general term cytokine in this book, but the term interleukin is used in the naming of specific cytokines such as interleukin-2 (abbreviated **IL-2**). The interleukins are listed in Appendix II.

When an antigen-specific antibody is used to immunize an individual, some of the antibodies elicited resemble the original antigen and are referred to as an **internal image**. Internal image antibodies can, in turn, be used to immunize other individuals to make antibodies to the original antigen.

The major histocompatibility complex (MHC) class II proteins are assembled in the endoplasmic reticulum with the **invariant chain** (abbreviated **Ii**), which is involved in shielding the MHC class II molecules from binding peptides and in delivering them to cellular vesicles. There Ii is degraded, leaving the MHC class II molecules able to bind peptide fragments of antigen.

ISCOMs are **i**mmune **s**timulatory **com**plexes of antigen held within a lipid matrix that acts as an adjuvant and enables the antigen to be taken up into the cytoplasm after fusion of the lipid with the plasma membrane.

Isoelectric focusing is an electrophoretic technique in which proteins migrate in a pH gradient until they reach the place in the gradient at which their net charge is neutral, their isoelectric point. Uncharged proteins no longer migrate so that each protein is focused at its isoelectric point.

Immunoglobulins are made in several distinct **isotypes** or classes, IgM, IgG, IgD, IgA, and IgE, each of which has a distinct heavy-chain constant region encoded by a distinct constant region gene. The isotype of an antibody determines what effector mechanisms it can engage upon binding antigen.

The first antibodies produced in a humoral immune response are IgM, but activated B cells subsequently undergo **isotype switching** to secrete antibodies of different isotypes: IgG, IgA, and IgE. Isotype switching does not affect antibody specificity significantly, but alters the effector functions an antibody can engage. Isotype switching occurs by a site-specific recombination involving deletion of the intervening DNA.

The **J gene segments**, or **joining gene segments** are immunological receptor gene segments found some distance 5′ to the C genes. A V and D gene segment must rearrange to a J gene segment to form a complete variable-region exon.

Junctional diversity is diversity in immunological receptors created during the process of joining V, D, and J gene segments.

Killer T cell is another commonly used term for **cytotoxic T cell**.

Kit is a cell-surface receptor found on developing B cells and other developing white blood cells for the **stem cell factor** borne on bone marrow stromal cells. Kit has protein tyrosine kinase activity.

Kupffer cells are phagocytes lining the hepatic sinusoids; they remove debris and dying cells from the blood, but are not known to elicit immune responses.

Langerhans' cells are phagocytic dendritic cells found in the epidermis. They can migrate from the epidermis to regional lymph nodes via the lymphatics. In the lymph node they differentiate into dendritic cells.

In type 1 immediate hypersensitivity reactions, the **late phase reaction** persists and is resistant to anti-histamine treatment.

Some viruses can enter a cell but not replicate, a state known as **latency**. Latency can be established in various ways; when the virus is reactivated and replicates, it can produce disease.

Late pro-B cell: see pro-B cell.

LCMV: see **lymphocytic choriomeningitis virus**.

The **lectin pathway** of complement activation is initiated by collectins, carbohydrate-binding proteins with collagen-like domains found in serum.

Lentiviruses area group of retroviruses, which includes the human immundeficiency virus (HIV), that cause disease after a long incubation, which may take years to become apparent.

Leprosy is caused by *Mycobacterium leprae* and occurs in a variety of forms. There are two polar forms, **lepromatous leprosy** which is characterized by abundant replication of leprosy bacilli and abundant antibody production without cell-mediated immunity, and **tuberculoid leprosy** in which few organisms are seen in the tissues, there is little or no antibody, but cell-mediated immunity is very active. The other forms of leprosy are intermediate between the polar forms.

Leukemia is the unrestrained proliferation of a malignant white blood cell characterized by very high numbers of the malignant cells in the blood. Leukemias can be lymphocytic, myelocytic, or monocytic.

Leukocyte is a general term for a white blood cell. Leukocytes include lymphocytes, polymorphonuclear leukocytes, and monocytes.

Leukocyte adhesion deficiency is an immunodeficiency disease in which the common β chain of the leukocyte integrins is not produced. This mainly affects the ability of leukocytes to enter sites of infection with extracellular pathogens, so that infections cannot be effectively eradicated.

The **leukocyte common antigen** is found on all leukocytes. It is also known as **CD45** and is a transmembrane tyrosine phosphatase that can be produced in a variety of isoforms depending on the cell type on which it appears.

Leukocyte integrins: see **lymphocyte function-associated antigens**.

Leukocytosis is the presence of increased numbers of leukocytes in the blood. It is commonly seen in acute infection.

LFA-1, LFA-3: see **lymphocyte function-associated antigen**.

The immunoglobulin **light (L) chain** is the smaller of the two chains that make up all immunoglobulins. It consists of one V and one C domain, and is disulfide-bonded to the heavy chain. There are two classes of light chain, known as κ and λ.

Linear epitope: see **continuous epitope**.

Alleles at linked loci within the major histocompatibility complex are said to be in **linkage disequilibrium** if they are inherited together more frequently than predicted from their individual frequencies.

Epitopes recognized by B cells and helper T cells must be physically linked in order for the helper T cell to activate the B cell. This is called **linked recognition**.

Low-zone tolerance: see **high-zone tolerance**.

L-selectin is an adhesion molecule of the selectin family found on lymphocytes. L-selectin binds to CD34 and GlyCAM-1 on high endothelial venules to initiate the migration of naive lymphocytes into lymphoid tissue.

Lyme disease is a chronic infection with *Borrelia burgdorferi*, a spirochete that can evade the immune response.

Lymphatic vessels or **lymphatics** are thin-walled vessels that carry **lymph**, the extracellular fluid that accumulates in tissues, back through the lymph nodes to the thoracic duct.

Lymph nodes are secondary lymphoid organs where adaptive immune responses are initiated. They are found in many locations where lymphatic vessels come together, delivering antigen to antigen-presenting cells which display it to the many recirculating lymphocytes that migrate through the lymph node. Some of these can recognize the antigen and respond to it, triggering an adaptive immune response.

A **lymphoblast** is a lymphocyte that has enlarged and increased its rate of RNA and protein synthesis.

Lymphocyte function-associated antigen-1 (LFA-1) is one of the **leukocyte integrins**, which are heterodimeric molecules involved in the interaction of leukocytes with other cells, such as endothelial cells and antigen-presenting cells. LFA-1 is particularly important in T-cell adhesion to these cells. The other leukocyte integrins are also known as Mac-1 and gp150,95.

Lymphocyte function-associated antigen-3 (LFA-3) is a molecule found on many cells that is the ligand for CD2 (also known as LFA-2). It is a member of the immunoglobulin superfamily.

All adaptive immune responses are mediated by **lymphocytes**. Lymphocytes have cell-surface receptors for antigen that are encoded in rearranging gene segments. There are two main classes of lymphocyte, B lymphocytes (B cells) and T lymphocytes (T cells), which mediate humoral and cell-mediated immunity respectively. Small lymphocytes have little cytoplasm and condensed nuclear chromatin; upon antigen recognition, the cell enlarges to form a lymphoblast and then proliferates and differentiates into an antigen-specific effector cell.

Lymphocytic choriomeningitis virus (LCMV) is a virus that causes a non-bacterial meningitis in mice and occasionally humans. It is used extensively in experimental studies.

Lymphoid organs are organized tissues characterized by very large numbers of lymphocytes interacting with a non-lymphoid stroma. The primary lymphoid organs, where lymphocytes are generated, are the thymus and bone marrow. The main secondary lymphoid organs, where adaptive immune responses are initiated, are the lymph nodes, spleen, and mucosal-associated lymphoid tissues such as tonsils and Peyer's patches.

Lymphokines are **cytokines** produced by lymphocytes.

Lymphomas are tumors of lymphocytes that grow in lymphoid and other tissues but do not enter the blood in large numbers. There are many types of lymphoma which represent the transformation of various classes of lymphoid cells.

Lymphotoxin (LT, TNF-β): Also known as tumor necrosis factor-β, a cytokine secreated by inflammatory CD4 T cells, which is directly cytotoxic for some cells.

Macroglobulin describes plasma proteins that are globulins of high molecular weight, including immunoglobulin M (IgM).

Macrophages are large mononuclear phagocytic cells important in innate immunity, in early non-adaptive phases of host defense, as antigen-presenting cells, and as effector cells in humoral and cell-mediated immunity. They are migratory cells deriving from bone marrow precursors and are found in most tissues of the body. They play a critical role in host defense.

Resting macrophages will not destroy certain intracellular bacteria unless the macrophage is activated by a T cell. **Macrophage activation** is important in controlling infection and also causes damage to neighboring tissues.

Macrophage chemoattractant and activating protein is a chemokine and is described in Appendix II.

MadCAM-1 is the mucosal cell adhesion molecule-1 or mucosal addressin that is recognized by the lymphocyte surface proteins L-selectin and VLA-4, allowing specific homing of lymphocytes to mucosal tissues.

The **major histocompatibility complex (MHC)** is a cluster of genes on human chromosome 6 or mouse chromosome 17 that encodes the **MHC molecules**. These are the **MHC class I molecules** or proteins that present peptides generated in cytosol to CD8 T cells, and the **MHC class II molecules** or proteins that present peptides degraded in cellular vesicles to CD4 T cells. The MHC also encodes proteins involved in antigen processing and host defense. The MHC is the most polymorphic gene cluster in the human genome, having large numbers of alleles at several different loci. Because this polymorphism is usually detected using antibodies or specific T cells, the MHC proteins are often called **major histocompatibility antigens**.

The MHC contains MHC class I, MHC class II, and **MHC class IB** molecules. The MHC class IB molecules are able to present a restricted set of antigens and are not highly polymorphic like the class I and class II genes.

The **mannose-binding protein (MBP)** is an acute phase protein that binds to mannose residues. It can opsonize pathogens bearing mannose on their surfaces and can activate the complement system. It has an important role in innate immunity.

The follicular **mantle zone** is a rim of B lymphocytes that surrounds lymphoid follicles. The precise nature and role of mantle zone lymphocytes has not yet been determined.

Mast cells are large cells found in connective tissues throughout the body, most abundantly in the submucosal tissues and the dermis. They contain large granules that store a variety of mediator molecules including the vasoactive amine histamine. Mast cells have high-affinity Fcε receptors (FcεRI) that allow them to bind IgE monomers. Antigen binding to this IgE triggers mast cell degranulation and mast cell activation, producing a local or systemic immediate hypersensitivity reaction. Mast cells play a crucial role in allergic reactions.

Mature B cells are B cells that have acquired surface IgM and IgD and have become able to respond to antigen.

The **medulla** is usually a central or collecting point of organs. The thymic medulla is the central area of each thymic lobe, rich in bone marrow derived antigen-presenting cells and cells of a distinctive medullary epithelium. The medulla of the lymph node is a site of macrophage and plasma cell concentration through which the lymph flows on its way to the efferent lymphatics.

The **membrane-attack complex** is made up of the terminal complement components which assemble to generate a membrane-spanning hydrophilic pore, damaging the membrane.

MHC: see **major histocompatibility complex**.

Antigen recognition by T cells is **MHC restricted**, which means that a given T cell will recognize antigen only when its peptide fragments are bound to a particular MHC molecule. Normally, as T cells are stimulated only in the presence of self MHC molecules, antigen is recognized only as peptides bound to self MHC molecules. However, experimental manipulations can produce T cells that recognize antigen only when its peptide fragments are bound to non-self MHC molecules. Thus, MHC restriction defines T-cell specificity both in terms of the antigen recognized and in terms of the MHC molecule that binds its peptide fragments.

Microorganisms are microscopic organisms, unicellular except for some fungi, which include bacteria, yeasts and other fungi, and protozoa, all of which can cause human disease.

Anti-carbohydrate antibodies can bind either the ends or the middles of polysaccharide chains; the latter antibodies are called **middle-binders**.

Minor histocompatibility antigens, or **minor H antigens**, are peptides of polymorphic cellular proteins bound to MHC molecules that can lead to graft rejection when they are recognized by T cells.

Minor lymphocyte stimulatory (Mls) loci are non-MHC loci that provoke strong primary mixed lymphocyte responses. The Mls loci are endogenous mammary tumor viruses integrated in the mouse genome. They produce their effects by making a viral superantigen encoded in the 3′ long terminal repeat of the integrated virus. The superantigen stimulates a large number of T lymphocytes by binding to the V_β domain of the T-cell receptor.

When lymphocytes from two unrelated individuals are cultured together, the T cells proliferate in a **mixed lymphocyte reaction** to the allogeneic MHC molecules on cells of the other donor. This **mixed lymphocyte culture** is used in testing for histocompatibility.

MMTV: see **mouse mammary tumor virus**.

It has been proposed that infectious agents could provoke autoimmunity by **molecular mimicry**, the induction of antibodies and T cells that react against the pathogen but also cross-react with self antigens.

Monoclonal antibodies are antibodies produced by a single clone of B lymphocytes. Monoclonal antibodies are usually produced by making hybrid antibody-forming cells from fusion of myeloma cells with immune spleen cells.

Monocytes are white blood cells with a bean-shaped nucleus which are precursors to macrophages.

Monokines are cytokines secreted by **macrophages**.

Some antibodies recognize all allelic forms of a polymorphic molecule such as an MHC class I protein; these antibodies are thus said to recognize a **monomorphic** epitope.

Lymphocytes have only one receptor and thus have the property of **monospecificity** in response to antigen.

Mouse mammary tumor virus (MMTV) is a retrovirus that encodes a viral superantigen; integrated copies of related viruses encode the endogenous superantigens known as minor lymphocyte stimulatory loci (Mls).

Mucins are highly glycosylated cell-surface proteins. Mucin-like molecules are bound by L-selectin in lymphocyte homing.

The **mucosal-associated lymphoid tissue** or **MALT**, comprises all lymphoid cells in epithelia and in the lamina propria lying below the body's **mucosal surfaces**. The main sites of mucosal associated lymphoid tissues are the **gut-associated lymphoid tissues**, or **GALT**, and the **bronchial-associated lymphoid tissues**, or **BALT**.

Multiple myeloma is a tumor of plasma cells, almost always first detected as multiple foci in bone marrow. Myeloma cells produce a monoclonal immunoglobulin called a myeloma protein which is detectable in the patient's plasma.

Multiple sclerosis is a neurological disease characterized by focal demyelination in the central nervous system, lymphocytic infiltration in the brain, and a chronic progressive course. It is believed to be an autoimmune disease.

Myasthenia gravis is an autoimmune disease in which autoantibodies to the acetylcholine receptor on skeletal muscle cells cause a block in neuromuscular junctions, leading to progressive weakness and eventually death.

Myeloid progenitors are cells in bone marrow that give rise to the granulocytes and macrophages of the immune system.

Myeloma proteins are the secreted immunoglobulin products of myeloma tumors that are found in the patient's plasma.

Myelopoiesis is the production of monocytes and polymorphonuclear leukocytes in bone marrow.

Naive lymphocytes are lymphocytes that have never encountered their specific antigen and thus have never responded to it, as distinct from memory or effector lymphocytes. All lymphocytes leaving the central lymphoid organs are naive lymphocytes, those from the thymus being **naive T cells** and those from bone marrow being **naive B cells**.

Natural killer cells or **NK cells** are non-T, non-B lymphocytes usually having granular morphology, that kill certain tumor cells. NK cells are important in innate immunity to viruses and other intracellular pathogens as well as in **antibody-dependent cell-mediated cytotoxicity (ADCC)**.

Necrosis is the death of cells or tissues due to chemical or physical injury, as opposed to apoptosis, which is a biologically programmed form of cell death. Necrosis leaves extensive cellular debris that needs to be removed by phagocytes, while apoptosis does not.

During intrathymic development, thymocytes that recognize self are deleted from the repertoire, a process known as **negative selection**. Autoreactive B cells undergo a similar process in bone marrow.

Antibodies that can inhibit the infectivity of a virus or the toxicity of a toxin molecule are said to **neutralize** them. Such antibodies are known as **neutralizing antibodies** and the process of inactivation as **neutralization**.

Neutrophils, also known as **neutrophilic polymorphonuclear leukocytes**, are the major class of white blood cell in human peripheral blood. They have a multilobed nucleus and neutrophilic granules. Neutrophils are phagocytes and have an important role in engulfing and killing extracellular pathogens.

NK cells: see **natural killer cells**.

Nodular sclerosis: see **Hodgkin's disease.**

Recombination signal sequences (RSS) consist of a seven nucleotide **heptamer** and a nine-nucleotide **nonamer** of conserved sequence, separated by 12 or 23 nucleotides. RSS forms the target for the site-specific recombinase that joins the gene segments.

When T- and B-cell receptor gene segments rearrange, they often form **non-productive rearrangements** that cannot encode a protein because the coding sequences are in the wrong translational reading frame.

N regions are made up of nucleotides that are inserted into the junctions between gene segments of T-cell receptor and immunoglobulin heavy-chain V-region genes during gene segment joining. These **N-nucleotides** are not encoded in either gene segment, but are inserted by the enzyme terminal deoxynucleotidyl transferase (TdT). They markedly increase the diversity of these receptors.

The *nude* mutation of mice produces hairlessness and defective formation of the thymic stroma, so that nude mice, which are homozygous for this mutation, have no mature T cells.

Oncogenes are genes involved in regulating cell growth. When these genes are defective in structure or expression, they can cause cells to grow continuously to form a tumor.

An **opportunistic pathogen** is a microorganism that causes disease only in individuals with compromised host defense mechanisms, as occurs in AIDS.

Opsonization is the alteration of the surface of a pathogen or other particle so that it can be ingested by phagocytes. Antibody and complement **opsonize** extracellular bacteria for destruction by neutrophils and macrophages.

Organ-specific autoimmune diseases are autoimmune diseases targeted at a particular organ, such as the thyroid in Graves' disease. They contrast with systemic autoimmune diseases that do not show organ specificity.

Original antigenic sin describes the tendency of humans to make antibody responses to those epitopes shared between the original strain of a virus and subsequent related viruses, while ignoring other highly immunogenic epitopes on the second and subsequent viruses.

Lymphocyte subpopulations can be isolated by **panning** on petri dishes coated with monoclonal antibodies against cell-surface markers, to which the lymphocytes bind.

The **paracortical area,** or **paracortex,** is the T cell area of lymph nodes, lying just below the follicular cortex that is primarily B cells.

Parasites are organisms that obtain sustenance from a live host. In medical practice, the term is restricted to worms and protozoa, the subject matter of parasitology.

Paroxysmal nocturnal hemoglobinuria (PNH) is a disease in which complement regulatory proteins are defective, so that complement activation leads to episodes of spontaneous hemolysis.

Partial agonist peptides, or **altered peptide ligands,** are able to stimulate a partial response from a cloned T-cell line, such as induction of cytokine secretion but not proliferation.

Passive hemagglutination is a technique for detecting antibody in which red blood cells are coated with antigen and the antibody is detected by agglutination of the coated red blood cells.

The injection of antibody or immune serum into a naive recipient is called **passive immunization,** as opposed to active immunization, the induction of an immune response by injection of antigen.

Pathogenic microorganisms, or **pathogens,** are microorganisms that can cause disease when they infect a host.

Pathology is the scientific study of disease. The term **pathology** is also used to describe detectable damage to tissues.

Pentadecacatechol is the chemical substance in the leaves of the poison ivy plant that causes the cell-mediated immunity associated with allergy to poison ivy.

Pentraxins are a family of **acute phase proteins** formed of five identical subunits, to which **C-reactive protein** and serum amyloid protein belong.

Perforin is a protein that can polymerize to form the membrane pores that are an important part of the killing mechanism in cell-mediated cytotoxicity. Perforin is produced by cytotoxic T cells and NK cells and is stored in granules that are released by the cell when it contacts a specific target cell.

The **periarteriolar lymphoid sheath (PALS)** is part of the inner region of the white pulp of the spleen, and contains mainly T cells.

Peripheral blood mononuclear cells are lymphocytes and monocytes isolated from peripheral blood, usually by Ficoll Hypaque density centrifugation.

Peripheral lymphoid organs are the lymph nodes, spleen, and mucosal-associated lymphoid tissues where immune responses are induced, as opposed to the central lymphoid organs where lymphocytes develop.

Peripheral tolerance is tolerance acquired by mature lymphocytes in the peripheral tissues, as opposed to central tolerance that is acquired by immature lymphocytes during their development.

Peyer's patches are aggregates of lymphocytes along the small intestine, especially the ileum.

Antibody-like phage can be produced by cloning immunoglobulin V-region genes in filamentous phage, which thus express antigen-binding domains on their surfaces, forming a **phage display library.** Antigen-binding phage can be replicated in bacteria and used like antibodies. This technique is being used to develop novel antibodies of any specificity.

Phagocytosis is the internalization of particulate matter by cells. Usually, the **phagocytic cells** or **phagocytes** are macrophages or neutrophils, and the particles are bacteria that are taken up and destroyed. The ingested material is contained in a vesicle called a **phagosome,** which then fuses with one or more lysosomes to form a **phagolysosome.** The lysosomal enzymes play an important role in pathogen destruction and degradation to small molecules.

Phospholipase C-γ is a key enzyme in signal transduction. It is activated by protein tyrosine kinases that are themselves activated by receptor ligation, and activated phospholipase C-γ cleaves inositol phospholipid into inositol trisphosphate and diacylglycerol.

Plasma is the fluid component of blood containing water, electrolytes, and the plasma proteins.

A **plasmablast** is a B cell in a lymph node that already shows some features of a **plasma cell.**

Plasma cells are terminally differentiated B lymphocytes. Plasma cells are the main antibody-secreting cells of the body. They are found in the medulla of the lymph nodes, in splenic red pulp, and in bone marrow. Malignant plasma cells form multiple tumors in bone marrow and are called **multiple myeloma.**

Platelets are small cell fragments found in the blood and are crucial for blood clotting. They are formed from megakaryocytes.

P-nucleotides are nucleotides found in junctions between gene segments of the rearranged V-region genes of immunological receptors. They are an inverse repeat of the sequence at the end of the adjacent gene segment, being generated from a hairpin intermediate during recombination, and hence are called palindromic or P-nucleotides.

Poison ivy is a plant whose leaves contain pentadecacatechol, a potent contact sensitizing agent and a frequent cause of contact hypersensitivity.

Antigen activates specific lymphocytes while all mitogens, by definition, activate most or all lymphocytes, a process known as **polyclonal activation** because it involves multiple clones of diverse specificity. Such mitogens are known as **polyclonal mitogens**.

The major histocompatibility complex is both **polygenic**, containing several loci encoding proteins of identical function, and **polymorphic**, having multiple alleles at each locus.

The **poly-Ig receptor** binds polymeric immunoglobulins, especially IgA, at the basolateral membrane of epithelia and transports them across the cell where they are released from the apical surface. This transcytotic process transfers IgA from its site of synthesis to its site of action at epithelial surfaces.

The **polymerase chain reaction (PCR)** is a technique for amplifying a specific sequence in DNA by repeated cycles of synthesis driven by pairs of reciprocally oriented primers.

Polymorphism literally means existing in a variety of different shapes. Genetic polymorphism is variability at a gene locus where the variants occur at a frequency of greater than 1%. The major histocompatibility complex is the most polymorphic gene cluster known in humans.

Polymorphonuclear leukocytes are white blood cells with multilobed nuclei and cytoplasmic granules. There are three types of polymorphonuclear leukocytes, the neutrophils with granules that stain with neutral dyes, the eosinophils with granules that stain with eosin, and the basophils with granules that stain with basic dyes.

Some antibodies show **polyspecificity**, the ability to bind to many different antigens.

Only those developing T cells whose receptors can recognize antigens presented by self MHC molecules can mature in the thymus, a process known as **positive selection**. All other developing T cells die before reaching maturity.

During B-cell development, **pre-B cells** are cells that have rearranged their heavy-chain genes but not their light-chain genes.

The **precipitin reaction** was the first quantitative technique for measuring antibody production. The amount of antibody is determined from the amount of precipitate obtained with a fixed amount of antigen. The precipitin reaction also can be used to define antigen valence and zones of antibody or antigen excess in mixtures of antigen and antibody.

Prednisone is a synthetic steroid with potent anti-inflammatory and immunosuppressive activity used in treating acute graft rejection and autoimmune disease.

During T-dependent antibody responses, a **primary focus** of B-cell activation forms in the vicinity of the margin between T and B cell areas of lymphoid tissue. Here, the T and B cells interact and B cells can differentiate directly into antibody-forming cells or migrate to lymphoid follicles for further proliferation and differentiation.

Lymphoid tissues contain lymphoid follicles made up of follicular dendritic cells and B lymphocytes. The **primary follicles** contain resting B lymphocytes and are the site at which germinal centers form when they are entered by activated B cells, forming **secondary follicles**

The **primary immune response** is the adaptive immune response to an initial exposure to antigen. **Primary immunization**, also known as **priming**, generates both the primary immune response and immunological memory.

The binding of antibody molecules to antigen is called a **primary interaction**, as distinct from **secondary interactions** in which binding is detected by some associated change such as precipitation of soluble antigen or agglutination of particulate antigen.

One speaks of **priming** when antigen is presented to T or B cells in an immunogenic form; the consequence is priming of cells that can respond as memory cells in a second and subsequent immune response.

During B-cell development **pro-B cells** are cells that have displayed B-cell surface marker proteins but have not yet completed heavy-chain gene rearrangement. They are divided into **early pro-B cells** and **late pro-B cells**.

Professional antigen-presenting cells or **APCs** are cells that normally initiate the responses of naive T cells to antigen. To date, only dendritic cells, macrophages, and B cells have been shown to have this capacity. A professional antigen-presenting cell must be able to display peptide fragments of antigen on appropriate MHC molecules and also have co-stimulatory molecules on its surface.

Progenitors are the more differentiated progeny of stem cells that give rise to distinct subsets of mature blood cells and that lack the self-renewal capacity of true stem cells.

Programmed cell death or **apoptosis** is cell death triggered from within the dying cell. Apoptosis eliminates developing T cells that fail positive or negative selection, excess effector cells, and mature lymphocytes that do not encounter antigen. It plays a critical role in maintaining the numbers of lymphocytes at appropriate levels.

Properdin, or factor P, is a positive regulatory component of the alternative pathway of complement activation. It acts by stabilizing the C3/C5 convertase of the alternative factor (comprising C3b,Bb) on the surface of bacterial cells.

Cytosolic proteins are degraded by a large catalytic multisubunit protease called a **proteasome**. It is thought that peptides that are presented by MHC class I molecules are generated by the action of proteasomes, and two subunits of some proteasomes are encoded in the MHC.

Protective immunity is the resistance to specific infection that follows infection or vaccination.

Protein A is a cell membrane component of *Staphylococcus aureus* which binds to the Fc region of IgG, and is thought to protect the bacteria from IgG antibodies by inhibiting their interactions with complement and Fc receptors. It is useful for purifying IgG antibodies.

Enzymes that add phosphate groups to tyrosine residues are called **protein tyrosine kinases**. These enzymes play crucial roles in signal transduction and regulation of cell growth.

Proto-oncogenes are cellular genes that regulate growth control. When mutated or aberrantly expressed, they can contribute to malignant transformation of cells leading to cancer.

Provirus is the DNA form of a retrovirus when it is integrated into the host cell genome, where it can remain transcriptionally inactive for a long period of time.

P-selectin: see **selectins**.

Purine nucleotide phophorylase deficiency is an enzyme defect that results in severe combined immunodeficiency (SCID). This enzyme is important in purine metabolism, and its deficiency causes accumulation of purine nucleosides which are toxic for developing T cells, causing the immune deficiency.

Radiation bone marrow chimeras are mice that have been heavily irradiated and then reconstituted with bone marrow cells of a different strain of mouse, so that the lymphocytes differ genetically from the environment in which they develop. Such chimeric mice have been important in studying lymphocyte development.

Antigen:antibody interaction can be studied by **radioimmunoassay (RIA)** in which antigen or antibody is labeled with radioactivity. An unlabeled antigen or antibody is attached to a solid support like a plastic surface, and the fraction of the labeled antibody or antigen retained on the surface is determined in order to measure binding.

The recombination activating genes *RAG-1* and *RAG-2* encode the proteins **RAG-1** and **RAG-2** that are critical to receptor gene rearrangement. Mice lacking either of these genes cannot form receptors and are severely immunodeficient.

Rapamycin is an immunosuppressive drug that blocks cytokine action.

IgE antibodies responsible for immediate hypersensitivity reactions were originally called **reagins** or **reaginic antibodies**.

Receptor expression requires variable region gene segment **rearrangement** in developing lymphocytes. Expressed V-region genes are composed of **rearranged** gene segments.

The distinguishing characteristic of lymphocytes is the expression of cell-surface **receptors** for antigen. Each lymphocyte bears a receptor of unique structure generated during lymphocyte development through rearrangement of receptor gene segments to produce a complete gene.

The replacement of a light chain of a self-reactive antigen receptor on immature B cells with a light chain that does not confer autoreactivity is known as **receptor editing**.

Receptor-mediated endocytosis is internalization into endosomes of molecules bound to cell-surface receptors. Antigens bound to B lymphocyte receptors are internalized by this process.

The totality of lymphocyte receptors is known as the lymphocyte **receptor repertoire**. It is made up of many millions of different receptors, with all the receptors on a single lymphocyte being identical in structure.

In any situation where cells or tissues are transplanted, they come from a donor and are placed in a **recipient** or host.

Recombination activating genes: see **RAG-1** and **RAG-2**.

Strains of mice derived from intra-strain crosses that have undergone recombination within the MHC are called **recombinant inbred strains**.

Recombination signal sequences (RSS) are short stretches of DNA that flank the gene segments that are rearranged to generate a V-region exon. They always consist of a conserved heptamer and nonamer separated by 12 or 23 base pairs. Gene segments are only joined if one is flanked by an RSS containing a 12 base pair spacer and the other is flanked by an RSS containing a 23 base pair spacer, the **12/23 rule** of gene segment joining.

The non-lymphoid area of the spleen in which red blood cells are broken down is called the **red pulp**.

The **rev** protein is the product of the *rev* gene of the human immunodeficiency virus (HIV). The rev protein promotes the passage of viral RNA from nucleus to cytoplasm during HIV replication.

The enzyme **reverse transcriptase** is an essential component of retroviruses, as it translates the RNA genome into DNA prior to its integration into host cell DNA. Reverse transcriptase also allows RNA sequences to be converted into complementary DNA (cDNA), and so to be cloned, and thus is an essential reagent in molecular biology.

The **Rhesus** or **Rh blood group antigen** is a red cell membrane antigen that is also detectable on the cells of rhesus monkeys. Anti-Rh antibodies do not agglutinate human red blood cells, so antibody to Rh antigen must be detected using a **Coombs test**.

Rheumatoid arthritis is a common inflammatory joint disease that is probably due to an autoimmune response. The disease is accompanied by the production of **rheumatoid factor**, an IgM anti-IgG antibody that may also be produced in normal immune responses.

The technique of **sandwich ELISA** uses antibody on a surface to trap a protein by binding to one of its epitopes. The trapped protein is then detected by an enzyme-linked antibody specific for a different epitope on the protein's surface. This gives the assay a high degree of specificity.

Scatchard analysis is a mathematical analysis of equilibrium binding that allows affinity and valence of a receptor–ligand interaction to be determined.

SCID, *scid*: see **severe combined immunodeficiency**.

SDS-PAGE is the common abbreviation for polyacrylamide gel electrophoresis (PAGE) of proteins dissolved in the detergent sodium dodecyl sulfate (SDS). This technique is widely used to characterize proteins, especially after labeling and immunoprecipitation.

A **secondary antibody response** is the antibody response induced by a **secondary** or **booster injection** of antigen, or **secondary immunization**. The secondary response starts sooner after antigen injection, reaches higher levels, is of higher affinity than the primary response, and is dominated by IgG antibodies.

Secondary interactions: see **primary interactions**.

When the recipient of a first tissue or organ graft has rejected that graft, a second graft from the same donor is rejected more rapidly and vigorously in what is called a **second set rejection**.

The co-stimulatory signal required for lymphocyte activation is often called a **second signal**, with the first signal coming from binding of antigen by the antigen receptor. Both signals are required to activate most lymphocytes.

The **secretory component** attached to IgA antibodies in body secretions is a fragment of the **poly-Ig receptor** left attached to the IgA after transport across epithelial cells.

A cell is said to be **selected** by antigen when its receptors bind that antigen. If the cell enters proliferation as a result, then this is called clonal selection, and the cell founds a clone; if the cell is killed by binding antigen, this is called negative selection or clonal deletion.

Selectins are a family of cell-surface adhesion molecules of leukocytes and endothelial cells that bind to sugar moieties on specific glycoproteins with mucin-like features.

Tolerance is the failure to respond to an antigen; when that antigen is borne by self tissues, then tolerance is called **self tolerance**. See also: **tolerance**.

Allergic reactions require prior immunization, called **sensitization**, by the allergen that elicits the acute response. Allergic reactions only occur in **sensitized** individuals.

Sepsis is infection of the bloodstream. This is a very serious and frequently fatal condition. Infection of the blood with Gram negative bacteria triggers **septic shock** through the release of the cytokine TNF-α.

A **sequence motif** is a pattern of nucleotides or amino acids shared by different genes or proteins that often have related functions. Sequence motifs observed in peptides that bind a particular MHC glycoprotein are based on the requirements for particular amino acids to achieve binding to that MHC molecule.

Seroconversion is the phase of an infection when antibodies against the infecting agent are first detectable in the blood.

Serology is the use of antibodies to detect and measure antigens using **serological assays**, so called because these assays were originally carried out with **serum**, the fluid component of clotted blood, from immunized individuals.

Serotonin is the principal vasoactive amine found in mast cell granules of rodents.

Serum is the fluid component of clotted blood.

Serum sickness occurs when foreign serum or serum proteins are injected into a person. It is caused by the formation of immune complexes between the injected protein and the antibodies formed against it. It is characterized by fever, arthralgias, and nephritis.

Severe combined immune deficiency or **SCID** is an immune deficiency disease in which neither antibody nor T-cell responses are made. It is usually the result of T-cell deficiencies. The *scid* mutation in mice causes severe combined immune deficiency in mice.

A **signal joint** is formed by the precise joining of recognition signal sequences in the process of somatic recombination that generates T-cell receptor and immunoglobulin genes.

During T-cell maturation in the thymus, mature T cells are detected by the expression of either the CD4 or the CD8 co-receptor and are therefore called **single-positive thymocytes**.

Smallpox is an infectious disease caused by the virus variola that once killed at least 10% of infected people. It has now been eradicated by vaccination.

During B-cell responses to antigen, the V-region genes undergo **somatic hypermutation** to generate variant antibodies, some of which bind with a higher affinity. This allows the affinity of the antibody response to increase. These mutations affect only somatic cells and are not inherited through germline transmission.

Somatic mutation theories of antibody diversity proposed that a single gene encoding all antibody molecules underwent mutation in somatic cells to generate the diversity of secreted antibodies.

During lymphocyte development, receptor gene segments undergo **somatic recombination** to generate intact V-region exons that encode the variable region of each antibody and T-cell receptor chain. These events occur only in somatic cells and the changes are not inherited.

The **spleen** is an organ containing a red pulp involved in removing senescent blood cells and a white pulp of lymphoid cells that respond to antigens delivered to the spleen by the blood.

Staphylococcal enterotoxins cause food poisoning and also stimulate many T cells by binding to MHC class II molecules and the Vβ domain of the T-cell receptor; the staphylococcal enterotoxins are thus **superantigens**.

Stem-cell factor (SCF) is a transmembrane protein found on bone marrow stromal cells that binds to **Kit**, a signaling receptor carried on developing B cells and other developing white blood cells.

Superantigens are molecules that stimulate a subset of T cells by binding to MHC class II molecules and Vβ domains of T-cell receptors, stimulating the activation of T cells expressing particular Vβ gene segments.

Suppressor T cells are T cells which, when mixed with naive or effector T cells, suppress their activity. The precise nature of suppressor T cells and their modes of antigen recognition and activation remain mysterious.

The membrane-bound immunoglobulin that acts as the antigen receptor on B cells is often known as **surface immunoglobulin**.

When isotype switching occurs, the active heavy-chain V-region exon undergoes somatic recombination with a 3′ constant-region gene at a **switch region** of DNA. These DNA joints do not need to occur at precise sites, since they occur in intronic DNA. Thus, all switch recombinations are productive.

When one eye is damaged, there is often an autoimmune response that damages the other eye, a syndrome known as **sympathetic ophthalmia**.

A **syngeneic graft** is a graft between two genetically identical individuals. It is accepted as self.

Systemic anaphylaxis is the most dangerous form of immediate hypersensitivity reaction. It involves antigen in the blood stream triggering mast cells all over the body. The activation of these mast cells causes widespread vasodilation, tissue fluid accumulation, epiglottal swelling, and often death.

Systemic autoimmunity or **systemic autoimmune disease** involves the production of antibodies to common self constituents. The major cause of pathology in systemic autoimmunity is deposition of immune complexes. The classical example of a systemic autoimmune disease is **systemic lupus erythematosus**, in which autoantibodies to DNA, RNA, and proteins associated with nucleic acids form immune complexes that damage small blood vessels.

The transporters associated with antigen processing, or **TAP-1** and **TAP-2**, are ATP-binding cassette proteins involved in transporting short peptides from the cytosol into the lumen of the endoplasmic reticulum. Here, the peptides may bind newly synthesized MHC class I molecules to complete their structure. TAP-1 and TAP-2 are required for proper expression of MHC class I molecules.

Effector T cell function is always assayed by changes they produce in antigen-bearing **target cells**. These can be B cells that are activated to produce antibody, macrophages that are activated to kill bacteria or tumor cells, or labeled cells that are killed by cytotoxic T cells.

The **tat** protein is a product of the *tat* gene of human immunodeficiency virus. It is produced when latently infected cells are activated, and it binds to a transcriptional enhancer in the long terminal repeat of the provirus, increasing transcription of the proviral genome.

T cells, or **T lymphocytes**, are a subset of lymphocytes defined by their development in the thymus and by heterodimeric receptors associated with the proteins of the CD3 complex. Most T cells have α:β heterodimeric receptors but γ:δ T cells have a γ:δ heterodimeric receptor.

T-cell clones: see **cloned T cell lines**.

T-cell hybrids are formed by fusing a specific, activated T cell with a T-cell lymphoma. The hybrid cells bear the receptor of the specific T cell parent and grow progressively like the lymphoma.

T cell lines are cultures of T cells grown by repeated cycles of stimulation, usually with antigen and antigen-presenting cells. When single T cells from these lines are propagated, they give rise to **T-cell clones** or **cloned T cell lines**.

The **T-cell receptor** consists of a disulfide-linked heterodimer of the highly variable α and β **chains** expressed at the cell membrane as a complex with the CD3 chains. T cells carrying this type of receptor are often called $\alpha{:}\beta$ T cells. An alternative receptor made up of variable γ and δ chains is expressed with CD3 on a subset of T cells.

The complement system can be activated directly or by antibody, but both pathways converge with the activation of the **terminal complement components** which assemble to form the membrane-attack complex.

The enzyme **terminal deoxynucleotidyl transferase (TdT)** inserts non-templated or N-nucleotides into the junctions between gene segments in T-cell receptor and immunoglobulin heavy-chain V-region genes. The N-nucleotides contribute greatly to junctional diversity in V regions.

When antigen is injected a third time, the response elicited is called a **tertiary response** and the injection a **tertiary immunization**.

T$_H$1 cells is an alternative name for inflammatory CD4 T cells.

T$_H$2 cells is an alternative name for helper CD4 T cells.

The term **T$_H$3 cell** has been used to describe unique cells that produce mainly transforming growth factor-β in response to antigen; they develop predominantly in the mucosal immune response to antigens that are presented orally.

The lymph from most of the body, except for the head, neck, and right arm, is gathered in a large lymphatic vessel, the **thoracic duct**, that runs parallel to the aorta through the thorax and drains into the left subclavian vein. The thoracic duct thus returns the lymphatic fluid and lymphocytes back into the peripheral blood circulation.

Surgical removal of the thymus is called **thymectomy**.

The **thymic anlage** is the tissue from which the thymic stroma develops during embryogenesis.

The **thymic cortex** is the outer region of each **thymic lobule** where thymic progenitor cells proliferate, rearrange their T-cell receptor genes, and undergo thymic selection, especially positive selection on **thymic cortical epithelial cells**.

The **thymic stroma** consists of epithelial cells and connective tissue that form the essential microenvironment for T-cell development.

Thymocytes are lymphoid cells found in the thymus. They consist mainly of developing T cells, although a few thymocytes have achieved functional maturity.

The **thymus**, the site of T-cell development, is a lymphoepithelial organ in the anterior superior mediastinum or upper part of the middle of the chest, just behind the breastbone.

Some antigens only elicit responses in animals or people that have T cells; they are called **thymus-dependent** or **TD antigens**. Other antigens can elicit antibody production in the absence of T cells and are called **thymus-independent** or **TI antigens**. There are two types of TI antigen, the **TI-1 antigens** which have intrinsic B-cell activating activity, and the **TI-2 antigens** that appear to activate B cells by having multiple identical epitopes that crosslink the B-cell receptor.

T cell and T lymphocyte are shortened designations for **thymus-dependent T lymphocyte**, the lymphocyte population that does not develop in the absence of a functioning thymus.

During the process of germinal center formation, cells called **tingible body macrophages** appear. These are phagocytic cells engulfing apoptotic B cells, which are produced in large numbers during the height of the germinal center response.

Almost all tissues have resident **tissue dendritic cells** that can take up antigen but only achieve effective co-stimulatory activity if they migrate to local lymphoid organs. Graft rejection is triggered by tissue dendritic cells that migrate from the graft to local lymph nodes to trigger an anti-graft response.

Transplantation of organ or **tissue grafts** such as skin grafts is used medically to repair organ or tissue deficits.

Some autoimmune diseases attack particular tissues, such as connective tissue, resulting in **tissue-specific autoimmune disease**.

T lymphocytes: see **T cells**.

Tolerance is the failure to respond to an antigen. Tolerance to self antigens is an essential feature of the immune system; when tolerance is lost, the immune system can destroy self tissues, as happens in autoimmune disease. See also: **central tolerance**, **peripheral tolerance**, and **self tolerance**.

The palatine **tonsils** that lie on either side of the pharynx are large aggregates of lymphoid cells organized as part of the mucosal or gut-associated immune system.

The recombination activating genes, *RAG-1* and *RAG-2*, seem to be related to **topoisomerases**, enzymes involved in cleaving and sealing DNA molecules to allow DNA replication and repair.

The toxic shock syndrome is caused by a bacterial superantigen, the **toxic shock syndrome toxin-1 (TSST-1)**, which is secreted by *Staphylococcus aureus*.

Inactivated toxins called **toxoids** are no longer toxic but retain their immunogenicity so that they can be used for immunization.

The active transport of molecules across epithelial cells is called **transcytosis**. Transcytosis of IgA molecules involves transport across intestinal epithelial cells in vesicles that originate on the baso-lateral surface and fuse with the apical surface in contact with the intestinal lumen.

The insertion of small pieces of DNA into cells is called **transfection**. If the DNA is expressed without integrating into host cell DNA, this is called a transient transfection; if the DNA integrates into host cell DNA, then it replicates whenever host cell DNA is replicated, producing a stable transfection.

Foreign genes can be placed in the mouse genome by **transgenesis**. This generates **transgenic mice** that are used to study the function of the inserted gene, the **transgene**, and the regulation of its expression.

The grafting of organs or tissues from one individual to another is called **transplantation**. The **transplanted organs** or grafts can be rejected by the immune system unless the host is tolerant to the graft antigens or immunosuppressive drugs are used to prevent rejection.

Transporters associated with antigen processing: see **TAP-1** and **TAP-2**.

The **tuberculin test** is a clinical test in which a purified protein derivative (called PPD) of *Mycobacterium tuberculosis*, the causative agent of tuberculosis, is injected subcutaneously. PPD elicits a delayed-type hypersensitivity reaction in individuals who have had tuberculosis or have been immunized against it.

Tuberculoid leprosy; see **leprosy.**

Tumor immunology is the study of host defenses against tumors, usually studied by tumor transplantation. Tumors transplanted into syngeneic recipients can grow progressively or can be rejected through T-cell recognition of **tumor-specific transplantation antigens (TSTA)**. TSTA are peptides of mutant or overexpressed cellular proteins bound to MHC class I molecules on the tumor cell surface.

Tumor necrosis factor-α (TNF-α) is a cytokine that is produced by macrophages and T cells and which has multiple functions in the immune response. It is the defining member of the TNF family of cytokines.

Tumor necrosis factor-β (TNF-β): see **lymphotoxin.**

The TdT-dependent dUTP–biotin nick end labeling or **TUNEL assay** identifies apoptotic cells *in situ* by the characteistic fragmentation of their DNA. Biotin-tagged dUTP added to the free 3' ends of the DNA fragments by the enzyme TdT can be detected by immunohistochemical staining with enzyme-linked streptavidin.

In **two-dimensional gel electrophoresis**, proteins are separated by isoelectric focusing in one dimension, followed by SDS-PAGE on a slab gel at right-angles to the first dimension. This can separate and identify large numbers of distinct proteins.

Hypersensitivity reactions are classified by mechanism: **type I hypersensitivity reactions** involve IgE antibody triggering of mast cells; **type II hypersensitivity reactions** involve IgG antibodies against cell surface or matrix antigens; **type III hypersensitivity reactions** involve antigen:antibody complexes; and **type IV hypersensitivity reactions** are T-cell mediated.

Urticaria is the specific term for hives, which are red, itchy skin welts usually brought on by an allergic reaction.

Vaccination is the deliberate induction of adaptive immunity to a pathogen by injecting a **vaccine**, a dead or attenuated (non-pathogenic) form of the pathogen.

The first effective vaccine was **vaccinia**, a cowpox virus that causes a limited infection in humans which leads to immunity to the human smallpox virus, variola.

The **valence** of an antibody or antigen is the number of different molecules it can combine with at one time.

The **variability** of a protein is a measure of the difference between the amino acid sequences of different variants of that protein. The most variable proteins known are antibodies and T-cell receptors.

Variability plot: see **Wu and Kabat plot.**

Variable gene segments: see **V gene segments.**

The **variable region** or **V region** of an immunological receptor is the most amino-terminal domain which is formed by recombination of V, D, and J gene segments during lymphocyte development.

Vascular addressins are molecules on endothelial cells to which leukocyte adhesion molecules bind. They play a key role in selective homing of leukocytes to particular sites in the body.

The **very late antigens**, or **VLA**, are members of the β_1 family of integrins involved in cell–cell and cell–matrix interactions. Some VLA are important in leukocyte and lymphocyte migration.

Vesicles are small membrane-bounded compartments within the cytosol.

The first 95 amino acids or so of immunoglobulin and T-cell receptor variable domains are encoded in inherited **V gene segments**. One V gene segment must rearrange to a J or DJ gene segment to produce an intact V domain exon so that the receptor chain can be synthesized. The **variable** or **V region** of a receptor chain pairs with a different V region or **V domain** to form the complete immunoglobulin or T cell receptor.

Virgin or **naive lymphocytes** are mature lymphocytes that have never been stimulated by antigen.

Virions are virus particles, the form in which some viruses spread from cell to cell or from one individual to another.

Viruses are particles with a nucleic acid genome that must replicate in a living cell, as viruses cannot carry out metabolic processes on their own.

Weibel-Palade bodies are granules within endothelial cells that contain **P-selectin** and activation of the endothelial cell by mediators like histamine and C5a leads to rapid translocation of P-selectin to the cell surface.

Western blotting is a technique for detecting proteins in a mixture using labeled antibodies, after the proteins have been separated, usually by gel electrophoresis, and transferred by blotting to nitrocellulose.

When small amounts of allergen are injected into the dermis of an allergic individual, a **wheal and flare reaction** is observed. This consists of a raised area of skin containing fluid and a spreading, red, itchy circular reaction.

The discrete areas of lymphoid tissue in the spleen are known as the **white pulp**.

The **Wiskott–Aldrich syndrome** is a congenital abnormality in which antibodies to polysaccharide antigens are defective. The underlying genetic defect is not known. Patients with the Wiskott-Aldrich syndrome are susceptible to infection with pyogenic bacteria.

A **Wu and Kabat plot** or **variability plot** is generated from the amino acid sequences of related proteins by plotting the variability of the sequence against amino acid residue number. Variability is the number of different amino acids observed at a position divided by the frequency of the most common amino acid.

Animals of different species are **xenogeneic.**

X-linked agammaglobulinemia is a genetic disorder in which B-cell development is arrested at the pre-B cell stage and no mature B cells or antibodies are formed. The disease is due to a defect in the gene encoding the protein tyrosine kinase btk.

X-linked hyper IgM syndrome is a disease in which little or no IgG, IgE, or IgA antibody is produced and even IgM responses are deficient, but serum IgM levels are normal to high. It is due to a defect in the gene encoding the CD40 ligand, the cell-surface protein gp39.

X-linked severe combined immunodeficiency (X-linked SCID) is a disease in which T-cell development fails at an early intrathymic stage and no mature T cells or T-cell dependent antibody production occurs. It is due to a defect in a gene that encodes part of the receptors for several different cytokines.

INDEX

How to use this index. All numbers are page numbers. Those in **bold** refer to a major text discussion; those followed by F refer to a figure; and those followed by FF refer to more than one consecutive figure.

How to use this index. All numbers are page
numbers. Those in **bold** refer to a major text
discussion; those followed by F refer to a figure;
and those followed by FF refer to more than one
consecutive figure.

How to use this index. All numbers are page numbers. Those in **bold** refer to a major text discussion; those followed by F refer to a figure; and those followed by FF refer to more than one consecutive figure.

Evolution, CD5 B cells and γ:δ T cells in, 9:24-9:25
  of MHC alleles, 4:30-4:31, 4:30FF
Exocytosis, in CD8 T cell-mediated apoptosis,
  7:30-7:31, 7:31F
Exotoxins, 8:21F
  tissue damage by, examples, diseases, 9:6F
Experimental allergic encephalomyelitis, see EAE
Experimental autoimmune encephalomyelitis,
  see EAE
Extracellular matrix, autoimmunity to, 11:18, 11:19F
Extravasation, diapedesis, 9:14F, 9:15
  steps, mechanisms, 9:13-9:15, 9:14F

Fab fragment, 3:4, 3:5F
  as antigen-binding site, 3:7, 3:8F
  T-cell receptor, comparison, 4:32-4:33, 4:32F
FACS, 2:31
  methods and uses, 2:28, 2:29F, 2:30
FACS analysis, of T cells in development, 6:7F
Factor D, 9:8F, 9:9, 9:10F
Factor H, 9:8F, 9:9, 9:10F
Factor I, 8:47, 8:47FF
Factor P, see Properdin
Farmer's lung, 11:11, 11:11F
Fas, 7:25, 7:25F
  in CD8 T cell-induced apoptosis, 7:32
Fas ligand, 7:25, 7:25F, 11:13F
  in suppression of B-cell activation, 12:8, 12:8F
Fc fragment, 3:4, 3:5F
  in complement fixation, 3:25, 3:26F
  effector Ig functions and, 3:25
  in IgG transport, 8:19-8:20, 8:19F
  in transcytosis of Ig A, 8:18-8:19, 8:19F
Fc receptors, 8:1, 8:2F
  activation, by bound Ig's, 8:24-8:25, 8:25F
    by opsonized pathogens, 8:25-8:26, 8:26F
    on natural killer cells, 8:27-8:28, 8:28F
  in allergy, 11:2F, 11:9
    type II, 11:2F, 11:4, 11:9-11:10
  in autoimmune diseases, 11:18, 11:19F
  defined, 8:23
  discrimination between free and bound Ig's,
    8:24-8:25, 8:25F
  exocytosis, triggered by, 8:27
  functions, 8:24
  in humoral immunity, **8:23-8:31**, 8:24FF
  on mast cells, 8:28
  phagocytosis, enhancement by, 8:25-8:26, 8:26FF
  structure, 8:24, 8:24F
  types and properties of each, 8:23, 8:24F
Fcγ receptor II (FcγRII), 12:3, 12:3F
FcRn, IgG transport by, 8:19-8:20, 8:19F
Fetal liver, B-cell development in, 5:3
Fetal tolerance, **11:33**, 11:33F
Fetus, anti-idiotype antibody effects, 12:6
  B cell types, 5:21-5:22, 5:21FF
  maternal IgG for, 8:18-8:20, 8:19FF
Fever, 10:8
FK binding proteins (FKBP), 12:12-12:13, 12:12FF
FK506, 4:42-4:43, 11:32
  mechanism of action, 7:16, 12:11-12:13, 12:12F
  structure, 12:13F
FKBP, see FK-binding protein (FKBP)
Flagellin, 10:4
Flow cytometer, lymphocyte subpopulation studies
  with, 2:28, 2:29F, 2:30
Fluorescence-activated cell sorter, see FACS
Follicles, see Lymphoid follicles

Follicular dendritic cells, 5:13, 9:32, 9:32F
  in B-cell activation, 3:38
  centrocyte contact with, 8:9F, 8:11
  properties for B-cell proliferation, 8:9-8:10, 8:9F
  in secondary antibody response of B cells, 9:38-
    9:40, 9:39F
  in selection of centrocytes, 8:11-8:12, 8:12F
Food allergy, 11:5F
Fragmentins, in apoptosis, 7:31
  mechanism of action, distribution, release, 7:30-
    7:31, 7:30F
Freund's adjuvant, 2:5F
  complete, EAE induction, 11:26, 11:26F, 11:41,
    11:42FF
  complete and incomplete on CD4 subset activa-
    tion, 12:16
Fungi, 1:2, 1:20F
  effector mechanisms, summary, 9:34F
  list, 9:4F, 9:5

G₀ phase of cell cycle, 2:31
G proteins, C5a receptor, coupling to, 8:40-8:41, 8:42F
  chemokines and, 9:18
gag gene and product, 10:23-10:24, 10:24F
GALT, on immunogenicity of antigens, 2:6-2:7, 2:7F
  structure and role, 1:8-1:9, 1:10F
γ chain, of IL-2 and IL-4 receptors, defect in
  X-linked SCID, 10:18
γ globulins, defined, 2:16
γ heavy chain, 3:24, 3:25F, 3:27, 3:27F
Gancyclovir, resistance, 2:51, 2:52F
Gene, recessive lethal, study methods, 2:53-2:54, 2:55F
  study in culture, by mutagenesis and transfec-
    tion, 2:50-2:52, 2:52FF
  study in vivo, by transgenesis and gene knock-
    out, 2:52-2:54, 2:53FF
Gene conversion, in immunoglobulin diversifica-
    tion, 5:17-5:18, 5:17F
  MHC polymorphism generation, 4:30-4:31, 4:30FF
Gene expression, control, Ig gene rearrangement
    and, 5:10
Gene knock-out, to get immunodeficient states, 10:10
  methods and uses, 2:53-2:54, 2:54FF
  P1 bacteriophage recombination system, 2:54, 2:55F
  to study cytokine defects, 10:18
Gene rearrangement, of Ig genes, see Immuno-
    globulin genes, rearrangement
  regulation of gene expression, 5:10
  in S. typhimurium and N. gonorrhoeae, 10:4
  in trypanosomes, 10:3-10:4, 10:4F
Gene-regulatory proteins, somatic recombination
    in B-cell development, 5:9-5:10, 5:9F
Gene therapy, to correct genetic defects, 10:19-10:20
Genetic engineering, to produce monoclonal
    antibodies, 2:19-2:20, 2:19F
Genetic immunization, 12:31-12:32, 12:31F
Germinal center, 1:8, 1:8F, 9:32, 9:32F
  centrocytes in, 8:9F, 8:10-8:11
  defined, 5:23, 5:23F, 8:10, 8:9F
  formation, 8:9-8:10, 8:9F
  in secondary responses, 9:38-9:40, 9:39FF
  somatic hypermutation of immunoglobulin V
    genes, 8:10-8:11
  tingible body macrophages in, 8:11
Germline configuration, of Ig genes, 3:14, 3:13F
Germline theory, defined, 3:13
GlyCAM-1, 7:4, 7:5FF
  in specific homing of armed effector T cells,

  9:30-9:31, 9:31F
Glycan receptor, on macrophages, 9:11, 9:11F
GM-CSF, dendritic cell development and, 7:12
  to enhance tumor immunogenicity, 12:25, 12:24F
  on macrophage differentiation, 7:37, 7:37F
  major actions, sources, 7:25FF, 7:27
  in type IV hypersensitivity reactions, 11:13F
Golgi apparatus, 7:24F
Gonorrhea, 10:4
Goodpasture's syndrome, 11:15F, 11:18, 11:19F
Gowans, James, 1:13
gp100, 12:20, 12:20F
gp75, 12:20, 12:20F
Graft, allo-, auto-, syngeneic, defined, 11:28
  fetus as tolerated allograft, 11:33, 11:33F
Graft rejection, 11:1
  acute, treatments for, 12:11
  alloreactivity and, 4:28-4:29, 4:29F
  donor APCs to initiate, 11:36, 11:37F
  in donor APC-depleted grafts, 11:36-11:37
  effector mechanism, summary, 11:45F
  first set rejection, 11:28-11:29, 11:29F
  genetic basis, discovery, 2:37, 2:37F
  harmful immune response in, 1:27, 1:28, 1:28F
  host APC role, 11:36-11:37
  hyperacute, antibody-mediated, 11:32, 11:32F
  in vitro correlates, 2:39-2:40, 2:40F
  MHC discovery from, 1:25
  of MHC-identical grafts, minor H antigens,
    11:30-11:31, 11:31F
  non-self MHC molecules on graft and, 11:30, 11:29F
  prevention by active tolerance (suppressor
    T cells), 11:38
  second set rejection, 11:29-11:30, 11:29F
  T-cell mediated, 11:28-11:30, 11:29F
  therapy, CD4 antibody to induce tolerance,
    12:14, 12:15F
    cyclosporin A, 4:42-4:43
    FK506 4:42-4:43
    monoclonal antibodies, 12:14-12:15, 12:15F
  tissue dendritic cells and, 7:13
  of xenografts, 11:32, 11:33
Graft-versus-host (GVH) disease, 10:19, 10:20F
Granulocyte-macrophage colony stimulating fac-
    tor, see GM-CSF
Granulocytes, 1:2, 1:3
Granuloma, 7:37, 7:38F, 10:15
Granzyme A, 7:24F
Granzymes, 7:25F
  in ADCC, 8:27
  mechanism of action, distribution, release,
    7:30-7:31, 7:30F
Graves' disease, 11:15F, 11:19-11:20, 11:20F
Growth, of tumors, experimental murine, 12:18-
    12:19, 12:18FF
    monoclonal antibodies to control, 12:22-
      12:23, 12:23F
Growth factors, in B-cell activation, 3:36
Gut-associated-lymphoid tissues, see GALT

How to use this index. All numbers are page
numbers. Those in **bold** refer to a major text
discussion; those followed by F refer to a figure;
and those followed by FF refer to more than one
consecutive figure.

How to use this index. All numbers are page numbers. Those in **bold** refer to a major text discussion; those followed by F refer to a figure; and those followed by FF refer to more than one consecutive figure.

How to use this index. All numbers are page numbers. Those in **bold** refer to a major text discussion; those followed by F refer to a figure; and those followed by FF refer to more than one consecutive figure.

How to use this index. All numbers are page numbers. Those in **bold** refer to a major text discussion; those followed by F refer to a figure; and those followed by FF refer to more than one consecutive figure.

How to use this index. All numbers are page numbers. Those in **bold** refer to a major text discussion; those followed by F refer to a figure; and those followed by FF refer to more than one consecutive figure.

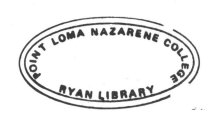